I0038711

Medical Herbalism

Medical Herbalism

Edited by George Moore

hayle
medical

New York

Hayle Medical,
750 Third Avenue, 9ᵗʰ Floor,
New York, NY 10017, USA

Visit us on the World Wide Web at:
www.haylemedical.com

© Hayle Medical, 2019

This book contains information obtained from authentic and highly regarded sources. Copyright for all individual chapters remain with the respective authors as indicated. All chapters are published with permission under the Creative Commons Attribution License or equivalent. A wide variety of references are listed. Permission and sources are indicated; for detailed attributions, please refer to the permissions page and list of contributors. Reasonable efforts have been made to publish reliable data and information, but the authors, editors and publisher cannot assume any responsibility for the validity of all materials or the consequences of their use.

ISBN: 978-1-63241-805-0

Trademark Notice: Registered trademark of products or corporate names are used only for explanation and identification without intent to infringe.

Cataloging-in-Publication Data

Medical herbalism / edited by George Moore.
   p. cm.
Includes bibliographical references and index.
ISBN 978-1-63241-805-0
1. Herbs--Therapeutic use. 2. Medicinal plants. 3. Materia medica, Vegetable.
4. Botany, Medical. I. Moore, George.
RM666.H33 M43 2019
615.321--dc23

Table of Contents

Preface..IX

Chapter 1 Phenolic profile and biological properties of the leaves of *Ficus vasta* Forssk.
(Moraceae) growing...1
Maria Fernanda Taviano, Khaled Rashed, Angela Filocamo, Francesco Cacciola,
Paola Dugo, Luigi Mondello, Carlo Bisignano, Rosaria Acquaviva,
Manuela D'Arrigo and Natalizia Miceli

Chapter 2 Comparison of the main components and bioactivity of *Rhus verniciflua Stokes
extracts* by different detoxification processing methods......................................12
Seon-Ok Lee, Sung-Ji Kim, Ju-Sung Kim, Hyuk Ji, Eun-Ok Lee and Hyo-Jeong Lee

Chapter 3 Anti diabetic property of aqueous extract of *Stevia rebaudiana* Bertoni leaves
in Streptozotocin-induced diabetes in albino rats..22
Uswa Ahmad and Rabia Shabir Ahmad

Chapter 4 Antioxidant and anticancer activities of *Trigonella foenum-graecum, Cassia
acutifolia* and *Rhazya stricta* 33
Bayan Al-Dabbagh, Ismail A. Elhaty, Ala'a Al Hrout, Reem Al Sakkaf,
Raafat El-Awady, S. Salman Ashraf and Amr Amin

Chapter 5 Dendritic cells pulsed with generated tumor cell lysate from *Phyllanthus
amarus* Schum. & Thonn. induces anti-tumor immune response 45
Shimaa Ibrahim Abdelmenym Mohamed, Ibrahim Jantan, Mohd Azlan Nafiah,
Mohamed Ali Seyed and Kok Meng Chan

Chapter 6 GLP-I secretion in healthy and diabetic Wistar rats in response to aqueous
extract of *Momordica charantia* 59
Gulzar Ahmad Bhat, Haseeb A. Khan, Abdullah S. Alhomida, Poonam Sharma,
Rambir Singh and Bilal Ahmad Paray

Chapter 7 Antibacterial mechanism of chelerythrine isolated from root of *Toddalia
asiatica* (Linn) Lam 67
Nan He, Peiqing Wang, Pengyu Wang, Changyang Ma and Wenyi Kang

Chapter 8 Anti-inflammatory effects of *Phyllanthus amarus* Schum. & Thonn. through
inhibition of NF-κB, MAPK, and PI3K-Akt signaling pathways in LPS-induced
human macrophages 75
Hemavathy Harikrishnan, Ibrahim Jantan, Md. Areeful Haque and
Endang Kumolosasi

Chapter 9 Antioxidant and skin-whitening effects of aerial part of *Euphorbia supina*
Raf. Extract 87
Sa-Haeng Kang, Yong-Deok Jeon, Ji-Yoon Cha, Sung-Woo Hwang,
Hoon-Yeon Lee, Min Park, Bo-Ri Lee, Min-Kyoung Shin, Su-Jeong Kim,
Sang-Min Shin, Dae-Ki Kim, Jong-Sik Jin and Young-Mi Lee

Chapter 10   **Water/ethanol extract of *Cucumis sativus* L. fruit attenuates
lipopolysaccharide-induced inflammatory response in endothelial cells**................................95
Chiara Bernardini, Augusta Zannoni, Martina Bertocchi, Irvin Tubon,
Mercedes Fernandez and Monica Forni

Chapter 11   **Phenolics from *Barleria cristata* var. Alba as carcinogenesis blockers against
menadione cytotoxicity through induction and protection of quinone reductase** 104
Ali M. El-Halawany, Hossam M. Abdallah, Ahmed R. Hamed,
Hany Ezzat Khalil and Ameen M. Almohammadi

Chapter 12   **Antidiabetic activity, glucose uptake stimulation and α-glucosidase inhibitory
effect of *Chrysophyllum cainito* L. stem bark extract** 111
Hau Van Doan, Siriporn Riyajan, Roongtip Iyara and Nuannoi Chudapongse

Chapter 13   ***Ipomoea batatas* L. Lam. ameliorates acute and chronic inflammations
by suppressing inflammatory mediators, a comprehensive exploration using
in vitro and in vivo models**...121
Muhammad Majid, Bakht Nasir, Syeda Saniya Zahra, Muhammad Rashid Khan,
Bushra Mirza and Ihsan-ul Haq

Chapter 14   **Phenolic contents, antimicrobial and antioxidant activity of *Olea ferruginea*
Royle (Oleaceae)** 141
Ansar Mehmood and Ghulam Murtaza

Chapter 15   **Protective effects and mechanisms of *Terminalia catappa* L. methenolic extract
on hydrogen-peroxide-induced oxidative stress in human skin fibroblasts** 147
Ya-Han Huang, Po-Yuan Wu, Kuo-Ching Wen,
Chien-Yih Lin and Hsiu-Mei Chiang

Chapter 16   **Anti-cancer effects of *Kaempferia parviflora* on ovarian cancer SKOV3 cells** 156
Suthasinee Paramee, Siriwoot Sookkhee, Choompone Sakonwasun,
Mingkwan Na Takuathung, Pitchaya Mungkornasawakul,
Wutigri Nimlamool and Saranyapin Potikanond

Chapter 17   **Post-marketing safety surveillance and re-evaluation of Xueshuantong
injection**...169
Chunxiao Li, Tao Xu, Peng Zhou, Junhua Zhang, Ge Guan, Hui Zhang,
Xiao Ling, Weixia Li, Fei Meng, Guanping Liu, Linyan Lv, Jun Yuan,
Xuelin Li and Mingjun Zhu

Chapter 18   ***Croton gratissimus* leaf extracts inhibit cancer cell growth by inducing
caspase 3/7 activation with additional anti-inflammatory and antioxidant
activities**..178
Emmanuel Mfotie Njoya, Jacobus N. Eloff and Lyndy J. McGaw

Chapter 19   **Aloe-emodin induces apoptosis in human oral squamous cell carcinoma
SCC15 cells**...189
Qihong Li, Jun Wen, Kaitao Yu, Yao Shu, Wulin He, Hongxing Chu,
Bin Zhang and Cheng Ge

Chapter 20   **Study of the anti-allergic and anti-inflammatory activity of *Brachychiton rupestris* and *Brachychiton discolor* leaves (Malvaceae) using in vitro models**............................194
Amany A. Thabet, Fadia S. Youssef, Michal Korinek, Fang-Rong Chang,
Yang-Chang Wu, Bing-Hung Chen, Mohamed El-Shazly,
Abdel Nasser B. Singab and Tsong-Long Hwang

Chapter 21   **Evaluation of the effect of *Lactobacillus reuteri* V3401 on biomarkers of inflammation, cardiovascular risk and liver steatosis in obese adults with metabolic syndrome**..208
Carmen Tenorio-Jiménez, María José Martínez-Ramírez,
Mercedes Tercero-Lozano, Carmen Arraiza-Irigoyen,
Isabel Del Castillo-Codes, Josune Olza, Julio Plaza-Díaz,
Luis Fontana, Jairo H. Migueles, Mónica Olivares,
Ángel Gil and Carolina Gomez-Llorente

Permissions

List of Contributors

Index

Preface

It is often said that books are a boon to mankind. They document every progress and pass on the knowledge from one generation to the other. They play a crucial role in our lives. Thus I was both excited and nervous while editing this book. I was pleased by the thought of being able to make a mark but I was also nervous to do it right because the future of students depends upon it. Hence, I took a few months to research further into the discipline, revise my knowledge and also explore some more aspects. Post this process, I begun with the editing of this book.

The study of botany associated with the use of plants for therapeutic and medicinal purposes, is known as medical herbalism. It is a popular form of alternative medicine. Sometimes, the use of bee products, minerals, fungal products, shells and some animal parts, for medicinal purposes, also fall under the scope of herbalism. It also includes phytotherapy, which is concerned with the use of alternative practices of using unrefined plant or animal extracts as medicinal components. Herbal medicine can be administered orally, topically or by inhalation. Oral herbal remedies may include herbal teas, infusions, tinctures and decoctions. This book provides significant information on medical herbalism to help develop a good understanding of herbalism and related fields. It attempts to understand the multiple branches that fall under herbalism and how such concepts have practical applications. Researchers and students actively engaged in this field will find this book full of crucial and unexplored concepts.

I thank my publisher with all my heart for considering me worthy of this unparalleled opportunity and for showing unwavering faith in my skills. I would also like to thank the editorial team who worked closely with me at every step and contributed immensely towards the successful completion of this book. Last but not the least, I wish to thank my friends and colleagues for their support.

Editor

Phenolic profile and biological properties of the leaves of *Ficus vasta* Forssk. (Moraceae) growing in Egypt

Maria Fernanda Taviano[1*†], Khaled Rashed[2], Angela Filocamo[3,1], Francesco Cacciola[4], Paola Dugo[1,5,6], Luigi Mondello[1,5,6], Carlo Bisignano[4], Rosaria Acquaviva[7], Manuela D'Arrigo[1] and Natalizia Miceli[1†]

Abstract

Background: *Ficus vasta* Forssk. (Moraceae) is traditionally used for the treatment of various ailments; nonetheless, this species has been poorly studied to date. This work aimed to characterize the phenolic profile and to evaluate the antioxidant and antimicrobial properties of a hydroalcoholic extract obtained from *F. vasta* leaves collected in Egypt.

Methods: The phenolic profile of the extract was characterized by HPLC-PDA/ESI-MS. The antioxidant properties were examined by different in vitro systems: DPPH test, reducing power and metal chelating activity assays. Moreover, the ability of the extract to protect *Escherichia coli* growth and survival from H_2O_2-induced oxidative stress was evaluated. The potential toxicity was investigated using *Artemia salina* lethality bioassay. Finally, the antimicrobial properties against a representative set of Gram-positive and Gram-negative bacterial strains and the yeast *C. albicans* were assayed by standard methods.

Results: By HPLC-PDA/ESI-MS analysis 12 compounds belonging to the groups of phenolic acids and flavonoids were identified. The extract exhibited strong radical scavenging activity in DPPH test ($IC_{50} = 0.0672 \pm 0.0038$ mg/mL), reducing power (3.65 ± 0.48 ASE/mL) and chelating activity ($IC_{50} = 0.801 \pm 0.007$ mg/mL). A total protection against H_2O_2-induced damage on *E. coli* was observed. No toxicity against *A. salina* was found ($LC_{50} > 1000$ μg/mL). The extract exhibited bacteriostatic activity against almost all the bacteria tested (MICs: 250–62.5 μg/mL).

Conclusions: The obtained results demonstrate the potential of *F. vasta* leaves as safe sources of natural antioxidant and antimicrobial compounds.

Keywords: *Ficus vasta* Forssk., Phenolic profile, Antioxidant activity, Oxidative stress in *Escherichia coli*, Antimicrobial activity, *Artemia salina* Leach

Background

Medicinal plants are considered as potential sources for drug development and many novel products. Nonetheless, such plants should be investigated to better understand their properties, safety, and efficiency. Currently, many researchers are looking for newer, effective, and safe antioxidants, in order to use them in foods and pharmaceutical preparations to replace the synthetic ones, which have been reported to be dangerous for human health. Medicinal plants are the major source of chemical compounds exhibiting antioxidant activity. Particularly, a direct relationship between antioxidant activity and phenolic compounds has been demonstrated in many studies [1–4].

Recently, there is an increased frequency of multiple drug resistance in human pathogenic microorganism due to indiscriminate use of commercial antimicrobial drugs commonly used to treat various diseases. Therefore, there is an interest in developing alternative antimicrobial drugs for the treatment of infections obtained from various sources such as medicinal plants. Phytochemicals have

* Correspondence: mtaviano@unime.it
†Equal contributors
[1]Dipartimento di Scienze Chimiche, Biologiche, Farmaceutiche ed Ambientali, University of Messina, Polo Annunziata, Viale Annunziata, 98168 Messina, Italy
Full list of author information is available at the end of the article

become the target of a great number of researches focused on the discovery of potentially safe and effective antimicrobials. Plant based antimicrobials either unaided or in combination with antibiotics may be an effective approach to deal with the global antimicrobial resistance. Among plant bioactive compounds, polyphenols are well documented to have microbicide activities against a great number of pathogenic bacteria [5].

The genus *Ficus* L. (Moraceae) comprises about 800 species and 2000 varieties of woody trees, shrubs and vines known as fig trees [6]. Several members of this genus are being used in folk medicine all over the world for a wide range of ailments of the gastrointestinal tract, central nervous, endocrine, and reproductive systems, as well as infectious disorders like tuberculosis, respiratory and skin diseases [7–9].

Ficus vasta Forssk. is a very large tree growing over 25 m tall, with spreading rounded crown. Leaves are alternate, spirally arranged, quite stiff, rough to the touch, almost circular (8–25 × 4–23 cm), margin entire, tip rounded but often with a blunt point, base rounded, heart shaped; usually glabrescent above, glabrescent, puberulous, hirsute or velutinous below [10].

This species is widespread throughout the dry north and eastern Africa, Sudan, Ethiopia, Saudi Arabia, Uganda and Tanzania. In Sudan the poultice of burned *F. vasta* leaves and barks was used as anti-tumor [11]. The leaves are traditionally used for the treatment of rheumatisms, pains and intestinal worms [12].

Although many species from the genus *Ficus* were subjected to phytochemical and pharmacological investigations, to the best of our information *F. vasta* has been poorly studied to date. Qualitative preliminary phytochemical analysis of Egyptian *F. vasta* leaves, using standard chemical tests, revealed the presence of carbohydrates, tannins, flavonoids, coumarins, and triterpenes [12]. Moreover, various phytoconstituents such as β-sitosterol, stigmasterol, lupeol, ursolic acid and some flavonoids were isolated and identified from *F. vasta* aerial parts [13]. Concerning biological activities, very few studies have been carried out on the leaves of this species [10, 14].

Thus, the present work was undertaken to characterize the phenolic profile and to investigate the antioxidant and antimicrobial properties of a hydroalcoholic extract obtained from the leaves of *F. vasta* collected in Egypt, never studied before.

Methods
Chemicals and reagents
LC-MS grade water (H_2O), acetonitrile (ACN), gallic acid, catechin, naringenin, chlorogenic acid, apigenin, rutin, kaempferol and quercetin were obtained from Merck KGaA (Darmstadt, Germany). LC-MS grade acetic acid

was attained from Riedel-de Haën (Seelze, Germany); methanol (MeOH) from Baker Analysed Reagent; Ferrous chloride ($FeCl_2$) was obtained from Carlo Erba (Milan, Italy). Müeller Hinton Broth (MHB), Sabouraud Dextrose Agar (SDA), and Luria-Bertani (LB) broth medium were supplied from Oxoid (Basingstoke, UK), RPMI 1640 from Gibco Laboratories (Grand Island, NY). Unless indicated otherwise, all chemicals were purchased from Sigma-Aldrich (Milan, Italy).

Plant material and extraction procedure
Ficus vasta leaves were collected in May from Al-Zohiriya garden, Giza, Egypt. The plant was identified by Dr. Mohammed El-Gebaly, Department of Botany, National Research Centre (NRC) and by Mrs. Tereeza Labib, consultant of Plant Taxonomy at the Ministry of Agriculture and director of Orman Botanical Garden, Giza, Egypt. A voucher specimen was deposited in the herbarium of Al-Zohiriya garden, Giza, Egypt, under accession number n° FN-2604.

The air dried and powdered *F. vasta* leaves (200 g) were extracted with 80% MeOH at room temperature several times under continuous shaking until exhaustion by maceration process. The extractive solutions were pooled, filtrated, and evaporated to dryness by rotary evaporator (40°C). The yield of *F. vasta* extract, referred to 100 g of dried leaves, was 13.00%.

Phytochemical investigations
Identification of flavonoid compounds by paper chromatography
F. vasta hydroalcoholic extract was subjected to paper chromatography (Whatman No.1) using three different solvent systems as n-butanol:acetic acid:water (BAW 4:1: 5, upper layer), 15% acetic acid, and water. By comparison with standard compounds some flavonoids were identified. Then, each band was cut, and the compounds were dissolved in a mixture of MeOH/H_2O, purified over Sephadex LH-20 and identified by UV, ^{1}H-NMR and MS analyses [15, 16].

Identification of phenolic compounds by HPLC-PDA/ESI-MS
HPLC-PDA/ESI-MS analyses were performed on a Prominence LC system (Shimadzu, Milan, Italy) equipped with photo diode array (PDA) and mass spectrometry (MS) (LCMS-2020, Shimadzu) detection. Data acquisition was performed by Shimadzu LabSolution software ver. 5.53.

For chromatographic separations, an Ascentis Express C18 column (15 cm × 4.6 mm I.D.) packed with 2.7 μm partially porous particles, was employed (Supelco, Bellefonte, PA, USA). The injection volume was 5 μL, and the mobile phase consisted of water/acetic acid (0.1%) at pH = 3 (solvent A) and ACN/acetic acid (0.1%) (solvent B)

, respectively in the following linear gradient mode: 0 min, 0% B; 5 min, 5% B; 15 min, 10% B; 30 min, 20% B; 60 min, 50% B; 70 min, 100% B; 71 min, 0% B. The mobile phase flow rate was 1.0 mL/min, and it was splitted to 0.3 mL/min prior to MS detection. PDA wavelength range was 210–400 nm and the chromatograms were extracted at 280 and 350 nm.

The extract (10 mg) was dissolved in DMSO (1 mL) and filtered through a 0.45 μm membrane filters (Whatman, Clifton, USA).

Phenolics identification was carried out by the complementary information provided by chromatographic retention times, PDA and mass spectra, and further supported by comparison to existing literature data [13].

The quantitative determination of each compound was carried out by means of the external standard method using gallic acid ($\lambda = 270$), catechin ($\lambda = 278$), naringenin ($\lambda = 283$), chlorogenic acid ($\lambda = 325$), apigenin ($\lambda = 330$), rutin ($\lambda = 355$), kaempferol ($\lambda = 365$) and quercetin ($\lambda = 370$) as reference compounds in a concentration range of 1–100 ppm. With three different concentration levels. Triplicate injections were made for each level, and a linear regression was generated. The calibration curves with the external standards were obtained using concentration (mg/L) with respect to the area obtained from the integration of the PDA peaks at a wavelength of 270 nm for benzoic acid-like, 278 nm for flavan-3-ol-like, 283 nm for flavanone-like, 325 nm for cinnamic acid-like, 330 nm for flavone-glycoside-like, 354 nm for flavonol-glycoside-like and flavanone-glycoside-like, 365 nm for flavone-like and 370 nm for flavonol-like compounds. The results were obtained from the average of three determinations and are expressed as mg/g dried extract ± percent relative standard deviation (%RSD).

Antioxidant activity

Free radical scavenging activity

The free radical scavenging activity of *F. vasta* extract was evaluated using the DPPH (2,2-diphenyl-1-picrylhydrazyl) test, according to the protocol previously reported [17]. An aliquot (0.5 mL) of 80% MeOH solution containing different amounts of the extract (0.0125–0.2 mg/mL) was added to 3 mL of daily prepared methanol DPPH solution (0.1 mM). The optical density change at 517 nm was measured, 20 min after the initial mixing, with a model UV-1601 spectrophotometer (Shimadzu). Butylated Hydroxytoluene (BHT) was used as reference. The scavenging activity was measured as the decrease in absorbance of the samples versus DPPH standard solution. The results were obtained from the average of three independent experiments, and are reported as mean radical scavenging activity percentage (%) ± SD. The results are also expressed as mean 50% Inhibitory Concentration

(IC_{50}) ± standard deviation (SD), determined graphically by interpolation of the dose-response curve; lower IC_{50} value indicates higher antioxidant activity.

Measurement of reducing power

The reducing power of *F. vasta* extract was evaluated by spectrophotometric detection of Fe^{3+}-Fe^{2+} transformation method, as previously reported [18]. Different amounts of the extract (0.0125–0.2 mg/mL) in 1 mL solvent were mixed with 2.5 mL of phosphate buffer (0.2 M, pH 6.6) and 2.5 mL of 1% potassium ferrycyanide [$K_3Fe(CN)_6$]. The mixture was incubated at 50 °C for 20 min. The resulting solution was cooled rapidly, mixed with 2.5 mL of 10% trichloroacetic acid, and centrifuged at 3000 rpm for 10 min. The resulting supernatant (2.5 mL) was mixed with 2.5 mL of distilled water and 0.5 mL of 0.1% fresh ferric chloride ($FeCl_3$), and the absorbance was measured at 700_{nm} after 10 min; the increased absorbance of the reaction mixture indicates an increase in reducing power. As blank, an equal volume (1 mL) of water was mixed with a solution prepared as described above. Ascorbic acid and BHT were used as reference standards. The results were obtained from the average of three independent experiments, and are expressed as mean absorbance values ± SD. The reducing power was also expressed as ascorbic acid equivalent (ASE/mL); when the reducing power is 1 ASE/mL, the reducing power of 1 mL extract is equivalent to 1 μmol ascorbic acid.

Ferrous ions (Fe^{2+}) chelating activity

The Fe^{2+} chelating activity of *F. vasta* extract was estimated by measuring the formation of the Fe^{2+}-ferrozine complex, according to the method previously reported [18]. Briefly, different concentrations of the extract (0.0125–0.2 mg/mL) in 1 mL solvent were mixed with 0.5 mL of methanol and 0.05 mL of 2 mM $FeCl_2$. The reaction was initiated by the addition of 0.1 mL of 5 mM ferrozine. Then the mixture was shaken vigorously and left standing at room temperature for 10 min. The absorbance of the solution was measured spectrophotometrically at 562 nm. The control contains $FeCl_2$ and ferrozine, complex formation molecules. Ethylenediaminetetraacetic acid (EDTA) was used as reference standard The results were obtained from the average of three independent experiments and are reported as mean inhibition of the Fe^{2+}-ferrozine complex formation (%) ± SD and IC_{50} ± SD.

Protective effect on Escherichia coli under peroxide stress

The ability of *F. vasta* extract to protect bacterial growth and survival from the oxidative stress induced by hydrogen peroxide (H_2O_2) was evaluated according the protocol described by Smirnova et al. [19], with some modifications.

Escherichia coli ATCC 25922 was obtained from the Department of Scienze Chimiche Biologiche Farmaceutiche ed Ambientali, University of Messina, in-house culture collection (Messina, Italy). Bacteria were grown overnight in LB medium. The overnight suspension was centrifuged (10 min at 3500 rpm), resuspended in LB fresh medium to obtain a final optical density at 600 nm (OD_{600}) = 0.1, and then grown aerobically at 37 °C with shaking at 150 rpm. In mid-log phase (OD_{600} = 0.6) bacteria were centrifuged and the OD_{600} adjusted to 0.2 value with fresh medium. The bacteria suspension was then aliquoted and *F. vasta* extract (1 mg/mL) and reference standard quercetin (0.2 mM) were added. Two control groups (Ctr), with and without H_2O_2 treatment, were included. After 30–40 min, when OD_{600} reached a value equal to 0.4, in order to establish the ability of *F. vasta* extract to exert protection against *E. coli* growth inhibition induced from oxidative stress bacteria were treated with H_2O_2 (2 mM), and the growth was monitored every 20 min for 3 h.

For survival studies, the bacteria (OD_{600} = 0.4) were exposed for 30 min to a higher concentration of H_2O_2 (10 mM), which caused bactericidal effect. Then an aliquot of each sample was diluted in 0.9% NaCl to obtain serial dilutions (1:10). Each sample was poured onto LB-agar plates and incubated at 37 °C; after 24 h the number of viable colonies was counted to estimate the cell survival. The percentage (%) of survival was calculated according to the formula: (colony forming units (CFU) of H_2O_2 treated culture/ CFU of untreated Ctr) × 100 [20].

The results were obtained from the average of three independent experiments and are expressed as mean absorbance ± SD and surviving (%) ± SD for protective effect on *E. coli* growth and survival, respectively. Statistical comparisons of the data were performed by Student's t-test for unpaired data. *P*-values lower than 0.05 were considered statistically significant.

Artemia salina lethality bioassay

The potential toxicity of *F. vasta* extract was investigated using brine shrimp (*Artemia salina* Leach) lethality bioassay, according to the method previously reported [21]. The extract was tested at different concentrations (10–1000 µg/mL). Ten brine shrimp larvae, taken 48 h after initiation of hatching in artificial seawater, were transferred to each sample vial, and artificial seawater was added to obtain a final volume of 5 mL. After 24 h of incubation at 25–28 °C, the vials were observed using a magnifying glass, and surviving larvae were counted. The assay was carried out in triplicate, and median lethal concentration (LC_{50}) values were determined using the probit analysis method. Extracts with LC_{50} higher than 1000 µg/ mL are considered non-toxic.

Antimicrobial activity
Microbial strains and culture conditions
The following strains were used as indicators for the antimicrobial testing and were obtained from the Department of Scienze Chimiche Biologiche Farmaceutiche ed Ambientali, University of Messina (Italy), in-house culture collection: *Bacillus subtilis* ATCC 6633, *Escherichia coli* ATCC 10536, *Escherichia coli* ATCC 25922, *Listeria monocytogenes* ATCC 13932, *Pseudomonas aeruginosa* ATCC 15442, *Salmonella typhimurium* ATCC 13311, *Salmonella enterica* (Wild type), *Staphylococcus aureus* ATCC 29213, and *Staphylococcus epidermidis* ATCC 12228 were grown at 37 °C in MHB; the yeast *Candida albicans* ATCC 10231 was grown at 35 °C on SDA.

Antimicrobial testing
The minimum inhibitory concentration (MIC) and minimum bactericidal and fungicidal concentration (MBC and MFC) values of *F. vasta* extract were determined using the in broth microdilution method according to the protocols recommended by the Clinical and Laboratory Standards Institute [22, 23].

Cultures of bacterial strains and *C. albicans* were prepared overnight in MHB and RPMI 1640, respectively; microorganism suspensions were therefore adjusted with sterile medium to give 1×10^6 for bacteria and 1×10^4 CFU/mL for *C. albicans*. The extract was dissolved in dimethyl sulfoxide (DMSO) (1%) and MHB to obtain a final concentration of 1 mg/mL. Two-fold serial dilutions were prepared in a 96-well plate. The tested concentrations ranged from 500 to 0.49 µg/mL. The MIC was defined as the lowest concentration (µg/mL) of extract which completely inhibit the visible growth of microorganisms in broth after 24 h of incubation for bacteria and 48 h for *C. albicans*. All experiments were performed in triplicate on three independent days. Positive and negative controls were also included.

Results
Phytochemical investigations
Identification of flavonoid compounds by paper chromatography
Chromatographic separation of *F. vasta* extract allowed the identification of some flavonoid compounds, namely luteolin, quercetin, vitexin, quercetin-3-O-β-galactoside and rutin. Their structures were elucidated on the basis of, UV, ¹H-NMR, and MS analyses. The spectral information is summarized in Table 1.

Identification of phenolic compounds by HPLC-PDA/ESI-MS
The quali-quantitative characterization of the phenolic compounds present in the *F. vasta* leaves extract was accomplished by HPLC-PDA/ESI-MS. Baseline compound separation was achieved on the employed fused-core

Table 1 Spectroscopic analyses of the flavonoid compounds isolated from *F. vasta* leaves hydroalcoholic extract

Compound	Physical state	¹H-NMR data	UV data	MS data
Luteolin	Yellow powder	¹H-NMR (DMSO-d₆, 400 MHz): δ ppm 12.9 (1H, s, 5-OH), 7.4 (1H, d, *J* = 8 Hz, H-6′), 7.38 (1H, d, *J* = 2 Hz, H-2′), 6.85 (1H, d, *J* = 8 Hz, H-5′), 6.6 (1H s, H-3), 6.4 (1H, d, *J* = 2 Hz, H-8), 6.15 (1H, d, *J* = 2 Hz, H-6)..		EI-MS: m/z 286
Quercetin	Yellow powder		UV λmax (MeOH): 255, 267, 371; (NaOMe): 270, 320, 420; (AlCl₃): 270, 455; (AlCl₃/HCl): 264, 303sh, 315sh, 428; (NaOAc): 257, 274, 318, 383; (NaOAc/H₃BO₃): 259, 387.	EI-MS: m/z 302.
Vitexin	Yellow amorphous powder	¹H-NMR (DMSO-d₆, 400 MHz): δ 8.04 (d, *J* = 8.5 Hz, 2H, H-2′,6′), 6.88 (d, *J* = 8.5 Hz, 2H, H-3′,5′), 6.42 (s, 1H, H-3), 6.74 (s, 1H, H-6), 4.65 (d, *J* = 9.6 Hz,1H, H-1′).	UV λmax (MeOH): 269, 331; (NaOMe): 279, 325 (sh), 391; (AlCl₃): 276, 303 (sh), 346, 382; (AlCl₃/HCl): 277; 303, 343, 380 (NaOAc): 278, 387 (NaOAc/H₃BO₃): 270, 319, 346.	ESI-MS *m/z:* 433 [M + H]⁺.
Quercetin 3-*O*-β-galactoside	Yellow crystals	¹H-NMR (DMSO-d₆, 400 MHz): δ 7.78 (1H, dd, *J* = 2, 8.5 Hz, H-6′), 7.54 (1H, d, *J* = 2 Hz, H-2′), 6.82 (1H, d, *J* = 8.5 Hz, H-5′), d 6.42 (1H, d, *J* = 2 Hz, H-8), 6.24 (1 H,d, *J* = 2 Hz, H-6), 5.5 (1H, d, *J* = 7.5 Hz, H-1″).		(−)ESI-MS: m/z 463 [M-H]⁻.
Quercetin 3-O-rutinoside (Rutin)	Yellow powder	¹H-NMR (400 MHz, DMSO-d₆): δ ppm 7.54 (2H, m, H-2′/6′), 6.85 (1H, d, *J* = 9 Hz, H-5′), 6.38 (1H, d, *J* = 2.5 Hz, H-8), 6.19 (1H, *J* = 2.5 Hz, H-6), 5.35 (1H, d, *J* = 7.5 Hz, H-1‴), 4.39 (1H, s, H-1‴′), 3.90–3.20 (m, remaining sugar protons), 0.99 (3H, d, *J* = 6 Hz, H-6‴).	UV λmax (MeOH): 258, 269, 361; (NaOMe): 276, 322, 416; (AlCl₃): 232, 276, 302, 366; (AlCl₃/HCl): 232, 276, 302, 366; (NaOAc): 284, 306, 381; (NaOAc/H₃BO₃): 261, 312, 376.	

C18 stationary phase; as far as detection is concerned on-line coupling to PDA and MS detection provided complementary information for reliable identification purposes. The analysis revealed the presence of 12 compounds, 2 out of them belonging to the group of phenolic acids (77.09 mg/g extract) and 10 to flavonoids (135. 98 mg/g extract). The flavonol quercetin-3-galactoside was found to be the main phenolic compound detected in the extract (81.5 mg/g ± 0.88% RSD), followed by gallic acid (76.36 mg/g ± 2.70% RSD) and isoquercitrin (22.5 mg/g ± 2.02% RSD) (Fig. 1, Table 2).

Antioxidant activity
Free radical scavenging activity
The results of DPPH assay are shown in Fig. 2a. *F. vasta* extract displayed strong radical scavenging effect, dose-dependent, which reached about 90% inhibition at the concentration of 0.15 mg/mL. The activity of the extract was higher than that of the standard BHT, as indicated also by the IC_{50} values (0.0672 ± 0.0038 mg/mL and 0. 0821 ± 0.0009 mg/mL, respectively).

Measurement of reducing power
F. vasta extract exhibited reducing power, that increased in a dose-dependent manner; the activity resulted lower than that of BHT, as confirmed by ASE/mL values (3.65 ± 0.48 ASE/mL and 1.97 ± 0.08 ASE/mL) (Fig. 2b).

Ferrous ions (Fe²⁺) chelating activity
In the Fe^{2+} chelating activity assay *F. vasta* extract showed mild, dose-dependent, effect (data not shown). As confirmed by the IC_{50} values, the chelating ability of the extract resulted much lower than that of the standard EDTA (0.801 ± 0.007 mg/mL and 0.0067 ± 3.98 E-05 mg/mL, respectively).

Protective effect on Escherichia coli under peroxide stress
In a preliminary experiment we established that *F. vasta* extract does not inhibit the growth of *E. coli* at the dose of 1 mg/mL under the experimental conditions utilized in this protocol, thus we tested the extract at the concentration of 1 mg/mL to evaluate its protective ability against the bacteriostatic and bactericidal effects of H_2O_2. As shown in Fig. 3, *F. vasta* extract displayed noticeable protective effect on *E. coli* growth under oxidative stress. Addition of 2 mM H_2O_2 resulted in a 60-min growth arrest of *E. coli* into the Ctr group. In the culture pretreated with quercetin (0.2 mM), addition of H_2O_2 did not inhibit bacterial growth. The pretreatment with *F. vasta* extract (1 mg/mL) provoked a strong protection against H_2O_2-induced damage, statistically significant at all time points compared to Ctr group treated with H_2O_2 ($P < 0.001$ and $P < 0.0001$). Further, the cell growth

of the culture treated with *F. vasta* extract notably exceeded that of quercetin group at 20, 40 and 60 min.

The results of protective effect on *E. coli* survival are shown in Fig. 4. After 30 min, an elevated loss of viability in the Ctr culture treated with 10 mM H_2O_2 (approximately 68% survival) compared to untreated Ctr was observed. In the culture pretreated with *F. vasta* extract, high survival (approximately 110%) was maintained in the presence of 10 mM H_2O_2, statistically significant compared to Ctr culture treated with H_2O_2 ($P < 0.0001$); even in this case the observed effect was higher than that of quercetin.

Artemia salina lethality bioassay
F. vasta extract did not display any toxicity against brine shrimp larvae ($LC_{50} > 1000$ µg/mL).

Antimicrobial activity
The antimicrobial properties of *F. vasta* extract were tested against a representative set of Gram-positive and Gram-negative bacterial strains and the yeast *C. albicans*, according to the protocols recommended by the Clinical and Laboratory Standards Institute [19, 20]. The MIC values of *F. vasta* extract are shown in Table 3.

After 24 h of exposure [20], the extract was effective against almost all the bacteria tested, with the exception of *B. subtilis* and *P. aeruginosa* (MIC > 500 µg/mL). The extract showed higher efficacy towards Gram-positive than Gram-negative bacteria, with *S. aureus* and *S. epidermidis* being the most sensitive strains (MIC: 62.5 µg/mL). None of the tested strains were inhibited by DMSO (maximum 0.5% v/v), used as negative control (data not shown). The MBC values indicated that the inhibitory effect of *F. vasta* extract was bacteriostatic within the concentrations tested (MBC > 500 µg/mL). Finally, no activity was detected against *C. albicans* (MIC > 500 µg/mL).

Discussion
In this work we report for the first time the quali-quantitative characterization of the phenolic compounds present in the hydroalcoholic extract obtained from *F. vasta* leaves collected in Egypt. HPLC-PDA/ESI-MS analysis revealed the presence of phenolic acids and flavonoids.

Phenolic compounds are well known for their antioxidant properties by acting either as free radical scavengers, reducing agents or metal chelators [24]. Flavonoids and phenolic acids represent the largest classes of plant phenolics; phytochemicals from these classes were found to have excellent antioxidant activity in both in vitro and in vivo investigations [25].

Antioxidant activity, especially of phytocomplexes, cannot be evaluated satisfactorily by a simple antioxidant test, but it is strongly suggested the use of various methods in order to acquire a more complete antioxidant profile. In

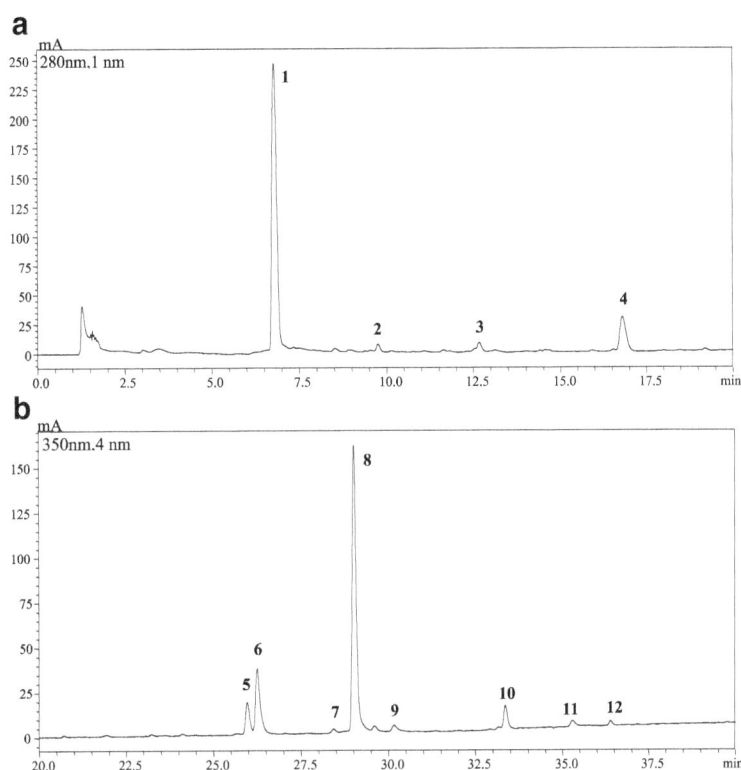

Fig. 1 HPLC-PDA chromatograms of the phenolic compounds, extracted at 280 nm (**a**) and 350 nm (**b**) wavelengths, of *F. vasta* leaves hydroalcoholic extract. For peak identification, see Table 2

these assays, plant extracts are generally assessed for their function as reducing agents, hydrogen donors, singlet oxygen quenchers or metal chelators, after which they are classified as primary (chain-breaking) and secondary (preventive) antioxidants [25]. Thus, three in vitro assays based on fundamentally different approaches and mechanisms were used to screen the antioxidant potential of *F.* *vasta* extract: the primary antioxidant properties were examined using the DPPH and the reducing power assays, and the secondary antioxidant ability was determined by measuring the Fe^{2+} chelating activity. Antioxidants can deactivate radicals by two major mechanisms: hydrogen atom transfer (HAT) and single electron transfer (SET); for DPPH test recently a combination of these two

Table 2 HPLC-PDA/ESI-MS (negative ionization mode) polyphenolic fingerprint of *Ficus vasta* leaves extract

No.	$t_{R\ (min)}$	Molecular Formula	$[M-H]^-$	UV/Vis (nm)	Compound	Class	mg/g extract	RSD (%)
1	6.8	$C_7H_6O_5$	169, 125	210, 270	Gallic acid	Benzoic acid-like acid	76.36	2.70
2	9.7	$C_{15}H_{14}O_6$	289	205, 278	Catechin	Flavan-3-ol-like	6.53	1.87
3	12.6	$C_{16}H_{18}O_9$	353, 191	215, 325	Chlorogenic acid	Cinnamic acid-like	0.73	1.73
4	16.8	$C_{15}H_{12}O_5$	271	283	Naringenin	Flavanone-like	5.84	1.30
5	26.0	$C_{27}H_{30}O_{16}$	601, 301	254, 354	Rutin	Flavonol-glycoside-like	9.33	1.38
6	26.2	$C_{21}H_{20}O_{12}$	463, 301	254, 354	Isoquercitrin	Flavonol-glycoside-like	22.50	2.02
7	28.4	$C_{27}H_{32}O_{14}$	579, 271	254, 354	Naringin	Flavanone-glycoside-like	1.20	3.56
8	29.0	$C_{21}H_{20}O_{12}$	463, 301	257, 354	Quercetin-3-galactoside	Flavonol-glycoside-like	81.75	0.88
9	30.2	$C_{21}H_{20}O_{10}$	431, 269	270, 330	Vitexin	Flavone-glycoside-like	0.64	2.95
10	33.4	$C_{21}H_{20}O_{11}$	447, 285	256, 346	Kaempferol-3-glucoside	Flavonol-glycoside-like	6.72	4.93
11	35.3	$C_{15}H_{10}O_7$	301	370	Quercetin	Flavonol-like	0.98	0.81
12	36.4	$C_{15}H_{10}O_7$	285	265, 365	Luteolin	Flavone-like	0.49	3.31

Column: Ascentis Express C_{18}, 15 cm × 4.6 mm, 2.7 μm d.p. (ESI, negative ionization mode; when observed, secondary fragment ions are reported).Values are expressed as the mean ± S.D. (n = 3)

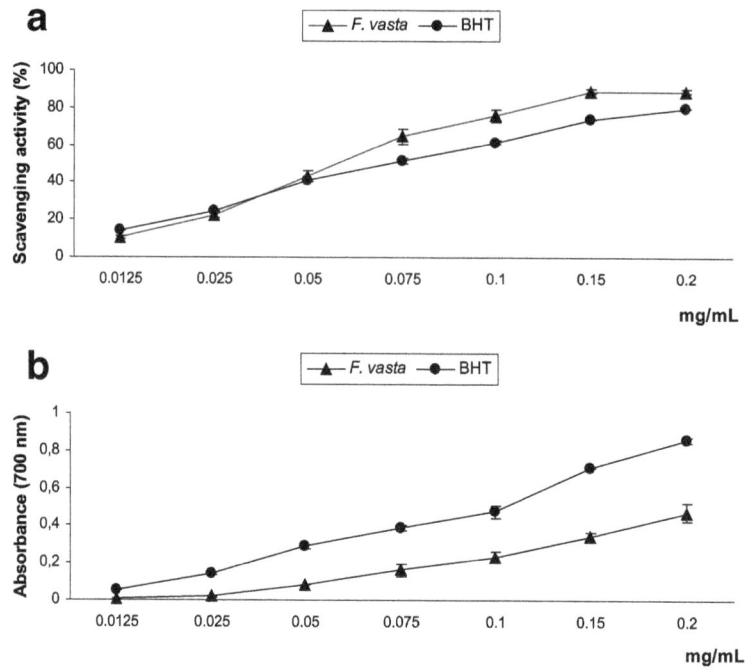

Fig. 2 Free radical scavenging activity (DPPH test) (**a**) and reducing power (**b**) of *F. vasta* leaves hydroalcoholic extract. Values are expressed as the mean ± SD (*n* = 3)

reactions, HAT and SET, was suggested to occur, whereas reducing power is recognized as electron transfer based method [25–27].

The results of antioxidant tests showed that *F. vasta* extract possesses primary antioxidant properties; these effects could depend mainly on the presence of flavonoids and phenolic acids, particularly quercetin-3-galactoside and gallic acid, which are present in high amounts in the extract. Previous studies demonstrated the strong radical scavenging properties of these compounds, as well as their ferric reducing ability [28–30]. Abdelwahed et al. [31] demonstrated that gallic acid adopt a hydrogen donating mechanism to scavenge the DPPH radical and it is even more effective than Vitamin E.

In order to investigate the antioxidant efficacy of *F. vasta* extract in a biological setting, the ability to protect bacterial growth and survival from the oxidative stress induced by hydrogen peroxide (H_2O_2) was evaluated on *Escherichia coli*. This microbial model is utilized as an effective system to establish the antioxidant properties of medicinal plant extracts or pure compounds [32]; it is easier in terms of experimental operation, lower in cost compared to cellular antioxidant activity assays, and more biologically relevant than the in vitro measurements of antioxidant activity.

The obtained results showed that *F. vasta* extract displayed noticeable protective effects on *E. coli* growth under oxidative stress. These results are similar to those previously reported for different extracts of *Potentilla*

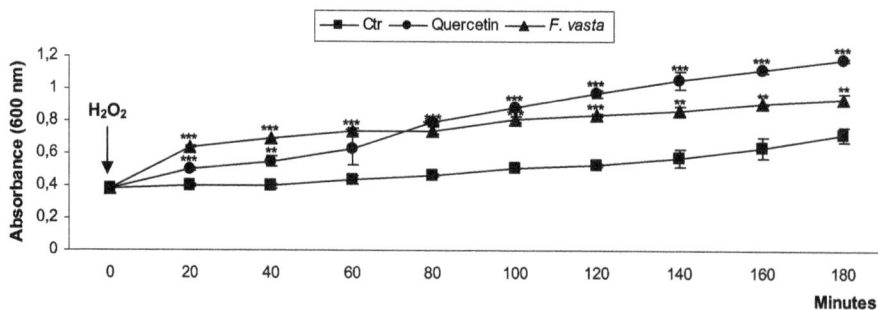

Fig. 3 Protective effect of *F. vasta* leaves hydroalcoholic extract on *Escherichia coli* growing under peroxide stress. Values are expressed as the mean ± SD (n = 3). Statistical differences compared to control group with H_2O_2 treatment (Ctr + H_2O_2) are noted with asterisk (**$P < 0.001$, ***$P < 0.0001$)

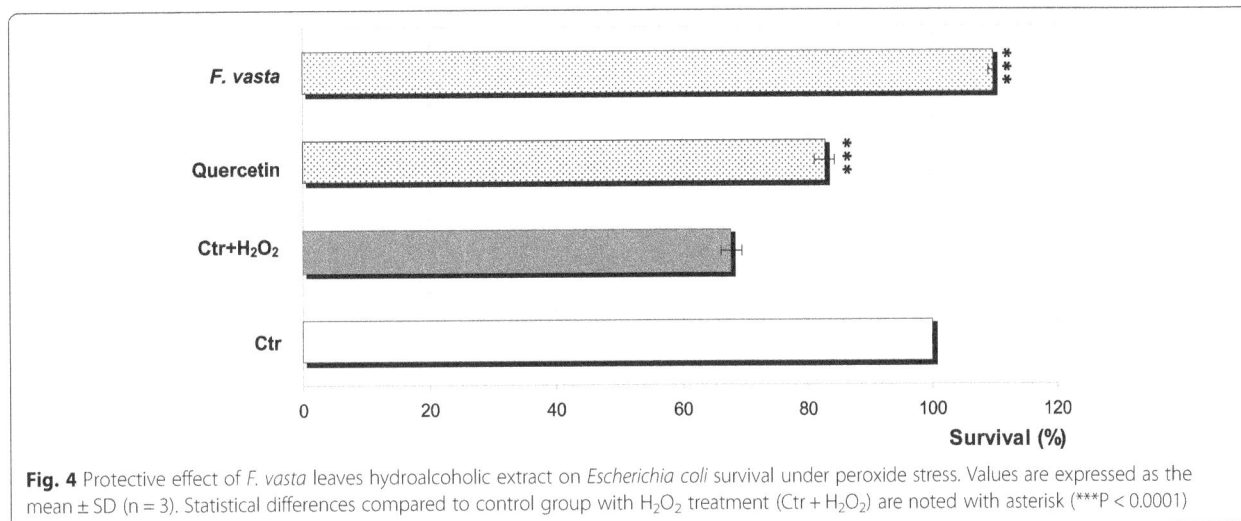

Fig. 4 Protective effect of *F. vasta* leaves hydroalcoholic extract on *Escherichia coli* survival under peroxide stress. Values are expressed as the mean ± SD (n = 3). Statistical differences compared to control group with H_2O_2 treatment (Ctr + H_2O_2) are noted with asterisk (***P < 0.0001)

fruticosa L., tested at the same concentration of *F. vasta* extract and under the same experimental conditions [33]. Oktyabrsky et al. [34] previously demonstrated the protective effect of several plant extracts on *E. coli* survival in the presence of high concentrations of H_2O_2 (10 mM); from a comparison of the results *F. vasta* extract showed a greater activity, displaying total protection against oxidative damage.

The protective effects of some polyphenols, as quercetin and catechin, on growth and survival of *E. coli* under peroxide stress has been previously reported [19]; thus, it can be hypothesized that the polyphenols contained in *F. vasta* extract are the main responsible for the observed activities.

In order to achieve a safe treatment with plant products, numerous research studies have recently been focused on the toxicity of medicinal plants. The brine shrimp (*Artemia salina* Leach) lethality bioassay has been established as a safe, practical and cheap method

Table 3 The MIC values of *F. vasta* leaves extract

Gram positive bacteria	MIC (µg/mL)
Bacillus subtilis ATCC 6633	> 500
Listeria monocytogenes ATCC 13932	125.0
Staphylococcus aureus ATCC 29213	62.5
Staphylococcus epidermidis ATCC 12228	62.5
Gram negative bacteria	
Escherichia coli ATCC 10536	250.0
Escherichia coli ATCC 25922	250.0
Pseudomonas aeruginosa ATCC 15442	> 500
Salmonella typhimurium ATCC 13311	250.0
Salmonella enterica (Wild type)	250.0
Yeast	
Candida albicans ATCC 10231	> 500

employed for preliminary assessment of toxicity and have been used for detection of fungal toxins, plant extract toxicity, heavy metals and pesticides [21]. According to Clarkson's toxicity criterion for the toxicity assessment of plant extracts, those with LC_{50} above 1000 µg/mL are considered as non-toxic [35]. *F. vasta* extract was found to be non-toxic against brine shrimps.

In the last decade, there has been growing interest in the use of plant extracts with low toxicity as sources of natural antimicrobial substances; particularly, the antimicrobial properties of plant extracts containing phenolic compounds were described [36–38].

F. vasta extract extract exhibited bacteriostatic activity against almost all the Gram-positive and Gram-negative bacteria tested, particularly against *S. aureus* and *S. epidermidis*.

Our results disagree with those of a previous work, which reported the lack of antibacterial properties of a 80% MeOH extract of *F. vasta* aerial parts against *S. aureus*, *S. epidermidis*, *E. coli* and *P. aeruginosa*, as evaluated by the disk-diffusion method [13]; nonetheless, the extract was tested at the dose of 1.19 µg only, and this could explain the disaccording results.

It can be hypothesized that the antimicrobial properties of *F. vasta* extract could depend on the presence of phenolic compounds. Gram-positive and Gram-negative bacterial species might have different sensitivities against the phenolics contained in *F. vasta* extract because of the difference in their membrane structure and associated cell wall differences. Many of the phenolic compounds were found to be effective against Gram-positive bacteria, whereas they showed no activity or negligible activity against Gram-negative bacteria. The partial hydrophobicity of some phenolic compounds allows them to act efficiently at the membrane-interface of Gram-positive bacteria, this causes the loss of membrane integrity and the dissipation of the proton motive force [39].

It is known that both flavonoids and phenolic acids are effective antimicrobial agents against a wide array of microorganisms [5, 40]. Liu et al. [41] previously reported that quercetin and luteolin showed a broad antimicrobial spectrum of activity on microorganisms including bacteria and fungi, whereas the glycoside derivatives such as quercetin 3-O-β-D-glucoside (isoquercitrin) exhibited relatively weak antimicrobial activity. Other authors showed that quercetin 3-O-glucoside didn't display any antibacterial efficacy [42].

The antibacterial activity of some phenolic acids such as gallic against Gram-positive (*S. aureus* and *L. monocytogenes*) and Gram-negative bacteria (*E. coli* and *P. aeruginosa*) was demonstrated; these compounds were found to be more efficient against the reported bacteria than conventional antibiotics such as gentamicin and streptomycin [43]. It was reported that gallic acid could restrain the growth of many bacteria, including methicillin-sensitive *S. aureus*, MRSA, *E. coli*, *P. aeruginosa*, and *S. typhi* [44]. Based on these statements, gallic acid, contained in high amount in the extract, could be the main component responsible of the observed effects.

Conclusions

This study is the first report on the characterization of the phenolic profile and the evaluation of antioxidant and antimicrobial activities of the leaves of *Ficus vasta* Forssk. growing in Egypt. The results of our investigations showed that *F. vasta* extract possesses strong primary antioxidant properties, as well as antibacterial efficacy, particularly against the Gram-positive tested strains. Besides, the extract showed no toxicity against brine shrimp larvae.

These findings contribute to an increase in knowledge about this species, demonstrating the potential of *Ficus vasta* leaves as safe sources of natural antioxidant and antimicrobial compounds.

Abbreviations

ACN: acetonitrile; ASE: ascorbic acid equivalent; BHT: Butylated Hydroxytoluene; CFU: colony forming unit; DMSO: dimethyl sulfoxide; DPPH: 2,2-diphenyl-1-picrylhydrazyl; EDTA: Ethylenediaminetetraacetic acid; H_2O_2: hydrogen peroxide; IC_{50}: mean 50% Inhibitory Concentration; LB: Luria-Bertani; LC_{50}: median lethal concentration; MBC: minimum bactericidal concentration; MeOH: methanol; MFC: minimum fungicidal concentration; MHB: Müeller Hinton Broth; RSD: relative standard deviation; SDA: Sabouraud Dextrose Agar

Acknowledgements

The authors wish to thank the Foundation "Prof. Antonio Imbesi". The authors also gratefully thank Dr. Mohammed El-Gebaly, Department of Botany, National Research Centre (NRC) and by Mrs. Tereeza Labib, consultant of Plant Taxonomy at the Ministry of Agriculture and director of Orman Botanical Garden, Giza, Egypt, for identification of plant material.

Authors' contributions

MFT and NM designed the study and wrote the manuscript. KR, FC, PD, and LM carried out the phytochemical studies; MFT, NM, and RA performed the antioxidant and toxicity experiments; AF, CB, and MD the antimicrobial experiments. All the authors revised the article critically and gave approval of the final version.

Competing interests

The authors declare that they have no competing interests.

Author details

[1]Dipartimento di Scienze Chimiche, Biologiche, Farmaceutiche ed Ambientali, University of Messina, Polo Annunziata, Viale Annunziata, 98168 Messina, Italy. [2]Pharmacognosy Department, National Research Centre, 33 El-Bohouth st. Dokki, P.O.12622, Giza, Egypt. [3]Foundation "Prof. Antonio Imbesi", University of Messina, Piazza Pugliatti 1, 98122 Messina, Italy. [4]Dipartimento di Scienze Biomediche, Odontoiatriche e delle Immagini Morfologiche e Funzionali, University of Messina, Via Consolare Valeria, 98125 Messina, Italy. [5]Scienze dell'Alimentazione e della Nutrizione Umana, Università Campus Biomedico di Roma, via Àlvaro del Portillo 21, 00128 Rome, Italy. [6]Chromaleont s.r.l., c/o Dipartimento di Scienze Chimiche, Biologiche, Farmaceutiche ed Ambientali, University of Messina, Polo Annunziata, Viale Annunziata, 98168 Messina, Italy. [7]Dipartimento di Scienze del Farmaco, sezione Biochimica, Viale Andrea Doria 6, 95123 Catania, Italy.

References

1. Acquaviva R, Menichini F, Ragusa S, Genovese C, Amodeo A, Tundis R, Loizzo MR, Iauk. Antimicrobial and antioxidant properties of *Betula aetnensis* Rafin. (Betulaceae) leaves extract. Nat Prod Res 2013a;27(4–5):475–479.
2. Acquaviva R, Di Giacomo C, Vanella L, Santangelo R, Sorrenti V, Barbagallo L, Genovese C, Mastrojeni S, Ragusa S, Iauk L. Antioxidant activity of extracts of *Momordica foetida* Schumach. Et Thonn. Molecules. 2013b;18(3):3241–9.
3. Hatami T, Emami SA, Miraghaee SS, Mojarrab M. Total phenolic contents and antioxidant activities of different extracts and fractions from the aerial parts of *Artemisia biennis* Willd. Iran J Pharm Res. 2014;13(2):551–9.
4. Dai J, Mumper RJ. Plant phenolics: extraction, analysis and their antioxidant and anticancer properties. Molecules. 2010;15(10):7313–52.
5. Cowan MM. Plant products as antimicrobial agents. Clin Microbiol Rev. 1999;12(4):564–82.
6. Ahmed F, MKK A, Abedin Z, Karim AA. Traditional uses and pharmacological potential of *Ficus exasperata* Vahl. Sys Rev Pharm. 2012;3(1):15–23.
7. Abdel-Hameed E-SS. Total phenolic contents and free radical scavenging activity of certain Egyptian *Ficus* species leaf samples. Food Chem. 2009; 114(4):1271–7.
8. Alqasoumi SI, Basudan OA, Al-Rehaily AJ, Abdel-Kader MS. Phytochemical and pharmacological study of *Ficus palmata* growing in Saudi Arabia. Saudi Pharm J. 2014;22(5):460–71.
9. Tkachenko H, Buyun L, Terech-Majewska E, Osadowski Z. *In vitro* antimicrobial activity of ethanolic extracts obtained from *Ficus* spp. leaves against the fish pathogen *Aeromonas hydrophila*. Arch Pol Fish. 2016;24:219–30.
10. Raju NJ, Yesuf EA, Bekele M, Wabe NT. Investigation of in vitro anthelmintic activity of *Ficus vasta* leaves. Asian J pharm Biol Res. 2011;1(4):454–8.
11. Mosa EO, Justin DD, Hamam SB, Mohamed EAO, Saad MHA. Evaluation of phytochemical and antimicrobial activities of some sudanese medicinal plants. World. J Pharm Pharm Sci. 2014;3(12):1769–76.
12. Rashed K, Anthonissen R, Cappoen D, Verschaeve L. Phytochemical composition and potential genotoxic effects of important Egyptian medicinal plants. Phcog Commn. 2015;5(3):207–16.
13. Rashed K, Ono L. Evaluation of cytotoxicity, anti-herpes simplex virus type 1 (HSV-1) and antibacterial activities of *Ficus vasta* and phytoconstituents. Int Curr Pharm J. 2013;3(1):211–8.

14. Osman ME, Yassen HH, Deng JD, Mustafa RO, Hussein SM. General phytochemical screening and antioxidant activity of some Sudanese medicinal plants. J Forest Prod Ind. 2014;3(6):292–5.
15. De Souza KC, Schapoval EE, Bassani VL. LC determination of flavonoids: separation of quercetin, luteolin and 3-O-methylquercetin in Achyrocline satureioides preparations. J Pharm Biomed Anal. 2002;28(3–4):771–7.
16. Fathiazad F, Delazar A, Amiri R, Sarker SD. Extraction of flavonoids and quantification of rutin from waste tobacco leaves. Iran J Pharm Res. 2006;3:222–7.
17. Taviano MF, Filocamo A, Ragusa S, Cacciola F, Dugo P, Mondello L, et al. Phenolic profile, antioxidant and cytotoxic properties of polar extracts from leaves and flowers of Isatis tinctoria L. (Brassicaceae) growing in Sicily. Plant Biosyst. 2017; https://doi.org/10.1080/11263504.2017.1338629.
18. Miceli N, Filocamo A, Ragusa S, Cacciola F, Dugo P, Mondello L, et al. Chemical characterization and biological activities of phenolic-rich fraction from cauline leaves of Isatis tinctoria L. (Brassicaceae) growing in Sicily, Italy. Chem Biodivers. 2017;14(8):1–11.
19. Smirnova GV, Samoylova ZY, Muzyka NG, Oktyabrsky ON. Influence of polyphenols on Escherichia coli resistance to oxidative stress. Free Rad Biol Med. 2009;46:759–68.
20. Schurig-Briccio LA, Farías RN, Rodríguez-Montelongo L, Rintoul MR, Rapisarda VA. Protection against oxidative stress in Escherichia coli stationary phase by a phosphate concentration-dependent genes expression. Arch Biochem Biophys. 2009;483:106–10.
21. Taviano MF, Marino A, Trovato A, Bellinghieri V, Melchini A, Dugo P, et al. Juniperus oxycedrus L. subsp. oxycedrus and Juniperus oxycedrus L. subsp. macrocarpa (Sibth. & Sm.) ball. "Berries" from Turkey: comparative evaluation of phenolic profile, antioxidant, cytotoxic and antimicrobial activities. Food Chem Toxicol. 2013;58:22–9.
22. Clinical and Laboratory Standards Institute (CLSI). Reference method for broth dilution antifungal susceptibility testing of Yeasts, 3rd ed. Approved standard M27-A3. In: Wayne (PA): clinical and laboratory standards institute; 2008.
23. Clinical and Laboratory Standards Institute (CLSI). Methods for dilution antimicrobial susceptibility tests for bacteria that grow aerobically, 9th ed. Approved standard M07-A9. In: Wayne (PA): clinical and laboratory standards institute; 2012.
24. Chua LS, Hidayathulla S. Phytochemical profile of fresh and senescent leaves due to storage for Ficus deltoidea. Plant Biosyst. 2017;151(1):74–83.
25. Kasote DM, Katyare SS, Hegde MV, Bae H. Significance of antioxidant potential of plants and its relevance to therapeutic applications. Int J Biol Sci. 2015;11(8):982–91.
26. Prior RL, Wu X, Schaich K. Standardized methods for the determination of antioxidant capacity and phenolics in foods and dietary supplements. J Agric Food Chem. 2005;53:4290–302.
27. Csepregi K, Neugart S, Schreine M, Hideg É. Comparative evaluation of total antioxidant capacities of plant polyphenols. Molecules. 2016;21(2), 208:1–16.
28. Parejo I, Viladomat F, Bastida J, Schmeda-Hirschmann G, Burillo JS, Codina C. Bioguided isolation and identification of the non-volatile antioxidant compounds from fennel (Foeniculum vulgare mill.) waste. J Agric Food Chem. 2004;52(7):1890.
29. Zhang Y, Wang D, Yang L, Zhou D, Zhang J. Purification and characterization of flavonoids from the leaves of Zanthoxylum bungeanum and correlation between their structure and antioxidant activity. PLOS ONE. 2014;9(8):e105725. 1–11
30. Badhani B, Sharma N, Kakkar R. Gallic acid: a versatile antioxidant with promising therapeutic and industrial applications. RSC Adv. 2015;5:27540–57.
31. Abdelwahed A, Bouhlel I, Skandrani I, Valenti K, Kadri M, Guiraud P, et al. Study of antimutagenic and antioxidant activities of Gallic acid and 1,2,3,4,6-pentagalloylglucose from Pistacia lentiscus. Confirmation by microarray expression profiling Chem Biol Interact. 2007;165(1):1–13.
32. Smirnova GV, Vysochina GI, Muzyka NG, Samoylova ZY, Kukushkina TA, Oktyabrsky ON. Evaluation of antioxidant properties of medical plants using microbial test systems. World J Microbiol Biotechnol. 2010;26(12):2269–76.
33. Yu D, Pu W, Li D, Wang D, Liu Q, Wang Y. Phenolic compounds and antioxidant activity of different organs of Potentilla fruticosa L. from two main production areas of China. Chem Biodivers. 2016;13(9):1140–8.
34. Oktyabrsky O, Vysochina G, Muzyka N, Samoilova Z, Kukushkina T, Smirnova G. Assessment of anti-oxidant activity of plant extracts using microbial test systems. J Appl Microbiol. 2009;106(4):1175–83.
35. Clarkson C, Maharaj VJ, Crouch NR, Grace OM, Pillay P, Matsabisa MG, Bhagwandin N, Smith PJ, Folb PI. In vitro antiplasmodial activity of medicinal plants native to or naturalized in South Africa. J Ethnopharmacol. 2004;92(2–3):177–91.
36. del Carmen Villalobos M, Serradilla MJ, Martín A, Ordiales E, Ruiz-Moyanoa S, de Guía Córdoba M. Antioxidant and antimicrobial activity of natural phenolic extract from defatted soybean flour by-product for stone fruit postharvest application. J Sci Food Agric. 2016;96(6):2116–24.
37. dos Reis Albuquerque AdJ, de Freitas e Silva PM, de Almeida Cavalcante ALF, Sampaiop FC. Polyphenols as a source of antimicrobial agents against human pathogens. In: Extracts P, editor. Giordano A, Costs A. New York (USA): Nova Science Publishers, Inc.; 2013. p. 275–94.
38. Bisignano C, Filocamo A, Faulks RM, Mandalari G. In vitro antimicrobial activity of pistachio (Pistacia vera L.) polyphenols. FEMS Microbiol Lett. 2013;341(1):62–7.
39. Davidson PM. Chemical preservatives and natural antimicrobial compounds. In: Beuchat LR, Montville TJ, editors. Doyle MP. Food Microbiology. Fundamentals and Frontiers. Washington DC (USA): ASM Press; 2001. p. 611–6.
40. Cushnie TPT, Lamb AJ. Recent advances in understanding the antibacterial properties of flavonoids. Int J Antimicrob Agents. 2011;38(2):99–107.
41. Liu H, Mou Y, Zhao J, Wang J, Zhou L, Wang M, et al. Flavonoids from Halostachys caspica and their antimicrobial and antioxidant activities. Molecules. 2010;15(11):7933–45.
42. Razavi SM, Zahri S, Zarrini G, Nazemiyeh H, Mohammadi S. Biological activity of quercetin-3-O-glucoside, a known plant flavonoid. Bioorg Khim. 2009;35(3):414–6.
43. Daglia M. Polyphenols as antimicrobial agents. Curr Opin Biotechnol. 2012;23(2):174–81.
44. Fu L, Lu W, Zhou X. Phenolic compounds and in vitro antibacterial and antioxidant activities of three tropic fruits: persimmon, guava, and sweetsop. Biomed Res Int. 2016;2016:1–9.

Comparison of the main components and bioactivity of *Rhus verniciflua Stokes extracts* by different detoxification processing methods

Seon-Ok Lee[1], Sung-Ji Kim[2], Ju-Sung Kim[4], Hyuk Ji[1], Eun-Ok Lee[1,2,3] and Hyo-Jeong Lee[1,2,3*]

Abstract

Background: *Rhus verniciflua* Stokes is an Asian tree species that is used as a food supplement and traditional medicine in Korea. However, its use is restricted by its potential to cause allergy. Thus, allergen-free *R. verniciflua* extracts are currently being marketed as a functional health food in Korea. In the present study, three different allergen-free *R. verniciflua* extracts (DRVE, FRVE, and FFRVE) were produced by detoxification of *R. verniciflua,* and their properties and constituents were compared.

Methods: The main components and properties (antibacterial, antioxidant, anticancer, and hepatic lipogenesis inhibitory effects) of the three allergen-free extracts were compared. Moreover, the major phenolic constituents of *R. verniciflua,* including gallic acid, fustin, fisetin, and quercetin, were analyzed in the three extracts.

Results: DRVE was superior to the two other extracts with regard to antioxidant activity, while FRVE was superior with regard to antimicrobial activity and suppression of hepatic lipogenesis. FRVE exhibited lipid-lowering effects by lowering sterol regulatory element-binding protein 1 and triglyceride levels, and promoting the activation of peroxisome proliferator-activated receptor and AMP-activated protein kinase in an in vitro model of non-alcoholic fatty liver.

Conclusions: Overall, our findings demonstrate various differences among the three extracts. This suggests that functional and bioactive compounds present in *R. verniciflua* could be altered by the detoxification process, and this property could be considered in the development of functional health foods in the future.

Keywords: *Rhus verniciflua* Stokes, Detoxification, Fermentation, Fustin, Fisetin

Background

Rhus verniciflua Stokes (RVS), the lacquer tree, has been used as a traditional medicine and food supplement for a long time in Eastern Asia. In Korea, RVS has been used as a herbal medicine for the treatment of abdominal pain, including pain caused by stomach disorders such as gastritis, and as a hemostatic agent [1]. RVS has been reported to exhibit anticancer, antioxidant, antimicrobial, and anti-inflammatory activities [2–6]. Moreover, RVS contains a wide variety of flavonoids and polyphenols, including fustin, fisetin, quercetin, butein, p-coumaric acid, kaempferol, sulfuretin, catechol, and ethyl gallate. However, despite the various biological activities of RVS, its use has been limited because of a component called urushiol, which is known to cause allergies. Therefore, urushiol should be removed before using RVS as a food supplement or medicine. Several detoxification methods have been developed to produce urushiol-free RVS, such as heat treatment, solvent extraction, and enzyme treatment by microbial or mushroom mycelium fermentation [7–9]. Currently, allergen-free RVS extracts are being marketed as health functional food in Korea. However, there are no comparative studies on the

* Correspondence: strong79@khu.ac.kr
[1]Department of Science in Korean Medicine, Graduate School, Kyung Hee University, Hoegi-dong, Dongdaemun-gu, 130-701 Seoul, Republic of Korea
[2]Department of Cancer Preventive Material Development, Graduate School, Kyung Hee University, Hoegi-dong, Dongdaemun-gu, 130-701 Seoul, Republic of Korea
Full list of author information is available at the end of the article

components and bioactivities of RVS extracts obtained by various detoxification methods. It is important to develop efficient and cost-effective food processing methods in order to enhance the content of bioactive components.

We previously reported that RVS detoxified via a microbial method could alleviate oleic acid (OA)-induced steatosis in HepG2 cells, and that it contained phenolics and cosanols with lipid-lowering potential. In the present study, we compared the effects of three RVS extracts detoxified by different methods with regard to their antioxidant, antimicrobial, and anticancer properties, their suppressive effect on hepatic lipogenesis, and their main components.

Methods

Preparation of DRVE, FRVE, and FFRVE powders

The three types of detoxified RVS extracts used in this study are products that are commercially available in Korea, and were purchased from Okkane (Seoul, Korea). The following three extracts were used: an allergen-free RVS extract detoxified by hot air drying (dried *R. verniciflua* extract, DRVE), an allergen-free RVS extract fermented with *Saccharomyces carlsbergensis* (fermented *R. verniciflua* extract, FRVE), and an allergen-free RVS extract fermented with mushroom mycelium (*Fomitella fraxinea*-fermented *R. verniciflua* extract, FFRVE). The extracts (one bottle = 1.5 L) were dried to a powder by freeze-drying.

Determination of antimicrobial activity by agar diffusion method

The antimicrobial activities of the three RVS extracts were determined via modified Kirby-Bauer disk diffusion method [10, 11]. The test microorganisms used in this experiment were *Propionibacterium acnes* (ATCC 6919) and *Trichophyton rubrum* (ATCC 22402), and were obtained from the Korean Culture Center of Microorganisms. *P. acnes* was cultured anaerobically at 37 °C in Mueller Hinton broth (Difco, USA) and Mueller Hinton agar (0.75% agar), while *T. rubrum* was cultured at 26 °C in Sabouraud Dextrose broth and Sabouraud Dextrose agar (0.75% agar). The three powdered extracts, DRVE, FRVE, and FFRVE, were dissolved in water to obtain concentrations of 100 and 1000 mg/mL for each extract. Fifty microliters of each extract was injected into a sterile disk of 6-mm diameter (Toyo Roshi Kaisha Ltd., Tokyo, Japan), and the solvent was allowed to dry off in an aseptic hood. Accordingly, disks were loaded with 5 and 50 mg of each crude extract. Standard disks containing distilled water served as negative controls for the antimicrobial test.

After 24 h, *P. acnes* or *T. rubrum* cultures were adjusted to 1×10^8 CFU/mL using 0.5 McFarland standards and inoculated into Mueller Hinton agar and Sabouraud Dextrose agar, respectively. Next, disks containing the extracts were placed on a plate and incubated at 37 and 26 °C, respectively. *P. acnes* and *T. rubrum* plates were incubated for 2 and 5 days, respectively. The antimicrobial activities of the extracts were then determined by measuring the diameter of the clear zones around the disks in millimeters. This measurement was carried out in triplicate.

Cell culture

Human hepatocellular carcinoma (HepG2, ATCC HB-8065) and murine normal hepatocyte (AML12, ATCC CRL-2254) cell lines were maintained in Dulbecco's modified Eagle's medium (DMEM) containing 10% fetal bovine serum (FBS, Welgene, Daegu, Korea) with 1% antibiotics (Welgene). Human prostate cancer (PC3, ATCC CRL-1435), breast cancer (MDA-MB-231, ATCC HTB-26), and colon cancer (HCT116, ATCC CCL-247) cell lines were maintained in RPMI 1640 containing 10% FBS (Welgene) with 1% antibiotics (Welgene).

Cell viability assay

HepG2, PC3, MDA-MB-231, HCT116, and AML12 cells were incubated in 96-well plates (5×10^4 cells/well) and treated with various doses of DRVE, FRVE, and FFRVE (0, 50, 100, 200, and 400 μg/mL) for 24 h. Next, 50 μL of 3-(4−5-dimethylthiazol-2-yl)-2,5-diphenyl tetrazolium bromide (MTT, 1 mg/mL, Sigma-Aldrich, St. Louis, MO, USA) was added. After 2 h, formazan crystals in viable cells were dissolved in dimethyl sulfoxide (DMSO), and cell viability was calculated by measuring the optical density (OD) at 570 nm using a microplate reader (Molecular Devices Co, Sunnyvale, CA, USA).

High-performance liquid chromatography

Urushiol in the three extracts was analyzed by high-performance liquid chromatography (HPLC, Agilent Technologies, Santa Clara, CA, USA) using Hichrome HPLC columns (5 μm, 250 mm × 4.6 mm, Hichrome, Ltd., Theale, UK). A flow rate of 0.3 mL/min and an injection volume of 10 μL were used. The solvent used was 100% methanol, and the detection wavelength was set to 254 nm.

Moreover, the polyphenols gallic acid, fustin, fisetin, quercetin, butein, and sulfuretin were analyzed in the three RVS extracts via HPLC. The mobile phases were composed of 0.1% formic acid in water (solvent A) and 100% methanol (solvent B), delivered at a flow rate of 0.7 mL/min. The following gradient conditions were used: 0–17 min, 100% B; 17–20 min, 100% B; 20–23 min, 0% B; and 23–30 min, 0% B. The detection wavelength was set to 254 nm, and an injection volume of 10 μL was used.

Oil red O staining

HepG2 cells were incubated in a 6-well plate (5×10^5 cells/well) for 24 h. The cells were then treated with DRVE, FRVE, and FFRVE (400 μg/mL), and stimulated with OA (200 μM) for a further 24 h. After incubation, the supernatants were discarded and cells were washed with phosphate-buffered saline (PBS). Cell fixation was done by treating with 4% formalin for 10 min, followed by washing with PBS and staining with Oil Red O (ORO). ORO stain was extracted using isopropanol and the OD was measured at 510 nm using a microplate reader (Molecular Devices Co).

Western blot analysis

HepG2 cells were incubated in a 6-well plate (5×10^5 cells/well) for 24 h. The cells were then treated with DRVE, FRVE, and FFRVE (400 μg/mL), and stimulated with OA (200 μM) for a further 24 h at 37 °C. Next, cells were harvested and lysed with radioimmunoprecipitation assay (RIPA) buffer (50 mM Tris-HCl (pH 7.4), 150 mM NaCl, 1% NP-40, 0.25% sodium deoxycholate, 1 M EDTA, 1 mM Na_3VO_4, 1 mM NaF, and protease-inhibitor cocktail). Protein samples were quantitated using a Bio-Rad DC protein assay kit II (Bio-Rad, Hercules, CA, USA), resolved via sodium dodecyl sulfate-polyacrylamide gel electrophoresis (SDS-PAGE) on 8% polyacrylamide gel, and electrotransferred onto a BioTrace NT transfer membrane (Pall, Gelman Laboratory, Port Washington, NY, USA). After electrotransfer, membranes were blocked with 5% skimmed milk (BD, NJ, USA) and probed with primary antibodies for sterol regulatory element-binding protein 1 (SREBP-1, Santa Cruz Biotechnology, Santa Cruz, CA, USA), peroxisome proliferator-activated receptor alpha (PPAR-α, Santa Cruz Biotechnology), AMP-activated protein kinase (AMPK, Cell Signaling, Denvers, MA, USA), phosphorylated AMPK (p-AMPK, Cell Signaling), and β-actin (Sigma-Aldrich) overnight, and exposed to horseradish peroxidase-conjugated secondary anti-mouse or anti-rabbit antibodies. Protein expression levels were detected using an EZ-Western Lumi Pico kit (DOGEN, Seoul, Korea).

Measurement of cellular triglyceride levels

HepG2 cells were incubated in a 6-well plate (5×10^5 cells/well) for 24 h. The cells were then treated with DRVE, FRVE, and FFRVE (400 μg/mL), and stimulated with OA (200 μM) for a further 24 h. To measure cellular triglyceride (TG) levels, a chloroform-methanol extraction method was applied with some modifications, as described in a previous protocol [12, 13]. Cells were collected and mixed with 1 mL of a 2:1 chloroform:methanol mixture at room temperature for 20 min. After centrifugation at 500×g for 10 min, the lower layers were collected and dried overnight at 4 °

C, and TG levels were measured using a TG assay kit (Asan Pharm, Hwaseong-si, Korea). The OD was measured at 550 nm using a microplate reader (Molecular Devices Co).

Determination of the antioxidant capacity of the three extracts

The 1,1-diphenyl-2-picrylhydrazyl (DPPH) radical scavenging activity was measured by the Blois method [14]. The extracts were mixed with DPPH and stabilized at room temperature for 30 min. The OD was then measured at 515 nm using a microplate reader (Molecular Devices Co).

Statistical analysis

Results are presented as means ± standard deviation of triplicates. Data were analyzed via Student's t-test. Differences among groups were considered statistically significant if $p < 0.05$.

Results

Confirmation of DRVE, FRVE, and FFRVE detoxification

To confirm detoxification of the three RVS extracts, the presence of the allergen urushiol was investigated by HPLC. Urushiol (Fig. 1a) was not detected in any of the three extracts (Fig. 1b, c, and d), thus confirming successful detoxification. The urushiol peak in the standard appeared at 13.62 min.

DRVE demonstrated the strongest antioxidant activity among the three extracts

The antioxidant activities of DRVE, FRVE, and FFRVE were evaluated via a DPPH radical scavenging assay. Quercetin, tannic acid, and ascorbic acid were used as standards to analyze DPPH scavenging capacity.

The half-maximal effective concentration (EC_{50}) of any antioxidant compound is inversely related to its antioxidant activity, as it is the concentration of the antioxidant needed to decrease the radical concentration by 50%. Thus, lower EC_{50} values indicate higher antioxidant activities. DRVE and FRVE exhibited EC_{50} values of 48.7 and 111.3 μg/mL, respectively, while the DPPH radical scavenging activity of FFRVE was 28.6% at its high concentration (200 μg/mL, Table 1). The radical scavenging activity of DRVE was stronger than that of the two other extracts (Table 1).

FRVE demonstrated the strongest antimicrobial activity among the three extracts

The antimicrobial activities of the three RVS extracts were investigated against two different microbes that cause skin diseases (*P. acne*, an acne-causing bacterium, and *T. rubrum*, a fungus that affects hands and nails and causes athlete's foot) using an agar diffusion

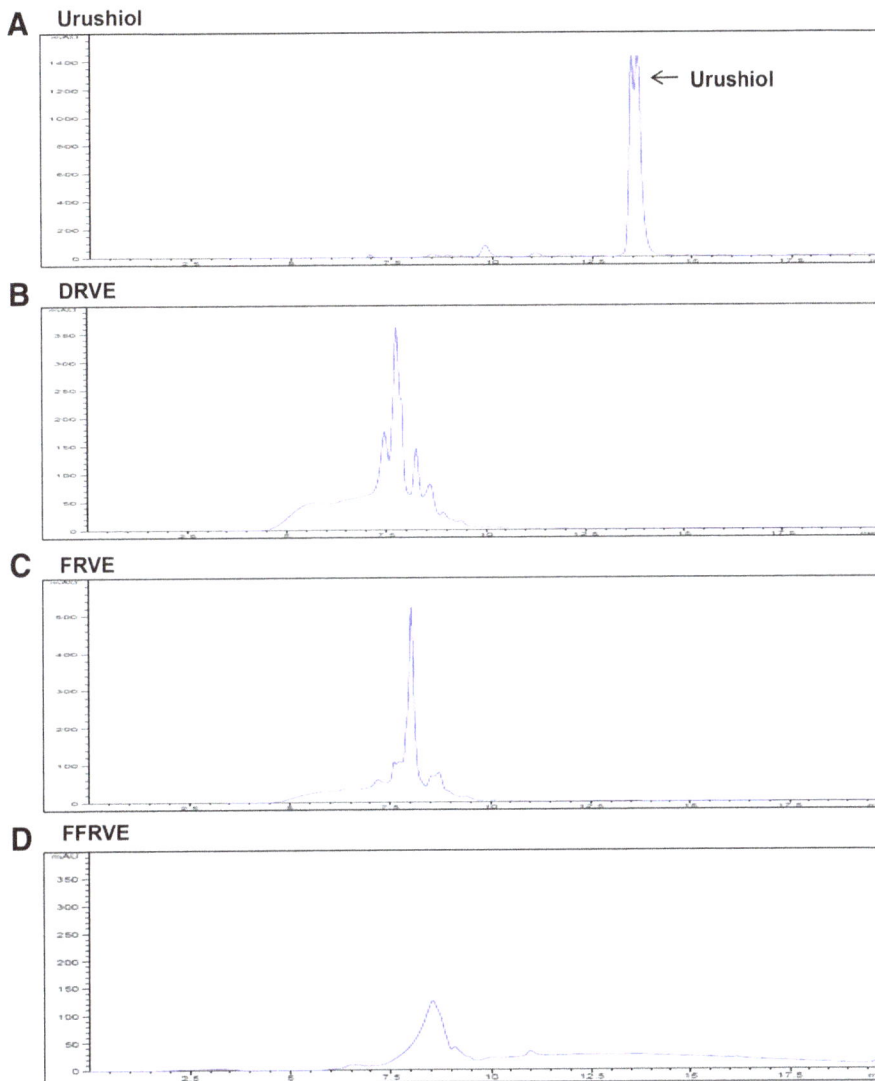

Fig. 1 Determination of allergen-free *Rhus verniciflua Stokes* extracts (DRVE, FRVE, FFRVE) by HPLC analysis. HPLC analysis identified urushiol as an allergen of *Rhus verinciflua Stokes*. **a** Urushiol standard **b** DRVE **c** FRVE **d** FFRVE

method at doses of 5 and 50 mg/disk. Only the 50 mg/disk dose of FRVE demonstrated a strong antimicrobial activity against *P. acnes* (Fig. 2a) and *T. rubrum*

cultures (Fig. 2b), producing 42- and 25-mm inhibition zones, respectively.

The anticancer effects of DRVE, FRVE, and FFRVE
DRVE and FRVE inhibit cancer cell viability without affecting normal cells

We tested the effects of DRVE, FRVE, and FFRVE on the viability of four human cancer cell lines (HepG2, PC3, MDA-MB-231, and HCT116) and of normal cells (AML-12). The concentrations of FRVE and DRVE tested were 0, 50, 100, 200, and 400 µg/mL.

As shown in Fig. 3a, the viability of HepG2 cells was reduced to 29, 22, and 12% when incubated with 400 µg/mL DRVE, FRVE, and FFRVE, respectively, for 24 h (Fig. 3a). Similarly, treatment with 400 µg/mL DRVE, FRVE, and FFRVE reduced prostate cancer cell

Table 1 Antioxidant capacity of the DRVE, FRVE, and FFRVE by DPPH scavenging assay

Sample	DPPH, EC50 (µg/ml)
DRVE	48.7 ± 2.1
FRVE	111.3 ± 1.3
FFRVE	> 200 (28.6%)
Quercetin	7.7 ± 0.1
Tannic acid	8.4 ± 0.5
Ascorbic acid	11.8 ± 1.1

Each value represents mean ± SD ($n = 3$)

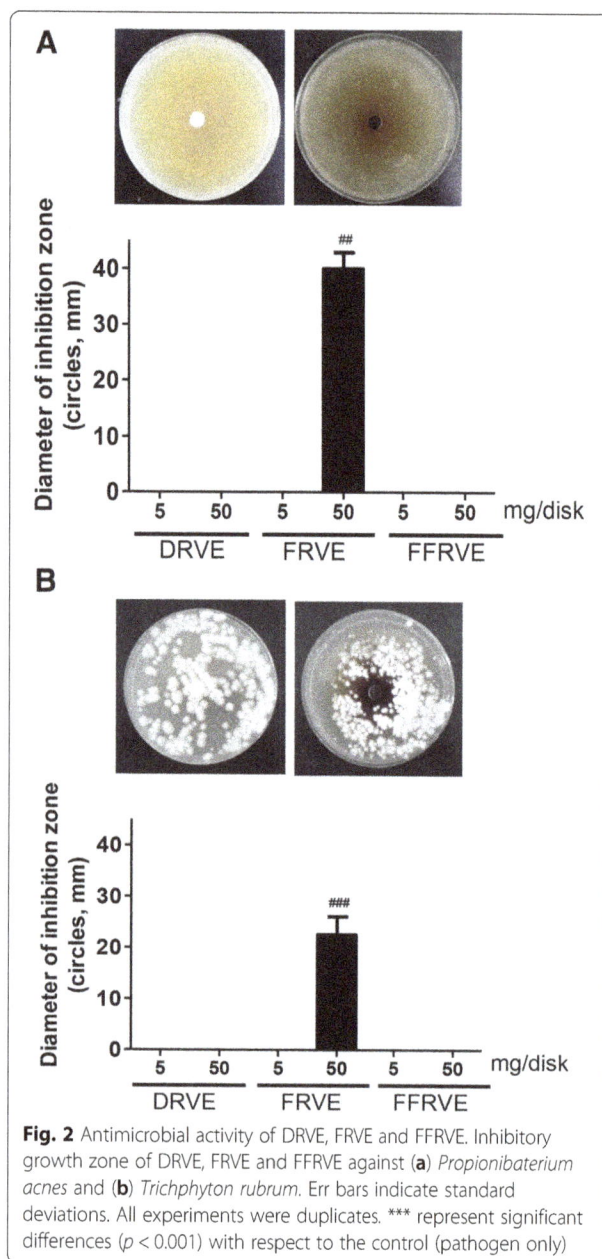

Fig. 2 Antimicrobial activity of DRVE, FRVE and FFRVE. Inhibitory growth zone of DRVE, FRVE and FFRVE against (**a**) *Propionibaterium acnes* and (**b**) *Trichphyton rubrum*. Err bars indicate standard deviations. All experiments were duplicates. *** represent significant differences ($p < 0.001$) with respect to the control (pathogen only)

FFRVE inhibited the growth of AML-12 cells by 8% (Fig. 3e).

The three RVS extracts suppressed hepatic lipogenesis in an in vitro model of non-alcoholic fatty liver

We previously reported that FRVE could inhibit hepatic lipogenesis in OA-treated HepG2 cells. In order to investigate whether DRVE and FFRVE could alleviate OA-induced cellular steatosis, OA-treated HepG2 cells were stained with ORO. As shown in Fig. 4a, DRVE decreased the number and size of lipid droplets in OA-treated HepG2 cells. DRVE, FRVE, and FFRVE treatments decreased the fat deposits by 22, 34, and 11%, respectively, compared with that in OA-treated HepG2 cells not treated with extracts (Fig. 4a).

To evaluate the regulatory effect of the extracts on lipogenesis and fatty acid oxidation, the levels of SREBP-1, PPAR-α, and AMPK in HepG2 cells were determined via western blotting. Our results showed that the three RVS extracts downregulated OA-induced elevation of SREBP-1 levels in HepG2 cells. FRVE and DRVE increased the expression of PPAR-α and p-AMPK, while FFRVE increased PPAR-α but not p-AMPK expression levels (Fig. 4b). In order to assess OA-induced TG accumulation, and the effects of the extracts on it, cellular TG levels were measured. OA-treated cells exhibited elevated TG levels compared to non-treated cells. However, treatment with DRVE, FRVE, and FFRVE lowered TG levels to 28, 35, and 17%, respectively (Fig. 4c).

Although the three extracts demonstrated lipid-lowering effects in the in vitro model of non-alcoholic fatty liver, DRVE and FRVE were more effective than FFRVE at the same concentration.

Comparison of the polyphenol content in the three RVS extracts

Gallic acid, fustin, fisetin, quercetin, butein, and sulfuretin are the main active constituents of *R. verniciflua*. We compared the contents of four phenolic compounds (gallic acid, fustin, fisetin, and quercetin) as marker compounds in DRVE, FRVE, and FFRVE via HPLC. The retention times of gallic acid, fisetin, fustin, and quercetin were 10.045, 13.033, 16.751, and 17.631 min, respectively (Fig. 5a).

These polyphenols were detected in DRVE, FRVE, and FFRVE eluents (Fig. 5b, c, and d, respectively). Gallic acid levels in DRVE, FRVE, and FFRVE were 170, 33, and 4 mg/g, respectively, and gallic acid content in DRVE was therefore 42.5 times greater than that in FFRVE (Table 2). Fustin levels in DRVE, FRVE, and FFRVE were 34.5, 129, and 10.7 mg/g, respectively, and fustin content in FRVE was therefore 12 times higher than that in FFRVE (Table 2). Fisetin levels in DRVE, FRVE, and FFRVE were 15, 59, and 1 mg/g, respectively,

viability by 39, 37, and 21%, respectively (Fig. 3b). Of all the cancer cell lines studied, the breast cancer cell line MDA-MB-231 showed the lowest viability (11%) after treatment with 400 μg/mL DRVE (Fig. 3c). With regard to colorectal cancer cells, DRVE and FRVE treatments showed similar effects on the viabilities of HCT116 cells (28 and 31%, respectively), whereas viability was approximately twice greater after FFRVE treatment (67%, Fig. 3d). Overall, DRVE exhibited the strongest cytotoxic effect against cancer cells.

In contrast, DRVE and FRVE did not affect the viability of normal cells (AML-12), even at the highest concentration tested (Fig. 3e), while 400 μg/mL

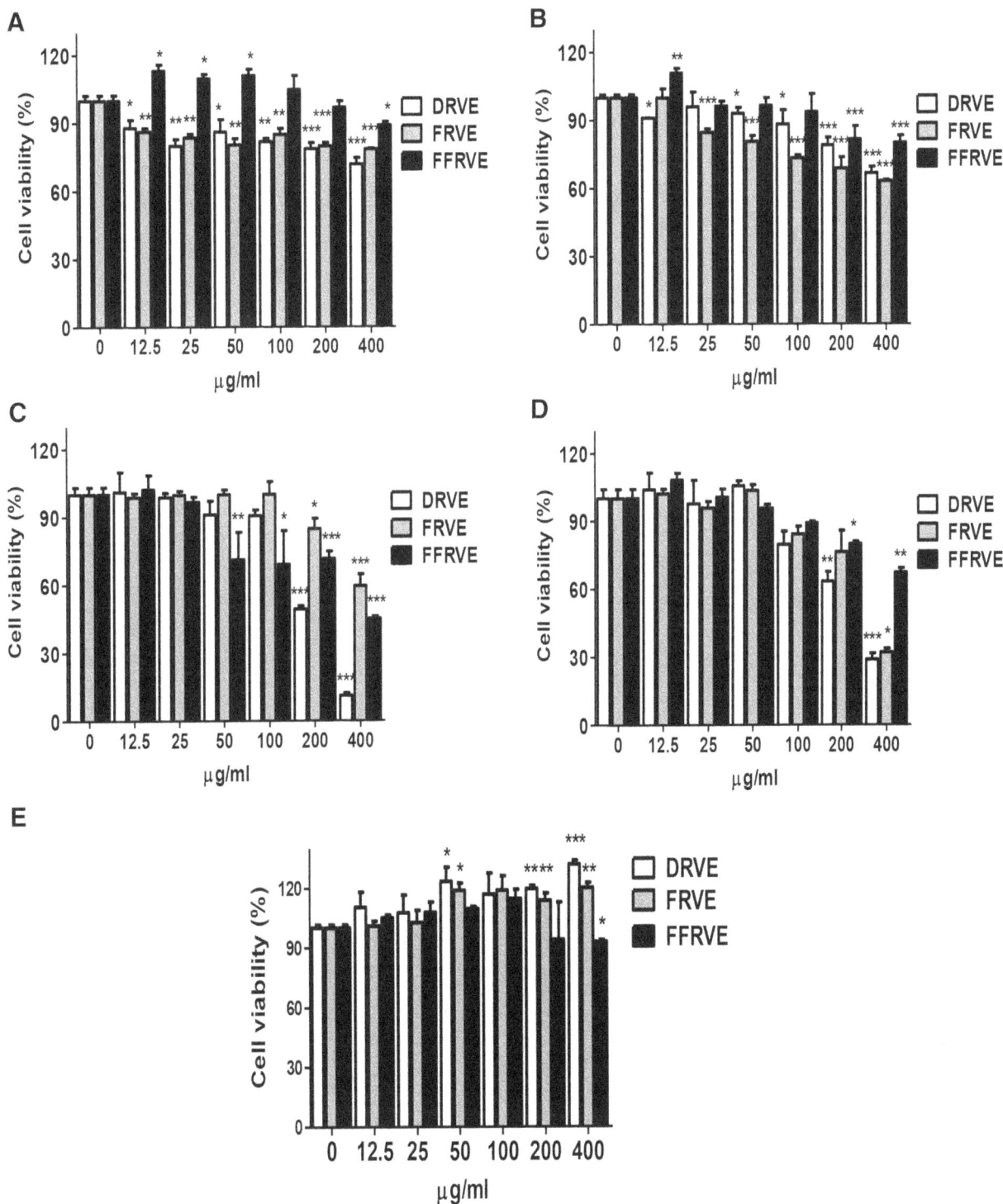

Fig. 3 Cell viability of DRVE, FRVE and FFRVE against various cancer cells. Cells were treated with various concentrations of DRVE, FRVE and FFRVE (0, 12.5, 25, 50, 100, 200, and 400 µg/ml) for 24 h. **a** HepG2, **b** PC-3, **c** MDA-MB-231, **d** HCT-116, **e** AML-12 cells. Data are represented as the mean ± SD for three experiments. * $p < 0.05$, ** $p < 0.01$, and *** $p < 0.001$ (in comparison to the control)

and fisetin content was therefore 59 times greater in FRVE than in FFRVE. Finally, quercetin levels in DRVE, FRVE, and FFRVE were 1.5, 4, and 19 mg/g, respectively (Table 2).

The four marker compounds of DRVE, FRVE, and FFRVE possess antioxidant activities

According to the DPPH scavenging assay, the antioxidant activities of the evaluated compounds could be

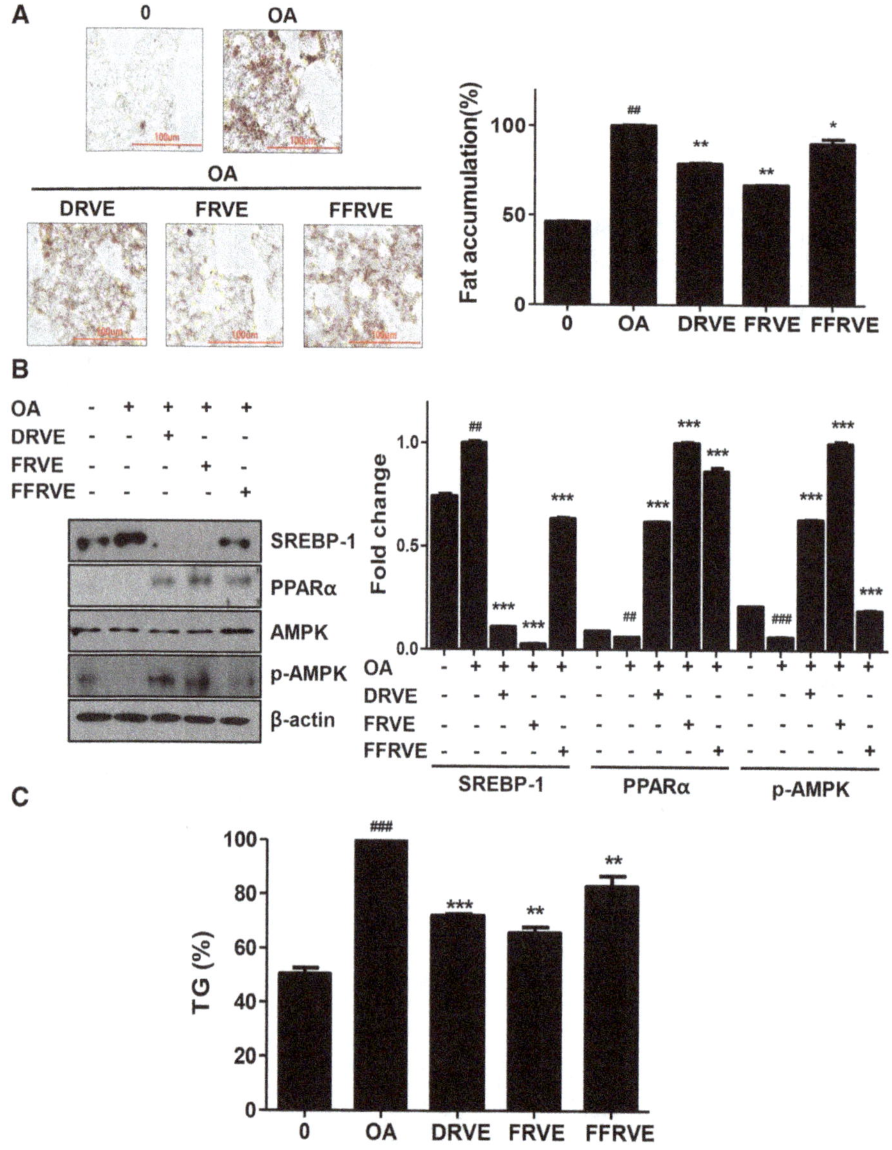

Fig. 4 Effect of DRVE, FRVE, FFRVE on cellular lipid accumulation and lipogenesis in OA-induced HepG2 cells. Cells were co-treated with OA and 400 µg/ml of DRVE, FRVE, FFRVE for 24 h. **a** Cells were stained with ORO as described in the materials and methods and then quantitatively analyzed. ORO staining image (magnification 400×), (##) $p < 0.01$ (in comparison to the non-OA treated control), * and ** represent significant differences ($p < 0.05$ and $p < 0.01$, respectively) with respect to the OA-treated control. **b** Determination of the expression of AMPK, SREBP-1 and PPARα by western blotting analysis. Quantitative protein levels were shown. (##) $p < 0.01$, and (###) $p < 0.001$ (in comparison to the non-OA-treated control). (**) $p < 0.01$ and (***) $p < 0.001$ (in comparison to the OA-treated control). **c** Total intracellular TG was analyzed by an enzymatic colorimetric method. Data are represented as the mean ± SD of three experiments. (###) $p < 0.001$ (in comparison to the non-OA treated control). (**) $p < 0.01$ and (***) $p < 0.001$ (in comparison to the OA-treated control)

ordered as follows: fisetin > gallic acid > ascorbic acid > quercetin > fustin (Table 3).

Fisetin showed the strongest radical scavenging activity and the lowest EC_{50} value (1 ± 0.01 µg/mL), whereas fustin exhibited the lowest DPPH scavenging activity and the highest EC_{50} value (15.1 ± 0.04 µg/mL, Table 3).

The relative antioxidant capacities of DRVE and FRVE (Table 1) were similar to those of gallic acid and fustin, respectively.

Discussion

Despite the various benefits of RVS, it is known to cause allergy, which may be due to the presence of urushiol. Nevertheless, due to its numerous biological activities, RVS is of high importance in the development of functional food and medicine. Therefore, various detoxification methods have been developed for the removal of allergens from RVS. In Korea, the Ministry of Food and Drug Safety permitted the use of

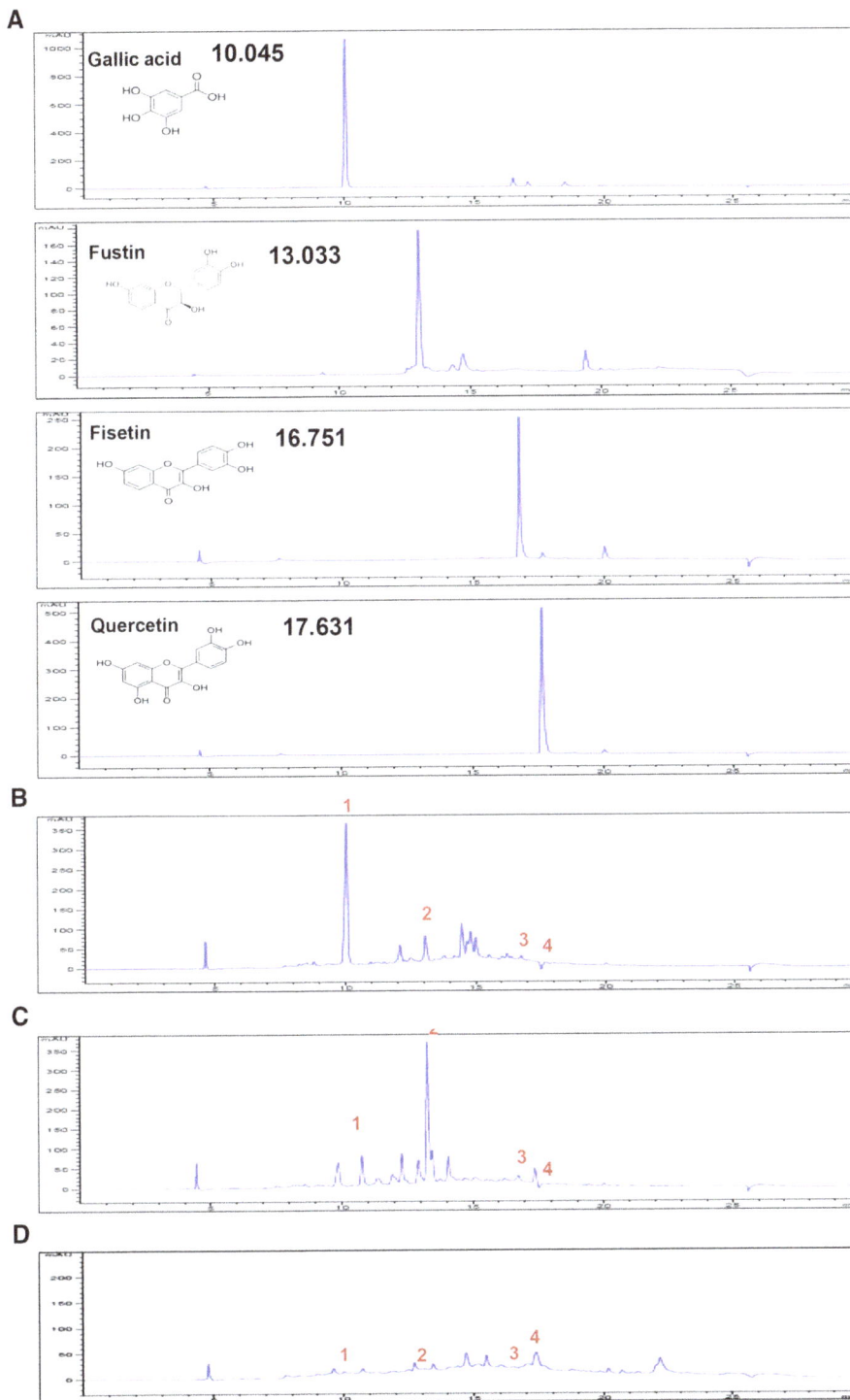

Fig. 5 HPLC chromatograms of the DRVE, FRVE, and FFRVE. Peaks of four main components (**a**) are gallic acid (1), fustin (2), fisetin (3), quercetin (4) and DRVE (**b**), FRVE (**c**), FFRVE (**d**). Mobile phase: 0.1% (v/v) Formic acid in water (solvent A) and 100% (v/v) Methanol (solvent B) at a flow rate of 0.7 ml/min, with gradient as follows: 0–17 min, 100%B; 17–20 min, 100%B; 20–23 min, 0%B; 23–30 min, 0%B. and detected at 254 nm

detoxified RVS extracts in 2012. Since then, the types of functional foods containing detoxified RVS extracts have been steadily increasing on a yearly basis. Detoxification methods include the removal of allergens from

RVS using solvents [15], electron beam radiation [16], high temperature [17], and microorganisms [9, 13]. However, RVS extracts detoxified by solvents and irradiation are not suitable for use in food.

Table 2 Contents of Phenolic acids in DRVE, FRVE, and FFRVE

Sample	Compound (mg/g)			
DRVE	Gallic acid	Fustin	Fisetin	Quercetin
FRVE	170	34.5	15	1.5
FFRVE	33	129	59	4
Sample	4.3	10.7	19	7

We have been studying the biological activities of RVS along with many other researchers, and to date, several bioactivities have been reported. However, studies on detoxified RVS extracts are still inadequate.

To the best of our knowledge, there are no studies comparing RVS extracts prepared by different detoxification methods. Thus, the present study was conducted to compare the bioactive constituents and biological activities of three RVS extracts prepared by different detoxification methods. The investigated extracts (DRVE, FRVE, and FFRVE) are commercially available as allergen-free functional food in Korea.

The antioxidant activities of the three extracts were assessed via DPPH scavenging assay. Among the three extracts, DRVE was found to possess a superior antioxidant activity. Regarding antimicrobial activity, FRVE was the most effective, and inhibited the growth of both *P. acnes* and *T. rubrum*. The three extracts successfully suppressed hepatic lipogenesis in an in vitro model of non-alcoholic fatty liver. However, DRVE and FRVE were more effective than FFRVE at the same concentration. These results suggest that the different detoxification methods may induce alterations in the major components of RVS, leading to differences in their activities. Therefore, we analyzed the polyphenolic constituents of RVS in the three extracts.

Polyphenols are bioactive compounds present at high concentrations in various plants [18]. Many studies have reported that phenolics such as a fustin, fisetin, gallic acid, and quercetin are highly abundant compounds in *R. verniciflua* [3, 19, 20].

According to a previous report, RVS extracts detoxified via heating methods show high gallic acid contents [17]. This is consistent with our finding that DRVE, an allergen-free RVS extract detoxified by heating to a high

temperature, possesses the highest gallic acid content. Moreover, another study reported that an allergen-free RVS extract detoxified by heating (by roasting in an iron pot at 240 °C for 50 min and extracting with water) contains higher amounts of fustin (130 mg/g) than fisetin (20 mg/g) [21]. Similar to these data, our results demonstrated that DRVE contained three times more fustin than fisetin. However, FFRVE, the RVS extract detoxified by fermentation with *F. fraxinea* mushroom, was found to contain more fisetin than fustin. This result is in agreement with that reported in a previous study [7]. Finally, FRVE, the RVS extract detoxified by fermentation with the yeast *S. carlsbergensis*, contained higher levels of fustin than fisetin or gallic acid, unlike DRVE or FFRVE. As shown in Tables 2 and 3, DRVE was found to contain the highest amount of gallic acid among the three extracts, and gallic acid was found to be the second most effective antioxidant after fisetin. Therefore, gallic acid was considered to be a marker compound reflecting the antioxidant effect of DRVE, while fustin was considered to be a marker compound reflecting the bioactivity of FRVE. However, the contents of all marker compounds, including fisetin, were low. Therefore, FFRVE seems to have a low biological activity when compared to DRVE or FRVE.

Conclusions

The present study reports a comparison between the components and biological activities of three different kinds of commercially available allergen-free RVS extracts in Korea. Our findings suggest that the components may vary according to the detoxification method used. Accordingly, by altering the detoxification method, it is possible to maximize the concentrations of components that exert specific effects for application in the health food or cosmetic product industry.

Abbreviations
AMPK: AMP-activated protein kinase; D.W: Distilled Water; DMSO: Dimethyl sulfoxide; DPPH: 1,1-diphenyl-2-picrylyhdrazyl; DRVE: Dried *Rhus verniciflua* STOKES extract; EC$_{50}$: Half maximal effective concentration; FBS: Fetal Bovine Serum; FFRVE: Fermented with Fomitella *fraxinea Rhus verniciflua* STOKES extract; FRVE: Fermented *Rhus verniciflua* STOKES extract; HRP: Horseradish peroxidase; MTT: 3-(4–5-dimethylthiazol-2-yl)-2,5-diphenyle tetrazolium bromide; O.D: Optical density; OA: Oleic acid; PBS: Phosphate-buffered saline; milk; PPARPα: Peroxisome proliferator-activated receptor alpha; RVS: *Rhus verniciflua* STOKES; SD: Standard deviation; SREBP-1: Sterol regulatory element-binding protein 1; TG: Triglyceride

Funding
This work was supported by grants (No. 2013R1A1A1008431) from the National Research Foundation of Korea (NRF) (MSIP, Ministry of Science, ICP and Future Planning) and "Cooperative Research Program for Agriculture Science and Technology Development (Project No. PJ01313501)" Rural Development Administration, Republic of Korea.

Table 3 Antioxidant effect of four main compounds by DPPH scavenging assay

Sample	DPPH, EC50 (μg/ml)
Ascorbic acid	8.1 ± 0.6
Gallic acid	1.8 ± 0.1
Fustin	15.1 ± 0.0
Fisetin	1 ± 0.0
Quercetin	7.9 ± 0.2

Each value represents mean ± SD (*n* = 3)

Authors' contributions

HJL conceived and designed the experiments; SOL, SJL, and HJL performed the experiments; EOL analyzed the data; and JSK contributed reagents/analysis tools. All authors contributed in validating, writing and approving the final version of the manuscript.

Competing interests

The authors declare that they have no competing interests.

Author details

[1]Department of Science in Korean Medicine, Graduate School, Kyung Hee University, Hoegi-dong, Dongdaemun-gu, 130-701 Seoul, Republic of Korea. [2]Department of Cancer Preventive Material Development, Graduate School, Kyung Hee University, Hoegi-dong, Dongdaemun-gu, 130-701 Seoul, Republic of Korea. [3]College of Korean Medicine, Kyung Hee university, 1 Hoegi-dong, Dondaemun-gu, 130-701 Seoul, Republic of Korea. [4]Major of Plant Resources and Environment, College of Applied Life Sciences, 102 Jeju National University, Jeju-si, Jeju-do 690-756, Korea.

References

1. Yoo H, Roh J. Compendium of Prescriptions From the Countryside (Hyangyakjipseongbang), vol. 1433. Seoul: Hangrimchulpansa; 1977.
2. Kim J-S, Kwon Y-S, Chun W-J, Kim T-Y, Sun J, Yu C-Y, Kim M-J. Rhus verniciflua Stokes flavonoid extracts have anti-oxidant, anti-microbial and α-glucosidase inhibitory effect. Food Chem. 2010;120:539–43.
3. Kim KH, Moon E, Choi SU, Kim SY, Lee KR. Polyphenols from the bark of Rhus verniciflua and their biological evaluation on antitumor and anti-inflammatory activities. Phytochemistry. 2013;92:113–21.
4. Kim M-O, Kim J-S, Sa Y-J, Jeong H-J, Chun W-J, Kwon Y-S, Kim T-Y, Choi H-S, Yu C-Y, Kim M-J. Screening of extraction solvent condition of fermented Rhus verniciflua stem bark by antioxidant activities. Korean J Med Crop Sci. 2010;18:217–23.
5. Kim M-J, Choi W-C, Barshinikov A, Kobayashi A. Anticancer and antioxidant activity of allergen-removed extract in Rhus verniciflua Stokes. Korean J Med Crop Sci. 2002;10:288–93.
6. M-o K, Yangb J, Kwonc YS, Kima MJ. Antioxidant and anticancer effects of fermented Rhus verniciflua stem bark extracts in HCT-116 cells. SCIENCEASIA. 2015;41:322–8.
7. Choi H-S, Yeo S-H, Jeong S-T, Choi J-H, Park H-S, Kim M-K. Preparation and characterization of urushiol free fermented Rhus verniciflua stem bark (FRVSB) extracts. Korean J Food Sci Technol. 2012;44:173–8.
8. Kobayashi S, Ikeda R, Oyabu H, Tanaka H, Uyama H. Artificial Urushi: design, synthesis, and enzymatic curing of new urushiol analogues. Chem Lett. 2000;29:1214–5.
9. Choi H-S, Kim M-K, Park H-S, Yun S-E, Mun S-P, Kim J-S, Sapkota K, Kim S, Kim T-Y, Kim S-J. Biological detoxification of lacquer tree (Rhus verniciflua Stokes) stem bark by mushroom species. Food Sci Biotechnol. 2007;16:935–42.
10. Bauer A, Kirby W, Sherris JC, Turck M. Antibiotic susceptibility testing by a standardized single disk method. Am J Clin Pathol. 1966;45:493.
11. Rios J, Recio M, Villar A. Screening methods for natural products with antimicrobial activity: a review of the literature. J Ethnopharmacol. 1988;23:127–49.
12. Folch J, Lees M, Sloane Stanley GH. A simple method for the isolation and purification of total lipides from animal tissues. J Biol Chem. 1957;226:497–509.
13. Lee MS, Kim JS, Cho SM, Lee SO, Kim SH, Lee HJ. Fermented Rhus verniciflua Stokes extract exerts an Antihepatic Lipogenic effect in oleic-acid-induced HepG2 cells via Upregulation of AMP-activated protein kinase. J Agric Food Chem. 2015;63:7270–6.
14. Blois MS. Antioxidant determinations by the use of a stable free radical. Nature. 1958;181:1199–200.
15. Choi WC, Park SJ, Kwon SP. Process for preparation of rhus verniciflua extracts having excellent anti-cancer activity and anti-cancer pharmaceutical composition containing the same. U.S. patent US7618661B2, November 17, 2009.
16. Kim B. The effect of irradiation and peroxyacetic acid treatment on the reduction of urushiol of Rhus verniciflua Stokes and the physiological activities. Gwangju: MS thesis, Chonbuk National University; 2010.
17. Liu C-S, Nam T-G, Han M-W, Ahn S-M, Choi HS, Kim TY, Chun OK, Koo SI, Kim D-O. Protective effect of detoxified Rhus verniciflua stokes on human keratinocytes and dermal fibroblasts against oxidative stress and identification of the bioactive phenolics. Biosci Biotechnol Biochem. 2013;77:1682–8.
18. Agrawal M. Natural polyphenols based new therapeutic avenues for advanced biomedical applications. Drug Metab Rev. 2015;47:420–30.
19. Im WK, Park HJ, Lee KS, Lee JH, Kim YD, Kim K-H, Park S-J, Hong S, Jeon SH. Fisetin-rich extracts of Rhus verniciflua Stokes improve blood flow rates in mice fed both normal and high-fat diets. J Med Food. 2016;19:120–6.
20. Chen H, Wang C, Zhou H, Tao R, Ye J, Li W. Antioxidant capacity and identification of the constituents of ethyl acetate fraction from Rhus verniciflua Stokes by HPLC-MS. Nat Prod Res. 2017;31:1573–7.
21. Cheon SH, Kim KS, Kim S, Jung HS, Choi WC, Eo WK. Efficacy and safety of Rhus verniciflua stokes extracts in patients with previously treated advanced non-small cell lung cancer. Complement Med Res. 2011;18:77–83.

3

Anti diabetic property of aqueous extract of *Stevia rebaudiana* Bertoni leaves in Streptozotocin-induced diabetes in albino rats

Uswa Ahmad[1] and Rabia Shabir Ahmad[1,2]*

Abstract

Background: Stevia (*Stevia rebaudiana*) natural, non-caloric sugar substitute is rich source of pharmacologically important glycoside stevioside that is linked to the pathology and complications of diabetes.

Methods: The current research was carried out to explore the anti-diabetic effect of aqueous extract of *Stevia rebaudiana* leaves in albino rats. For this purpose, diabetes was induced by administration of streptozotocin (40 mg/kg body weight, intraperitoneally). The diabetic rats were administered with aqueous stevia extract at different dose levels (200, 300, 400 and 500 ppm/kg b.w) for 8 weeks; the control rats were fed basal diet during this period.

Results: Stevia aqueous extract improved caloric management and weight control by decreasing the feed intake and body weight gain. Furthermore, intake of stevia extract resulted in significant ($P < 0.05$) decrease in the random blood glucose level (-73.24%) and fasting blood glucose (-66.09%) and glycosylated (HbA1c) hemoglobin (5.32%) while insulin (17.82 μIU/mL) and liver glycogen (45.02 mg/g) levels significantly improved in the diabetic rats, compared with the diabetic and non-diabetic control rats after 8 weeks study period.

Conclusions: It is concluded that aqueous extact of stevia has anti-diabetic effects in albino rats, and therefore could be promising nutraceutical therapy for the management of diabetes and its associated complications.

Keywords: Diabetes, Fasting blood glucose, Insulin, HbA1c, Liver glycogen, Random blood glucose, *Stevia rebaudiana* bertoni, Stevioside

Background

Diabetes mellitus is a group of metabolic diseases characterized by chronic hyperglycemia resulting from defects in insulin secretion, insulin action, or both [1]. According to World Health Organization Diabetes mellitus will become the seventh leading cause of death worldwide in 2030 [2]. Through proper diet, exercise and pharmacologic interventions, the incidence of diabetes can be overcome [3]. The pharmacological drugs used for the treatment of diabetes, are either too expensive or have certain adverse side effects. Therefore, for the treatment of diabetes mellitus many traditional plants have been preferred as natural source of drugs [4] because they are considered to be safe, less toxic than synthetic ones [5] and have strong antioxidant activities due to which these plants become more effective against diabetes [6]. *Stevia rebaudiana* Bertoni as a traditional plant is famous due to its sweet taste and beneficial effects in blood glucose regulation. *Stevia rebaudiana* Bertoni (family Asteraceae) popularly known as stevia, sweet weed, honey leaf and sweet herb of Paraguay [7]. Stevia leaves contained complex mixture of diterpene glycosides including stevioside, steviolbioside, rebaudiosides (A, B, C, D, E) and dulcoside A but the major sweet constituents are stevioside and rebaudioside A [8, 9]. Natural

* Correspondence: rabiaahmad@gcuf.edu.pk
[1]Department of Food Science, Nutrition & Home Economics, Government College University, Allama Iqbal Road, Faisalabad 38000, Pakistan
[2]Institute of Home and Food Sciences, Government College University, Faisalabad 38000, Pakistan

non-caloric sweetener stevioside (a major component of stevia) is 100–300 times sweeter than sucrose and have been extensively used as a non-caloric sugar substitute in many kinds of foods, medicine, beverage, cosmetics, wine making, household chemical industry and other food industries [10]. It possesses anti-hyperglycaemic, anti-hypertensive, anti-oxidant, anti-tumor, anti-diarrheal, diuretic, gastro and renal-protective and immunomodulatory properties [11]. The anti-hyperglycemic effect of S. rebaudiana was investigated in both rats and humans by [12, 13]. They mentioned that stevioside demonstrates a positive effect on hyperglycemia through decreasing the absorption of glucose in duodenum, glycogenolysis and gluconeogenesis.

As the synthetic drugs used for the treatment of diabetes result in many complications. Hence the use of natural source (Stevia rebaudiana Bertoni) for the treatment of diabetes is safe and non-carcinogenic [8, 9]. Hence, the present experiment was undertaken to study the antidiabetic effect of S. rebaudiana in albino rats.

Methods

Plant material

Stevia (Stevia rebaudiana Bertoni) leaves were collected from Ayub Agricultural Research Institute (AARI), Faisalabad (Reference no. 606/8). Stevia leaves were washed to remove the dirt, dust and foreign material adhered to the surface. After washing, leaves of stevia were air-dried under shade at room temperature and finely powdered with the help of grinder (MJ-176-NR-3899) [14].

Stevia aqueous extract preparation

Stevioside was extracted from the dried ground leaves of stevia plant by using water extraction. The dried ground leaves of stevia were mixed with hot water (65 °C) at the ratio of 1:45 (w/v) [15]. The mixture was shaken properly and kept at room temperature for 24 h. It was stirred 2–3 times a day. After 24 h, mixture was filtered through What man filter paper and the filtrate was evaporated using rotary vacuum evaporator (EYELA N-1110S 115V) at 40–45 °C [14].

Experimental animals

Sixty adult male albino rats of average weight 152.53 g were purchased from National Institute of Health, Islamabad, Pakistan, after getting permission from Institution of Animal Ethics Committee (IAEC). The rats were kept in stainless steel wire bottom cages under standard conditions (temperature 25 ± 2 °C and $60 \pm 5\%$ relative humidity with 12 h light-dark cycle) in environmentally controlled animal house of College of Pharmacology, Faculty of Science and Technology, Government College University, Faisalabad Pakistan. The rats were fed on the freshly prepared basal diet containing 65% starch, 10% casein, 10% corn oil, 4%

salt mixture, 1% vitamins mixture and 10% cellulose [16] and distilled water for two week that meets their requirements for growing ad libitum.

Induction of diabetes

The diabetes was induced in the rats by a single intraperitonial injection of STZ (40 mg/kg of body weight) freshly prepared in citrate buffer (0.1 M, pH 4.5), into the femoral vein of rats after an overnight fasting [17]. STZ-injected animals were given 20% glucose solution for 24 h to prevent initial drug-induced hypoglycemic mortality [5]. The normal control rats received only distilled water and standard diet.

Development of diabetes mellitus in the rats was confirmed by testing fasting blood glucose (FBG), after 72 h of STZ injection. The rats with FBG higher than 200 mg/dL were considered diabetic and were selected for the study [18].

Animal groups and experimental design

Sixty male albino rats were divided into six groups of ten animals each. 1st and 2nd groups included normal (non-diabetic) and diabetic control rats respectively that received only distilled water that was free from impurities like dissolved salts and colloidal particles that can affect the results of the present research and standard diet throughout the whole trial. Diabetic rats consumed Stevia rebaudiana Bertoni aqueous extract dissolved at the levels of 200, 300, 400 and 500 ppm/kg b.w of albino rats in distilled water and administered orally as a daily dose for 8 weeks were included in 3rd, 4th, 5th and 6th groups respectively as shown in Table 1.

Feed and water intake

Net feed intake of individual rat was calculated on daily basis by excluding left-over and collected spilled diet during the entire period to determine the effect of individual experimental diet. Water was provided with the help of graduated drinking bottles and its consumption was also measured on daily basis.

Gain in body weight

Gain in body weight of individual rat in each group was estimated on weekly basis throughout the experimental period to find out the effect of individual diet on body weight using electronic weighing balance (KERN 440-35 N).

Collection of serum of rats

For the serum, overnight fasted albino rats were killed using 0.4 mL of urethane anesthesia (25%) /100 g of body weight. Then blood was collected by cardiac puncture. After that serum was separated by centrifugation in the centrifuge machine (LABCENT 5000) at 3000 rpm for

Table 1 Addition of aqueous Stevia extract in the distilled water of rats at different substitution levels

Non-diabetic rats	Diabetic rats				
N_0	D_0	D_1	D_2	D_3	D_4
Control (Basal diet+ distilled water)	Control (Basal diet+ distilled water)	Basal diet + 200 ppm SAE	Basal diet+ 300 ppm SAE	Basal diet+ 400 ppm SAE	Basal diet+ 500 ppm SAE

N_0 = Basal diet and distilled water
D_0 = Basal diet and distilled water
D_1 = Basal diet and distilled water with 200 ppm Stevia leaf Aqueous extract
D_2 = Basal diet and distilled water with 300 ppm Stevia leaf Aqueous extract
D_3 = Basal diet and distilled water with 400 ppm Stevia leaf Aqueous extract
D_4 = Basal diet and distilled water with 500 ppm Stevia leaf Aqueous extract

15 min after allowing the blood to stand for at least 30 min at room temperature as per standard protocols [19].

Analysis of serum biochemical profile of rats
Following analysis were made from the collected serum samples.

Random blood glucose and fasting blood glucose levels
Fasting as well as random levels of glucose were estimated within 3 hours of sample collection by "GOD PAP Enzymatic Colorimetric Test Method" [20] on Humalyzer, 3000 ("Semi-automatic chemistry analyzer by Human, Germany, Model no. 16700") by the use of standard kits. Effect of stevia aqueous extract on fasting blood glucose level as well as random blood glucose levels were observed at 1st, 2nd, 3rd, 4th, 5th, 6th, 7th and 8th week of drug treatment in order to observe the variation in fasting and random blood glucose levels. For it blood was be taken by making a small cut at terminal tail vein of rats.

Glycosylated hemoglobin (HbA1c) level
HbA1c in the blood was estimated by the method Nayak and Pattabiraman [21]. First lysed 5.5 mL of water with saline washed erythrocytes (0.5 mL), mixed and incubated for 15 min at 37 °C. The supernatant was discarded after the centrifugation of contents, then for the further process for estimation of HbA1c, 0.5 mL of saline was added and mixed. The contents were heated for 4 h at 100 °C after the addition of 0.02 mL of aliquot and 4 mL of oxalate hydrochloric solution. The solution was cooled and precipitated with 2 mL of 40% TCA. 0.5 mL of supernatant, 0.05 mL of 80% phenol and 3.0 mL of concentrated H_2SO_4 were added, after the centrifugation of the mixture. After 30 min, the color was developed that was read at 480 nm.

Insulin level
The plasma insulin was assayed by Enzyme Linked Immunosorbent Assay (ELISA) method using Boehringer-Mannheim kit [22]. 0.1 mL of plasma was injected into the plastic tubes coated with monoclonal anti-insulin antibodies. To form anti-insulin antibody–POD conjugate, phosphate buffer and

anti-insulin POD conjugate was added. Indicators reaction was formed by the addition of substrate chromogen solution. Then in the similar manner, a set of standards were also treated. The absorbance was read after the development of color at 420 nm.

Liver glycogen
Liver glycogen level was measured according to the standard protocol [23]. Liver of both diabetic and non-diabetic rats was removed immediately at the end of the experiment and washed using ice-cold saline solution. Then hepatic tissues were minced and homogenized in hot ethanol (80%) at a tissue concentration of 100 mg/mL and centrifuged in the centrifuge machine (LABCENT 5000) at 9500 rpm for 20 min. 5 mL water and 6 mL of 52% perchloric acid were added. From it the residue was collected, dried and extracted. The collected material was centrifuged at 9500 rpm for 15 min for the recovery of supernatant. In the graduated test tube, 0.2 mL of supernatant, 1 mL distilled water and anthrone reagent (4 mL) was added, heated, cooled at room temperature and at 630 nm the intensity of the green to dark green color of the solution was recorded. From a standard curve prepared with standard glucose solution, glycogen content of the sample was determined.

Statistical analysis
Results are expressed as mean ± standard deviation (SD). Analysis of variance (ANOVA) and least significance difference (LSD) were carried out on the result data at 95% confidence level using SPSS statistical software package, version 17 (SPSS Inc., Chicago).

Results
Means values for feed and water intakes in different groups of rats (per rat/day) have been shown graphically in Figs. 1 and 2. The results demonstrated that administration of stevia sweetener reduced the feed and water intakes in diabetic rats than N_0 and D_0. The highest feed and water intakes 14.57 g/rat/day, 29.82 mL/day and 13.14 g/rat/day, 28.95 mL/day respectively were observed in N_0 (non-diabetic control) and D_0 (diabetic control). While stevia sweetener at

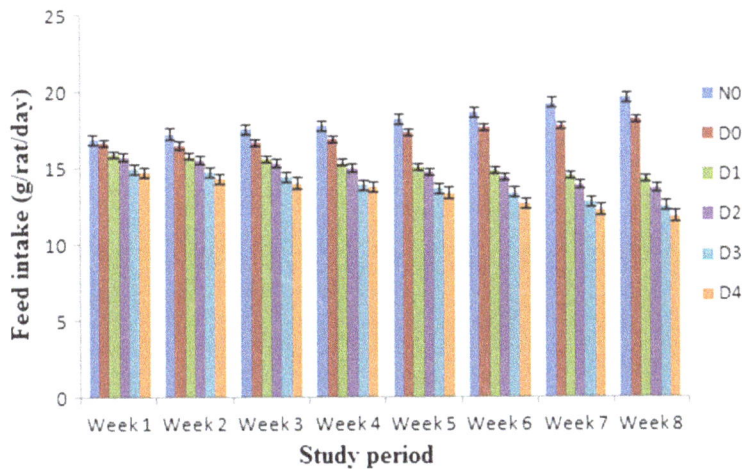

Fig. 1 Feed intake (g) in normal and diabetic rats during 8 weeks (rat/week). Results are expressed as amount of feed intake levels of diabetic and non-diabetic rats (mean ± standard deviation (SD). $n = 10$). The feed intake of diabetic rats (D_1, D_2, D_3 and D_4) received stevia aqueous extract in different concentrations (200, 300, 400 and 500 ppm) respectively significantly ($P < 0.05$) decreased from non-diabetic (N_0) and diabetic (D_0) control groups

dose of 500 ppm/kg b.w showed the lowest amounts of feed and water intake (13.38 ± 0.98 g/rat/day) and (24.38 ± 0.58 mL/day) followed by 200 ppm/kg b.w (15.20 ± 1.00 g/day), (26.26 ± 0.53 mL/day), 300 ppm/kg b.w (14.81 ± 0.97 g/rat/day), (25.68 ± 0.60 mL/day) and 400 ppm/kg b. wt (13.82 ± 0.99 g/rat/day), (25.10 ± 0.64 mL/day) of stevia extracts respectively (Figs. 1 & 2).

Effect of administration of stevioside on the body weight of rats has been shown in Table 2. It is apparent from the results that the highest body weights (154.60 ± 4.02–185.90 ± 5.87 g/rat) and (153.22 ± 4.22–179.32 ± 4.55 g/rat) were observed in N_0 (normal control) and D_0 (diabetic control). While the lowest body weight was recorded in D_4 (diabetic rats received 500 ppm/kg

b.w aqueous stevia extract) (148.60 ± 7.02–120.81 ± 7.80 g/rat) as followed by D_1 (152.12 ± 5.01–132.78 ± 4.32 g/rat), D_2 (150.30 ± 6.33–128.70 ± 4.54 g/rat) and D_3 (149.82 ± 6.88–124.32 ± 6.10 g/rat) during study period from 1st week to 8 weeks.

Regarding the body weight gain %, highest percentage (23.27%) and (19.48%) was observed in N_0 and D_0. When diabetic rats were given stevia sweetener then their body weight gain % decreased by -13.84, -15.89, -18.75 and -20.55% respectively after 8 weeks (Table 2).

Table 3 represents the random blood glucose levels of normal and diabetic rats, affected by different levels of stevia aqueous extracts. From the results, it was observed that random blood glucose (RBG) levels of N_0

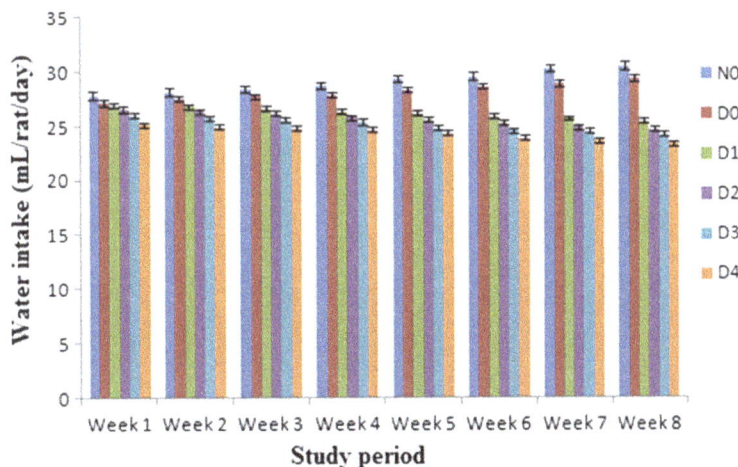

Fig. 2 Water intake (mL) in normal and diabetic rats during 8 weeks (rat/week). Results are expressed as amount of water intake levels of diabetic and non-diabetic rats (mean ± standard deviation (SD). n = 10). The water intake of diabetic rats (D_1, D_2, D_3 and D_4) received stevia aqueous extract in different concentrations (200, 300, 400 and 500 ppm) respectively significantly (P < 0.05) decreased from non-diabetic (N_0) and diabetic (D_0) control groups

Table 2 Effect of *Stevia* aqueous extract on body weight of diabetic and non-diabetic rats

Diet groups	Week 0	Week 1	Weeks 2	Weeks 3	Weeks 4	Weeks 5	Weeks 6	Weeks 7	Weeks 8	Body weight gain (%)
N_0	150.08 ± 9.02Ai	154.60 ± 4.02 Ah	158.15 ± 6.75Ag	161.18 ± 9.04Af	165.62 ± 9.22Ae	170.44 ± 9.33Ad	175.25 ± 9.21Ac	180.49 ± 5.43Ab	185.90 ± 5.87Aa	23.27
D_0	150.06 ± 8.22Ai	153.22 ± 4.22 Ah	157.41 ± 5.43Ag	160.1 ± 9.32Af	164.00 ± 8.76Ae	167.30 ± 9.09ABd	171.54 ± 7.99Bc	175.82 ± 4.32Bb	179.32 ± 4.55Ba	19.48
D_1	154.04 ± 9.44Ba	152.12 ± 5.01ABb	150.33 ± 6.22Bc	146.4 ± 8.02 Bd	143.21 ± 8.21Bf	140.22 ± 9.21Bf	137.68 ± 8.76Cg	134.22 ± 4.87Ch	132.73 ± 4.32 Ci	−13.84
D_2	153.02 ± 7.04Ba	150.30 ± 6.33Bb	147.32 ± 4.32BCc	143.2 ± 8.42Cd	140.00 ± 7.66Ce	137.40 ± 7.65Cf	134.68 ± 9.20Dg	131.60 ± 3.44CDh	128.70 ± 4.54CDi	−15.89
D_3	153.05 ± 9.32Ba	149.82 ± 6.88Bb	146.56 ± 4.87BCc	143.9 ± 5.01Cd	140.90 ± 5.02Ce	136.32 ± 6.54Cf	133.95 ± 8.90Dg	129.53 ± 3.78Dh	124.32 ± 6.10Di	−18.75
D_4	152.07 ± 9.11Ca	148.60 ± 7.02Bb	144.21 ± 3.21Cc	140.6 ± 5.11Dd	136.42 ± 6.05De	133.56 ± 5.65Df	130.21 ± 5.65Eg	125.87 ± 4.65Eh	120.81 ± 7.80Ei	−20.55

Values are mean ± standard deviation (SD) (n = 10)

Mean followed by different upper case letters (A, B, C, D) in the same columns represent significant difference ($P < 0.05$) treatment wise

Mean followed by different lower case letters (a, b, c, d) in the same rows represent significant difference ($P < 0.05$) among study periods (8 weeks)

N_0 = Non-diabetic rats given basal diet and distilled water

D_0 = Diabetic rats given basal diet and distilled water

D_1 = Diabetic rats given basal diet and distilled water with 200 ppm Stevia leaf aqueous extract

D_2 = Diabetic rats given basal diet and distilled water with 300 ppm Stevia leaf aqueous extract

D_3 = Diabetic rats given basal diet and distilled water with 400 ppm Stevia leaf aqueous extract

D_4 = Diabetic rats given basal diet and distilled water with 500 ppm Stevia leaf aqueous extract

Table 3 Random blood glucose levels (mg/dL) of normal and diabetic rats

Diet groups	Week 0	Week 1	Weeks 2	Weeks 3	Weeks 4	Weeks 5	Weeks 6	Weeks 7	Weeks 8	RBG %
N_0	80.72 ± 3.82Ec	82.73 ± 2.91Dc	83.4 ± 2.62Ebc	83.7 ± 2.44Fbc	84.9 ± 2.54Fb	85.4 ± 2.66Fb	87.3 ± 2.86Fa	88.4 ± 2.77Fa	89.25 ± 2.76Ca	7.88
D_0	340.1 ± 2.32Dd	342.1 ± 1.22Ad	348.7 ± 1.32Ad	354.3 ± 1.43Acd	360.9 ± 1.66Ac	366.2 ± 1.55Ac	273.3 ± 1.54Ac	381.2 ± 2.89Ab	391.22 ± 1.65Aa	15.04
D_1	334.23 ± 1.99Ca	332.23 ± 1.34Bb	320.22 ± 1.44Bc	278.88 ± 1.65 Bd	256.66 ± 1.67Be	166.67 ± 1.43Bf	143.33 ± 1.87Bg	122.23 ± 1.78Bh	94.43 ± 1.23Bi	−71.74
D_2	336.23 ± 2.94Ba	330.23 ± 1.44BCb	312.22 ± 1.43Cc	262.22 ± 1.34Cd	240.44 ± 1.88Ce	153.32 ± 1.77Cf	130.98 ± 1.65Cg	118.87 ± 1.54Ch	93.29 ± 1.54Bi	−72.25
D_3	338.88 ± 3.77ABa	327.88 ± 1.23Cb	310.88 ± 1.65CDc	251.42 ± 1.23Dd	232.22 ± 1.98De	140.98 ± 1.87Df	122.21 ± 1.87Dg	112.32 ± 1.56Dh	91.22 ± 1.87BCi	−73.08
D_4	339.22 ± 4.32Aa	326.44 ± 1.65Cb	308.65 ± 1.23Cc	243.32 ± 1.77Ed	221.32 ± 1.80Ee	127.76 ± 1.45Ef	116.54 ± 1.98Eg	107.65 ± 1.32Eh	90.77 ± 1.27Ci	−73.24

Values are mean ± standard deviation (SD) (n = 10)

Mean followed by different upper case letters (A, B, C, D) in the same columns represent significant difference ($P < 0.05$) treatment wise

Mean followed by different lower case letters (a, b, c, d) in the same rows represent significant difference ($P < 0.05$) among study periods (8 weeks)

and D_0 increased from $(82.73 \pm 2.91$ to 89.25 ± 2.76 mg/dL) and $(342.1 \pm 1.22$ to 391.22 ± 1.65 mg/dL) respectively at the beginning of the study to end of trail respectively. However, the RBG levels of D_1, D_2, D_3 and D_4 decreased from 332.23 ± 1.34, 330.23 ± 1.44, 327.88 ± 1.23 and 326.44 ± 1.65 mg/dL at 1st week to 94.43 ± 1.23, 93.29 ± 1.54, 91.22 ± 1.87 and 90.77 ± 1.27 mg/dL respectively at 8th week (Table 3). Stevia extract decreased the random blood glucose % levels of groups D_1, D_2, D_3 and D_4 by -71.74, -72.25, -73.08 and -73.24% respectively after 8 weeks (Table 3).

As presented in Table 4, there was significant ($P < 0.05$) increase in the fasting blood glucose level of the diabetic control group rats, relative to the normal control group. However, this was significantly ($P < 0.05$) restored toward normal in the diabetic rats given stevia aqueous extract, as indicated by the decrease in their fasting blood glucose levels from the 1st week to the 8th week. According to results highest level of fasting blood glucose (306.4 ± 2.65 mg/dL) was recorded in D_0 (diabetic control group rats). While fasting blood glucose levels of diabetic rats received stevia aqueous extract significantly decreased from 90.70 ± 2.98 (D_1) to 88.22 ± 2.97 (D_4) mg/dL. The fasting blood glucose % levels of groups D_1, D_2, D_3 and D_4 decreased by -64.87, -65.28, -65.96 and -66.09% respectively after 8 weeks (Table 4).

The glycosylated hemoglobin (HbA1c) level of the rats is shown in Fig. 3. According to results HbA1c level ($9.27 \pm 1.09\%$) of D_0 significantly ($P < 0.05$) increased than N_0 ($5.92 \pm 1.02\%$). But as compared to the D_0, diabetic groups D_1, D_2, D_3 and D_4 received stevia aqueous extract had significantly ($P < 0.05$) lower HbA1c levels ($6.22 \pm 1.11\%$, $6.06 \pm 1.08\%$, $5.77 \pm 1.06\%$ and $5.32 \pm 1.00\%$) respectively; indicating that the stevia extract decrease the glycosylation of hemoglobin.

The insulin levels of diabetic and normal rats are shown in Fig. 4. According to results the insulin levels of diabetic D_0 (15.89 ± 1.22 μIU/mL) control group decreased as compared to N_0 (18.02 ± 1.44 μIU/mL). The results of this study concluded that diabetic rats given stevioside mixed in distilled water increased the levels of serum insulin. The results further demonstrated that given stevia aqueous extracts at different dose levels improved significantly ($P < 0.05$) from 16.04 ± 1.24 to 17.82 ± 1.33 μIU/mL (D_1 to D_4) (Fig. 4).

The liver glycogen level of the rats is shown in Fig. 5. In this study, glycogen level of D_0 (17.07 ± 1.35 mg/g) decreased significantly ($P < 0.05$) compared to the N_0 (45.22 ± 2.22 mg/g) (Fig. 5). However, the diabetic rats received stevia aqueous extracts (200, 300, 400 and 500 ppm/kg) significantly ($P < 0.05$) increased the liver glycogen levels (35.27 ± 2.12, 37.43 ± 2.14, 42.66 ± 2.20 and 45.02 ± 2.24 mg/g) (Fig. 5).

Discussion

In this study, we evaluated the anti-diabetic activity of aqueous extract of stevia in diabetic albino rats as previous researches confirmed its pharmacological importance due to presence of glycosides like stevioside in it. Administration of aqueous stevia extract orally at different concentrations (200, 300, 400 and 500 mg/kg) for 8 weeks, significantly decline the feed and water intakes of diabetic albino rats. Stevia a low-caloric sweetener may reduce the feed and water intake and not promote weight gain because they do not stimulate the appetite [24]. Similarly, stevia sweetener at doses of 25, 250, 500 and 1000 mg/kg b. w may also reduce the feed intake in adult female wistar strain rats [25].

The results indicated that aqueous extract from leaves of *Stevia rebaudiana*, produced a significant ($P < 0.05$) dose-dependent reduction in body weight (Table 2) and body weight gain percentage of the rats treated with Stevia extract (Table 3) as compared to N_0. The highest gain in body weight was noticed in N_0 while lowest was recorded in D_4. Stevioside in the diet lowered the blood glucose level. The body weight of rats might reduce due to lower metabolisation of diet glucose or decrease amount of rat's food consumption [26]. This reduction in weights of rats receiving stevia extract may be due to high amount of stevioside that reduced the food intake of rats [27]. This finding is collaborated with the previous researches which proved a positive association between the decrease of body weight gain percent and the decline in feed intake and dose of stevioside given to the rats [28–30].

This study depicted that different concentrations of stevia extract had a good efficacy in controlling diabetes with an excellent control of random and fasting blood glucose level in diabetic rats at study period of 8 weeks. Previous study showed that stevioside was able to regulate blood glucose levels by enhancing not only insulin secretion and sensitivity but also insulin utilization in insulin deficient rats which was due to decreased PEPCK gene expression in rat liver [31]. According to another study, stevia extract may contain some biomolecules that may sensitize the insulin receptor to insulin or stimulates the β-cells of islets of langerhans to release insulin which may finally lead to improvement of carbohydrate metabolizing enzymes towards the reestablishment of normal blood glucose level [32]. *Stevia rebaudiana* leaves extract decreased the random and fasting blood glucose levels of rats by revitalizing the β-cells of pancreas thus reactivated the glycogen synthase system by improving insulin secretion and liver glycogen level [25, 27, 33, 34]. These results are in agreement with Awney et al. [27]; Abo Elnaga et al. [25]; Assaei et al. [30] and Akbarzadeh et al. [34] who also observed that stevia aqueous extract lowered the random and fasting blood

Table 4 Fasting blood glucose levels (mg/dL) of normal and diabetic rats

Diet groups	Week 0	Week 1	Weeks 2	Weeks 3	Weeks 4	Weeks 5	Weeks 6	Weeks 7	Weeks 8	FBG %
N_0	80.20 ± 3.47Dc	80.23 ± 2.94Dc	81.22 ± 2.92Fc	82.32 ± 2.89Fbc	82.30 ± 2.86Fbc	83.44 ± 2.65Fb	84.55 ± 2.90Fb	86.65 ± 2.78Fa	87.77 ± 2.99Ca	9.39
D_0	262.3 ± 2.34Ai	266.4 ± 2.54 Ah	269.8 ± 2.87Ag	275.6 ± 2.67Af	280.8 ± 1.22Ae	286.6 ± 1.45Ad	292.3 ± 1.45Ac	298.6 ± 1.32Ab	306.4 ± 2.65Aa	16.81
D_1	258.22 ± 1.99Ca	255.32 ± 2.94Ba	245.45 ± 2.34Bb	221.73 ± 2.93Bc	212.99 ± 2.98 Bd	165.55 ± 1.34Be	132.22 ± 1.65Bf	112.55 ± 1.87Bg	90.70 ± 2.98Bh	−64.87
D_2	258.18 ± 2.94Ca	253.22 ± 2.91BCa	237.77 ± 2.97Cb	215.55 ± 2.76Cc	180.99 ± 2.94Cd	155.54 ± 2.87Ce	122.87 ± 2.91Cf	106.66 ± 1.87Cg	89.64 ± 2.81Bh	−65.28
D_3	259.88 ± 3.77Ba	242.21 ± 2.42Cb	220.88 ± 2.90Dc	212.34 ± 2.21Dd	160.66 ± 2.93De	134.44 ± 2.93Df	115.54 ± 1.22Dg	104.44 ± 1.89Dh	89.44 ± 2.88Bi	−65.96
D_4	260.02 ± 4.32Ba	240.22 ± 2.76Cb	215.55 ± 2.91Ec	180.88 ± 2.76Ed	145.55 ± 2.65Ee	122.32 ± 2.32Ef	108.78 ± 1.32Eg	102.22 ± 1.34Eh	88.22 ± 2.97BCi	−66.09

Values are mean ± standard deviation (SD) (n = 10)
Mean followed by different upper case letters (A, B, C, D) in the same columns represent significant difference ($P < 0.05$) treatment wise
Mean followed by different lower case letters (a, b, c, d) in the same rows represent significant difference ($P < 0.05$) among study periods (8 weeks)

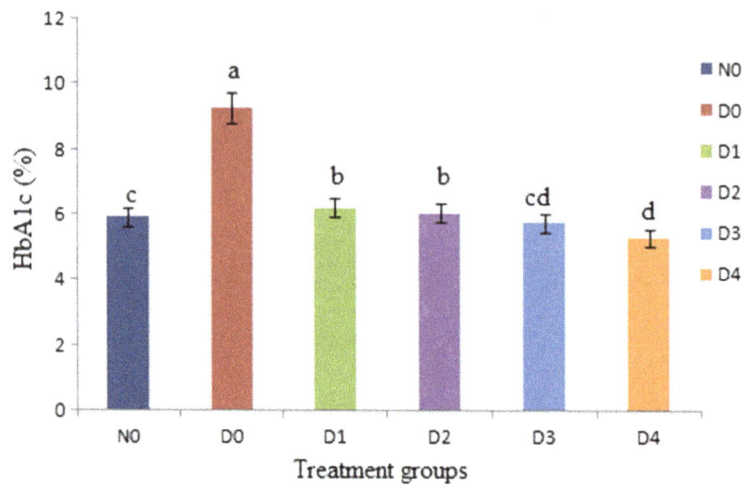

Fig. 3 Effect of Stevia aqueous extract on the glycosylated hemoglobin (HbA1c) level of the rats. Results are expressed as percentage of HbA1c levels of diabetic and non-diabetic rats (mean ± standard deviation (SD). n = 10). a, b, c, d represent significant difference ($P < 0.05$) in HbA1c levels treatment wise. HbA1c levels of diabetic rats (D_1, D_2, D_3 and D_4) received stevia aqueous extract in different concentrations (200, 300, 400 and 500 ppm) respectively significantly ($P < 0.05$) decreased as compared diabetic (D_0) control groups and near to N_0

glucose levels in diabetic rats due to more insulin secretion and increased glycogen level.

The diabetic rats treated with stevia aqueous extract exhibited HbA1c values near normal levels (≥6.5% (48 mmol/mol) as a result of improved glycemic control due to initiation of glycogen production framework of the extract. The decrease of HbA1c showed that the ability of extract to control the diabetes [33].

These results are in accordance with Prasad et al. [35] and Rao et al. [36] who demonstrated the anti-diabetic effects of ethanolic extract of the roots of *Chonemorpha fragrans* and combination of herbal product (*Curcuma longa* and *Eugenia jambolana*) in streptozotocin-

induced diabetic rats and concluded that both have a good efficacy in controlling diabetes.

The serum insulin level in the diabetic control group decreased due to STZ that resulted in diabetes by the rapid depletion of β-cells, which reduced the insulin release. An insufficient release of insulin causes hyperglycemia, which results in oxidative damage by the generation of reactive oxygen species and the development of diabetic complications [37]. When stevia aqueous extracts at different dose levels were given to the diabetic albino rats then their insulin levels improved significantly (Fig. 4) due to the presence of natural components (stevioside) in stevia leaves that are related to

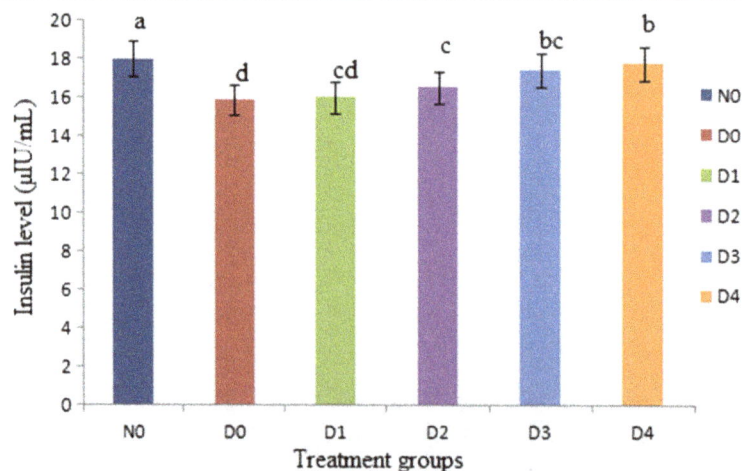

Fig. 4 Effect of Stevia aqueous extract on insulin levels of different groups of rats. Results are expressed as concentration of insulin levels of diabetic and non-diabetic rats (mean ± standard deviation (SD). n = 10). a, b, c, d represent significant difference ($P < 0.05$) in insulin levels treatment wise. The insulin levels of diabetic rats (D_1, D_2, D_3 and D_4) received stevia aqueous extract in different concentrations (200, 300, 400 and 500 ppm) respectively significantly ($P < 0.05$) increased as compared diabetic (D_0) control groups and near to N_0

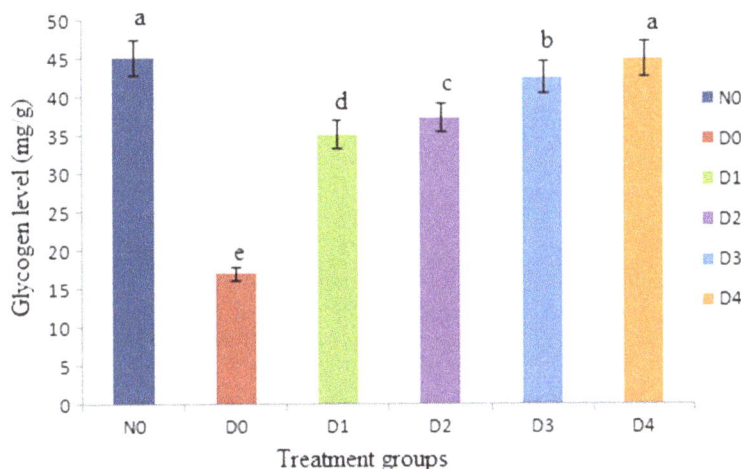

Fig. 5 Effect of Stevia aqueous extract on the glycogen level of the rats. Results are expressed as concentration of glycogen levels of diabetic and non-diabetic rats (mean ± standard deviation (SD). n = 10). a, b, c, d represent significant difference (P < 0.05) in insulin levels treatment wise. The glycogen levels of diabetic rats (D_1, D_2, D_3 and D_4) received stevia aqueous extract in different concentrations (200, 300, 400 and 500 ppm) respectively significantly (P < 0.05) increased as compared diabetic (D_0) control groups and near to N_0

inhibition of hepatic expression of phosphoenolpyruvate carboxykinase and gluconeogenesis coupled with stimulation of hepatic glycogen synthesis that resulted in increase of insulin secretion and insulin sensitivity [38]. Evidence from other studies revealed that stevia aqueous extract elevate the insulin level due to stevioside that acts on pancreatic tissue, exerts beneficial anti-hyperglycemic effects through the PPARγ-dependent mechanism [34, 30].

The results are in collaborations with the studies conducted by Shivanna et al. [39]; Saleh et al. [40] and Abou khalil et al. [41] who concluded that aqueous extracts of *Stevia rebaudiana* leaves and Desert date (*Balanites aegyptiaca*) and Parsley (*Petroselinum sativum*) stevioside normalize the pancreatic cell function by restoring the insulin immune reactivity in STZ-induced diabetic rats.

The reduction in insulin release and liver glycogen level of diabetic control group rats are due to STZ (a known diabetogen) used for induction of diabetes in rats that brings about the destruction of β- cells of the islets of Langerhans [42]. However, the diabetic rats received stevia aqueous extracts (200, 300, 400 and 500 ppm/kg) were able to significantly (P < 0.05) improve the liver glycogen levels (Fig. 5). Stevioside (sweetener) present in stevia extract acts directly on pancreatic beta cells and resulted in increase of insulin secretion [12]. Increased level of Insulin enhances intracellular glycogen deposition by stimulating activities of glycogen synthase and inhibiting glycogen phosphorylase [38].

Similar results were observed by previous researchers who found that *Plectranthus esculenthus* extracts and *Mangifera indica* kernel flour-supplemented diet restored the liver glycogen levels in STZ induced diabetic rats [42, 43].

Conclusions

The present study suggests that aqueous extract from stevia leaves may decrease the random blood glucose level and fasting blood glucose and glycosylated (HbA1c) hemoglobin while insulin and liver glycogen levels significantly increased of the diabetic rats, compared with the diabetic and non-diabetic control rats after 8 weeks study period. It is concluded that aqueous extact of stevia with concentration 500 ppm/kg body weight of rats showed best results of all the parameters determined. It is understood from the results that stevia extract has anti-diabetic effects in albino rats, and therefore could be used as natural anti-diabetic drug for the treatment of diabetes and its associated complications.

Acknowledgements
The authors are thankful to the Institute of Home and Food Sciences, Government College University Faisalabad Pakistan for providing research facilities to prepare this valuable document.

Authors' contributions
UA conceptualized and performed the study; RSA provided the technical assistance, guided in the data collection and also helped to analyze the data and drafting the manuscript. Both authors read and approved the final manuscript.

Competing interests
The authors declare that they have no competing interests.

References

1. American Diabetes Association. Diagnosis and classification of diabetes mellitus. Diabetes Care. 2014;37(Suppl 1):S81–90.

2. Mathers CD, Loncar D. Projections of global mortality and burden of disease from 2002 to 2030. PLoS Med. 2006;3(11):e442.

3. Li G, Zhang P, Wang J, Gregg EW, Yang W, Gong Q. The long- term effect of life style interventions to prevent diabetes in the China Da Qing diabetes prevention study: a 20-year follow-up study. Lancet. 2008;371:1783–9.

4. Dhasarathan P, Theriappan P. Evaluation of anti-diabetic activity of *Strychonous potatorum* in alloxan induced diabetic rats. J Med Sci. 2011;2(2):670–4.

5. Ramesh B, Pugalendi KV. Anti-hyperglycemic effect of Umbelliferone in Streptozotocin diabetic rats. J Med. Plants. 2006;9(4):562–6.

6. Loew D, Kaszkin M. Approaching the problem of bioequivalence of herbal medicinal products. Phytother Res. 2002;16:705–11.

7. Anbazhagan M, Kalpana M, Rajendran R, Natarajan V, Dhanavel D. In vitroproduction of Stevia rebaudiana Bertoni. EJFA. 2010;22(3):216–22.

8. Brahmachari G, Mandal LC, Roy R, Mondal S, Brahmachari AK. Stevioside and related compounds-molecules of pharmaceutical promise: a critical overview. Arch Pharm Chem Life Sci. 2011;1:5–19.

9. Lemus-Mondaca R, Vega-Galvez A, Zura-Bravo L, Ah-Hen K. Stevia rebaudiana Bertoni, source of a high-potency natural sweetener: a comprehensive review on the biochemical, nutritional and functional aspects. J Food Chem. 2012;132:1121–32.

10. Stoyanova S, Genus J, Heideg E, Den Ende VV. The food additives insulin and stevioside counteract oxidative stress. Int J Food Sci Nutr. 2011;62:207–14.

11. Ferrazzano GF, Cantile T, Alcidi B, Coda M, Ingenito A, Zarrelli A, Fabio GD, Pollio A. Is *Stevia rebaudiana* Bertoni a non cariogenic sweetener? A review. Molecules. 2016;21:1–38. https://doi.org/10.3390/molecules21010038.

12. Jeppesen PB, Gregersen S, Rolfsen SE, Jepsen M, Colombo M, Agger A, Xiao J, Kruhoffer M, Orntoff T, Hermansen K. Antihyperglycemic and blood pressure-reducing effects of stevioside in the diabetic Goto-Kakizaki rat. Metabolism. 2003;52:372–8.

13. Thomas JE, Stevia GMJ. It's not just about calories. The Open Obesity Journal. 2010;2:101–9.

14. Kujur RS, Singh V, Ram M, Yadava HN, Singh KK, Kumari S, Roy BK. Anti-diabetic activity and phytochemical screening of crude extract of Stevia rebaudiana in alloxan-induced diabetic rats. Pharm Res. 2010;2(4):258–63.

15. Abou-Arab AE, Abou-Arab AA, Abu-Salem MF. Physico-chemical assessment of natural sweeteners steviosides produced from Stevia rebaudiana Bertoni plant. Afr J Food Sci. 2010;4:269–81.

16. AOAC. Official Methods of Analysis of the Association of Official Analytical Chemists International. 17th ed. Arlington, VA, USA: Association of Official Analytical Chemists International; 2000.

17. Parveen K, Khan R, Siddiqui WA. Antidiabetic effects afforded by Terminalia arjunain high fat- fed and streptozotocin-induced type 2 diabetic rats. Int J Diab Metab. 2011;19:23–33.

18. Ashish B, Swapnil G, Baldi A. Hypoglycemic, effect of Polyherbal formulation in Alloxan induced diabetic rats. PhOL. 2011;13:764–73.

19. Uchida K, Satoh T, Ogura Y, Yamaga N, Yamada K. Effect of partial ileal bypass on cholesterol and bile acid metabolism in rats. Yanago. Acta Medica. 2001;44:69–77.

20. Trinder P. Determination of glucose in blood using glucose oxidase with an alternative.oxygen receptor. Ann Clin Biochem. 1969;6:24–7.

21. Nayak SS, Pattabiraman TN. A new calorimetric method for the estimation of glycosylated haemoglobin. Clin Chim Acta. 1981;109:267–74.

22. Andersen L, Dinesen B, Jorgesen PN, Poulsen F, Roder MF. Enzyme immuno assay for intact human insulin in serum or plasma. Clin Chim Acta. 1993;38:578–85.

23. Babu V, Gangadevi T, Subramoniam A. Antidiabetic activity of ethanol extract of Cassia kleinii leaf in streptozotocin-induced diabetic rats and

24. isolation of an active fraction and toxicity evaluation of the extract. Indian J Pharmacol. 2003;35(5):290–6.

24. Robarts MW, Wright JT. Sweetness without sugar. Dimeus Dental Hygiene. 2010;8:8–61.

25. Abo Elnaga NIE, Massoud Mona I, Yousef MI, Mohamed Hayam HA. Effect stevia sweetener consumption as non-caloric sweetening on body weight gain and biochemical parameters in over weight female rats. Annals Agri Sci. 2016;61(1):155–63.

26. Chang JC, Wu MC, Liu IM, Cheng JT. Increase of insulin sensitivity by stevioside in fructose-rich chow-fed rats. Horm Metab Res. 2005;37:610–6.

27. Awney H, Massoud M, El-Maghrabi S. Long-term feeding effects of stevioside sweetener on some toxicological parameters of growing male rats. J Appl Toxicol. 2010;31:431–8.

28. Bernal J, Mendiola J, Ibanez E, Cifuentes A. Advanced analysis of nutraceuticals. J Pharm Biomed Anal. 2011;55:758–74.

29. Abd El-Razek AM, Massoud MI. Biological evaluation of aqueous extract of *Stevia. rebaudiana* leaves. Egypt J Food Sci. 2012;40:47–61.

30. Assaei R, Mokarram P, Dastghaib S, Darbandi S, Darbandi M, Zal F, Akmali M, GHR O. Hypoglycemic effect of aquatic extract of Stevia in pancreas of diabetic rats: PPARγ-dependent regulation or antioxidant potential. Avicenna J med Biotech. 2016;8(2):65–74.

31. Geuns JMC, Buyse J, Vankeirsbilck A, Temme EHM. Metabolism of stevioside by healthy subjects. Exp Biol Med. 2007;232:164–73.

32. Hossain MS, Alam MB, Asadujjaman M, Islam MM, Rahman MA, Islam MA, Islam A. Antihyperglycemic and anti hyperlipidemic effects of different fractions of stevia rebaudiana leaves in alloxan-induced diabetic rats. Int J Pharm Sci Res. 2011;2(7):1722–9.

33. Shirwaikar A, Rajendran K, Punitha ISR. Antidiabetic activity of alcoholic stem extract of *Coscinium fenestratum* in streptozotocin-nicotinamide induced type 2 diabetic rats. J Ethnopharmacol. 2005;97(2):369–74.

34. Akbarzadeh S, Eskandari F, Tangestani H, Bagherinejad ST, Bargahi A, Bazzi P, Daneshi A, Sahrapoor A, O'Connor WJ, Rahbar AR. The effect of Stevia rebaudiana on serum omentin and visfatin level in stz-induced diabetic rats. J diet Suppl. 2015;12(1):1–12.

35. Prasad BS, Srinivasan KK, Harindran J. *Chonemorpha Fragrans* (moon) Alston-an effective Antihyperglycemic and anti hyperlipidemic agent in Streptozotocin nicotinamide induced diabetic rats. Int J Pharm Sci Res. 2016;7(3):1149–55.

36. Rao SS, Najam R. Efficacy of combination herbal product (curcuma longaand Eugenia jambolana) used for diabetes mellitus. Pak J Pharm Sci. 2016;29(1):201–4.

37. Kangralkar V, Shivraj A, Patil D, Bandivadekar RM. Oxidative stress and diabetes: a review. Inter J Pharmaceut Appl. 2010;1:38–45.

38. Yang PS, Lee JJ, Tsao CW, Wu HT, Cheng JT. Stimulatory effect of stevioside on peripheral muopioid receptors in animals. Neurosci Lett. 2009;454(1):72–5.

39. Shivanna N, Naika M, Khanum F, Kaul VK. Antioxidant, anti-diabetic and renal protective properties of Stevia rebaudiana. J Diab Compl. 2013;27:103–13.

40. Saleh OM, Awad NS, Soliman MM, Mansour AA, Nassan MA. Insulin-mimetic activity of stevioside on diabetic rats: biochemical, molecular and histopathological study. Afr J Tradit Complement Altern Med. 2016;13(2):156–63.

41. Abou Khalil NS, Abou-Elhamd Alaa S, Wasfy Salwa IA, El Mileegy Ibtisam MH, Hamed Mohamed Y, Ageely Hussien M. Antidiabetic and antioxidant impacts of desert date (Balanites aegyptiaca) and parsley (Petroselinum sativum) aqueous extracts: lessons from experimental rats. J Diab Res 2016; Article ID 8408326, 10 pages http://dx.doi.org/10.1155/2016/8408326, 2016.

42. Irondi EA, Oboh G, Akindahunsi AA. Antidiabetic effects of Mangifera indica kernel flour- supplemented diet in streptozotocin-induced type 2 diabetes in rats. J Food Sci Nutri. 2016;4(6):828–39.

43. Jayaprasad B, Sharavanan PS, Sivaraj R. Antidiabetic effect of *Chloroxylon swietenia* bark extracts on streptozotocin induced diabetic rats. Beni-Suef University J Basic. Appl Sci. 2016;5(1):61–9.

4

Antioxidant and anticancer activities of *Trigonella foenum-graecum*, *Cassia acutifolia* and *Rhazya stricta*

Bayan Al-Dabbagh[1*], Ismail A. Elhaty[1], Ala'a Al Hrout[2], Reem Al Sakkaf[1], Raafat El-Awady[4], S. Salman Ashraf[1] and Amr Amin[2,3*]

Abstract

Background: Here, we determined in vitro antioxidant activity, total phenols and flavonoids and evaluated antiproliferative activity of three medicinal plant extracts: *Trigonella foenum-graecum* (Fenugreek), *Cassia acutifolia* (Senna) and *Rhazya stricta* (Harmal).

Methods: The leaves of the three medicinal plants were extracted with 70% ethanol. Antioxidant activities of the extracts were determined by using DPPH (1,1-diphenyl-2-picrylhydrazyl) assay. Total flavonoid and phenolic contents were determined using colorimetric assays. MTT assay was used to estimate the antiproliferative activities of the extracts against human hepatoma (HepG2) cancer cell line. In addition, the effects of *R. stricta* extract on cell cycle, colony formation, and wound healing of HepG2 cells and tube formation of HUVEC cells were assessed.

Results: Percentage inhibition of DPPH scavenging activity were dose-dependent and ranged between (89.9% ± 0.51) and (28.6% ± 2.07). Phenolic contents ranged between (11.5 ± 0.013) and (9.7 ± 0.008) mg GAE/g while flavonoid content ranged between (20.8 ± 0.40) and (0.12 ± 0.0.01) mg QE/g. Antiproliferative results of the extracts were found to be consistent with their antioxidant activity. Among the extracts evaluated, that of *R. stricta* showed the best antioxidant, antiproliferative and antimetastatic activities at low concentration. It also inhibited the colony-formation capacity of HepG2 cells and exhibited antiangiogenic activity. Cell cycle analysis showed significant arrest of cells at G2/M phase 12 and 48 h after treatment and significant arrest at G1/S phase after 24 h of treatment. Consistent data were observed in western blot analysis of protein levels of Cdc2 and its cyclin partners.

Conclusions: These findings introduce *R. stricta* as a potentially useful anti-metastatic agent and a novel potential anti-tumour agent for hepatocellular carcinoma (HCC) treatment.

Keywords: Antioxidants, Anticancer, Medicinal plants, Traditional medicine, *Rhazya stricta*

Background

Free radicals are mainly produced by oxidation processes and they have an important role in the processes of food spoilage and chemical materials degradation. They also contribute to human disorders such as aging-associated diseases, cardiovascular diseases, cancer and inflammatory diseases [1, 2]. Free radicals may also cause a depletion of the immune system antioxidants, a change in the gene expression and may induce the synthesis of abnormal proteins. About 5% or more of the inhaled oxygen (O_2) is converted to reactive oxygen species (ROS) such as O_2^-, H_2O_2, and OH radicals. ROS represents the major type of free radicals in any biological system. They are produced through the mitochondrial electrons transport chain [2, 3].

Antioxidants are used to neutralize the effects of free radicals. Thus, they protect humans against infection and degenerative diseases. Antioxidants can be classified into two major categories, natural and synthetic. Synthetic antioxidants include butylated hydroxy anisole (BHA), butylated hydroxyl toluenes (BHT), tertiary butylated hydroquinone and gallic acid esters. These antioxidants effectively inhibit

* Correspondence: bayan.al-dabbagh@uaeu.ac.ae; a.amin@uaeu.ac.ae
[1]Department of Chemistry, College of Science, UAE University, PO Box 15551, Al Ain, UAE
[2]Department of Biology, College of Science, UAE University, PO Box 15551, Al Ain, UAE
Full list of author information is available at the end of the article

oxidation, may serve as chelating agents such as ethylene diamine tetra acetic acid (EDTA), and can bind metals reducing their contribution to the process [4]. However, antioxidants are thought to cause or promote negative health effects such as mutagenesis and carcinogenesis in humans [5]. Therefore, there is a strong trend to replace the synthetic with naturally occurring antioxidants that can prevent free radical-related diseases [4, 6].

Natural antioxidants help in controlling the formation of free radicals and activated oxygen species or they can inhibit their reaction with biological structures [7]. These antioxidants include antioxidative enzymes, such as superoxide dismutase, catalase, and glutathione peroxidase, and small nonenzymatic antioxidant molecules, such as glutathione and vitamins C and E [8]. Many herbs and spices (rosemary, thyme, oregano, sage, basil, pepper, clove, cinnamon, nutmeg, and saffron), and plant extracts (tea, grapeseed, and lemon balm) contain antioxidant components [9–11].

In this study, three hydroalcoholic extracts of traditionally medicinal plants used in the United Arab Emirates (UAE) were evaluated for their antioxidant activities, phenol and flavonoid contents. These plants are, *Trigonella foenum-graecum*, locally known as "Helba", *Cassia acutifolia*, commonly known as "Holoul" and *Rhazya stricta* which is locally called "Harmal".

T. foenum-graecum seeds are traditionally used as herbal medicine for their carminative, tonic, aphrodisiac and anticancer effects [12–14]. The leaves of *C. acutifolia* is frequently used in folk medicine as a purgative for a long time [15]. The extracts of *R. stricta* leaves are traditionally used for the treatment of various disorders such as diabetes, sore throat, helminthiasis, inflammatory conditions and rheumatism [16].

Available treatment for hepatocellular carcinoma are mainly limited to invasive hepatectomy or chemotherapy. However, the attention has shifted in recent years to natural-based products for candidate anticancer therapeutics. In the present study, the antiproliferative effects of *Trigonella foenum-graecum*, *Cassia acutifolia*, and *Rhazya stricta* on hepatoma cell line HepG2 were investigated. The use of HepG2 cells to test the cytotoxic effects of a wide range of drugs has been well documented, due to their wide availability, well-differentiation, and drug metabolizing activity [17].

Despite playing a key role in cellular processes, free radicals pose a threat to cells by damaging DNA, proteins, and cellular membranes, leading to onset of many diseases including cancer [18, 19]. Thus, by decreasing free radicals and oxidative stress, antioxidants play a role in ameliorating DNA damage, reducing the rate of abnormal cell division, and decreasing mutagenesis [20]. Therefore, many antioxidant-rich plants possess anticancer activity [21–23].

Vascular endothelial growth factor (VEGF) has been recognized to be involved in several stages of angiogenesis in malignant diseases by its multi-functional effects in activating and integrating signalling pathway networks [24]. VEGF signalling blockade reduces new vessel growth and leads to endothelial cell apoptosis. Therefore, using tyrosine kinase inhibitors or VEGF/VEGF receptor (VEGFR) antibodies to inhibit crucial angiogenic steps is a practical therapeutic strategy when treating neovascularisation diseases [25]. A potent angiogenesis inhibitor known as E7820, has been shown to reduce integrin α 2 mRNA expression and inhibit basic fibroblast growth factor/VEGF-induced HUVEC proliferation and tube formation [26, 27]. Integrin α 2β 1/α 1β 1 expression is reportedly regulated by VEGF and an inhibitory antibody against α 2β 1/α 1β 1 has been shown to inhibit angiogenesis and tumour growth in VEGF-overexpressing tumour cells [28, 29]. Therefore, we investigated here the effect of *R. stricta* leaves extract on angiogenesis utilizing HUVEC tube formation assay; as it showed the most promising antiproliferative activity. In addition, this work was set to determine the in vitro antioxidant activity, total phenols and flavonoids, anticancer activities of tested plants with special interest in *R. stricta*.

Methods

Chemicals

All solvents were analytical grade. Agilent Cary 60 UV-Vis Spectrophotometer was used in all spectrophotometric measurements. Ascorbic acid, ferric chloride, aluminium chloride, potassium acetate, quercetin, DPPH reagent, Folin-Ciocalteau reagent, gallic acid, sodium carbonate, methanol and ethanol were obtained from Sigma Chemical Co. (St. Louis, MO, USA). Millipore deionized water was used throughout. Thiazolyl Blue Tetrazolium Bromide (Sigma Aldrich, USA), Dimethyl Sulfoxide (Sigma Aldrich, USA).

Plant samples

Dried leaves of *C. acutifolia*, *R. stricta* and *T. foenum-graecum* were purchased from the local market. The taxonomic authentication of all the plants was carried out by Dr. Fatima Al-Ansari at the Biology Department, College of Science, United Arab Emirates University. Voucher specimens were deposited at the herbarium of the Biology Department (voucher reference numbers: BA2018–1, BA2018–2, BA2018–3).

Preparation of plant extracts

The leaves of the medicinal plants were crushed separately in a grinder. A sample of 10 g of each plant was extracted with 150 mL of 70% ethanol and 30% water as it showed the best extraction yield [30]. The crushed plants were macerated for 48 h at 4 °C. The resulting mixture was then filtered under vacuum and concentrated under reduced pressure in a rotary evaporator at 40 °C. The extracts were further dried using a TELSTAR

CRYODOS freeze dryer machine then kept at − 20 °C for further analysis. A solution of 30 mg/mL of each plant was prepared in 50% ethanol for the following tests.

Determination of total polyphenol content

The total phenolic content (TPC) was determined by using the Folin-Ciocalteau reagent [31]. A 10% solution was prepared from the stock solution (30 mg/mL) using 50% ethanol. 100 µl of this solution was mixed with 200 µl of the Folin-Ciocalteau reagent and 2 mL of de-ionized water then incubated at room temperature for 3 min. A sample of 20% aqueous sodium carbonate (w/w, 1 mL) was then added to the mixture. The total polyphenols were determined after 1 h of incubation at room temperature. A negative control sample was also prepared using the same procedure. The absorbance of the resulting blue colour was measured at 765 nm. Results were expressed in mg gallic acid equivalents (GAE) per g dry weight of plant material using an equation obtained from gallic acid calibration curve. The samples were analyzed in triplicate.

Free-radical scavenging activity

The antioxidant activity of the extracts was assessed based on their ability to scavenge the stable 1,1-diphenyl-2-picrylhydrazyl (DPPH) radical as described previously [32]. Various concentrations of the three extracts in methanol were prepared (0.15 to 1.5 mg/mL). A methanolic solution of DPPH (3.8 mL, 60 µg/mL) was rapidly mixed with the plant extract (200 µl, 30 mg/mL) in a test tube, with methanol serving as the blank sample and a control was also assayed simultaneously. The contents of the tubes were swirled then allowed to stand for 30 min at room temperature in the dark. The absorbance was measured at 517 nm in a spectrophotometer. The scavenging ability of the plant extract was calculated using this equation: DPPH Scavenging activity (%) = [(Abs control−Abs sample)]/ (Abs control)] × 100, where Abs control is the absorbance of DPPH + methanol; Abs sample is the absorbance of DPPH radical + sample (sample or standard). The EC_{50} value (µg/mL), the effective concentration at which DPPH· radicals are scavenged by 50%, was determined graphically. The total antioxidant activity was expressed as ascorbic acid equivalent/g dry extract. The assay was done in triplicates.

Determination of total flavonoids

The total flavonoids content in the extracts was determined using the aluminium chloride colorimetric method [33]. A known concentration (600 µg/mL) of each extract in methanol was prepared. A 500 µl of the extracts were mixed separately with 0.1 mL of 10% (w/v) aluminium chloride solution, 0.1 mL of 1 M potassium acetate solution, 1.5 mL of methanol and 2.8 mL of distilled water. The solutions were thoroughly mixed and incubated at room temperature for 30 min. The absorbance of the reaction mixture was measured at 415 nm using a spectrophotometer. The total flavonoids content was determined using a standard curve with quercetin (1 to 25 µg/mL) as the standard. The mean of three readings was used and expressed as mg of quercetin equivalents (QE)/ g of the dry extract.

Cell culture

A human hepatocellular carcinoma (HCC)-derived cell line (HepG2) was cultured in RPMI 1640 medium containing 1% antibiotic cocktail and supplemented with 10% fetal bovine serum. Cells were incubated at 37 °C in 5% CO_2 humidified incubator. Cells were passaged every 2–3 days using 0.25% trypsin-EDTA.

Cytotoxicity assay

HepG2 were seeded at a density of 5000 cells/well in a 96-well plate, and were allowed to attach overnight. Thereafter, cells were treated with various concentrations of the plants extracts for 24 h. To assess the cytotoxic effect of the three plants extracts, MTT (3-[4,5-dimethylthiazol-1-2-yl]-2,5-diphenyltratrazolium bromide) assay was carried out. Briefly, cells treated with the plant extracts were exposed to tetrazolium MTT at a concentration of 5 mg/mL. Viable active cells reduced yellow MTT salt to insoluble purple formazan, which was dissolved using DMSO. The absorbance of the coloured solution was measured at a wavelength of 570 nm using Epoch microplate spectrophotometer (BioTek). The obtained absorbance at 570 nm of both control and treated cells was used to calculate percentage of cell viability. Assuming 100% viability in control cells, percentage of treated cells viability will be calculated accordingly:

Percent of viable cells
$$= (\text{Abs. of treated cells}/\text{Abs. of control cells}) \times 100$$

Assessment of morphological changes

HepG2 were seeded at a density of 0.25×10^6 cells/ well in a 6-well plate, and were allowed to attach overnight. After which, cells were treated without (0 µg, control) or with increasing concentrations of R. stricta (10, 20, 30, 50, 70 µg) for 24 h. The morphology of the cells was assessed after being fixed and stained with 0.5% crystal violet using bright-field microscopy (200 x magnification, scale = 200 µm).

Colony formation assay

To assess the effects of R. stricta on cell survival, the colony formation assay was carried out in vitro. Briefly, HepG2 cells were seeded at a density of 1000 cells/ well in a 6-well plate, and were incubate for 24 h to allow attachment. The second day, the cells were treated without (0 μg, control) or with increasing concentrations (10, 20, 30 μg) of the extract for 24 h. After which, the media was replaced with fresh complete growth media without the extract, and cells were left to incubate until visible colonies were formed; while changing the media every 3–4 days. The experiment was carried out in triplicates. Colonies were fixed with absolute methanol, then stained with 0.5% crystal violet. Results are represented as the percentage of the well area that is covered by colonies (colony area percentage). Analysis has been carried out using ImageJ plugin ColonyArea [34]. In addition, an absorption-based method was carried out to validate the earlier results, by which the absorption of the crystal violet dye in each well is measured after being dissolved. Briefly, the samples that had been analysed using ImageJ were subjected to 10% acetic acid solution, then were placed on an orbital shaker for 15 min. After which, 100 μL of each triplicate sample was transferred to a 96-well plate (in triplicates), and absorbance was measured using Epoch microplate spectrophotometer (BioTek).

Wound-healing assay

To assess the ability of HepG2 to migrate after the treatment with R. stricta, wound-healing assay was carried out in vitro. Cells were seeded at a density of 0.5×10^6/ well in 6-well plate, and were allowed to attach overnight. A scratch in the cell monolayer was made using a sterile plastic pipetting tip, and then the monolayer was washed with PBS. The cells were treated without (0 μg) or with 20, 30 μg of the extract. Images were taken at 0, 24, 48, 72 h using bright-field microscopy (40 x magnification). Analysis was carried out using ImageJ, percent of open area was calculated according to the following formula [$T_x = T_{24}$, T_{48}, or T_{72} (at time 24, 48, or 72 h, respectively]: Percent of open area = (open area at T_x/ open area at T_0) X 100.

Experiment was carried out in triplicates, data is representative of 3 random regions in each triplicate of each sample.

Cell cycle analysis

Effect of R. stricta extract on cell cycle progression of HepG2 cells was analysed as previously described [35]. Cells were treated without or with 30 μg of R. stricta extract at different time intervals (6 – 48 h), collected by trypsinization, washed twice with PBS, fixed in 70% ethanol, treated with RNase, stained with propidium iodide and then cell cycle distribution was analysed in BD Accuri C6 cytometer and software (BD Biosciences, USA).

Western blotting

HepG2 were seeded at a density of 1×10^6 in 60 mm dish and allowed to attach overnight. Cells were treated without or with 30 μg of extract for 6, 12, 24, 48 h. Cells were lysed and total protein was quantified using BCA. 20 μg of total protein was separated on SDS-PAGE, transferred onto nitrocellulose membranes that were blocked using 5% BSA TBST. Primary antibodies against Cdc2 (1:000; cell signalling), p-Cdc2 (1:1000; cell signalling), Cyclin B1 (1:1000; cell signalling), Cyclin A1 (1:000; Abcam) were used. GAPDH (1:15000; Abcam) was used as loading control. Proteins were detected using LI-COR C-DiGit Chemiluminescence Western Blot Scanner.

Matrigel capillary tube formation

96-well plate was coated with Matrigel matrix (Corning, NY, USA) at 50 ul/well and allowed to polymerize for 60 min at 37 °C. HUVEC cells were then seeded on the Matrigel at a concentration of 2×10^4 cells/well without (0 μg) or with (10, 20, 30 μg) R. stricta extract. After incubation for 18 h, tubules were imaged using an inverted microscope and analyzed with ImageJ software.

Statistical analysis

All data were expressed as mean ± standard deviation (SD) of three independent experiments. Correlation analysis of antioxidants versus the total phenolic and flavonoid contents were carried out using the regression analysis, with GraphPad Prism 6.0 and Microsoft Excel 2016. $P < 0.05$ was considered to indicate a significant difference.

Results and discussion

Medicinal plants have been of great interest as a source of natural antioxidants used for health promotion. The therapeutic activity of plants is mostly due to their biologically active polyphenolic substances, mostly flavonoids and phenolic acids. These substances exhibit antioxidant, anti-lipoxygenase and anticancer activities. The present study elaborates on the antioxidant activity, polyphenolic and flavonoid contents of three folk plants from the UAE; T. foenum-graecum, C. acutifolia and R. stricta. The antiproliferative effect of such plants was studied against human cancer cells HepG2 in an attempt to find a correlation with the antioxidant activity of those extracts that are based on their phenolic and flavonoid contents.

Plant extraction

Different solvents have been used in the literature for the preparation of plant extracts [36]. In this study, we used 70% ethanol as the extraction solvent. The amorphous solid of the leave extracts under investigation was obtained by complete evaporation of ethanol/water. The yield of each extract was calculated as w/w percent yield. The yields of T. foenum-graecum, C. acutifolia and R. stricta extracts were 25, 23 and 30% respectively.

Total polyphenol content of the extracts

Polyphenols are aromatic secondary plant metabolites and are widely spread throughout plants. They have been associated with colour, sensory qualities, and nutritional and antioxidant properties of food [37]. It is reported that there is a strong relationship between total polyphenol contents and antioxidant activity. The hydroxyl groups in phenols have a strong scavenging ability for free radicals. Therefore, the total polyphenol contents of plants may directly contribute to their antioxidant activity [32, 38]. The Folin-Ciocalteau reagent is commonly used in the literature to determine phenolic compounds. This reagent reacts with phenolic compounds and gives a blue colour complex that absorbs radiation and allows quantification [39]. The total phenolic content for the ethanolic extracts of *C. acutifolia*, *R. stricta* and *T. foenum-graecum* was determined by the Folin-Ciocalteau method using gallic acid as a standard. The calibration curve showed linearity for gallic acid in the range of 0.5–26 µg/mL, with a correlation coefficient (R^2) of 0.984. *R. stricta* contained the highest total polyphenols (11.5 ± 0.013 mg GAE/g extract), followed by *C. acutifolia* (10.8 ± 0.025 mg GAE/g extract) and *T. foenum-graecum* (9.7 ± 0.008 mg GAE/g extract) (Fig. 1). Belguith-Hadriche et al. [40] reported the total phenolic content of various extracts of *T. foenum-graecum* ranged between 9.42 ± 0.50 in hexane and 78.1 ± 0.90 mg GAE/g dry weight extracts in methanol. A study conducted in Saudi Arabia showed the total phenolic content of *R. stricta* extracts ranged between 62.5 ± 0.2 and 66.63 ± 0.03 mg GAE/g extract [41].

The DPPH radical scavenging activity

The antioxidant activity of each plant was also assessed based on its ability to reduce the stable DPPH radical according to the method reported by Lim [32]. The DPPH radical (DPPH•) is a stable radical and has the ability to accept an electron or hydrogen radical and form a stable diamagnetic molecule producing a colour change from blue to yellow [42]. The colour change of DPPH has been widely used to measure the radical scavenging activity because of its stability, simplicity, and reproducibility [43]. The free radical scavenging capacity of the ethanolic extracts of the three plants were assayed based on the remaining amount (%) of DPPH• as a function of time (30 min). The total antioxidant activity was expressed as ascorbic acid equivalent/g dry extract.

The calibration curve of ascorbic acid showed linearity in the range of 5–20 µg/mL, with a correlation coefficient (R^2) of 0.994. The percentage inhibitions of DPPH scavenging activity in all the extracts were dose-dependent (Fig. 2). The DPPH scavenging activity by the *T. foenum-graecum* extract was (89.7% ± 1.54) at 1.5 mg/mL and (28.6% ± 2.07) at 0.15 mg/mL. DPPH of *C. acutifolia* was (86.3% ± 0.64) at 1.5 mg/mL and (30.0% ± 1.37) at 0.15 mg/mL while that of *R. stricta* was (89.9% ± 0.51) at 1.5 mg/mL and (28.7% ± 1.27) at 0.15 mg/mL. The results showed that there is no clear difference between the obtained DPPH scavenging activities of the three extracts. These results are almost in agreement with their total polyphenol contents. Consequently, the antioxidant activity of these plants might be related to their contents of phenolic compounds.

In addition, the DPPH radical scavenging ability of the extracts was evaluated as EC_{50} (µg/mL) value. The smallest EC_{50} values indicates the best free radical scavenging activity. The highest scavenging activity was exerted by *R. stricta* (EC_{50} = 241.8 µg/mL) which contained the highest amount of total polyphenol content (11.5 µg/mL), followed by *C. acutifolia* (EC_{50} = 244.8, TPC = 10.8 µg/mL). The lowest radical scavenging activity was exhibited by the *T. foenum-graecum* extract (EC_{50} = 245.9, TPC = 9.7 µg/mL). The relationship between total phenol content and free radical scavenging activity (using EC_{50}) was also studied using linear regression analysis (Fig. 3a). The results showed a

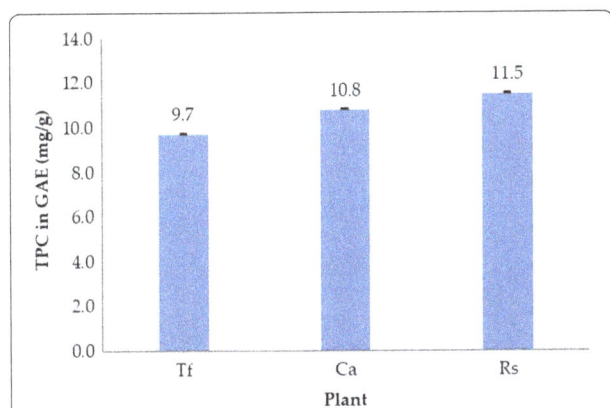

Fig. 1 Total phenolic content of *T. foenum-graecum* (Tf), *C. acutifolia* (Ca) and *R. stricta* (Rs) extracts determined by the Folin-Ciocalteau assay and calculated as mg GAE/g extract based on dry weight. Results are the average of triplicates ± SD

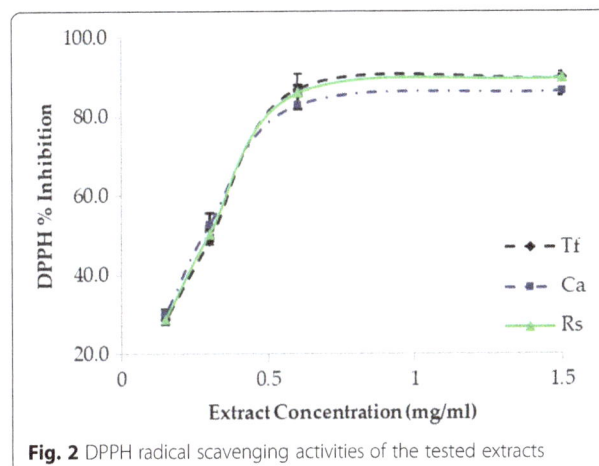

Fig. 2 DPPH radical scavenging activities of the tested extracts

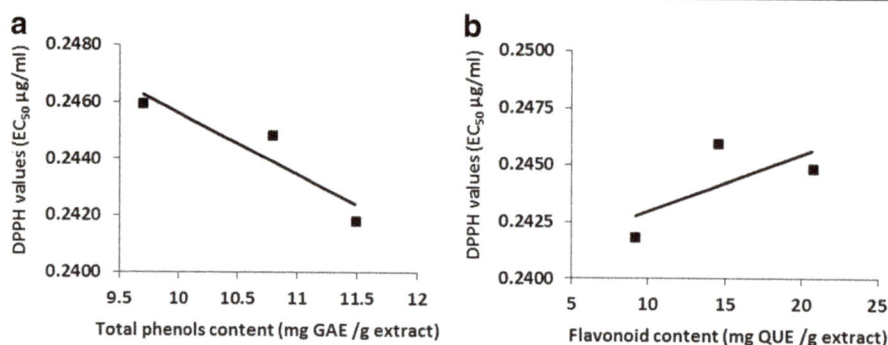

Fig. 3 Linear correlations between the amount of total phenols and DPPH· radical scavenging activity (**a**) and between the flavonoid content and DPPH· radical scavenging activity (**b**)

significant negative correlation ($R^2 = -0.856$, P-value < 0.05) between EC_{50} (DPPH· scavenging) and total phenolic content suggesting that the presence of the phenolic compounds contributed significantly to the antioxidant activity of the tested plants. These results are consistent with previous works that showed a liner correlation between the total phenolic content and the reducing antioxidant capacity of some plant extracts [32, 38, 44].

Total flavonoid contents

Flavonoids are a class of secondary plant phenolics. Flavonoids and their derivatives have a wide range of biological actions including anticancer activity. The anticancer activity of flavonoids is attributed to their potent antioxidant effects which include metal chelation and free-radical scavenging activities [45]. Flavonoids present in herbs were found to significantly contribute to their antioxidant properties [44]. The flavonoid content was obtained using aluminium chloride assay which based on the formation of a complex between the aluminium ion, Al (III), and the carbonyl and hydroxyl groups of flavones and flavonols that produce a yellow colour [46]. Flavonoid content was calculated from the regression equation of quercetin calibration curve and was expressed as quercetin equivalents. The calibration curve showed linearity in the range of 1–25 µg/mL, with a correlation coefficient (R^2) of 0.999.

Figure 4 shows the flavonoids contents in all the extracts. Using the standard curve generated by quercetin, the total flavonoids content of the *T. foenum-graecum* extract was (14.6 ± 0.21 mg QE/g), whereas, the *C. actutifolia* extract was (20.8 ± 0.40 mg QE/g) and finally that of *R. stricta* was (9.2 ± 0.22 mg QE/g).

The relationship between the total flavonoids content and the free radical scavenging activity (using EC_{50}) was studied using linear regression analysis (Fig. 3b). The results showed a positive correlation ($R^2 = 0.460$, P-value < 0.05) between EC_{50} (DPPH scavenging) and total flavonoids content. The obtained correlation was moderate

suggesting that other compounds maybe participating in the radical scavenging activity of these plant extracts.

Effects of extracts on cell viability in HepG2 cells

HCC remains among the leading cause of cancer-related death worldwide [47, 48]. Although therapeutic approaches for advanced HCC are limited to the use of multikinase inhibitors, such as sorafenib, only modest survival benefits have clinically been reported. Thus, identifying new compounds with promise antitumor activity against HCC is exceedingly needed [48, 49]. Natural products, especially from plants, are often better tolerated than their synthetic analogs used in cancer treatments [50]. They contain a wide spectrum of bioactive secondary metabolites that are the foundation of the recently introduced notion of broad-spectrum integrative approach for cancer prevention and treatment [51].

Effects of tested extracts were investigated against human hepatoma (HepG2) cancer cell line. A dose-dependent reduction in cell viability was reported in cells treated with all tested extracts (Fig. 5). The IC_{50} values of extracts ranged from 30 µg/mL to 200 µg/mL. Treatment with *R. stricta* significantly enhanced the mortality of cancer cells at the lowest concentration (30 µg/mL). *T. foenum-graecum* was

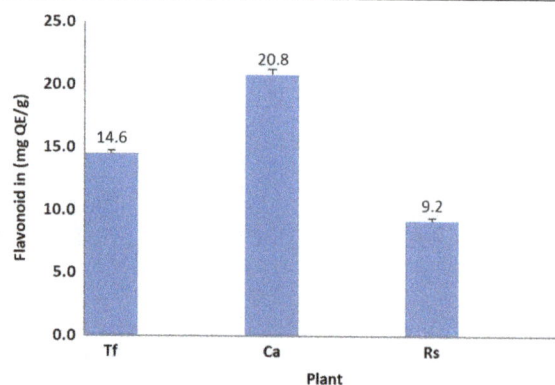

Fig. 4 Flavonoids content of the tested extracts

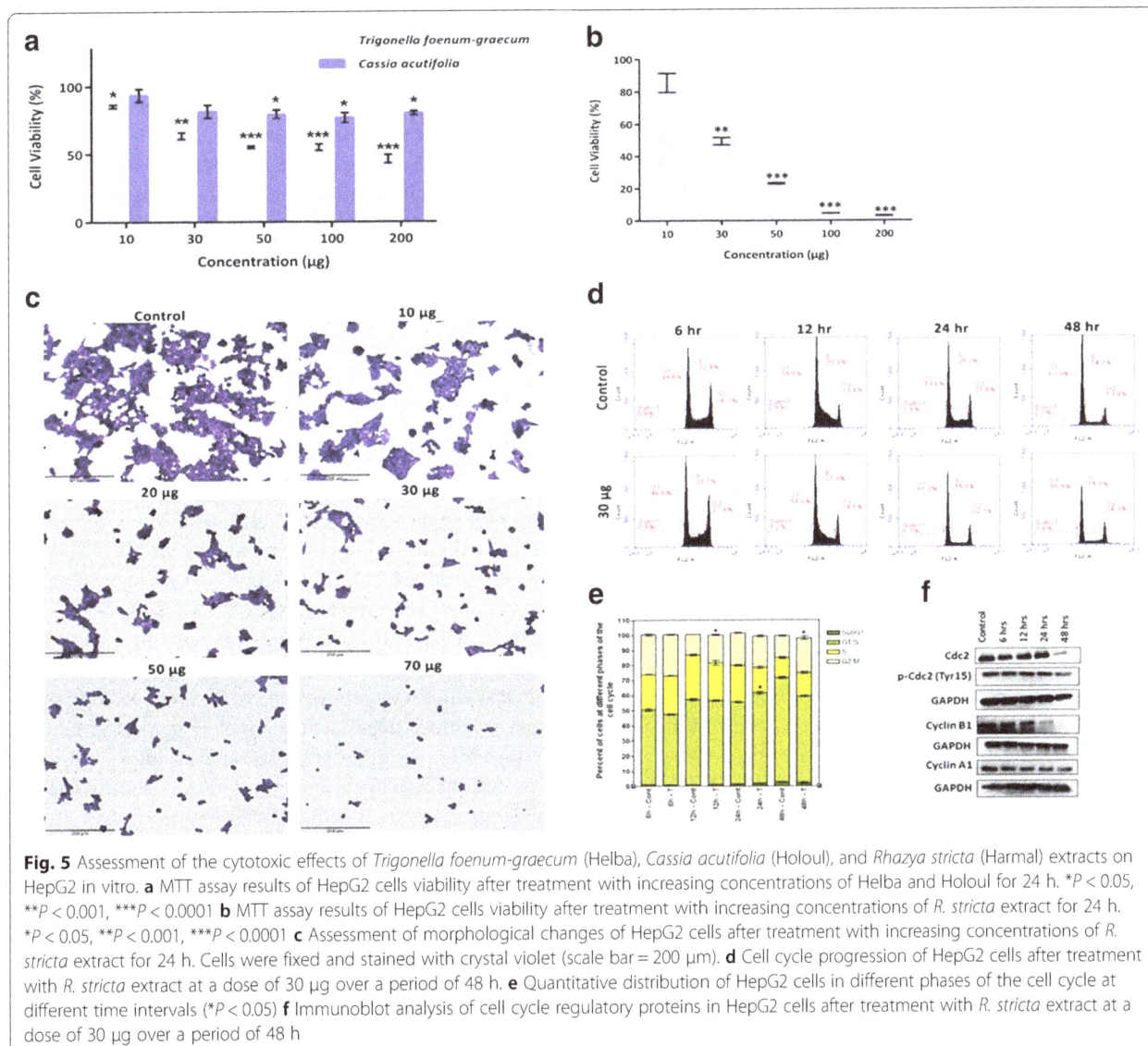

Fig. 5 Assessment of the cytotoxic effects of *Trigonella foenum-graecum* (Helba), *Cassia acutifolia* (Holoul), and *Rhazya stricta* (Harmal) extracts on HepG2 in vitro. **a** MTT assay results of HepG2 cells viability after treatment with increasing concentrations of Helba and Holoul for 24 h. *$P < 0.05$, **$P < 0.001$, ***$P < 0.0001$ **b** MTT assay results of HepG2 cells viability after treatment with increasing concentrations of *R. stricta* extract for 24 h. *$P < 0.05$, **$P < 0.001$, ***$P < 0.0001$ **c** Assessment of morphological changes of HepG2 cells after treatment with increasing concentrations of *R. stricta* extract for 24 h. Cells were fixed and stained with crystal violet (scale bar = 200 μm). **d** Cell cycle progression of HepG2 cells after treatment with *R. stricta* extract at a dose of 30 μg over a period of 48 h. **e** Quantitative distribution of HepG2 cells in different phases of the cell cycle at different time intervals (*$P < 0.05$) **f** Immunoblot analysis of cell cycle regulatory proteins in HepG2 cells after treatment with *R. stricta* extract at a dose of 30 μg over a period of 48 h

however less potent with IC_{50} of 200 μg/mL where 50% of HepG2 cancer cells were eradicated at 200 μg/mL. A fenugreek-enriched diet decreased colon tumour incidence and hepatic lipid peroxidation in liver cancer-induced rats in addition to increasing the endogenous antioxidant activities in liver [52]. Li et al. [53] showed that diosgenin, fenugreek's main active ingredient, down regulated the expression of various STAT3-regulated genes, inhibited proliferation and potentiated the apoptotic effects of paclitaxel and doxorubicin, suggesting that diosgenin could be a novel and potential treatment option for HCC and other cancers. Therefore, the role of fenugreek extract and its active principals as supplements in diet-based preventive/therapeutic strategies to improve health care continues to be a fast growing field of research. The correlation between the antioxidant activities (free radical scavenging activity) and the anticancer activities (cell viability) of *C. acutifolia*,

R. stricta and *T. foenum-graecum* extracts was studied using linear regression analysis. The results showed a significant positive correlation ($R^2 = - 0.933$, 0.997 and 0.797, *P*-value < 0.05) for *C. acutifolia*, *R. stricta* and *T. foenum-graecum* extracts respectively.

At a concentration range of (100–200 μg/mL) *Cassia acutifolia's* extract was similarly cytotoxic to HepG2 cells. Alkaloids extracted from Senna species reduced cell viability in a concentration-dependent manner of different tumour cell lines including HepG2 [49]. Senna alkaloids showed important antiproliferative activity on HepG2 cells that was mediated by ERK inactivation and down-regulation of cyclin D1 expression. Similarly, extracts of different cassia species were able to inhibit growth of colorectal (DLD1), among other, human cancer cell lines [54]. Thus, Senna's extract may represent a potential new antitumor and/or adjuvant treatment against liver and colorectal cancer and further investigations should be conducted to unravel its molecular mechanism. *R. stricta*'s extract was by far the most effective cytotoxic agent tested at the present study at as little as 30 μg/mL. The δ-tocopherol and alkaloid fraction of *R. stricta*'s leaves extract have been shown to delay many angiogenic and inflammatory activities and to inhibit cell viability of HepG2, hence potentially useful against cancer [55, 56]. As *R. stricta* extract showed the most promising antiproliferative activity, its antiproliferative effects were tested against other GI cell line. The present study also showed that *R. stricta* extract inhibited cell proliferation in colorectal cancer cells (HCT116), in a dose -dependent manner (Additional file 1: Figure S1). To get insight into the molecular effects of *R. stricta* on HepG2 cells, its effect on cell cycle progression was analysed. *R. stricta* treatment induced arrest of cells in the G2/M phase (12 and 48 h time points) and in G1/S phase (24 h time point) (Fig. 5d and e). This cell cycle arrest reflects the cytotoxic effects of *R. stricta* on HepG2 cells where the cells are arrested at these phases to repair the toxic lesions induced by *R. stricta* or to be removed by death pathways such as apoptosis. The significant increase of the fraction of cells in G2/M after long term treatment (48 h) may indicate permanent arrest of cells in this phase (quiescence). These findings are consistent with western blot data, where cell cycle promoting proteins cdc2 and its cyclin partners (cyclin A1 and cyclin B1) are down regulated post *R. stricta* treatment (Fig. 5f). Cdc2 activity is regulated through two mechanisms, first by binding to its cyclin partners [57], and second by being phosphorylated at Tyr15, and subsequently inhibited [58, 59]. Cdc2/cyclin complexes contribute to cell cycle progression through phosphorylation of target proteins [60]. As shown, Cdc2, and its partners cyclin A and cyclin B were downregulated in a time-dependent manner (Fig. 5f). In addition, treatment with *R. stricta* extract resulted in a slight increase in Tyr15 phosphorylated Cdc2 (Fig. 5f).

R. stricta extract inhibited the colony formation of HepG2 cells

This assay measures the ability of tumour cells to survive and grow to form colonies after treatment with cytotoxic agents. To assess clonogenicity, cells were plated onto 6-well plates and incubated with 0.0, 10, 20, and 30 μg of *R. stricta* extract and treated cultures were maintained in culture for an additional 10 days to allow formation of colonies [61, 62]. The results from that assay showed that *R. stricta* extract inhibited the colony formation of HepG2 cells in a dose-dependent manner (0, 10, 20, 30 μg). ImageJ analysis results were consistent with results obtained from the absorption-based method where *R. stricta* extract also inhibited the survival of HepG2 cells in a dose-dependent manner (Fig. 6a and b).

R. stricta extract inhibits the migration ability of HepG2 cells

Many cancer patients die of tumour mobilization which often lead to metastatic foci in distant part/s of the body. Therefore, attempts to prevent or slowdown progression and metastasis of cancer cells are crucial [63]. Earlier study showed that *R. stricta* extract exerts potent anti-cancer ability against human breast cancer [64]. To date, however, limited information is available regarding *R. stricta* extract effect on cell migration in any cancer type. The potential role of *R. stricta* extract on HepG2 cells' migration was assessed using wound healing assay. Cell migration was inhibited in a dose-dependent manner (0, 20 and 30 μg) starting from 24 to 72 h post *R. stricta* extract treatments compared to the control (Fig. 6c).

R. stricta extract inhibits endothelial cell tube formation

Cell migration and invasion are crucial steps in various physiological processes such as morphogenesis, angiogenesis, wound healing and inflammation [65]. Invasion and migration are critical events for tumour progression and tumour recurrence [66, 67]. HUVEC cells had greater numbers of branching tube networks after 18 h of incubation with no *R. stricta* extract (Fig. 7a). This tube branching was attenuated by *R. stricta* extract treatments in a dose-dependent manner (Fig. 7b and c). Colony formation results demonstrate that colony numbers in all dose groups were decreased. These results suggest that *R. stricta* extract reduced cell migration and colony formation capacity in HepG2 cancer cells. *R. stricta* extract may, therefore, be introduced as a novel agent to treat/prevent HCC and as a single agent or in combination with other drugs. It would also be of interest to identify *R. stricta* extract bioactive molecules and assess their effects against cancer, particularly HCC. Further studies are currently underway to identify and characterize *R. stricta* extract bioactive ingredients and to unravel their molecular mechanism against cancer.

The obtained antiproliferative results of the three extracts against HepG2 cancer cell line were found to be consistent with their antioxidant activity, free radical scavenging ability and phenolic content. Out of the three extracts, *R. stricta* showed considerable antiprolifrative activity at low concentration and was the most potent among the tested plants with $IC_{50} = 30$ μg/mL. In addition, *R. stricta* showed the highest total polyphenols (11.5 ± 0.013 mg GAE/g extract). It has also the most percentage inhibitions of DPPH scavenging activity (89.9% ± 0.51) at 1.5 mg/ml and (28.7% ± 1.27) at 0.15 mg/ml. This indicates that the antiproliferative effect of the three extracts, in particular *R. stricta*, may be attributed to their antioxidant polyphenolic and flavonoid contents. Phenolic compounds have been found to counteract cancer either by means of

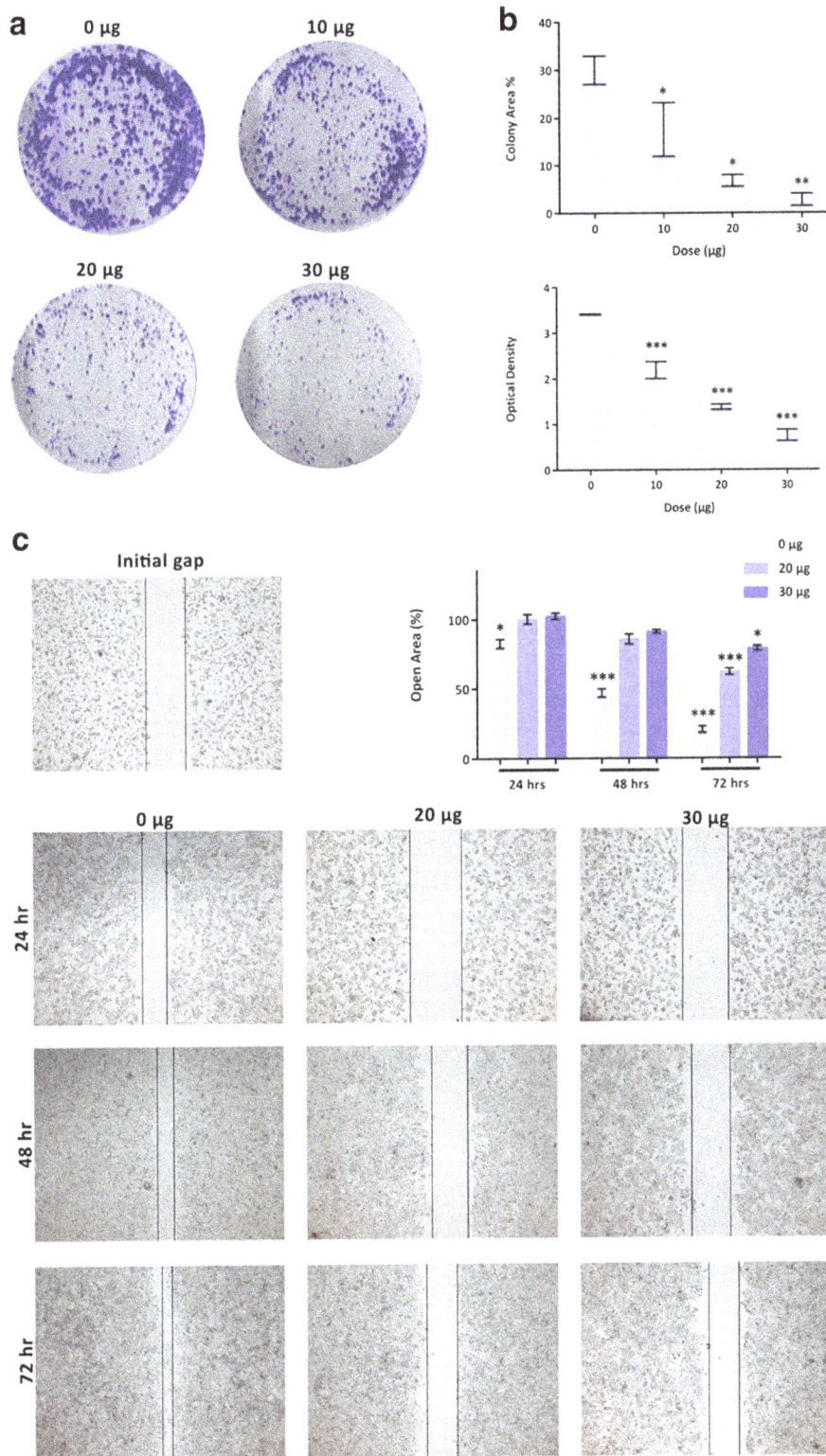

Fig. 6 *Rhazya stricta* extract inhibits colony forming ability and wound healing of HepG2 cells in a dose-dependent manner. **a** Representative images of HepG2 colonies after treatment with increasing concentrations of *R. stricta* extract. **b** Percent of area occupied by colonies in treated and non-treated wells (representative of triplicate samples; *$P < 0.05$, **$P < 0.005$, ***$P < 0.0001$) and absorbance of each treated and non-treated wells (representative of 3 biological triplicates, each in triplicate; *$P < 0.05$, **$P < 0.001$, ***$P < 0.0001$). **c** Representative images and quantification (three regions of three biological triplicates; *$P < 0.05$, **$P < 0.001$, ***$P < 0.0001$) of wound-healing assay results of HepG2 cells treated without or with 20 and 30 µg of *R. stricta* extract

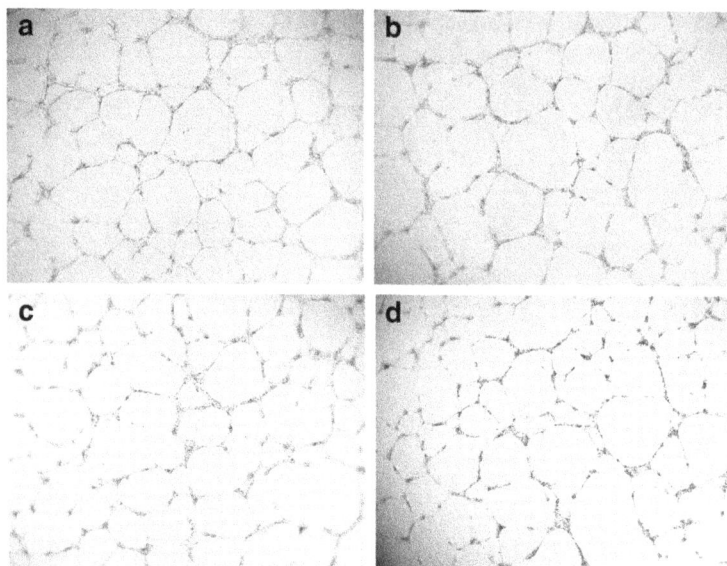

Fig. 7 *Rhazya stricta* extract inhibits tube formation in HUVECs on Matrigel in a dose-dependent manner. Photographs of tube formation in HUVECs on Matrigel after incubation with or without *R. stricta* extract at 18 h. Cells were treated with *R. stricta* extract at a series of concentrations (10 µg; **b**, 20 µg; **c**, 30 µg; **d**) or DMSO vehicle (control; **a**) for 18 h

antioxidant effect or by inhibiting the formation of carcinogenic metabolites that damage the vital biomolecules [68].

Finally, the investigated UAE plants have shown a strong reducing antioxidant capacity and free radical scavenging ability. These findings validate the use of these plants in folk medicine for the treatment of certain diseases. Oxidative cell damage events are frequently correlated with the oxidative stress. We show here that both of those properties are present in the ethanolic extract of *R. stricta*, which has significant antiproliferative activity and a great antioxidant activity. The results reported here are very promising indicators for the potential application of this plant for preventive and therapeutic purposes.

Conclusions

In conclusion, natural antioxidants have many important applications in health promotion, food preservation, food flavouring and cosmetics. They are preferred over synthetic antioxidants because they are safer for consumption and more environmentally friendly. The present study investigates the antioxidant activity and polyphenolic content of three medicinal plants from the UAE. We found extracts rich in antioxidants and in polyphenols, which merit further investigations. Of the extracts evaluated, that of *R. stricta* (Harmal) showed the greatest antioxidant, antiangiogenic and antiproliferative activities, a discovery that makes this species a promising source of anticancer agent development especially for colon and liver cancers, and

hence worthy of further investigation. Isolation of active compounds and exploring their mode of action against tumours by using in vivo experimental models would make an important future study.

Acknowledgments

This work was supported by a start-up grant (Grant 31S 215), Division of Research and Graduate Studies, UAEU and an individual research grant (Grant 31S 188), College of Science, UAEU to the PI: Dr. Bayan Al-Dabbagh and by Zayed Bin Sultan Centre for Health Sciences (ZCHS) grant number 31R050 for Dr. Amr Amin.

Funding

This work was supported by a start-up grant (Grant 31S 215), Division of Research and Graduate Studies, UAEU and an individual research grant (Grant 31S 188), College of Science, UAEU to the PI: Dr. Bayan Al-Dabbagh and by Zayed Bin Sultan Centre for Health Sciences (ZCHS) grant number 31R050 for Dr. Amr Amin.

Authors' contributions

BA and AA designed the research. BA, IAE, AAH, RA and RE performed the experiments. SSA participated in the interpretation of the results. BA and AA analyzed the data and wrote the paper. All authors read and approved the final manuscript.

Competing interests

The authors declare that they have no competing interests.

Author details

[1]Department of Chemistry, College of Science, UAE University, PO Box 15551, Al Ain, UAE. [2]Department of Biology, College of Science, UAE University, PO Box 15551, Al Ain, UAE. [3]Zoology Department, Cairo University, Giza, Egypt. [4]Department of Pharmacy Practice and Pharmacotherapeutics, Sharjah Institute for Medical Research and College of Pharmacy, University of Sharjah, Sharjah, UAE.

References

1. Aruoma OI. Free radicals, antioxidants and international nutrition. Asia Pac J Clin Nutr. 1999;8:53–63.
2. Gupta VK, Sharma SK. Plants as natural antioxidants. Nat Prod Rad. 2006;5:326–34.
3. Magder S. Reactive oxygen species: toxic molecules or spark of life? Crit Care. 2006;10:208.
4. Brewer MS. Natural antioxidants: sources, compounds, mechanisms of action, and potential applications. Compr Rev Food Sci Food Saf. 2011;10:221–47.
5. Lu LY, Ou N, Lu Q-B. Antioxidant induces DNA damage, cell death and mutagenicity in human lung and skin normal cells. Sci Rep. 2013;3:3169.
6. Soobrattee MA, Neergheen VS, Luximon-Ramma A, Aruoma OI, Bahorun T. Phenolics as potential antioxidant therapeutic agents: mechanism and actions. Mutat Res. 2005;579:200–13.
7. Chaudière J, Ferrari-Iliou R. Intracellular antioxidants: from chemical to biochemical mechanisms. Food Chem Toxicol. 1999;37:949–62.
8. Fridovich I. Fundamental aspects of reactive oxygen species, or what's the matter with oxygen? Ann N Y Acad Sci. 1999;893:13–8.
9. Hinneburg I, Damien Dorman HJ, Hiltunen R. Antioxidant activities of extracts from selected culinary herbs and spices. Food Chem. 2006;97:122–9.
10. Amin A, Hamza AA, Bajbouj K, Ashraf SS, Daoud S. Saffron: a potential candidate for a novel anticancer drug against hepatocellular carcinoma. Hepatology. 2011;54:857–67.
11. Hamza AA, Ahmed MM, Elwey HM, Amin A. Melissa officinalis protects against doxorubicin-induced cardiotoxicity in rats and potentiates its anticancer activity on MCF-7 cells. PLoS One. 2016;11:e0167049.
12. Xue WL, Li XS, Zhang J, Liu YH, Wang ZL, Zhang RJ. Effect of Trigonella foenum-graecum (fenugreek) extract on blood glucose, blood lipid and hemorheological properties in streptozotocin-induced diabetic rats. Asia Pac J Clin Nutr. 2007;16(Suppl 1):422–6.
13. Amin A, Alkaabi A, Al-Falasi S, Daoud SA. Chemopreventive activities of Trigonella foenum graecum (fenugreek) against breast cancer. Cell Biol Int. 2005;29:687–94.
14. El Bairi K, Ouzir M, Agnieszka N, Khalki L. Anticancer potential of Trigonella foenum graecum: cellular and molecular targets. Biomed Pharmacother. 2017;90:479–91.
15. Seethapathy GS, Ganesh D, Kumar JUS, Senthilkumar U, Newmaster SG, Ragupathy S, et al. Assessing product adulteration in natural health products for laxative yielding plants, Cassia, Senna, and Chamaecrista, in southern India using DNA barcoding. Int J Legal Med. 2015;129:693–700.
16. Elkady AI. Crude alkaloid extract of Rhazya stricta inhibits cell growth and sensitizes human lung cancer cells to cisplatin through induction of apoptosis. Genet Mol Biol. 2013;36:12–21.
17. Faqi AS. A comprehensive guide to toxicology in preclinical drug development: Academic Press; 2013.
18. Diplock AT, Charuleux JL, Crozier-Willi G, Kok FJ, Rice-Evans C, Roberfroid M, et al. Functional food science and defence against reactive oxidative species. Br J Nutr. 1998;80:S77–S112.
19. Valko M, Leibfritz D, Moncol J, Cronin MT, Mazur M, Telser J. Free radicals and antioxidants in normal physiological functions and human disease. Int J Biochem Cell Biol. 2007;39:44–84.
20. Shigenaga MK, Ames BN. Oxidants and mitogenesis as causes of mutation and cancer: the influence of diet. Basic Life Sci. 1993;61:419–36.
21. Greenwell M, Rahman P. Medicinal plants: their use in anticancer treatment. Int J Pharm Sci Res. 2015;6:4103.
22. Alam AHMK, Hossain ASMS, Khan MA, Kabir SR, Reza MA, Rahman MM, et al. The Antioxidative Fraction of White Mulberry Induces Apoptosis through Regulation of p53 and NFκB in EAC Cells. PLoS ONE. 2016;11:e0167536.
23. Islam S, Nasrin S, Khan MA, Hossain ASMS, Islam F, Khandokhar P, et al. Evaluation of antioxidant and anticancer properties of the seed extracts of Syzygium fruticosum Roxb. growing in Rajshahi, Bangladesh. BMC Complement Altern Med. 2013;13:142.
24. Carmeliet P. Angiogenesis in life, disease and medicine. Nature. 2005;438:932.
25. Bar J, Goss GD. Tumor vasculature as a therapeutic target in non-small cell lung cancer. J Thorac Oncol. 2012;7:609–20.
26. Keizer RJ, Funahashi Y, Semba T, Wanders J, Beijnen J, Schellens J, et al. Evaluation of α 2-integrin expression as a biomarker for tumor growth inhibition for the investigational integrin inhibitor E7820 in preclinical and clinical studies. AAPS J. 2011;13:230–9.
27. Mita M, Kelly KR, Mita A, Ricart AD, Romero O, Tolcher A, et al. Phase I study of E7820, an oral inhibitor of integrin α-2 expression with antiangiogenic properties, in patients with advanced malignancies. Clin Cancer Res. 2011;17:193–200.
28. Senger DR, Perruzzi CA, Streit M, Koteliansky VE, de Fougerolles AR, Detmar M. The α1β1 and α2β1 integrins provide critical support for vascular endothelial growth factor signaling, endothelial cell migration, and tumor angiogenesis. Am J Pathol. 2002;160:195–204.
29. Senger DR, Claffey KP, Benes JE, Perruzzi CA, Sergiou AP, Detmar M. Angiogenesis promoted by vascular endothelial growth factor: regulation through α1β1 and α2β1 integrins. Proc Natl Acad Sci U S A. 1997;94:13612–7.
30. Amzad Hossain M, Shah MD. A study on the total phenols content and antioxidant activity of essential oil and different solvent extracts of endemic plant Merremia borneensis. Arab J Chem. 2015;8:66–71.
31. Singleton VL, Orthofer R, Lamuela-Raventós RM. Analysis of total phenols and other oxidation substrates and antioxidants by means of folin-ciocalteu reagent: Methods Enzymol Academic Press; 1999. p. 152–78.
32. Lim YY, Quah EPL. Antioxidant properties of different cultivars of Portulaca oleracea. Food Chem. 2007;103:734–40.
33. Chang C-C, Yang M-H, Wen H-M, Chern J-C. Estimation of total flavonoid content in propolis by two complementary colorimetric methods. J Food Drug Anal. 2002;10:178–82.
34. Guzmán C, Bagga M, Kaur A, Westermarck J, Abankwa D. ColonyArea: an ImageJ plugin to automatically quantify Colony formation in Clonogenic assays. PLoS One. 2014;9:e92444.
35. Saleh E, El-Awady R, Anis N. Predictive markers for the response to 5-fluorouracil therapy in cancer cells: constant-field gel electrophoresis as a tool for prediction of response to 5-fluorouracil-based chemotherapy. Oncol Lett. 2013;5:321–7.
36. Khan MA, Rahman AA, Islam S, Khandokhar P, Parvin S, Islam MB, et al. A comparative study on the antioxidant activity of methanolic extracts from different parts of Morus alba L. (Moraceae). BMC Res Notes. 2013;6:24.
37. Robbins RJ. Phenolic acids in foods: an overview of analytical methodology. J Agric Food Chem. 2003;51:2866–87.
38. Wojdyło A, Oszmiański J, Czemerys R. Antioxidant activity and phenolic compounds in 32 selected herbs. Food Chem. 2007;105:940–9.
39. Pontis JA, LAMAd C, SJRd S, Flach A. Color, phenolic and flavonoid content, and antioxidant activity of honey from Roraima, Brazil. Food Sci. Technol (Campinas). 2014;34:69–73.
40. Belguith-Hadriche O, Bouaziz M, Jamoussi K, Simmonds MS, El Feki A, Makni-Ayedi F. Comparative study on hypocholesterolemic and antioxidant activities of various extracts of fenugreek seeds. Food Chem. 2013;138:1448–53.
41. Bukhari NA, Al-Otaibi RA, Ibhrahim MM. Phytochemical and taxonomic evaluation of Rhazya stricta in Saudi Arabia. Saudi J Biol Sci. 2017;24:1513–21.
42. Robards K, Prenzler PD, Tucker G, Swatsitang P, Glover W. Phenolic compounds and their role in oxidative processes in fruits. Food Chem. 1999;66:401–36.
43. Kitts DD, Wijewickreme AN, Hu C. Antioxidant properties of a north American ginseng extract. Mol Cell Biochem. 2000;203:1–10.
44. Shan B, Cai YZ, Sun M, Corke H. Antioxidant capacity of 26 spice extracts and characterization of their phenolic constituents. J Agric Food Chem. 2005;53:7749–59.
45. Amin A, Mousa M. Merits of anti-cancer plants from the Arabian gulf region. Cancer Ther. 2007;5:55–66.
46. Popova M, Bankova V, Butovska D, Petkov V, Nikolova-Damyanova B, Sabatini AG, et al. Validated methods for the quantification of biologically active constituents of poplar-type propolis. Phytochem Anal. 2004;15:235–40.
47. Amin A, Hamza AA, Daoud S, Khazanehdari K, Hrout AA, Baig B, et al. Saffron-based Crocin prevents early lesions of liver Cancer: in vivo, in vitro and network analyses. Recent Pat Anticancer Drug Discov. 2016;11:121–33.
48. Wu C-T, Tsai Y-T, Lai J-N. Demographic and medication characteristics of traditional Chinese medicine users among colorectal cancer survivors: a nationwide database study in Taiwan. J Tradit Complement Med. 2016;7:188–94.
49. Pereira RM, Ferreira-Silva GA, Pivatto M, Santos Lde A, Bolzani Vda S, Chagas de Paula DA, et al. Alkaloids derived from flowers of Senna spectabilis, (−)-cassine and (−)-spectaline, have antiproliferative activity on HepG2 cells for inducing cell cycle arrest in G1/S transition through ERK inactivation and downregulation of cyclin D1 expression. Toxicol In Vitro. 2016;31:86–92.
50. Newman DJ, Cragg GM. Natural products as sources of new drugs from 1981 to 2014. J Nat Prod. 2016;79:629 61.
51. Block KI, Gyllenhaal C, Lowe L, Amedei A, Amin ARMR, Amin A, et al. Designing a broad-spectrum integrative approach for cancer prevention and treatment. Semin Cancer Biol. 2015;35(Supplement):S276–304.

52. Devasena T, Venugopal MP. Fenugreek seeds modulate 1,2-dimethylhydrazine-induced hepatic oxidative stress during colon carcinogenesis. Ital J Biochem. 2007;56:28–34.

53. Li F, Fernandez PP, Rajendran P, Hui KM, Sethi G. Diosgenin: a steroidal saponin, inhibits STAT3 signaling pathway leading to suppression of proliferation and chemosensitization of human hepatocellular carcinoma cells. Cancer Lett. 2010;292:197–207.

54. Chandra P, Pandey R, Kumar B, Srivastva M, Pandey P, Sarkar J, et al. Quantification of multianalyte by UPLC–QqQLIT–MS/MS and in-vitro anti-proliferative screening in Cassia species. Ind Crop Prod. 2015;76:1133–41.

55. Nehdi IA, Sbihi HM, Tan CP, Al-Resayes SI. Seed oil from Harmal (Rhazya stricta Decne) grown in Riyadh (Saudi Arabia): a potential source of δ-tocopherol. J Saudi Chem Soc. 2016;20:107–13.

56. El Gendy MAM, Ali BH, Michail K, Siraki AG, El-Kadi AOS. Induction of quinone oxidoreductase 1 enzyme by Rhazya stricta through Nrf2-dependent mechanism. J Ethnopharmacol. 2012;144:416–24.

57. Brown NR, Noble ME, Endicott JA, Johnson LN. The structural basis for specificity of substrate and recruitment peptides for cyclin-dependent kinases. Nat Cell Biol. 1999;1:438–43.

58. McGowan CH, Russell P. Human Wee1 kinase inhibits cell division by phosphorylating p34cdc2 exclusively on Tyr15. EMBO J. 1993;12:75.

59. Wells NJ, Watanabe N, Tokusumi T, Jiang W, Verdecia MA, Hunter T. The C-terminal domain of the Cdc2 inhibitory kinase Myt1 interacts with Cdc2 complexes and is required for inhibition of G (2)/M progression. J Cell Sci. 1999;112:3361–71.

60. Enserink JM, Kolodner RD. An overview of Cdk1-controlled targets and processes. Cell Div. 2010;5:11–52.

61. Gach K, Grądzka I, Wasyk I, Męczyńska-Wielgosz S, Iwaneńko T, Szymański J, et al. Anticancer activity and radiosensitization effect of methyleneisoxazolidin-5-ones in hepatocellular carcinoma HepG2 cells. Chem Biol Interact. 2016;248:68–73.

62. Rafehi H, Orlowski C, Georgiadis GT, Ververis K, El-Osta A, Karagiannis TC. Clonogenic assay: adherent cells. J Vis Exp. 2011;49:2573.

63. Jiang WG, Sanders AJ, Katoh M, Ungefroren H, Gieseler F, Prince M, et al. Molecular, biological and clinical perspectives. Semin Cancer Biol. 2015;35(Supplement):S244–75.

64. Baeshen NA, Elkady AI, Abuzinadah OA, Mutwakil MH. Potential anticancer activity of the medicinal herb, Rhazya stricta, against human breast cancer. Afr J Biotechnol. 2012;11:8960–72.

65. Bozzuto G, Ruggieri P, Molinari A. Molecular aspects of tumor cell migration and invasion. Ann Ist Super Sanita. 2010;46:66–80.

66. Alur I, Dodurga Y, Secme M, Elmas L, Bagci G, Goksin I, et al. Anti-tumor effects of bemiparin in HepG2 and MIA PaCa-2 cells. Gene. 2016;585:241–6.

67. Lavictoire SJ, Parolin DA, Klimowicz AC, Kelly JF, Lorimer IA. Interaction of Hsp90 with the nascent form of the mutant epidermal growth factor receptor EGFRvIII. J Biol Chem. 2003;278:5292–9.

68. Hocman G. Chemoprevention of cancer: phenolic antioxidants (BHT, BHA). Int J BioChemiPhysics. 1988;20:639–51.

Dendritic cells pulsed with generated tumor cell lysate from *Phyllanthus amarus* Schum. & Thonn. induces anti-tumor immune response

Shimaa Ibrahim Abdelmenym Mohamed[1], Ibrahim Jantan[1,5]* (iD), Mohd Azlan Nafiah[2], Mohamed Ali Seyed[3] and Kok Meng Chan[4]

Abstract

Background: Dendritic cells (DCs) are unique antigen presenting cells (APC) which play a pivotal role in immunotherapy and induction of an effective immune response against tumors. In the present study, 80% ethanol extract of *Phyllanthus amarus* was used to generate tumor lysate (TLY) derived from HCT 116 and MCF-7 cancer cell lines via induction of apoptosis. Monocyte-derived DCs were generated ex vivo from the adherent population of peripheral blood mononuclear cells (PBMCs). The generated TLY were used to impulse DCs to investigate its effect on their cellular immune functions including antigen presentation capacity, phagocytic activity, chemotaxis capacity, T-cell proliferation and cytokines release.

Methods: The effect of *P. amarus*-generated TLY on DCs maturation was evaluated by determination of MHC class I, II and CD 11c expression as well as the co-stimulatory molecules CD 83 and 86 by using flow cytometry. The phagocytic capacity of TLY-pulsed DCs was investigated through FITC-dextran uptake by using flow cytometry. The effect on the cytokines release including IL-12, IL-6 and IL-10 was elucidated by using ELISA. The migration capacity and T cell proliferation activity of pulsed DCs were measured. The relative gene expression levels of cytokines were determined by using qRT-PCR. The major constituents of *P. amarus* extract were qualitatively and quantitatively analyzed by using validated reversed-phase high performance liquid chromatography (HPLC) methods.

Results: *P. amarus*-generated TLY significantly up-regulated the expression levels of MHC class I, CD 11 c, CD 83 and 86 in pulsed DCs. The release of interleukin IL-12 and IL-6 was enhanced by TLY-DCs at a ratio of 1 DC: 3 tumor apoptotic bodies (APO), however, the release of IL-10 was suppressed. The migration ability as well as allogeneic T-cell proliferation activities of loaded DCs were significantly enhanced, but their phagocytic capacity was highly attenuated. The gene expression profiles for IL-12 and IL-6 of DCs showed increase in their mRNA gene expression in TLY pulsed DCs versus unloaded and LPS-treated only DCs.

Conclusion: The effect of *P. amarus*-generated TLY on the immune effector mechanisms of DCs verified its potential to induce an in vitro anti-tumor immune response against the recognized tumor antigen.

Keywords: *Phyllanthus amarus*, Dendritic cells, Immunotherapy, Tumor lysate, Anti-tumor, Immune response

* Correspondence: profibj@gmail.com
[1]Drug and Herbal Research Centre, Faculty of Pharmacy, Universiti Kebangsaan Malaysia, Jalan Raja Muda Abdul Aziz, 50300 Kuala Lumpur, Malaysia
[5]School of Pharmacy, Taylor's University, Lakeside Campus, 47500 Subang Jaya, Selangor, Malaysia
Full list of author information is available at the end of the article

Background

There are several treatment modalities of cancer including surgery, radiation therapy, chemotherapy, hormonal therapy, and immunotherapy. Treatment modalities can be used alone or in combination based on the stage of the disease and also the general health condition of the patient. Most of cancer treatment modalities were proved to be ineligible in spite of their moderate progression. This was assumed due to the inadequate immune response against the progressive tumors mainly in the development of effector T cell responses. Cancer immunotherapy represents a novel approach that destroys the existing tumor cells as well as develops a long-lasting immunity which will prevent tumor relapse [1]. It aims to induce the immune system to target the tumor antigens and proteins that are specifically expressed by the tumor cells. Tumor associated antigens (TAA) are normal proteins but overexpressed on the tumor cells. Dendritic cells (DCs) are the most potent antigens presenting cells (APC) and act as a link between innate and adaptive immune systems [2]. Immature DCs possess the capacity to capture and uptake antigens which results in the maturation of dendritic cells and then followed by their migration to the lymphoid organs [3]. Mature DCs process and present the TAA to naïve T cells through major histocompatibility complex (MHC) class I and II that leads to activation and clonal expansion of T lymphocytes mainly into CD 4$^+$ helper T cell and CD8$^+$ cytotoxic T cells. Furthermore, mature DCs are characterized by the high expression level of MHC as well as co-stimulatory molecules such as CD 80, CD 83 and CD 86 that stabilize the interaction between DCs and naïve T lymphocytes for induction of antitumor immune response [4]. This is in addition to the release of pro-inflammatory cytokines such as interferon (IFN)-γ and interleukin (IL)-12 that activate Th1 response, which catalyzes the activation of cytotoxic T lymphocyte (CTL) [5]. Activated CTL can effectively migrate and infiltrate the tumor microenvironment to directly attack the tumor cells by induction of apoptosis as well as via release of perforin and granzymes [6]. Additionally, DCs possess the ability to induce NK cells and B cells. This dual role in both the innate and adaptive immune systems derived into the possibility of using DCs in immunotherapy in combination with alternative treatment modalities. The using of tumor lysate pulsed-DCs represents a new approach to boost the patient immunity and induces an effective cytotoxic immune response against the tumor cells, which can easily escape the immune surveillance [7]. The apoptotic cells were proved to be an efficient source of antigens that can be recognized by the immune system [8]. Moreover, the protein fragments derived from phagocytosed cells are well presented more than the processed by MHC II products of DCs [9].

In addition to the induction of antitumor immune response, the cancer immunotherapy functions through the alteration of tumor microenvironment by the release of pro-inflammatory cytokines such as IL-12, IL-6, and TNF-α. IL-12 is produced mainly by DCs and stimulates the cytotoxic activity of natural killer cells (NKs) as well as the clonal expansion of naïve T lymphocytes into CD4$^+$ helper and CD8$^+$ cytotoxic T cells (CTL) [10, 11]. Furthermore, the release of tumor necrosis factor (TNF)-α, IL-1α/β and IL-6, can induce an immune response against the tumor and increase the production of reactive oxygen species (ROS) and reactive nitrogen species (RNS) by the immune cells infiltrating the tumor microenvironment that have a destructive effect on the tumor cells [12, 13]. Several clinical studies have been conducted to evaluate the effectiveness of DCs based vaccines to induce tumor-antigen specific immune response against various types of cancer including prostate cancer [14], ovarian cancer [15], renal cell cancer [16], metastatic melanoma cell cancer [17], pancreatic cancer [18] and glioblastoma [19]. Moreover, there is a tendency in the recent trials to use tumor antigen obtained from patient's tumor sample.

Phyllanthus amarus has been widely used as a traditional and alternative medication in the treatment of various diseases including diarrhea, jaundice, kidney disorders, influenza, diabetes, liver ailment, fever, scabies, ulcers and wound [20–23]. The hairy root methanol extract of *P. amarus* was found to exhibit anti-proliferative effect on MCF-7 human breast cancer cells via induction of apoptosis by increasing ROS level as well as the reduction in mitochondrial membrane potential [24]. *P. amarus* induced strong cytotoxic and apoptotic activities on MCF-7 and human lung cancer A549 cells alongside with anti-metastasis effect [25]. Therefore, in the previous studies, the anticancer effect of *P. amarus* has been reported through anti-proliferative, apoptotic, anti-metastatic and anti-angiogenesis activities. However, there are no reports available on the effect of pulsing of DCs against tumor antigen generated by *Phyllanthus* spp. Thus, the rationale behind our proposed study was that using of *P. amarus* to elicit apoptosis in the tumor cells and create a collection of TAAs in the form of dead and dying cellular debris that could activate APC mainly DCs. Additionally, the cellular immune functions (i.e. antigen presentation capacity, phagocytic activity, chemotaxis, T-cell proliferation and cytokines release) were investigated by using *P. amarus*-generated tumor lysate on DCs grown ex vivo. This finding can contribute to the development of a novel DCs based vaccine strategy by using natural immunomodulators for colon and breast cancer.

Methods

All experiments by using human whole blood were carried out under a protocol approved by the Human

Ethical Committee of Universiti Kebangsaan Malaysia (Approval no: UKM PPI/111/8/JEP-2017-335).

Collection of plant material

The whole plant of *P. amarus* was obtained from Marang, Kuala Terengganu, Malaysia in the month of June 2012. The plant was authenticated by Dr. Abdul Latif Mohamad of the Faculty of Science and Technology, Universiti Kebangsaan Malaysia (UKM), and a voucher specimen (UKMB 30078) was deposited at the Herbarium of UKM, Bangi, Malaysia. The collection of plant samples did not involve endangered or protected species, and the study was carried out at the Drug and Herbal Research Centre, Faculty of Pharmacy, UKM. The whole plant of *P. amarus* (1 kg) was ground and extracted with 80% EtOH (3 × 3 L) at room temperature for 72 h, then filtered through Whatman® Grade1 filter paper (Sigma-Aldrich Corp). The filtrate was collected, and excess solvent was evaporated under reduced pressure using a rotary evaporator at temperature between 55 and 60 °C. The yield of extract obtained was 108 g (10.8% *w/w*). The extract was examined for the endotoxin contamination by using E-Toxate assay kit (Sigma-Aldrich Co. LLC) according to manufacturer's protocol.

High performance liquid chromatography analysis of 80% ethanol extract of *Phyllanthus amarus*

High performance liquid chromatography (HPLC) analysis and validation were performed based on the chromatographic conditions described by Jantan et al. [26]. Briefly, the HPLC analysis was performed using the following conditions: reverse-phase C-18 column (250 mm × 4.6 mm ID, 5 m, XBridge™; Waters Corporation, Milford, MA, USA), and photodiode array (PDA) detector (Waters 2998) of wavelength ranging from 205 to 270 nm. Identification and quantification of components of the extracts and standard compounds including gallic acid, ellagic acid, corilagin, geraniin, niranthin, phyltetralin, isolintetralin, phyllanthin, and hypophyllanthin were performed using two different chromatographic conditions; method 1 and method 2, as described in our previous study [26]. HPLC analyses of the extracts and standard solutions of compounds (gallic acid, ellagic acid, corilagin, geraniin, niranthin, phyltetralin and isolintetralin) were performed using method 1. The identification of each compound was carried out by comparing the retention times and ultraviolet-visible (UV-Vis) spectra of the peaks with those of the standard compounds. Identification and quantification of the phyllanthin and hypophyllanthin were carried out based on the chromatographic conditions described in method 2. The validation of HPLC for the standardization of the extract was carried out by determination of linearity, precision, and limits of quantification (LOQ) and detection (LOD).

Cell lines and culture

Cancerous cells MCF-7 human breast cancer and HCT 116 human colon cancer cell lines were obtained from American Type Culture Collection (USA). The cells were cultured and maintained in Dulbecco's modified Eagle's medium (DMEM) (Gibco Co. USA) supplemented by 10% fetal bovine serum (FBS) (Sigma, St. Louis, MO, USA) and 1% antibiotic (streptomycin 200 µg/mL and penicillin 100 units/mL) (Gibco Co. USA). Cells were incubated at 37 °C in 5% CO_2 environment and then detached and harvested at confluence 80–90% by trypsinization with trypsin-EDTA (Sigma, St. Louis, MO, USA).

Preparation of *Phyllanthus amarus* generated tumor lysate

Apoptotic bodies were prepared and purified. Briefly, the cells (passage # 5) were treated with 80% ethanol extract of *P. amarus* at a concentration of 1000 µg/mL. Floating dead cells were collected everyday by centrifugation at 125 xg for 10 min and stored at 4 °C until they were subjected for 5 cycles of freeze-thaw. Purified apoptotic bodies were stained with FITC- Annexine V apoptosis detection kit (BD Pharmingen, BD Bioscience, USA) for determination of apoptosis by FACScan analysis. The apoptotic cells were suspended in 2 mL of HBSS and lysed by 5 freezes (liquid nitrogen)–thaw (at room temperature) cycles. Total cell disruption was microscopically validated using trypan blue staining. After sonication for 10 min, lysate was centrifuged at 15000 xg for 15 min at 4 °C and stored in aliquots at – 80 °C until use.

Generation of monocyte-derived dendritic cells ex vivo

All experiments by using human blood were carried out under a protocol approved by the Universiti Kebangsaan Malaysia Research Ethics Committee (No. UKM PPI/ 111/8/JEP-2017-335). DCs were generated from freshly isolated peripheral blood monocytes (PBMCs). In brief, PBMCs were isolated from peripheral blood of healthy donors by Lymphoprep® separation medium (Axis- Shield Pc-AS, Oslo, Norway). Cells were allowed to adhere by incubation for 1 h at 5% CO_2 and 37 °C in an appropriate amount of PromoCell monocyte attachment medium (Promo-Cell GmbH, Heidelberg, Germany) at a density of 2–3 million/cm². The adherent cells were washed three times with warm monocyte attachment medium by swirling the vessel and aspirating the supernatant. The cells were cultured in an appropriate amount of PromoCell DCs generation medium DXF supplemented with GM-CSF (1000 units/mL) and IL-4 (1000 units/mL) (Promo-Cell GmbH, Heidelberg, Germany) then incubated at 37 °C and 5% CO_2. The generation of immature dendritic cells was characterized by CD14⁻, HLA-DR bright, CD83⁺, and CD 86⁺ phenotypical expression using flow cytometry analyses. On day 6, the cells were seeded in 6-well plates at a density of 1 × 10⁶ cells/mL and co-cultured with lysate generated from *P. amarus*-treated tumor cells at different ratios (1:1, 1:3, 1:5 and 1:7) DC: APO for 4 h. DCs were subsequently activated with LPS from *Escherichia coli* strain (Sigma, St. Louis, MO, USA) at 1 μg/mL for 48 h which results in the generation of mature tumor lysate pulsed dendritic cells (TLY-DCs). However, LPS-only stimulated DCs were generated by activation of immature DCs with LPS only at a concentration of 1 μg/mL for 48 h. The cell viability was evaluated by using by trypan blue exclusion method.

Determination of the phagocytosis of *Phyllanthus amarus*-treated damaged tumor cells by immature dendritic cells

For induction of an effective immune response, DCs need first to uptake tumor-derived material before processing and presenting the antigen to T lymphocytes. Therefore, we investigated whether monocytes-derived-DCs (mo-DCs) were able to endocytose *P.amarus*-treated damaged tumor cells remnants and fragments. To validate this, both HCT 116 (colon cancer) and MCF-7 (breast cancer) cells were stained with a fluorescent dye CFSE [5, 6-carboxyfluorescein diacetate succinimidyl ester] (BD Pharmingen, BD Bioscience, USA) that gives a strong and stable green fluorescence. CFSE-labeled tumor cells were seeded in 6 well plates and incubated with 80% ethanol extract of *Phyllanthus amarus* at a concentration of 1000 μg/mL. The tumor cells fragments were prepared by 5 freeze and thaw cycles. The CFSE-labeled tumor cells remnants were co-cultured with DCs at ratio 1: 3 (DCs: APO) in culture media and incubated for 24 h at 37 °C and 5% CO_2. The non-ingested debris was removed and the uptake of fluorescent labelled tumor cells remnants by DCs (stained with APC-H7 conjugated antihuman monoclonal antibody against HLA-DR) was determined by flow cytometer analysis.

Endocytic activity of tumor lysate pulsed dendritic cells

Endocytic activity of DCs was assessed by the uptake of fluorescein iso-thiocyanate FITC-dextran (Sigma, St. Louis, MO, USA). Immature, mature and LPS-only stimulated dendritic cells were cultured in the complete culture medium containing FITC-dextran at a concentration of 0.5 mg/mL and incubated for 30 min at 5% CO_2 and 37 °C (negative control was incubated on ice). After the incubation time, cells were extensively washed for 3 times using phosphate buffered saline (PBS) (Sigma, St. Louis, MO, USA) and the uptake of FITC-dextran was analyzed by flow cytometry analysis.

Phenotypic characterization

In order to determine the maturation and antigen presentation capacity of mo-DCs after engulfment of *P. amarus*- generated tumor lysate, 1×10^6 /mL cells were stained with anti-human monoclonal antibodies PE-Cy7-conjugated anti-CD11c, Per-CP conjugated anti-HLA-I, APC-conjugated anti-CD 86 and APC-H7- conjugated anti-HLA-DR and anti-CD 14 for 15 min at room temperature in PBS containing 2% FBS. After the incubation time, the cells were washed with 1 mL cold PBS and analyzed by flow cytometer BD FACS Canto II. All anti-human monoclonal antibodies against HLA-DR, HLA-I, CD 86, CD 83, CD 11c and CD 14 were acquired from BD Pharmingen (BD Bioscience, USA).

Cytokine release

For the measurements of IL-12 P40, IL-6, and IL-10, mo-DCs were pulsed first with PA generated tumor lysate. DCs were treated with tumor lysate at ratios 1:1 and 1:3 of DCs: APO for 4 h and then stimulated with LPS (1 μg /mL) for 48 h at 37 °C in 5% CO_2. The cytokines in the supernatants were determined using enzyme-linked immunosorbent (ELISA) kits (R&D System, Minneapolis, MN, USA) according to the manufacturer's instructions. The concentrations were calculated from the standard curves.

Migration assay

Chemotaxis activity of tumor lysate pulsed DCs (1:1 and 1:3) was assessed by using a commercially available 96-well cell migration assay kit (Cytoselect 96-Well Cell Migration Assay, Cell Biolabs, INC.) of 5 μm pore size. The cell suspension comprising of 1×10^6 cells/mL was prepared in serum-free media. One hundred and fifty μL of media containing CCL 21 (at a concentration of 250 ng/mL) was added to the membrane chamber. CCL21 (R&D System, Minneapolis, MN, USA) is a lymph node (LN) secreted chemokine and acts as chemoattractant agent for DCs. After covering the plate, it was placed in 37 °C incubator for 3 h. Prior to the end of the incubation time, 150 μL of cell detachment solution was transferred into the wells of a clean 96-well cell harvesting tray. The 96-well cell migration plate was then carefully removed from the incubator, followed by the separation of the membrane chamber from the feeder tray. The media from the top of the membrane chamber were removed by aspiration. The membrane chamber was then placed into the cell harvesting tray containing 150 μL of cell detachment solution, followed by incubation for 30 min at 37 °C. The cells from the underside of the membrane were dislodged by tilting the membrane chamber in the cell detachment solution. Fifty μL of 4X Lysis buffer/CyQuant GR dye solution was added to each well, followed by incubation at room temperature for 20 min. At the end, 150 μL of the mixture was transferred to the 96-well plate for measurement of fluorescence in the fluorescence plate reader at 480 nm/ 520 nm.

T cell proliferation assay

Allogeneic T cells enriched fractions were obtained as 1 h non-adherent cells of PBMCs prepared from the buffy coats. The capacity of mature DCs to induce the proliferation of allogeneic T-cells was assessed. DCs (2 × 10^5 cells/mL) were harvested and co-cultured with allogeneic non-adherent mononuclear in 96 well round bottom plates at different ratios 1:20, 1:40, 1:80 and 1:160 (DCs: T cells) in triplicates. Phytohaemagglutinin (PHA) (20 μg/mL) (Sigma, St. Louis, MO, USA) was used as positive control. After incubation at 37 °C and 5% CO_2 for 4 days, the cells were pulsed with 1 μCi/well of $[H]^3$ Thymidine and incubated for further 18 h at 37 °C and 5% CO_2. After incubation, the cells were harvested by using glass fiber filters. The harvested cells were dissolved in 2.5 mL of liquid scintillation cocktail and the thymidine incorporation was determined by using liquid scintillation counter.

Quantitative PCR

The effect *P. amarus* generated tumor lysate on the gene expression of IL-12, IL-6, IL-10 in dendritic cells was examined by real-time polymerase chain reaction (RT-PCR). Monocyte-derived dendritic cells were seeded in 24-well plates at a density of 1×10^6 cells/mL. Dendritic cells were pretreated with *P. amarus* generated tumor lysate at ratio 1DCs: 3 tumor cells for 4 h before stimulation with LPS at 1 mg/mL for 48 h. The total RNA from iDCs, TLY-DCs and LPS treated DCs was isolated and purified using RNeasy Micro Kit according to the manufacturer's protocol. The quantity and integrity of the extracted RNA were analyzed using Nano-Drop spectrophotometer (Thermo Scientific, Switzerland). Total RNA was reverse transcribed to cDNA by using Quantinova ™ Reverse Transcription kit according to the manufacture's protocol (Qiagen, UK). The cDNA was amplified by using the following primers IL-12 P40 (For- CGGTCATCTGCCGCAAA Rev-TGCCCATTC GCTCCAAGA), IL-10 (For-GGTGATGCCCCAAGCTGA Rev-TCCCCCAGGGAGTTCACA), IL-6 (For-AGCCACT CACCTCTTCAGAACGAA Rev-CAGTGCCTCTTTGC TGCTTTCACA), and GAPDH (For-AGCCTCAAGAT CATCAGCAATG Rev-CACGATACCAAAGTTGTCATG GA). Quantitative PCR was performed on cDNA by using SYPER GREEN MASTER MIX (Quanti-Nova ™ SYPER Green PCR Kit, Qiagen, UK) on Bio-Rad CFX- Real-Time PCR System Thermal Cyclers. A total of 40 cycles was performed. The relative fold change between samples was determined by using the comparative cycle threshold method ($2^{-\Delta\Delta Ct}$). The gene expression was normalized against the housekeeping gene GAPDH mRNA expression.

Statistical analysis

All the experiments were performed on three independent healthy donors and data presented as the mean ± standard error of mean (SEM). All the data were statistically analyzed using Graph Pad Prism 5 software (Graphpad Software, Inc., La Jolla, CA, USA) by one-way analysis of variance (ANOVA) to determine the mean difference between groups, followed by Dunnett's test $P \leq 0.05$ was considered statistically significant.

Results

HPLC qualitative and quantitative analyses of 80% ethanol extract of *Phyllanthus amarus*

The chromatograms of reversed-phase HPLC of the 80% ethanol extract of *P. amarus* showed nine major compounds (gallic acid, ellagic acid, geraniin, corilagin, niranthin, phyltetralin, isolintetralin, phyllanthin, and hypophyllanthin) (Fig. 1a and b). Quantitative determination of the major compounds by HPLC indicated that ellagic acid was the most abundant at concentration of 218.833 μg/mL followed by phyllanthin (170.69 μg/mL), and corilagin (138.689 μg/mL) (Table 1). The calibration curves were plotted for the standard solutions of different compounds showed correlation coefficients (r^2) of ≥0.996. The reproducibility of the results was confirmed by the relative standard deviations (% RSDs) of the mean area under the peak and mean retention time by inter day and intra-assay precision assays.

Generation and pulsing of immature DCs with tumor lysate

The induction of apoptosis after treatment with *P. amarus* in HCT 116 and MCF-7 at 1000 μg/mL for 24 h was determined by Annexin V-FITC/PI dual staining assay (Fig. 2a). Generation of monocyte-derived dendritic cells was highly reproducible. The generated dendritic cells were characterized microscopically as a cluster of cells with veil like-processes. Additionally, the immature dendritic cells expressed CD 14 ⁻, HLA-DR⁺ (57.7%), CD 86 ⁺ (54%), and CD 83 ⁺ (17.5%) that were determined by flow cytometry analyses (Fig. 2b). At day 6, immature dendritic cells were co-cultured with tumor lysate that was generated by five freeze and thaw cycles from *P. amarus*-treated HCT 116 human colon cells and MCF-7 adenocarcinoma breast cancer cells. The cell viability of tumor lysate dendritic cells was determined by trypan blue exclusion method and the cells were counted by hemocytometer. The treatment of DCs with tumor apoptotic bodies (APO) at ratios 1:1 and 1:3 (DCs: APO) was found to be non-toxic (cell viability ≥90%), however, at ratio 1:5 or more influenced the cell viability (Fig. 2c).

Phagocytic capacity of the generated DCs to uptake the tumor lysate

The phagocytic capacity of the generated DCs towards HCT 116 human colon and MCF-7 human breast cancer cell debris was studied. The uptake of the carboxyfluorescein succinimidyl ester (CFSE)-labelled tumor cell

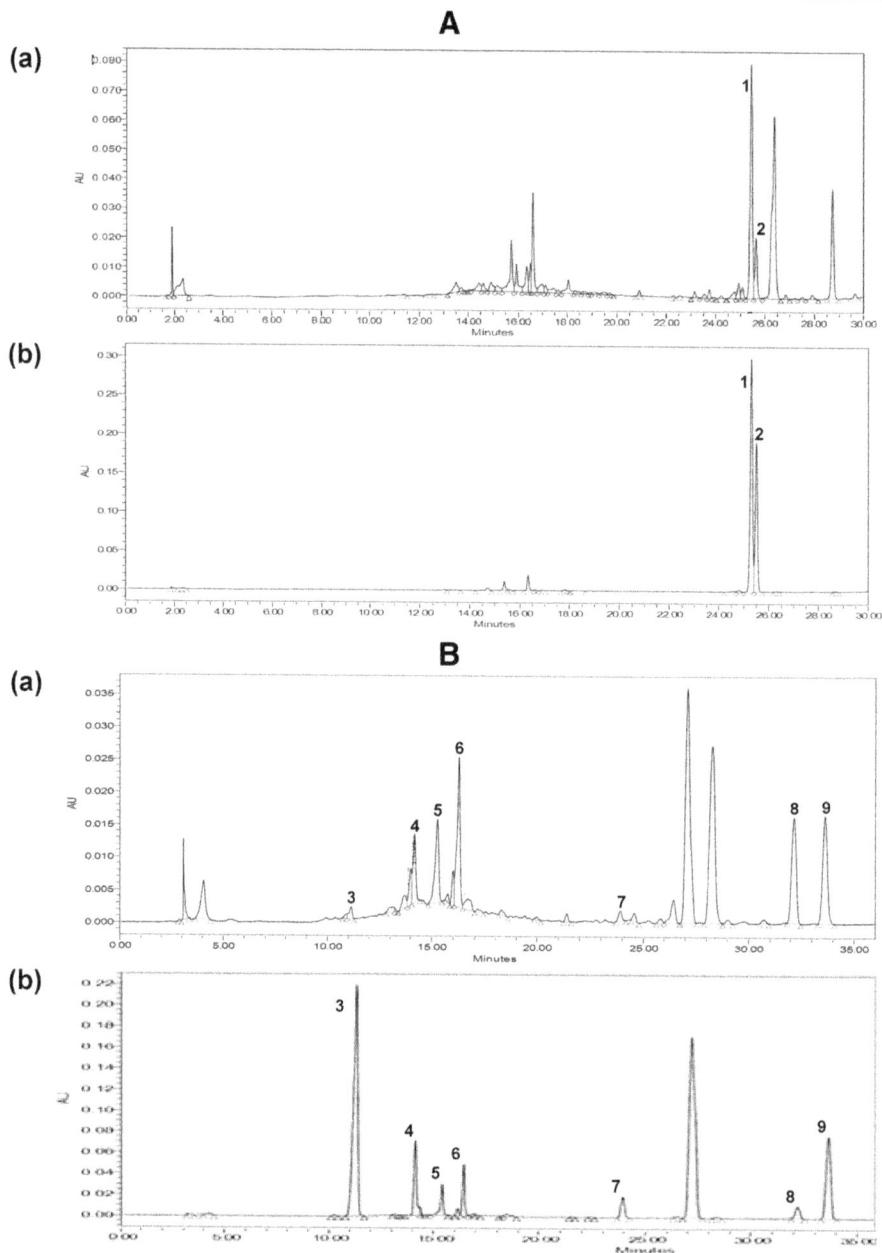

Fig. 1 HPLC analyses of 80% ethanol extract of *Phyllanthus amarus*. **a** Representative HPLC chromatograms of (a) 80% ethanol extract of *Phyllanthus amarus* (b) mixture of standards for identification and quantification of (1) phyllanthin (RT 25.354 min) and (2) hypophyllanthin (RT 25.547 min). **b** Representative HPLC chromatograms of (a) 80% ethanol extract of *Phyllanthus amarus* (b) mixture of standards for identification and quantification of (3) gallic acid at (RT 11.155 min), (4) geraniin at (RT 14.204 min), (5) corilagin at (RT 15.273 min), (6) ellagic acid at (RT 16.283 min), (7) niranthin at (RT 23.933), (8) phyltetralin at (RT 32.157), and (9) isolintetralin at (RT 33.628)

remnants was monitored by flow cytometry as a proportion of HLA-DR $^+$ DCs acquired green fluorescence. The data showed that DCs have a high capacity to endocytose the CFSE-labeled tumor debris with 88 and 85.3% for HCT 116 and MCF-7, respectively (Fig. 3a). The percentage of phagocytosis represented the proportion of viable DCs (HLA-DR $^+$) which obtained the green fluorescence (CFSE$^+$) (Fig. 3b).

Decrease in the endocytic capacity of tumor lysate pulsed DCs

Generally, DCs express mannose receptor on their surface that allows the dextran phagocytosis. This active uptake can reflect the antigen endocytic capacity of DCs. The data demonstrated that unloaded immature DCs exhibited the highest capacity to incorporate FITC-dextran up to 98.1 ± 1.6%. However, in mature

Table 1 Quantification of the major compounds found in *Phyllanthus amarus* (μg/mL) by using HPLC quantification assay

No.	Compound	Concentration (μg/mL)	Retention time (min)
Method 2			
1	Phyllanthin	170.69	25.354
2	Hypophyllanthin	76.863	25.547
Method 1			
3	Gallic acid	53.732	11.155
4	Geraniin	96.569	14.204
5	Corilagin	138.68	15.273
6	Ellagic acid	218.833	16.283
7	Niranthin	46.428	23.826
8	Phyltetralin	122.46	32.157
9	Isolintetralin	119.018	33.628

tumor lysate-pulsed DCs, the cells lost their endocytic capacity to incorporate dextran followed the maturation and uptake of tumor lysates (1.1 ± 0.65 for HCT 116 TLY-DCs and $0.7 \pm 0.15\%$ for MCF-7 TLY-DCs) as shown in Fig. 3c and d. LPS-stimulated dendritic cells showed moderate dextran uptake ($52 \pm 3.52\%$). The endocytic capacity of DCs was negatively correlated with the cell activation and uptake of CFSE-labeled tumor lysate.

Upregulation in the DCs surface marker expression

In the phenotypic characterization of tumor lysate pulsed DCs (TLY-DCs), the data showed that the surface expression of MHC molecules, HLA-DR and HLA-I, were markedly increased in comparison with the immature unloaded DCs and LPS-stimulated DCs at ratio 1:3 (DC: APO). Whereas, the mean HLA-DR surface expression rate upregulated from 64.07 ± 4.02 up to 93.8 ± 3.7 and $94.7 \pm 2.55\%$ in HCT 116-TLY–DCs and MCF-7-TLY-DCs, respectively (Fig. 4a). The results revealed that the immature DCs expressed low levels of

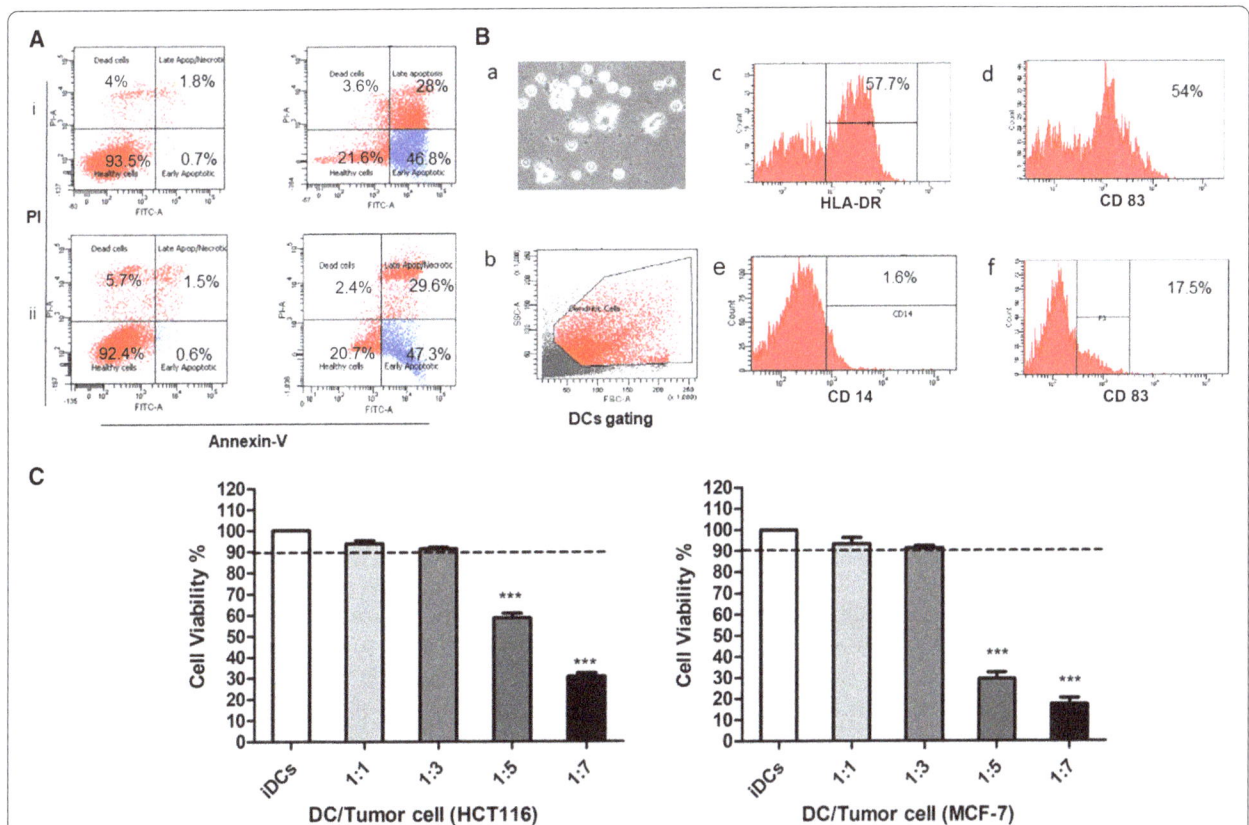

Fig. 2 Generation of tumor lysate and monocyte-derived dendritic cells. **a** Flow cytometric analysis of the apoptotic effect of 80% ethanol extract of *Phyllanthus amarus* on (i) HCT-116 and (ii) MCF-7. **b** Characterization of the generated immature monocyte-derived DCs ex vivo at day 6 (a) microscopically, (b) representative gating strategy, and (c-f) flow cytometric analysis of HLA-DR⁺, CD 83⁺, CD 14⁻ and CD 86⁺ expression by iDCs. **c** The cell viability assay of DCs treated with PA generated tumor lysate (HCT 116 and MCF-7 TLY) by trypan blue exclusion method after 48 h. The data are representative of three experiments comprising three different healthy donors and analyzed by one-way ANOVA followed by Dunnett's test. ***$P < 0.001$. Mean ± SEM. are shown. DCs, Dendritic cells; PA, *Phyllanthus amarus*; Ann V, Annexin V; PI, Propidium iodide

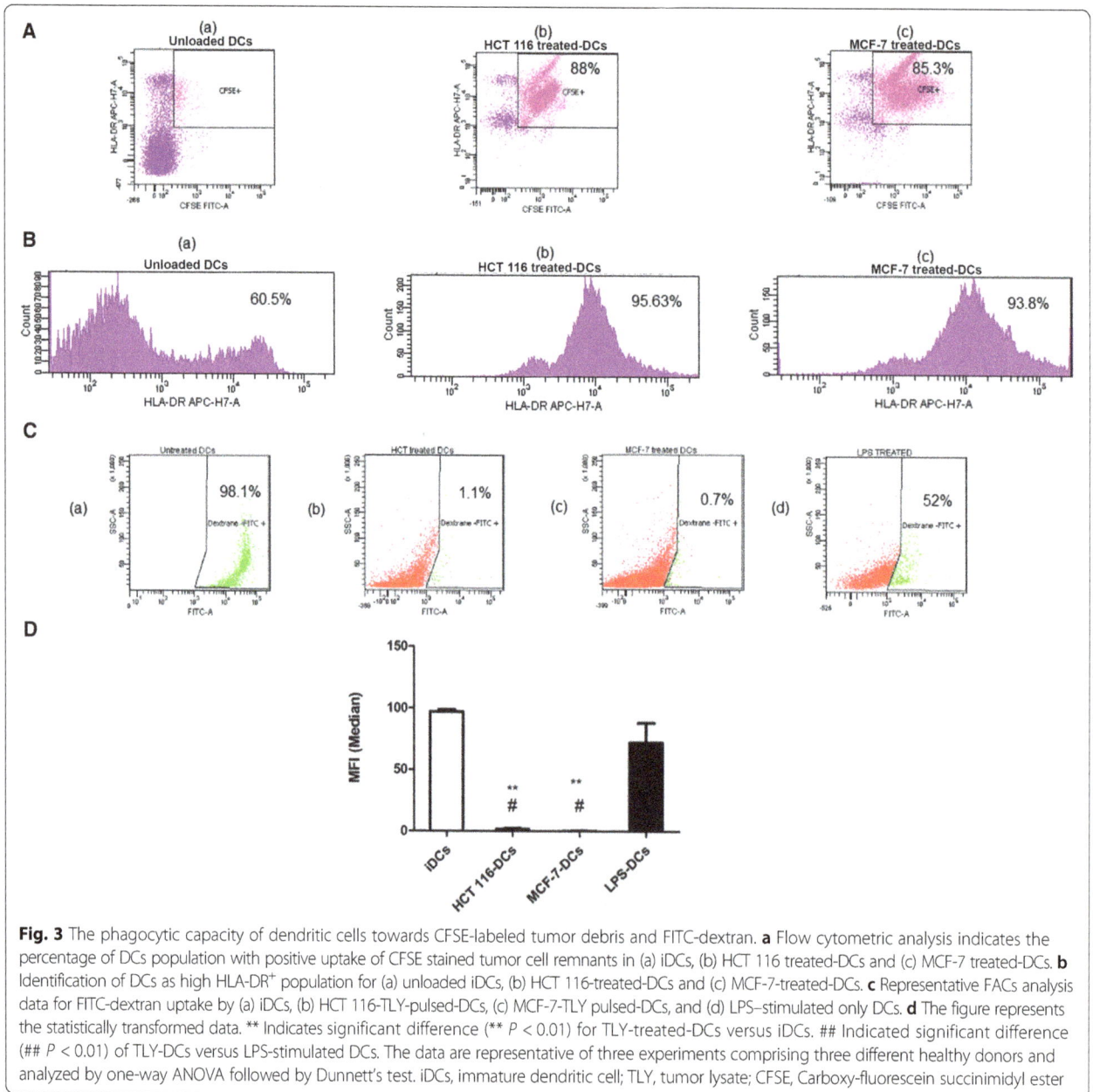

Fig. 3 The phagocytic capacity of dendritic cells towards CFSE-labeled tumor debris and FITC-dextran. **a** Flow cytometric analysis indicates the percentage of DCs population with positive uptake of CFSE stained tumor cell remnants in (a) iDCs, (b) HCT 116 treated-DCs and (c) MCF-7 treated-DCs. **b** Identification of DCs as high HLA-DR⁺ population for (a) unloaded iDCs, (b) HCT 116-treated-DCs and (c) MCF-7-treated-DCs. **c** Representative FACs analysis data for FITC-dextran uptake by (a) iDCs, (b) HCT 116-TLY-pulsed-DCs, (c) MCF-7-TLY pulsed-DCs, and (d) LPS–stimulated only DCs. **d** The figure represents the statistically transformed data. ** Indicates significant difference (** $P < 0.01$) for TLY-treated-DCs versus iDCs. ## Indicated significant difference (## $P < 0.01$) of TLY-DCs versus LPS-stimulated DCs. The data are representative of three experiments comprising three different healthy donors and analyzed by one-way ANOVA followed by Dunnett's test. iDCs, immature dendritic cell; TLY, tumor lysate; CFSE, Carboxy-fluorescein succinimidyl ester

HLA-I and CD 11c, however, in pulsed dendritic cells the surface expression levels of HLA-1 and adhesion molecule CD11c were significantly elevated. Moreover, the expression levels of co-stimulatory molecules, CD 83 and CD 86 that stabilize the interaction between dendritic cells and T lymphocytes, were dramatically increased in comparison with the immature DCs as well as LPS-only stimulated DCs. In HCT 116 TLY–DCs, the maturation and expression of co-stimulatory CD 86 ($88.35 \pm 6.45\%$) and CD 83 ($45.05 \pm 3.25\%$) molecules were more efficient than MCF-7 TLY-DCs with the mean expression values of CD 86 and CD 83 of $65.55 \pm 3.25\%$ and $40.15 \pm 1.05\%$, respectively (Fig. 4b).

IL-12, IL-6, and IL-10 productions by dendritic cells

High level of IL-12 P 40 was detected in the supernatant of HCT 116 and MCF-7 tumor lysate pulsed DCs whereas the IL-12 concentration showed significant difference (518.2 ± 3.88 and 485.8 ± 6.005 pg/mL in HCT 116 and MCF-7, respectively, $P < 0.001$) at ratio 1:3 (DC: APO) in comparison with the immature DCs. Furthermore, the results showed that the release of IL-6 was increased by HCT 116 (1167 ± 2.59 pg/mL) and MCF-TLY pulsed DC (1493 ± 1.24 pg/mL) at ratio 1:3 more than at 1:1 which was significantly different in comparison with the non-pulsed DCs and also from LPS-only stimulated DCs (1050 ± 3.19 pg/mL). In contrast, the most profound

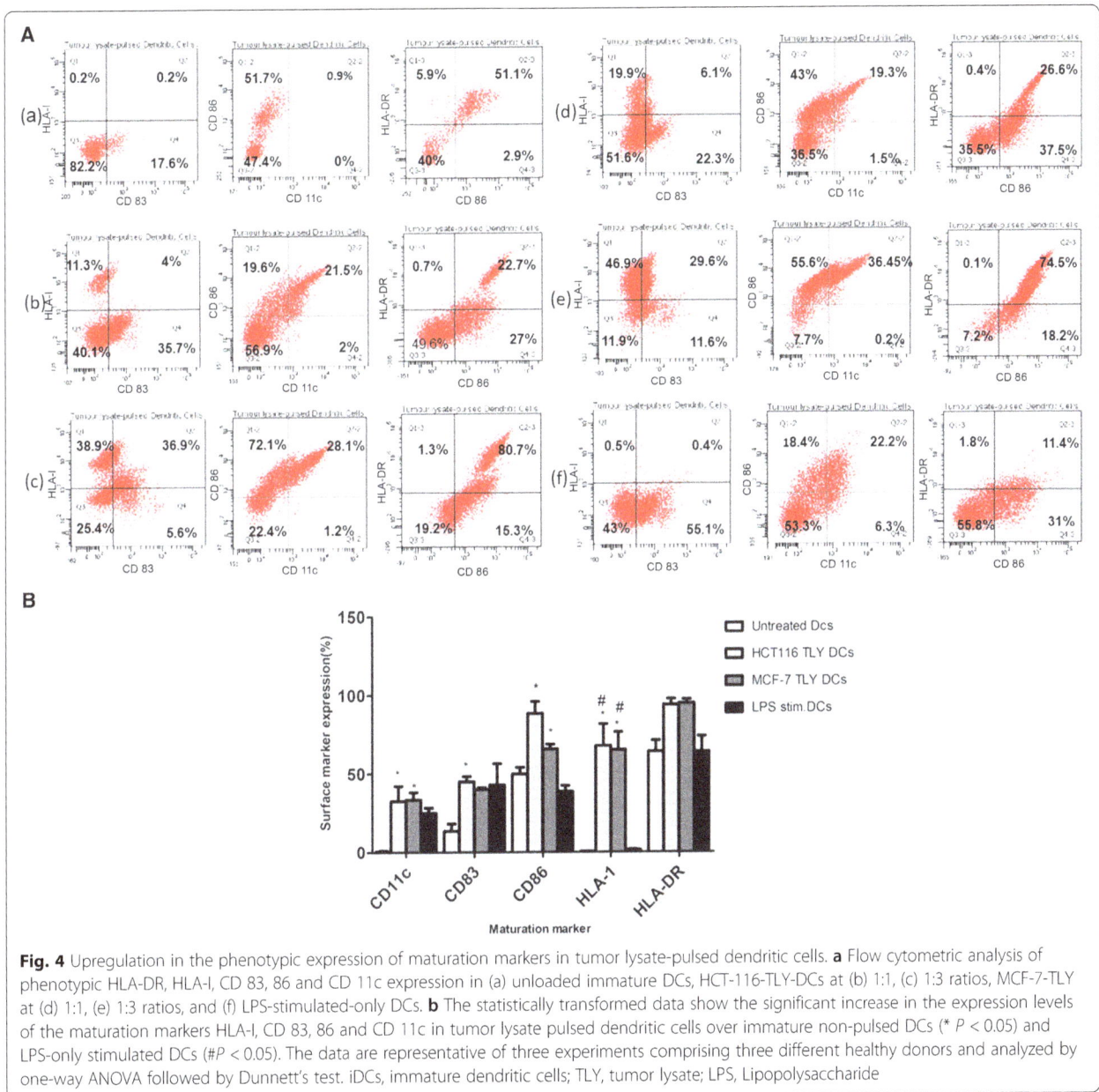

Fig. 4 Upregulation in the phenotypic expression of maturation markers in tumor lysate-pulsed dendritic cells. **a** Flow cytometric analysis of phenotypic HLA-DR, HLA-I, CD 83, 86 and CD 11c expression in (a) unloaded immature DCs, HCT-116-TLY-DCs at (b) 1:1, (c) 1:3 ratios, MCF-7-TLY at (d) 1:1, (e) 1:3 ratios, and (f) LPS-stimulated-only DCs. **b** The statistically transformed data show the significant increase in the expression levels of the maturation markers HLA-I, CD 83, 86 and CD 11c in tumor lysate pulsed dendritic cells over immature non-pulsed DCs (* $P < 0.05$) and LPS-only stimulated DCs (#$P < 0.05$). The data are representative of three experiments comprising three different healthy donors and analyzed by one-way ANOVA followed by Dunnett's test. iDCs, immature dendritic cells; TLY, tumor lysate; LPS, Lipopolysaccharide

effect was observed in the suppression of IL-10 release in 1:1 as well as 1:3 loaded DCs since the cells were matured and shifted towards the production of IL-12. Interestingly, the incorporation and uptake of tumor lysate influenced the cytokines release profile of DCs which then were stimulated with LPS. In particular, there was a statistically significant increase in IL-12 P40 as well as IL-6 production and a remarkable reduction in IL-10 release (Fig. 5).

Increase in the migration potential of tumor lysate pulsed DCs

Migration of matured DCs to lymph node is an essential step in the development of DCs–based vaccine. Thus, the migration potential of TLY-loaded DCs was evaluated at

1:1 and 1:3 ratios (DC: APO). The results demonstrated that both HCT 116 and MCF-7 TLY pulsed DCs displayed an enhanced migration capacity toward LN chemo-attractant CCL21 (250 ng/mL) up to 3–4 times in comparison with unloaded as well as LPS-stimulated DCs only. This finding indicated the DCs maturation. Stimulation of DCs with LPS alone did not improve the migration capacity of the cells; therefore, loading of DCs with tumor lysate dramatically induced the maturation and migration of the DCs towards the lymph node (Fig. 6).

Allogeneic T cell stimulation capacity

T cell proliferation assay was performed to determine the capacity of *P. amarus*-generated tumor lysate pulsed

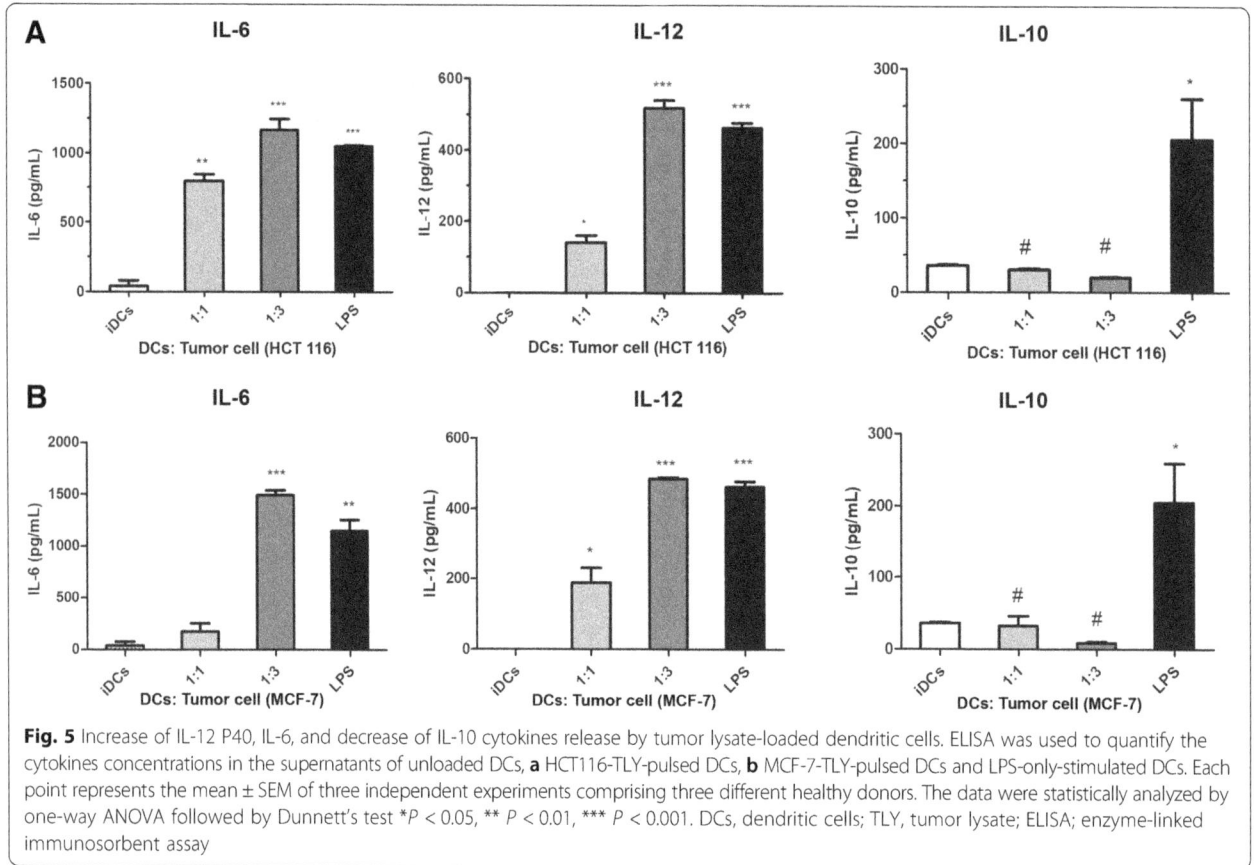

Fig. 5 Increase of IL-12 P40, IL-6, and decrease of IL-10 cytokines release by tumor lysate-loaded dendritic cells. ELISA was used to quantify the cytokines concentrations in the supernatants of unloaded DCs, **a** HCT116-TLY-pulsed DCs, **b** MCF-7-TLY-pulsed DCs and LPS-only-stimulated DCs. Each point represents the mean ± SEM of three independent experiments comprising three different healthy donors. The data were statistically analyzed by one-way ANOVA followed by Dunnett's test *$P < 0.05$, ** $P < 0.01$, *** $P < 0.001$. DCs, dendritic cells; TLY, tumor lysate; ELISA; enzyme-linked immunosorbent assay

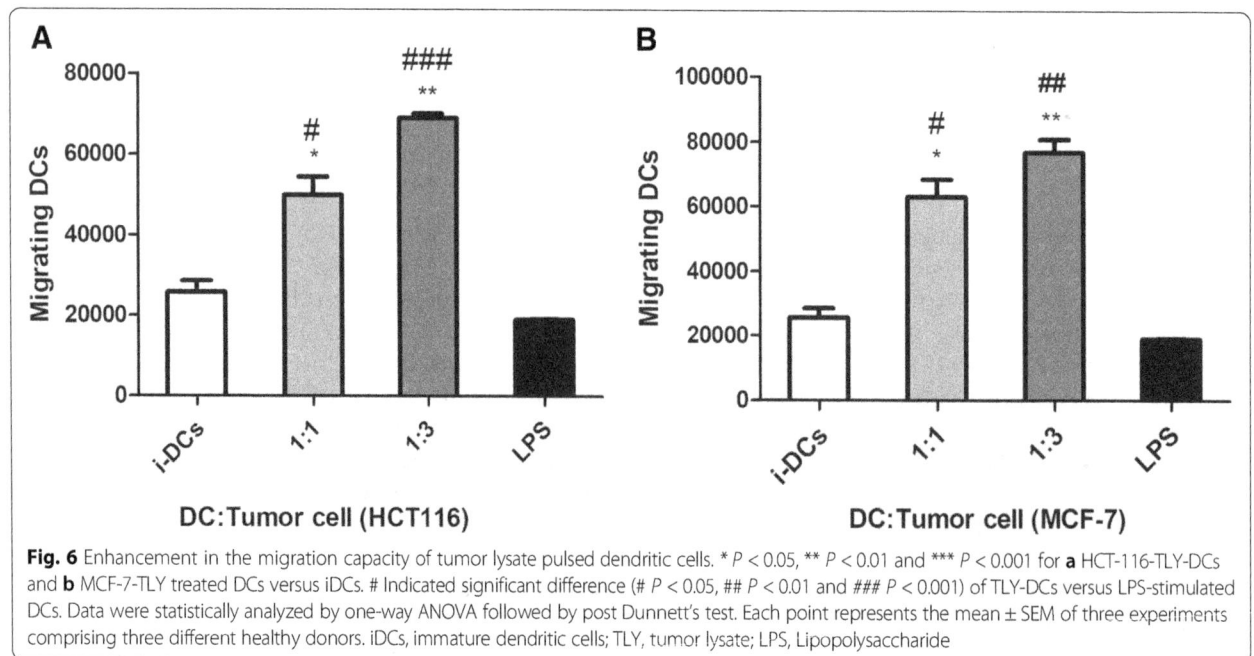

Fig. 6 Enhancement in the migration capacity of tumor lysate pulsed dendritic cells. * $P < 0.05$, ** $P < 0.01$ and *** $P < 0.001$ for **a** HCT-116-TLY-DCs and **b** MCF-7-TLY treated DCs versus iDCs. # Indicated significant difference (# $P < 0.05$, ## $P < 0.01$ and ### $P < 0.001$) of TLY-DCs versus LPS-stimulated DCs. Data were statistically analyzed by one-way ANOVA followed by post Dunnett's test. Each point represents the mean ± SEM of three experiments comprising three different healthy donors. iDCs, immature dendritic cells; TLY, tumor lysate; LPS, Lipopolysaccharide

DCs to stimulate allogeneic T cell proliferation. This assay was carried out to identify the stimulation capacity of tumor lysate loaded DCs (1:1 and 1:3) to T cell response as a marker of DCs stimulation and maturation. The lymphocyte proliferation was studied using liquid scintillation counter. The results demonstrated that T cell proliferation capacity of HCT-116 mature DCs was significantly increased in comparison with unloaded immature DCs as well as LPS-stimulated DCs. However, MCF-7 TLY showed inhibitory impact on T cell proliferation capacity of the loaded DCs. This finding indicated that in vitro loading of immature DCs with PA–HCT-116 TLY improved the T cell stimulation capacity that was attributed to the maturation and up-regulation in the surface expression of co-stimulatory molecules CD 86 and CD 83 mainly in HCT116 TLY-DCs (Fig. 7).

Effect of the tumor lysate on the gene expression profile of dendritic cells

Based on the above results, the ability of HCT116-PA-generated TLY to modulate the gene expression profile of the pulsed dendritic cells was elucidated. The mRNA expression of IL-12 P40, IL-6, and IL-10 were studied by RT-qPCR relative to GAPDH mRNA expression level. The result demonstrated the significant up-regulation in the gene expression level of both IL-12 P40 and IL-6 in HCT 116-TLY pulsed DCs at 1: 3 ratios in comparison with unloaded DCs as well as LPS-stimulated only DCs (Fig. 8). In contrast, the expression of IL-10 gene was undetectable in the non-pulsed as well as TLY pulsed DCs cells. This finding supported that TLY pulsed DCs retained their capacity to produce pro-inflammatory cytokines, which were able to trigger their migration into lymph nodes to induce an effective immune response against the recognized tumor antigens.

Discussion

Dendritic cells are the most commanding and professional APCs that implement a key role in cancer immunotherapy. Several studies referred that DCs pulsed with apoptotic tumor cells lysate have been used successfully to induce tumor vaccination [27]. Furthermore, the using of whole tumor cell lysate represents a rich source of antigens with epitopes for CD8[+] cytotoxic T cells (CTLs) as well as CD4[+] T helper cells that generate strong and a long-lasting antitumor immune response [28, 29]. There are several studies that demonstrated the effectiveness of different types of tumor cell death on the stimulation of DCs. Apoptosis is the programmed cell death that is characterized by the loss of the plasma membrane asymmetry and externalization of phosphatidylserine (PS) to the outer leaflet of the cell membrane [30]. DCs express PS receptors that were found to perform an essential role in the uptake of apoptotic cells [31]. However, irradiated tumor cells that showed approximately 30 to 35% of apoptosis, inhibited DCs maturation through the downregulation of MHC II and CD 86 expression as well as suppression of IL-12, TNF α and IL-6 release [32]. Although the danger theory suggests that the necrotic cell death elicits trigger signals to initiate an effective innate immune response [33], many studies reported the immunosuppressive effect of the necrotic cell material generated by freeze and thaw cycles on the immune system [34]. Therefore, the process of induction of mode of cell death can figure the immunogenicity of the generated tumor lysate. Accordingly, in this study we aimed to use *P. amarus* to induce programmed cell death in HCT 16 human colon cancer and MCF-7 human breast cancer cell lines, create a collection of tumor-associated antigens (TAAs) that could activate DCs and evaluate whether this priming process would induce the antigen presenting and processing as

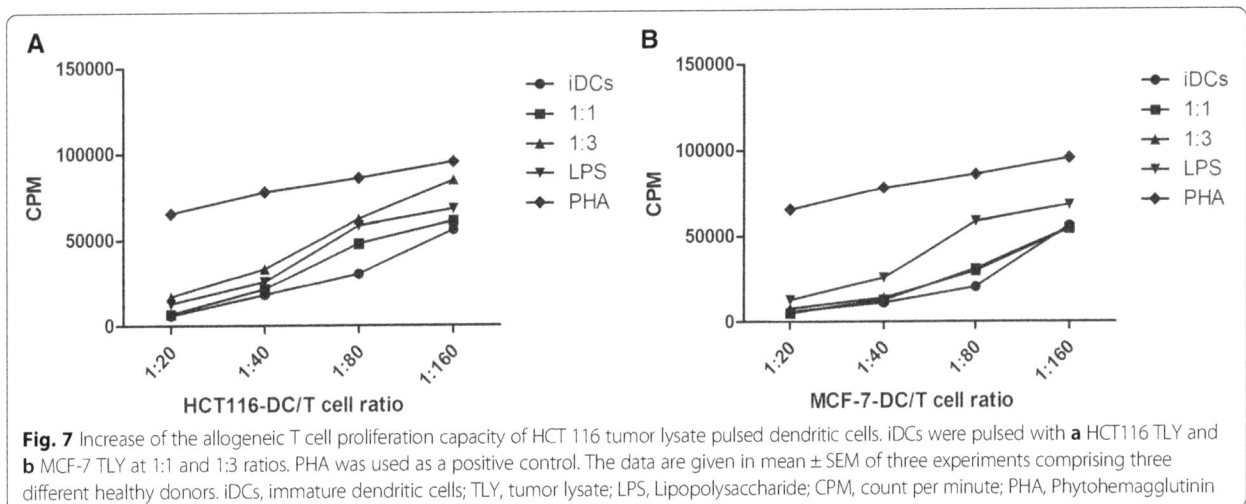

Fig. 7 Increase of the allogeneic T cell proliferation capacity of HCT 116 tumor lysate pulsed dendritic cells. iDCs were pulsed with **a** HCT116 TLY and **b** MCF-7 TLY at 1:1 and 1:3 ratios. PHA was used as a positive control. The data are given in mean ± SEM of three experiments comprising three different healthy donors. iDCs, immature dendritic cells; TLY, tumor lysate; LPS, Lipopolysaccharide; CPM, count per minute; PHA, Phytohemagglutinin

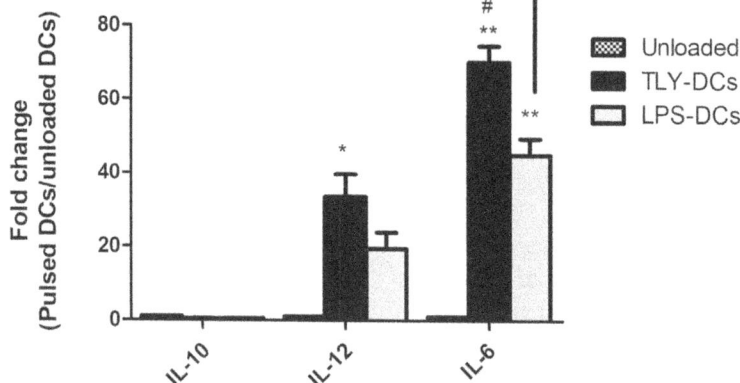

Fig. 8 Alteration in the gene expression profile of IL-10, IL-12 P40 and IL-6 before and after tumor lysate pulsing of dendritic cells. The data show the fold change between loaded /unloaded DCs. The data were normalized to GAPDH mRNA expression level. #$P < 0.05$ represents the significant difference from LPS -DCs. *$P < 0.05$, **$P < 0.01$, and ***$P < 0.001$ represent significance to unloaded DCs. The data are given in mean value ± SEM of three experiments comprising three different healthy donors. iDCs, immature dendritic cells; TLY, tumor lysate; LPS, Lipopolysaccharide

well as the cellular immune function of the primed dendritic cells.

HPLC analysis revealed the presence of lignans and polyphenolic compounds mainly gallic acid, ellagic acid and geraniin that have been reported by previous studies to inhibit the cell proliferation and induce apoptosis in different tumor cell types [35–37]. *P. amarus* successfully induced apoptosis in HCT 116 and MCF-7 at 1000 µg/mL with 80.55 ± 2.05% and 75.9 ± 0.6%, respectively, after 24 h and this was detected with Annexin V FITC dual staining kit.

The immature monocyte-derived DCs were generated ex vivo and pulsed with tumor lysate at ratios 1:1 and 1:3 (DCs: APO) that were found to be non-toxic to the DCs. It was clear from our data that ratio 1:1 showed lower stimulatory effect on the DCs activities. Furthermore, 1:3 ratio has been commonly used in the previous clinical trials [38, 39]. For complete maturation of DCs, the loaded cells were subsequently stimulated with LPS (1 µg/mL). The efficiency and safety of LPS as a maturation stimulus for DCs were already established in various clinical studies with almost no or limited side effects [40, 41]. The data showed that the loaded DCs with tumor lysates from human colon cancer HCT 116 and breast cancer MCF-7 upregulated the surface expression of maturation markers including, MHC I, MHC II as well as adhesion molecule CD 11c. The expression of co-stimulatory molecules CD 86 and CD 83 in HCT 116–TLY DCs was markedly increased and correlated with their high T-cell proliferation capacity. In contrast, MCF-7 tumor lysate reduced the T cell proliferation capacity of loaded DCs followed the engulfment of tumor lysate. Previous studies reported that soluble factors produced by the tumor cells may participate in the

attenuation of the DCs allostimulatory function such as transforming growth factor β and other tumor-derived lipids without affecting the DCs phenotypic expression of MHC II [42]. Therefore, T cell proliferation activity of tumor lysate-challenged DCs is an important determinant in development of an effective DCs-based vaccine that should be monitored before the clinical studies. In order to confirm that the generated DCs ex vivo were fully functioning as an APC, we studied their antigen uptake capacity towards HCT 116 and MCF-7 cancer cells debris stained with CFSE fluorescence dye. DCs were found to display a strong phagocytic activity towards tumor cell remnants up to 85 and 88% for both cell lines. Generally, mature DCs are characterized by reduced capacity of further antigen uptake [43], thus the endocytic activity of loaded DCs for FITC- dextran was evaluated, and it was impaired as a hallmark of DCs activation and maturation. However, immature DCs could strongly incorporate FITC-dextran up to 98.1 ± 1.6%.

The cytokines profile of DCs was studied by evaluation of their release in the supernatant in unloaded, tumor lysate pulsed DCs as well as LPS-stimulated only DCs. Our data showed the significant upregulation in IL-12 and IL-6 release in compare with unloaded and also LPS-stimulated DCs as a characteristic of DCs maturation. On the other hand, the production of the anti-inflammatory cytokine IL-10 in tumor lysate-pulsed DCs was strongly attenuated following the engulfment of tumor lysate. IL-12 is involved in the differentiation of naive T cell into Th1 phenotype [44], in addition to its ability to induce the proliferation and growth of T lymphocytes as well as the release of TNFα and INF γ. Besides, IL-12 enhances the cytotoxic activity of CD 8[+] T lymphocytes and natural killer cells (NK cells) against the tumor cells. Thus, this finding revealed that *P. amarus*-generated tumor lysate induced the release of IL-12 by pulsed DCs that possesses an important function in the regulation of T lymphocyte-induced antitumor immune response. IL-6 was reported to enhance CD8$^+$ T-cell proliferation in vitro [45, 46] and in vivo. Furthermore, IL-6 induced the survival of naïve T cells [47] and participated in a complete and effective in vivo cytotoxic CD8$^+$ T-cell response. In contrast, IL-10 is an anti-inflammatory cytokine that induces immunosuppressive response which enables the tumor cells to evade the immune control [48]. Additionally, it is associated with the generation of T $_{reg}$ lymphocytes that inhibit the antitumor immune response and support the tumor growth and propagation [49]. The results for the cytokines release have been confirmed by determination of their mRNA expression levels and the transcriptional change in their encoding genes before and after tumor lysate challenge. In this study, the effect of *P. amarus*-generated tumor lysate on the migration capacity of the DCs was investigated toward CCL21 LN-secreted chemokine. The data detected the obvious enhancement in the migration potential of the loaded DCs with tumor lysate in the presence of maturation signal from LPS, in comparison with unloaded DCs. However, LPS-stimulated only DCs demonstrated lower migration capacity than pulsed DCs since the earlier studies stated that the maturation of DCs using LPS as well as INF γ did not improve the migration ability of the cells and also could not migrate well [50]. Maturation of DCs mainly via antigen uptake and presentation is accompanied by their migration to lymphoid tissue in order to impulse naïve T-lymphocytes. Therefore, this finding suggested that TLY-pulsed DCs were activated and matured.

Conclusions

In conclusion, the present study demonstrated that *P. amarus*-generated tumor lysate induced the expression of maturation markers mainly MHC I, CD 86, CD 83 as well as the adhesion molecule CD11c in pulsed DCs. Furthermore, it induced IL-12 and Il-6 cytokines release and suppressed IL-10 production. Additionally, DCs migration and T cell proliferation allostimulatory capacities were highly stimulated. Taken together, our data revealed that whole tumor lysate generated by *P. amarus* induced the maturation of DCs and their capacity to stimulate an efficient in vitro antitumor immune response. Thus, we present a novel in-vitro DCs-based vaccine model that has been developed against colon and breast cancer by using a natural immunomodulatory, *P. amarus*-induced apoptotic

tumor cells. Nevertheless, further in vivo studies in different animal models, pharmacokinetic and pre-clinical investigations are needed before human studies can be carried out on the generated DCs based vaccine.

Abbreviation

APC: Antigen presenting cells; ATCC: American type culture collection; CFSE: 5, 6-carboxyfluorescein diacetate succinimidyl ester; CTLs: Cytotoxic T lymphocytes; DCs: dendritic cells; DMEM: Dulbecco's modified Eagle's medium; ELISA: enzyme-linked immunosorbent assay; FBS: fetal bovine serum; FITC: Fluorescein isothiocyanate; GM-CSF: Granulocytes-macrophage colony stimulating factor; HPLC: High performance liquid chromatography; IL-4: Interleukin 4; MHC: Major histocompatibility complex; NK: Natural killer cells; PA: *Phyllanthus amarus*; PBMC: peripheral blood monocytes; PHA: Phytohaemagglutinin; PS: Phosphatidylserine; TAA: Tumor associated antigens; TLY: Tumor lysate; TNF-α: Tumor necrosis factor-alpha

Acknowledgements

The work was supported by the Ministry of Agriculture and Agro-based Industry Malaysia, under the NKEA Research Grant Scheme (NRGS) (Grant no. NF-2015-004).

Funding

This study was funded by the Ministry of Agriculture and Agro-based Industry, Malaysia under the NKEA Research Grant Scheme (NRGS) (no. NF-2015-004).

Authors' contributions

SIAM performed the experiments, analyzed and interpreted the data, and drafted the manuscript. IJ, MAN and MAS designed the study. IJ coordinated the study, analyzed and interpreted the data, revised the manuscript and approved the final version to be submitted for publication. KMC participated in the analysis and interpretation of data. All authors read and approved the final manuscript.

Competing interests

The authors declare that they have no competing interests.

Author details

[1]Drug and Herbal Research Centre, Faculty of Pharmacy, Universiti Kebangsaan Malaysia, Jalan Raja Muda Abdul Aziz, 50300 Kuala Lumpur, Malaysia. [2]Department of Chemistry, Faculty of Science and Mathematics, Universiti Pendidikan Sultan Idris, 35900 Tanjung Malim, Perak, Malaysia. [3]Faculty of Medicine, University of Tabuk, Tabuk 71491, Saudi Arabia. [4]Faculty of Health Sciences, Universiti Kebangsaan Malaysia, Jalan Raja Muda Abdul Aziz, 50300 Kuala Lumpur, Malaysia. [5]School of Pharmacy, Taylor's University, Lakeside Campus, 47500 Subang Jaya, Selangor, Malaysia.

References

1. Palucka K, Banchereau J. Cancer immunotherapy via dendritic cells. Nat Rev Cancer. 2012;12(4):265–77.
2. Steinman RM. The dendritic cell system and its role in immunogenicity. Annu Rev Immunol. 1991;9:203–8.
3. Banchereau J, Steinman RM. Dendritic cells and the control of immunity. Nature. 1998;392:245–52.
4. Stockwin LH, McGonagle D, Martin IG, Blair GE. Dendritic cells: immunological sentinels with a central role in health and disease. Immunol Cell Biol. 2000;78(2):91–102.

5. Tugues S, Burkhard SH, Ohs I, Vrohlings M, Nussbaum K, Vom BJ. New insights into IL-12-mediated tumor suppression. Cell Death Differ. 2015;22(2):237–46.

6. Martínez-Lostao L, Anel A, Pardo J. How do cytotoxic lymphocytes kill cancer cells? Clin Cancer Res. 2015;21(22):5047–56.

7. Palucka K, Ueno H, Fay J, Banchereau J. Dendritic cells and immunity against cancer. J Intern Med. 2011;269(1):64–73.

8. Koh JS, Levine JS. Apoptosis and autoimmunity. Curr Opin Nephrol Hypertens. 1997;6(3):259–66.

9. Inaba K, Turley S, Yamaide F, Iyoda T, Mahnke K, Inaba M. Efficient presentation of phagocytosed cellular fragments on the major histocompatibility complex class II products of dendritic cells. J Exp Med. 1998;188(11):2163–73.

10. Trinchieri G. Interleukin-12: a proinflammatory cytokine with immunoregulatory functions that bridge innate resistence and antigen-specific adaptive immunity. Annu Rev Immunol. 1995;13:251–176.

11. Ma Y, Shurin GV, Peiyuan Z, Shurin MR. Dendritic cells in the cancer microenvironment. J Cancer. 2013;4(1):36–44.

12. Balkwill F. Tumour necrosis factor and cancer. Nat Rev Cancer. 2009;9(5):361–71.

13. Grivennikov SI, Karin M. Inflammatory cytokines in cancer: tumour necrosis factor and interleukin 6 take the stage. Ann Rheum Dis. 2011;70:104–8.

14. Podrazil M, Horvath R, Becht E, Rozkova D, Bilkova P, Hromadkova H. Phase I/II clinical trial of dendritic-cell based immunotherapy (DCVAC/PCa) combined with chemotherapy in patients with metastatic, castration-resistant prostate cancer. Oncotarget. 2015;6(20):18192–205.

15. Gray HJ, Benigno B, Berek J, Chang J, Mason J, Mileshkin L. Progression-free and overall survival in ovarian cancer patients treated with CVac, a mucin 1 dendritic cell therapy in a randomized phase 2 trial. J Immunother Cancer. 2016;4(1):34.

16. Amin A, Dudek AZ, Logan TF, Lance RS, Holzbeierlein JM, Knox JJ. Survival with AGS-003, an autologous dendritic cell–based immunotherapy, in combination with sunitinib in unfavorable risk patients with advanced renal cell carcinoma (RCC): phase 2 study results. J Immunother Cancer. 2015;3(1):14.

17. Dillman RO, Selvan SR, Schiltz PM, McClay EF, Barth NM, DePriest C. Phase II trial of dendritic cells loaded with antigens from self-renewing, proliferating autologous tumor cells as patient-specific antitumor vaccines in patients with metastatic melanoma: final report. Cancer Biother Radiopharm. 2009;24(3):311–9.

18. Mayanagi S, Kitago M, Sakurai T, Matsuda T, Fujita T, Higuchi H. Phase I pilot study of Wilms tumor gene 1 peptide-pulsed dendritic cell vaccination combined with gemcitabine in pancreatic cancer. Cancer Sci. 2015;106(3):397–406.

19. Polyzoidis S, Ashkan K. DCVax®-L - developed by northwest biotherapeutics. Hum Vaccines Immunother. 2014;10(11):3139–45.

20. Notka F, Meier GR, Wagner R. Inhibition of wild-type human immunodeficiency virus and reverse transcriptase inhibitor-resistant variants by Phyllanthus amarus. Antivir Res. 2003;58(2):175–86.

21. Yuandani, Ilangkovan M, Jantan I, Mohamad HF, Husain K, Abdul Razak AF. Inhibitory effects of standardized extracts of Phyllanthus amarus and Phyllanthus urinaria and their marker compounds on phagocytic activity of human neutrophils. Evidence-based Complement Altern Med. 2013;2013:603634.

22. Bhat SS, Hegde KS, Chandrashekhar S, Rao SN, Manikkoth S. Preclinical screening of Phyllanthus amarus ethanolic extract for its analgesic and antimicrobial activity. Pharm Res. 2015;7(4):378–84.

23. Lawson-Evi P, Eklu-Gadeg K, Agbonon A, Aklikokou K, Creppy E, Gbeassor M. Antidiabetic activity of Phyllanthus amarus Schum. And Thonn. (Euphorbiaceae) on alloxan induced diabetes in male wistar rats. J Appl Sci. 2011;11(16):2968–73.

24. Abhyankar G, Suprasanna P, Pandey BN, Mishra KP, Rao KV, Reddy VD. Hairy root extract of Phyllanthus amarus induces apoptotic cell death in human breast cancer cells. Innov Food Sci Emerg Technol. 2010;11(3):526–32.

25. Lee SH, Jaganath IB, Wang SM, Sekaran SD. Antimetastatic effects of Phyllanthus on human lung (A549) and breast (MCF-7) cancer cell lines. PLoS One. 2011;6(6):1–14.

26. Jantan I, Ilangkovan M, Mohamad HF. Correlation between the major components of Phyllanthus amarus and Phyllanthus urinaria and their inhibitory effects on phagocytic activity of human neutrophils. Evidence-based Complement Altern Med. 2014;14:1–12.

27. Henry F, Boisteau O, Bretaudeau L, Lieubeau B, Meflah K, Grégoire M. Antigen-presenting cells that phagocytose apoptotic tumor-derived cells are potent tumor vaccines. Cancer Res. 1999;59(14):3329–32.

28. Toes RE, Ossendorp F, Offringa R, Melief CJ. CD4 T cells and their role in antitumor immune responses. J Exp Med. 1999;189(5):753–6.

29. Zajac AJ, Blattman JN, Murali-Krishna K, Sourdive DJ, Suresh M, Altman JD. Viral immune evasion due to persistence of activated T cells without effector function. J Exp Med. 1998;188(12):2205–13.

30. Nicholson DW, Thornberry NA. Apoptosis. Life and death decisions. Science. 2003;299(5604):214–5.

31. Fadok VA, Bratton DL, Rose DM, Pearson A, Ezekewitz RAB, Henson PM. A receptor for phosphatidylserine-specific clearance of apoptotic cells. Nature. 2000;405(6782):85–90.

32. Idoyaga J, Moreno J, Bonifaz L. Tumor cells prevent mouse dendritic cell maturation induced by TLR ligands. Cancer Immunol Immunother. 2007;56(8):1237–50.

33. Scaffidi P, Misteli T, Bianchi ME. Release of chromatin protein HMGB1 by necrotic cells triggers inflammation. Nature. 2002;418(6894):191–5.

34. Strome SE, Voss S, Wilcox R, Wakefield TL, Tamada K, Flies D. Strategies for antigen loading of dendritic cells to enhance the antitumor immune response. Cancer Res. 2002;62(6):1884–9.

35. Parvathaneni M, Battu GR, Gray AI, Gummalla P. Investigation of anticancer potential of hypophyllanthin and phyllanthin against breast cancer by in vitro and in vivo methods. Asian Pacific J Trop Dis. 2014;4(S1):930–5.

36. Pang JHS, Huang ST, Wang CY, Yang RC, Wu HT, Yang SH. Ellagic acid, the active compound of Phyllanthus urinaria, exerts in vivo anti-angiogenic effect and inhibits MMP-2 activity. Evidence-based Complement Altern Med. 2011;2011:1–11.

37. Bin-Chuan JI, Hsu WH, Yang JS, Hsia TC, Lu CC, Chiang JH. Gallic acid induces apoptosis via caspase-3 and mitochondrion-dependent pathways in vitro and suppresses lung xenograft tumor growth in vivo. J Agric Food Chem. 2009;57(16):7596–604.

38. Hatfield P, Merrick AE, West E, O'Donnell D, Selby P, Vile R. Optimization of dendritic cell loading with tumor cell lysates for cancer immunotherapy. J Immunother. 2008;31(7):620–32.

39. Fields RC, Shimizu K, Mulé JJ. Murine dendritic cells pulsed with whole tumor lysates mediate potent antitumor immune responses in vitro and in vivo. Proc Natl Acad Sci U S A. 1998;95(16):9482–7.

40. Sharma A, Koldovsky U, Xu S, Mick R, Roses R, Fitzpatrick E. HER-2 pulsed dendritic cell vaccine can eliminate HER-2 expression and impact ductal carcinoma in situ. Cancer. 2012;118(17):4354–62.

41. Czerniecki BJ, Koski GK, Koldovsky U, Xu S, Cohen PA, Mick R. Targeting HER-2/neu in early breast cancer development using dendritic cells with staged Interleukin-12 burst secretion. Cancer Res. 2007;67(4):1842–52.

42. Bonham CA, Lu L, Banas RA, Fontes P, Rao AS, Starzl TE. TGF-β1 pretreatment impairs the allostimulatory function of human bone marrow-derived antigen-presenting cells for both naive and primed T cells. Transpl Immunol. 1996;4(3):186–91.

43. Sallusto F, Cella M, Danieli C, Lanzavecchia A. Dendritic cells use macropinocytosis and the mannose receptor to concentrate macromolecules in the major histocompatibility complex class II compartment: downregulation by cytokines and bacterial products. J Exp Med. 1995;182:389–400.

44. Hsieh CS, Macatonia SE, Tripp CS, Wolf SF, O'Garra A, Murphy KM. Development of TH1 CD4+ T cells through IL-12 produced by listeria-induced macrophages. Science. 1993;260(5107):547–9.

45. Vanden Bush TJ, Buchta CM, Claudio J, Bishop GA. Cutting edge: importance of IL-6 and cooperation between innate and adaptive immune receptors in cellular vaccination with B lymphocytes. J Immunol. 2009;183(8):4833–7.

46. Gagnon J, Ramanathan S, Leblanc C, Cloutier A, McDonald PP, Ilangumaran S. IL-6, in synergy with IL-7 or IL-15, stimulates TCR-independent proliferation and functional differentiation of CD8+ T lymphocytes. J Immunol. 2008;180(12):7958–68.

47. Teague TK, Marrack P, Kappler JW, Vella AT. IL-6 rescues resting mouse T cells from apoptosis. J Immunol. 1997;158(12):5791–6.

48. Mohamed SIA, Jantan I, Haque MA. Naturally occurring immunomodulators with antitumor activity: an insight on their mechanisms of action. Int Immunopharmacol. 2017;50:291–304.

49. Zhang X, Huang H, Yuan J, Sun D, Hou W-S, Gordon J. CD4-8- dendritic cells prime CD4+ T regulatory 1 cells to suppress antitumor immunity. J Immunol. 2005;175(5):2931–7.

50. Vopenkova K, Mollova K, Buresova I, Michalek J. Complex evaluation of human monocyte-derived dendritic cells for cancer immunotherapy. J Cell Mol Med. 2012;16(11):2827–37.

GLP-I secretion in healthy and diabetic Wistar rats in response to aqueous extract of *Momordica charantia*

Gulzar Ahmad Bhat[1], Haseeb A. Khan[2*], Abdullah S. Alhomida[2], Poonam Sharma[3], Rambir Singh[4] and Bilal Ahmad Paray[5]

Abstract

Background: Diabetes mellitus is one of the major global health disorders increasing at an alarming rate in both developed and developing countries. The objective of this study was to assess the effect of aqueous extract of *Momordica charantia* (AEMC) on fasting blood glucose (FBG), tissue glycogen, glycosylated haemoglobin, plasma concentrations of insulin and GLP-1 hormone (glucagon-like peptide 1) in healthy and diabetic wistar rats.

Methods: Male Wistar rats (both normal and diabetic) were treated with AEMC by gavaging (300 mg/kg body wt/day for 28 days).

Results: AEMC was found to increase tissue glycogen, serum insulin and GLP-1 non-significantly ($P > 0.05$) in normal, significantly ($P < 0.01$) in diabetic Wistar rats, whereas decrease in FBG and Glycosylated haemoglobin non-significantly ($P > 0.05$) in normal, significantly ($P < 0.01$) in diabetic Wistar rats. The elevation of GLP-1 level in normal and diabetic treated groups may be due to the L-cell regeneration and proliferation by binding with L-cell receptors and makes a conformational change, resulting in the activation of a series of signal transducers. The polar molecules of *M. charantia* also depolarize the L-cell through elevation of intracellular Ca^{2+} concentration and which in turn releases GLP-1. GLP-1 in turn elevates beta-cell proliferation and insulin secretion.

Conclusion: The findings tend to provide a possible explanation for the hypoglycemic action of *M. charantia* fruit extracts as alternative nutritional therapy in the management and treatment of diabetes.

Keywords: Diabetes mellitus, Glucagon-like peptide 1, Wistar rats, *Momordica charantia*

Background

Diabetes Mellitus (DM) is one of the most prevalent and serious metabolic disorders affecting about 200 million people worldwide [1]. Type 2 DM (T2DM) is the prevalent form of DM, which poses huge economic burden to all nations, especially the developing countries, which are accounting for more than 80% of reported cases of T2DM [2]. New generation antidiabetic drugs chiefly, α-glucosidase inhibitors, insulin sensitizers, GLP-1 agonists and DPP-4 inhibitors have been developed for effective control and management of T2DM [3].

Glucagon-like peptide (GLP-1) is physiologically important regulators of metabolic control and is an important hormone that stimulates the secretion of glucose-dependent insulin from pancreatic -cells. This endocrine hormone of 30-amino acids is produced in the enteroendocrine L-cells [4]. Is has been reported that the continuous GLP-1 treatment in T2DM improve β-cell function, normalizes blood glucose and restore first-phase insulin secretion and "glucose competence" to β-cells; hence, GLP-1/GLP-1Rs are therapeutic targets for treating T2DM [5]. Recently GLP-1 analogs such as Exenatide, Liraglutide, Metformin etc. have been introduced for therapeutic intervention. However, there are many side effects of these drugs like fluid retention, weight gain, headache, upper respiratory tract infection and urinary tract infection.

* Correspondence: haseeb@ksu.edu.sa
[2]Department of Biochemistry, College of Science, King Saud University, Riyadh 11451, Saudi Arabia
Full list of author information is available at the end of the article

The side effects and costly treatment associated with current day antidiabetic drugs, necessitated search for alternate remedy for the treatment of DM. Since ancient times, medicinal plants and their extracts have been effectively used as first line therapy to combat diabetes but are yet to be commercially formulated as modern medicines [6]. Traditional alternative medicine involves the use of herbs and their products as alternatives to chemical drugs.

Momordica charantia (MC) commonly known as bitter melon belongs to the family *Cucurbitaceae* is a tropical herbaceous vegatable used for management of DM throughout the world [7, 8]. The antidiabetic effects of MC have been extensively reviewed [9–11]. The possible mechanisms reported include protection of islet -cells [12], increasing insulin secretion [13], inhibition of intestinal -glucosidase [14], and glucose transport [15], activation of AMPK [16, 17], improving insulin resistance [18, 19] and increasing hepatic glucose disposal and decreasing gluconeogenesis [20, 21]. Charantin substance extracted from MC showed hypoglycaemic effect on normal and diabetic rabbits [22]. Bitter melon has been found to increase insulin sensitivity [23]. Decrease in blood glucose, cholesterol and triglycerides through a decrement in PKC-β activity was reported in diabetic rats induced by streptozotocin when MC juice was administered at 6 mL/kg [24]. At the dosage of 375 mg/kg, methanolic fruit extract of MC decreased the fasting blood glucose (FBG) after 12 h in alloxan-induced diabetic rats [25].

In this study, we probed the effects of oral administration of aqueous extract of *Momordica charantia* (AEMC) on fasting blood glucose (FBG), tissue glycogen, glycosylated haemoglobin, serum insulin and GLP-1 in diabetic Wistar rats.

Methods
Plant material and its extraction
The fruit of *M. charantia* was purchased from local market. The sample were taken to the Herbarium in Department of Botany, Bundelkhand University, Jhansi, where Dr. Rajdeep Kudesia, confirm its identification and a voucher specimen number (BU-MC- 00712) was placed in the Herbarium. The dried fruit was grinded into powder using grinder and extracted with double distilled water (1:3) by stirring whole night using homogenizer. The extract was filtered and then centrifuged (3000 x g, 10 min) for further purification. The supernatant was further lyophilized for complete dryness to obtain Aqueous Extract of *M. charantia*.

Chemicals
Streptozoticin (STZ) from Sigma Aldrich was used to induce diabetes. All chemicals and solvents used in this study were purchased from different companies like Merck, Himedia, Rankem, Qualikems, Loba, Sigma and other chemical companies of analytical grade.

Animals
Two to three months old adult male Wistar rats weighing about 200–250 g (average = 235.5 ± 4.27 g) were purchased from animal DRDE, Gawlior (India). Rats were individually housed in stainless steel wire cages in an animal room with a light: dark cycle (12:12) and temperature (22 ± 2 °C). The Animals were fed pellet diet and water ad-libitum. All procedures described in this study were performed in accordance to the guidelines of Institutional Animal Ethical Committee (BU/ Pharma/ IAEC/12/031).

Induction of diabetes
In overnight fasted animals, diabetes was induced at 7 am by a single intraperitoneal injection of a freshly prepared solution of streptozotocin (50 mg/kg b.w) in a 0.1 M citrate buffer (pH 4.5). On the third day of STZ-injection, the animals with signs of polyuria and polydipsia and with fasting glycemia (> 200 mg/dl) were considered to be diabetic and included in the study [26].

Treatment schedule
In the experiment, the rats were randomly divided into 4 groups ($n = 6$/group) as per treatment schedule given below.

Group I ($n = 6$) Normal Control

Group II ($n = 6$) Normal treated with AEMC @ 300mg/kg body weight

Group III ($n = 6$) Diabetic control

Group IV ($n = 6$) Diabetic treated with AEMC @ 300mg/kg body weight

The control group was given 0.9% normal saline, intramuscularly. Single dose of AEMC was given orally on daily basis for 28 days. Acute study of GLP-1 and serum insulin was done from blood serum in single dose administration of AEMC on first day of experiment. The blood samples were obtained from tail vein at the interval of 0, 20, 30, 40, 50, and 60 min, whereas the subchronic study was done following same procedure after 28 days' administration of AEMC. The 0 min reading indicates taking blood for the estimation of GLP-1 and serum insulin without giving the treatment of AEMC. At the end of the experimental period (after 28 days of treatment), the rats were anaesthetized by chloroform inhalation followed by cervical dislocation and sacrificed as per the guidelines of Institutional Animal Ethics Committee (IAEC). A midline incision was performed at the thoracic region on 29th day of treatment. Trunk blood was collected in heparinized tubes and the plasma was obtained by centrifugation at 5000 rpm for 5 min for the determination of biochemical parameters. The liver and muscle tissues were collected from each group of rats and used for estimation of free and fixed Glycogen.

Fasting Blood Glucose (FBG)

The blood glucose level of animals was estimated on 0, 14th and 28th day by Glucose Oxidase–Peroxidase Enzymatic Method using a digital glucometer (ACCU-CHEK brand active).

Glycosilated Haemoglobin (HbA1C)

Glycosylated haemoglobin was estimated by Euro diagnostic system kit based on photometric test at 415 nm using ion exchange resin [27–29].

Tissue glycogen

This estimation indicates the distinction between free and fixed glycogen content in tissues by using the Anthrone reagent. Immediately after the excision of liver and muscle tissues, 1 g of the tissue were digested within 2 mL of 30% boiling potassium hydroxide (KOH) solution and cooled, and following this 3 mL of 95% ethanol was added and heated until the tissues gets dissolved. Mixtures were cooled and centrifuged at 1000 rpm for 5 min, the supernatant was discarded. The residual material was dissolved in 2 mL of distilled water, and then 10 mL of Anthrone reagent was added and immersed in ice bath to prevent excessive healing. The Tubes were incubated at 100 °C for 4 min for color development and immersed in an ice bath. The absorbance was measured at 620 nm using spectrophotometer.

Serum insulin

The serum insulin concentrations were measured by an enzyme linked immunosorbent assay (ELISA) method using an ultrasensitive rat insulin ELISA kit (Mercodia, Uppsala, Sweden) in a multi plate ELISA reader (Biorad-680, BIORAD Ltd., Japan).

Glucagon-Like Peptide-1 (GLP-1)

GLP-1were determined by Ray Bio® Rat GLP-1 ELISA kit given by Toft-Neilsen [30] and Meier et al. [31].

Statistical analysis

All data were presented as the mean ± SEM. The groups were compared by one-way ANOVA analysis. Data were analyzed by using a statistical software package (SPSS for Windows, version 18) using Tukey's-HSD multiple range post hoc test. Values were considered significantly different at $p < 0.05$.

Results

Effect of *M. charantia* on FBG level in normal and diabetic rats

Oral administration of AEMC 300 mg/kg/day b.w. in normal rats showed non-significant ($P > 0.05$) decrease in FBG on 14 day (5.2%) and 28 day (10.46%) as compared to 0 day in group II, whereas, no change was observed in group I and group III. However, FBG levels showed significant ($P < 0.01$) decrease in group IV on 14 day (41.42%) and 28 day (69.57%) as compared to 0 day readings. On comparing group I with group III, significant increase ($P < 0.01$) in FBG was observed in group III on 14 day (176.16%) and 28 day (286%). However non-significant ($P > 0.05$) decrease in FBG was found on 14 day (23.35%), followed by significant ($P < 0.01$) decrease at 28 day (70.23%) in group IV as compared to group I. At the end of treatment, significant reduction was observed on 14 and 28 day in relation to diabetic control (Group III) (Table 1).

Effect of *M. charantia* on liver glycogen, muscle glycogen and glycosylated haemoglobin in normal and diabetic rats

The effect of AEMC on the Liver Glycogen, Muscle Glycogen and Glycosylated Haemoglobin level of normal and diabetic rats is presented in Table 2. After administration of AEMC in normal rats, liver glycogen level was non-significantly ($P < 0.05$) increased (3.97%) in group II, whereas, significant ($P < 0.01$) decrease was observed (65.16%) in group III compared to group I. However, level of liver glycogen increased significantly ($P < 0.01$) in Group IV (171.42%) when compared to group III. Non-significant ($P < 0.05$) increase in muscle glycogen was found (6.37%) in group II. On contrary, significant ($P < 0.01$) decrease in muscle glycogen was reported in group III (58.48%) when compared to group I. However, muscle glycogen in AEMC treated groups increased significantly ($P < 0.01$) in group IV (110.36%) as compared to group III. The level of HbA1C decreased (9.48%) non-significantly ($P > 0.05$) in group II, whereas in diabetic control the HbA1C showed

Table 1 The effect of *Momordica charantia* on FBG level in normal and diabetic rats

No. of days →	0	14	28
Group I	83.83 ± 2.701	82.5 ± 3.757	85.66 ± 2.929
Group II	82.83 ± 0.401	78.5 ± 0.619$^{\alpha *}$	74.16 ± 0.542$^{\alpha *}$
Group III	301.5 ± 9.570	299.16 ± 31.836$^{\gamma **}$	310.83 ± 11.652$^{\gamma **}$
Group IV	304.00 ± 9.292	177.93 ± 7.923$^{\gamma r}$	92.50 ± 13.200$^{\gamma r}$

The values represent as Mean ± SEM for 6 rats each. The results are expressed in mg/dl. α = ($P > 0.05$), β = ($P < 0.05$), γ = ($P < 0.01$) represents comparison of 0 day reading of each group with 14 and 28 days. * = ($P > 0.05$), ** = ($P < 0.05$), *** = ($P < 0.01$) represents comparison of Group-III with Group-I. ^{P} = $P > 0.05$), ^{q} = ($P < 0.05$), ^{r} = ($P < 0.01$) compared Group IV with Group III. Group-I Normal Control; Group-II Normal treated (AEMC); Group-III Diabetic control; Group-IV diabetic treated (AEMC)

Table 2 The effect of *Momordica charantia* on Liver Glycogen, Muscle Glycogen and Glycosylated Heamoglobin in normal and diabetic rats

Parameter	Group I	Group II	Group III	Group IV
Liver Glycogen (mg/g)	23.91 ± 1.74	24.86 ± 1.712*	8.33 ± 0.741***	22.61 ± 1.795r
Muscle Glycogen (mg/g)	19.75 ± 1.109	21.01 ± 1.19*	8.2 ± 0.958***	17.25 ± 0.909r
Glycosylated Hemoglobin (%)	5.06 ± 0.100	4.58 ± 0.170*	20.51 ± 5.154***	7.021 ± 0.187r

The values represent as Mean ± SEM for 6 rats each. * = ($P > 0.05$), ** = ($P < 0.05$), *** = ($P < 0.01$) represents comparison of Group-II, III with Group-I. p = $P > 0.05$), q = ($P < 0.05$), r = ($P < 0.01$) compared group IV with Group III. Group-I Normal Control; Group-II Normal treated (AEMC); Group-III Diabetic control; Group-IV diabetic treated (AEMC)

significant ($P < 0.01$) increase in group III (305.33%) as compared to group I. The diabetic rats when treated with AEMC, the HbA1C percentage significantly ($P < 0.01$) decreased in group IV (65.7%) when compared to group III.

Effect of single dose of AEMC on serum insulin level in normal and diabetic rats

Despite that the serum insulin levels were not significantly different ($P > 0.05$) at each time points (Table 3), except, 20 min where serum level was significantly higher in all groups, compared to that at 0 min. In group II, non-significant ($P > 0.05$) increase in serum insulin was observed on administration of AEMC at 20 min (6.41%), and tries to compensate towards normal at 60 min (1.41%). However, in group IV significant ($P < 0.05$) increase (85.36%) was observed at 20 min followed by non-significant increase ($P > 0.05$) at 30 min (75%), which again non-significantly falls towards normal at 60 mins (1.62%). Furthermore, significant ($P < 0.05$) change in serum insulin was observed at each time point (20 min 64.0%, 30 min 18.07%, 40 min 15.67%, 50 min 15.38%, and 60 min 0.0%) in group IV when compared to group III.

Effect of sub-chronic administration of *M. charantia* on serum insulin level in normal and diabetic rats

On sub-chronic administration of AEMC in normal rats, non-significant ($P > 0.05$) increase in serum insulin was also observed on administration of AEMC at 20 min (23.3 and 85.1%) and falls towards normal at 60 min (0.40 and 8.15%) in comparison to 0 min in group II and group IV respectively. Significant ($P < 0.01$) increase in serum

insulin level was observed (20 min 275.5%, 30 min 229.4%, 40 min 202.2%, 50 min 158.4% and 60 min 144%) in group IV as compared to group III (Table 4).

Effect of single dose of *M. charantia* on GLP-1 level in normal and diabetic rats

In the present investigation during short term administration of AEMC, GLP-1 level increased significantly ($P < 0.01$) at 20 min (64.6 and 111.46%) and non-significantly ($P > 0.05$) at 60 min (6.61 and 15.77%) in group II and group IV, respectively, when compared to 0 min readings (Table 5). The GLP-1 level showed significant ($P < 0.01$) decrease at 20 min (35.13%), 30 min (39.8%), 40 min (47.79%), 50 min (48.79%) and 60 min (51.4%) in group III as compared with group I. however, significant ($P < 0.05$) increase in GLP-1 was observed (20 min 19.67%, 30 min 19.52%, 40 min 19.41%, 50 min 18.26% and 60 min 14%) in group IV on comparison with group III.

Effect of long term exposure of *M. charantia* on GLP-1 level in normal and diabetic rats

Significant ($P < 0.01$) increase in GLP-1 in sub-chronic experiment was observed at 20 min (51.82%) and tends to be normalize at 60 min (6.61%) in comparison to 0 min in group II. However significant increase in GLP-1 level was depicted at 20 min (306.9%) and then falls towards normal at 60 min (16.5%) in comparison with 0 min in group IV. Long term administration of AEMC in diabetic rats results significant ($P < 0.05$) increase in GLP-1 level from (20mins 306.18%, 30mins 238.18%, 40mins 144.97%, 50mins 62.89%, and 60mins 16.50%) in group V, on comparison with group IV Table 6.

Table 3 The effect of single dose of *Momordica charantia* on Serum insulin level in normal and diabetic Wistar rats

Time in second	0 min	20 min	30 min	40 min	50 min	60 min
Group I	4.10 ± 0.217	4.20 ± 0.206	4.17 ± 0.210	4.16 ± 0.211	4.14 ± 0.211	4.12 ± 0.212
Group II	4.21 ± 0.288	4.48 ± 0.277a**	4.36 ± 0.260a*	4.30 ± 0.237a*	4.25 ± 0.258a*	4.22 ± 0.274a*
Group III	1.25 ± 0.239	1.39 ± 0.194a***	1.36 ± 0.205a***	1.34 ± 0.207a***	1.30 ± 0.219a***	1.25 ± 0.234a**
Group IV	1.23 ± 0.226	2.28 ± 0.399γr	1.66 ± 0.352βr	1.55 ± 0.236ar	1.50 ± 0.241ar	1.25 ± 0.227ar

The values represent as Mean ± SEM for 6 rats each. The results are expressed in ng/mL. α = ($P > 0.05$), β = ($P < 0.05$), γ = ($P < 0.01$) represents comparison of 0 min reading of each group with 20,30,40,50 and 60 min. * = ($P > 0.05$), ** = ($P < 0.05$), *** = ($P < 0.01$) represents comparison of Group-III with Group-I. p = $P > 0.05$), q = ($P < 0.05$), r = ($P < 0.01$) compared Group IV with Group III. Group-I Normal Control; Group-II Normal treated (AEMC); Group-III Diabetic control; Group-IV diabetic treated (AEMC)

Table 4 The effect of sub-chronic administration of *Momordica charantia* on Serum insulin level in normal and diabetic Wistar rats

Time in second	0 min	20 min	30 min	40 min	50 min	60 min
Group I	4.10 ± 0.217	4.20 ± 0.206	4.17 ± 0.210	4.16 ± 0.211	4.14 ± 0.211	4.12 ± 0.212
Group II	4.16 ± 0.301	5.60 ± 0.263$^{\alpha*}$	5.46 ± 0.278$^{\alpha*}$	4.37 ± 0.296$^{\alpha*}$	4.28 ± 0.292$^{\alpha*}$	4.18 ± 0.299$^{\alpha*}$
Group III	1.25 ± 0.239	1.39 ± 0.194$^{\alpha***}$	1.36 ± 0.205$^{\alpha***}$	1.34 ± 0.207$^{\alpha***}$	1.30 ± 0.219$^{\alpha***}$	1.25 ± 0.234$^{\alpha**}$
Group IV	2.82 ± 0.136	5.22 ± 0.273$^{\gamma r}$	4.48 ± 0.310$^{\gamma r}$	4.05 ± 0.310$^{\beta r}$	3.36 ± 0.204$^{\alpha r}$	3.05 ± 0.195$^{\alpha r}$

The values represent as Mean ± SEM for 6 rats each. The results are expressed in ng/mL. $\alpha = (P > 0.05)$, $\beta = (P < 0.05)$, $\gamma = (P < 0.01)$ represents comparison of 0 min reading of each group with 20,30,40,50 and 60 min. $* = (P > 0.05)$, $** = (P < 0.05)$, $*** = (P < 0.01)$ represents comparison of Group-II, III with Group-I. $^{p} = P > 0.05)$, $^{q} = (P < 0.05)$, $^{r} = (P < 0.01)$ compared Group IV with Group III. Group-I Normal Control; Group-II Normal treated (AEMC); Group-III Diabetic control; Group-IV diabetic treated (AEMC)

Discussion

Our hypothesis that AEMC might exert an incretin effect was supported by data obtained in this study. Fasting blood glucose levels in the normal control group remained unchanged throughout the experimental work. Administration of AEMC to normal rats showed reduction in blood sugar levels from day 1 to day 28. But in case of diabetic treated groups the blood sugar level reached near to normal control within 28 days of experiment. The antidiabetic effect of AEMC may be due to increased utilization of glucose, decreased absorption of glucose from GI tract, control on the insulin secretion or inhibition of the α-glucosidase activity.

AEMC has been reported to inhibit absorption of glucose by inhibiting α-glucosidase and suppressing the activity of disaccharidases in the intestine [32]. Whereas Lal et al. [33] experiment on diabetic rats, reported the hypoglycemic activity of AEMC. Results of other scientists [22, 34, 35] on AEMC treatment are also in conformity with the present work.

The Glycosylated hemoglobin (HbA1c) assay has become the most commonly used measure of chronic glycaemia in epidemiological studies, clinical trials and the management of diabetes. In the present study, the diabetic rats have shown significant increase in HbA1c level as compared to normal control which indicates that diabetic rats have poor glycemic control. The long term administration of aqueous extracts AEMC in diabetic rats results a significant decrease in the HbA1c levels in the diabetic rats, but no significant difference in HbA1c percentage found in normal treated groups. HbA1c levels which were noted in consistent with other reports may

be due to low plasma level of insulin or high glucose utilization in the peripheral tissues as reported in the present work. The various experimental reports obtained from recent papers on AEMC [22] and in *Elaeodendron glaucum* [36] concords with our results.

It is well known that in diabetes mellitus there will be marked depletion in glycogen storage in hepatic cells and muscle cells in diabetic rats. Liver glycogen and muscle glycogen is drastically reduced in diabetic group and on administration of AEMC for 28 days in the normal and diabetic rats corrects the glycogen level, but not equivalent to normal control group. The decrease in tissue glycogen may be due to enhanced catabolic process such as glycogenolysis, lipolysis and proteolysis, which are the outcomes of lack of insulin or oxidative stress by diabetes may inactive the oxygen synthase or decrease in GLUT4 transporter protein of muscles and cellular glucose in liver cells. Previous studies have validated that a number of plant materials induced an antidiabetic activity partly through stimulation of hepatic glycogenesis [37, 38]. Thus, the significantly higher liver glycogen content recorded in the Diabetic treated (Group IV) compared to the diabetic control (Group III) specified that AEMC was mediated by stimulating insulin secretion, retarding carbohydrates digestion, or by increasing hepatic glycogen synthesis.

In present investigation diabetic group showed low insulin level than control group which indicates the β-cell failure in diabetic rats. The insulin level increased nonsignificantly 20 to 60 min in short term administration of AEMC, but in diabetic AEMC treated serum insulin increased significantly. The possible mechanism behind

Table 5 The effect of single dose of *Momordica charantia* on GLP-1 level in normal and diabetic Wistar rats

Time in second	0 min	20 min	30 min	40 min	50 min	60 min
Group I	12.00 ± 0.288	15.20 ± 0.970	14.81 ± 0.788	13.81 ± 0.484	12.30 ± 0.463	12.08 ± 0.422
Group II	12.15 ± .669	20.00 ± 1.403$^{\beta***}$	17.28 ± 0.967$^{\alpha***}$	15.23 ± 0.871$^{\alpha*}$	14.75 ± 0.963$^{\alpha*}$	13.65 ± 1.007$^{\alpha*}$
Group III	5.10 ± 0.289	9.86 ± 0.603 $^{\gamma***}$	8.91 ± 0.534 $^{\gamma***}$	7.21 ± 0.391 $^{\beta***}$	6.35 ± 0.396$^{\alpha***}$	5.82 ± 0.311$^{\alpha***}$
Group IV	5.58 ± 0.733	11.80 ± 1.562$^{\gamma p}$	10.65 ± 1.327$^{\gamma p}$	8.61 ± 1.069$^{\alpha p}$	7.51 ± 0.938$^{\alpha p}$	6.46 ± 0.820$^{\alpha p}$

The values represent as Mean ± SEM for 6 rats each. The results are expressed in pg/mL. $\alpha = (P > 0.05)$, $\beta = (P < 0.05)$, $\gamma = (P < 0.01)$ represents comparison of 0 min reading of each group with 20,30,40,50 and 60 min. $* = (P > 0.05)$, $** = (P < 0.05)$, $*** = (P < 0.01)$ represents comparison of Group-III with Group-I. $^{p} = P > 0.05)$, $^{q} = (P < 0.05)$, $^{r} = (P < 0.01)$ compared Group IV with Group III. Group-I Normal Control; Group-II Normal treated (AEMC); Group-III Diabetic control; Group-IV diabetic treated (AEMC)

Table 6 The effect of long term exposure of *Momordica charantia* on GLP-1 level in normal and diabetic rats

Time in second	0 min	20 min	30 min	40 min	50 min	60 min
Group I	12.00 ± 0.288	15.20 ± 0.970	14.81 ± 0.788	13.81 ± 0.484	12.30 ± 0.463	12.08 ± 0.422
Group II	15.63 ± 0.841	23.73 ± 1.654$^{\gamma***}$	20.52 ± 1.090$^{\gamma***}$	18.66 ± 0.667$^{\alpha***}$	17.46 ± 0.507$^{\alpha***}$	16.33 ± 0.729$^{\alpha***}$
Group III	5.10 ± 0.289	9.86 ± 0.603$^{\gamma***}$	8.91 ± 0.534$^{\gamma***}$	7.21 ± 0.391$^{\beta***}$	6.35 ± 0.396$^{\alpha***}$	5.82 ± 0.311$^{\alpha***}$
Group IV	9.27 ± 0.638	37.72 ± 2.315$^{\gamma r}$	31.35 ± 1.704$^{\gamma r}$	22.71 ± 0.948$^{\gamma r}$	15.10 ± 0.276$^{\beta r}$	10.80 ± 0.600$^{\alpha r}$

The values represent as Mean ± SEM for 6 rats each. The results are expressed in pg/mL. $\alpha = (P > 0.05)$, $\beta = (P < 0.05)$, $\gamma = (P < 0.01)$ represents comparison of 0 min reading of each group with 20,30,40,50 and 60 min. $* = (P > 0.05)$, $** = (P < 0.05)$, $*** = (P < 0.01)$ represents comparison of Group-III with Group-I. $^{p} = P > 0.05)$, $^{q} = (P < 0.05)$, $^{r} = (P < 0.01)$ compared Group IV with Group III. Group-I Normal Control; Group-II Normal treated (AEMC); Group-III Diabetic control; Group-IV diabetic treated (AEMC)

the increase in insulin secretion in acute administration of AEMC might have increased the activity of β-cell receptors or showed insulin like activity, or decreases blood glucose concentrations by acting on GLUT-4. In sub-chronic administration of AEMC, the serum insulin level in diabetic treated groups increased as compared to diabetic group. Serum insulin was also increased in the normal AEMC treated rats. These results are in agreement with the findings of Rotshteyn and Zito [39] and Fernandes et al. [22]. This significant change in serum insulin level in long term exposure of AEMC might be due to increasing the number of β-cell receptors or β-cell proliferation. These results also suggest that AEMC increases the renewal and number of β cells in the pancreas as compared to untreated diabetic rats or may permit the recovery of STZ destroyed β cells and stimulates pancreatic insulin secretion [40]. In support with the present study the elevation of insulin levels was also observed with the administration of AEMC by other authors [36, 41].

Increase in GLP-1 level, from 0 to 60 min was observed in normal and diabetic rats in both short term and long term treatment with AEMC. In diabetic rats highest increase in GLP-1 level was at 20 min of AEMC administration, as compared to 0 min. The results also suggest that induction of GLP-1 on administration of AEMC was more pronounced in diabetic rats as compared to normal. It is possible that in normal rats high increase in GLP-1 is prohibited due to normal physiology and normal level of glucose regulating hormones including GLP-1. Since there is decrease in insulin as well as GLP-1 in diabetic rats, GLP-1 induction is more pounced to decrease enhanced glucose level. These findings indicate that the GLP-1 level is highly significant in sub-chronic administration of AEMC compared to acute administration of AEMC. The Mechanism of elevation of GLP-1 on sub-chronic administration of AEMC in normal and diabetic rats may be due to increased L-cell receptors or L-cell regeneration. The secretion of GLP-1 by AEMC may be due to the presence of sugars, amino acids, small peptides, water soluble alkaloids and plant secondary metabolites, which are known to stimulate GLP-1 secretion [42]. These nutrient molecules activate

the enteroendocrine cells of gut by G-protein coupled receptors [43].

In support with the present study Cicero and Tartagni [44] reported that administration of *Beriberis* plant at the dose of 500 mg/kg bw, showed that Berberine is an alkaloid present in *Beriberis* plant that affects glucose metabolism, increasing insulin secretion, stimulating glycolysis, Berberine also increases glucose transporter-4 (GLUT-4) and GLP-1 levels. Other results in support of increase in GLP-1 were observed in *Smallanthus sonchifolius* [45], *Agave tequilana* Gto. and *Dasylirion spp.* [46], *Ilex paraguariensis* [47], *Cinnamomum zeylanicum* [48], *Pinus koraiensis* [49], *Glycine max* [50] and *Berberis* [45].

Conclusion

Results of present study supported the traditional use of aqueous extract of *M. charantia* significantly for the hypoglycemic action in the management of diabetes.

Abbreviations

AEMC: Aqueous extract of *Momordica charantia*; AMPK: Adenosine monophosphate activated protein kinase; ANOVA: Analysis of variance; DM: Diabetes mellitus; DPP: Dipeptidyl peptidase; DRDE: Defence research & development establishment; ELISA: Enzyme linked immunosorbent assay; FBG: Fasting blood glucose; GI: Gastrointestinal; GLP-1: Glucagon like peptide; GLUT: Glucose transporter; HbA1C: Glycosilated haemoglobin; IAEC: Institutional animal ethics committee; KOH: Potassium hydroxide; PKC: Protein kinase-C; STZ: Streptozoticin; T2DM: Type 2 diabetes mellitus

Acknowledgements

We are thankful to Department of zoology, Hemvati Nandan Bahuguna Central University Garhwal Uttarakhand, India, for providing necessary facilities.

Funding

The authors would like to express their sincere appreciation to the Deanship of Scientific Research at the King Saud University, Riyadh, Saudi Arabia for funding this Research Group project no RGP-009.

Authors' contributions

GAB carried out the experiments and assisted with data analysis. HAK and ASA secured funding for project and help in manuscript preparation. PS participated in the design of the study. RS did extract preparation and assisted with manuscript preparation. BAP carried out subject recruitment, data collection, coordination of the study and compliance. All authors read and approved the final version of the manuscript.

Competing interests

The authors declare that they have no competing interests.

Author details

[1]Department of Zoology, HNB Central University Garhwal, Srinagar, Uttarakhand 249161, India. [2]Department of Biochemistry, College of Science, King Saud University, Riyadh 11451, Saudi Arabia. [3]Department of Zoology, Indira Gandhi National Tribal University, (A Central University), Amarkantak, M.P 484887, India. [4]Department of Biomedical Sciences, Bundelkhand University, Jhansi, India. [5]Zoology Department, College of Science, King Saud University, PO Box 2455, Riyadh 11451, Saudi Arabia.

References

1. Zimmet P, Alberti KG, Shaw J. Global and societal implications of the diabetes epidemic. Nature. 2001;414:782–7.
2. Unwin N, Whiting D, Gan D, Jacqmain O, Ghyoot G. IDF Diabetes Atlas. 4th ed. Brussels: International Diabetes Federation; 2009.
3. Raptis SA, Dimitriadis GD. Oral hypoglycemic agents: insulin secretagogues, alpha-glucosidase inhibitors and insulin sensitizers. Exp Clin Endocrinol Diabetes. 2001;109:265–87.
4. Huang TN, Lu KN, Pai YP, Chin H, Huan CJ. Role of GLP-1 in the hypoglycemi effects of wild bitter gourd. Evid Base Complement Alternat Med. 2013;625892:1-13.
5. Holz GG, Kühtreiber WM, Habener JF. Pancreatic beta-cells are rendered glucose-competent by the insulinotropic hormone glucagon-like peptide-1(7-37). Nature. 1993;361:362–5.
6. Wadkar KA, Magdum CS, Patil SS, Naikwade NS. Antidiabetic potential and Indian medicinal plants. J Herbal Med Toxicol. 2008;2:45–50.
7. Cefalu WT, Ye J, Wang ZQ. Efficacy of dietary supplementation with botanicals on carbohydrate metabolism in humans. Endocr Metab Immune Disord Drug Targets. 2008;8:78–81.
8. Joseph B, Jini D. Antidiabetic effects of Momordica charantia (bitter melon) and its medicinal potency. Asian Pac J Trop Dis. 2013;3:93–102.
9. Basch E, Gabardi S, Ulbricht C. Bittermelon (Momordica charantia): a review of efficacy and safety. Am J Health Syst Pharm. 2003;4:356–9.
10. Grover JK, Yadav SP. Pharmacological actions and potential uses of Momordica charantia: a review. J Ethnopharmacol. 2004;93(1):123–32.
11. Krawinkel MB, Keding GB. Bitter gourd (Momordica charantia): a dietary approach to hyperglycemia. Nutr Rev. 2006;64(7):331–7.
12. Ahmed I, Adeghate E, Sharma AK, Pallot DJ, Singh J. Effects of Momordica charantia fruit juice on islet morphology in the pancreas of the streptozotocin-diabetic rat. Diabetes Res Clin Pract. 1998;40(3):145–51.
13. Keller AC, Ma J, Kavalier A, He K, Brillantes AM, Kennelly EJ. Saponins from the traditional medicinal plant Momordica charantia stimulate insulin secretion in vitro. Phytomedicine. 2011;19(1):32–7.
14. Uebanso T, Arai H, Taketani Y, Fukaya M, Yamamoto H, Mizuno A, Uryu K, Hada T, Takeda E. Extracts of Momordica charantia suppress postprandial hyperglycemia in rats. J Nutr Sci Vitaminol. 2007;6:482–8.
15. Mahomoodally MF, Gurib-Fakim A, Subratty AH. Effect of exogenous ATP on Momordica charantia Linn.(Cucurbitaceae) induced inhibition of d-glucose, l-tyrosine and fluid transport across rat everted intestinal sacs in vitro. J Ethnopharmacol. 2007;110(2):257–63.
16. Tan MJ, Ye JM, Turner N, Hohnen-Behrens C, Ke CQ, Tang CP, Chen T, Weiss HC, Gesing ER, Rowland A, James DE, Ye Y. Antidiabetic activities of triterpenoids isolated from bitter melon associated with activation of the AMPK pathway. Chem Biol. 2008;15(3):263–73.
17. Cheng HL, Huang HK, Chang CI, Tsai CP, Chou CH. A cell-based screening identifies compounds from the stem of Momordica charantia that overcome insulin resistance and activate AMP-activated protein kinase. J Agric Food Chem. 2008;56(16):6835–43.
18. Shih CC, Lin CH, Lin WL, Wu JB. Momordica charantia extract on insulin resistance and the skeletal muscle GLUT4 protein in fructose-fed rats. J Ethnopharmacol. 2009;1:82–90.
19. Wang ZQ, Zhang XH, Yu Y. Bioactives from bitter melon enhance insulin signaling and modulate acyl carnitine content in skeletal muscle in high-fat diet-fed mice. J Nutr Biochem. 2011;22(11):1064–73.
20. Sarkar S, Pranava M, Marita RA. Demonstration of the hypoglycemic action of Momordica charantia in a validated animal model of diabetes. Pharmacol Res. 1996;33(1):1–4.
21. Fernandes NPC, Lagishetty CV, Panda VS, Naik SR. An experimental evaluation of the antidiabetic and antilipidemic properties of a standardized Momordica charantia fruit extract. BMC Complement Altern Med. 2007;7:29.
22. Lolitkar MM, Rao MRR. Note on a Hypoglycaemic principle isolated from the fruits of Momordica charantia. J Uni Bombay. 1962;29:223–4.
23. Sridhar MG, Vinayagamoorthi R, Suyambunathan VA, Bobby Z, Selvaraj N. Bitter gourd (Momordica charantia) improves insulin sensitivity by increasing skeletal muscle insulin-stimulated IRS-1 tyrosine phosphorylation in high-fat-fed rats. British J Nutr. 2008;99:806–12.
24. Kolawole OT, Ayankunle AA. Seasonal variation in the anti-diabetic and hypolipidemic effects of Momordica charantia fruit extract in rats. EJMP. 2012;2:177–85.
25. Nkambo W, Anyama NG, Onegi B. In vivo hypoglycemic effect of methanolic fruit extract of Momordica charantia. L. Afr Health Sci. 2013;13:933–9.
26. Vasconcelos CFB, Maranhão HML, Batista TM, Carneiro EM, Ferreira F, Costa J, Soares LAL, Sá MDC, Souza TP, Wanderley AG. Hypoglycaemic activity and molecular mechanisms of Caesalpinia ferrea Martius bark extract on streptozotocin-induced diabetes in Wistar rats. J Ethnopharmacol. 2011;137:1533–41.
27. Trivelli LA, Ranney HM, Lai HT. Hemoglobin components in patients with diabetes mellitus. New Eng J Med. 1971;284:357.
28. Nathan DM, Singer DE, Hurxthal K, Goodson JD. The clinical information value of the glycosylated hemoglobin assay. N Engl J Med. 1984;310:341–6.
29. Bunn HF. Evaluation of glycosylated hemoglobin in diabetic patients. Diabetes. 1981;30:613–7.
30. Toft-Nielsen M, Madsbad S, Holst J. Determints of the effectiveness of glucagon-like peptide-1 in type 2 diabetes. J Clin Endocrinol Metab. 2001;86:3853–60.
31. Meier J, Weyhe D, Michaely M, Senkal M, Zumtobel V, Nauck M, Holst J, Schmidt W, Gallwitz B. Intervenous glucagon-I-like peptide 1 normalizes blood glucose after major surgery in patients with type 2 diabetes. Crit Care Med. 2004;32:848–51.
32. Chaturvedi P. Antidiabetic potentials of Momordica charantia: multiple mechanisms behind the effects. J Med Food. 2012;15:101–7.
33. Lal VK, Gupta PP, Tripathi P, Pandey A. Interaction of aqueous extract of Momordica charantia fruits with Glibenclamide in Streptozotocin induced diabetic rats. American. J Pharmacol Toxicol. 2011;6:102–6.
34. Matheka DM, Alkizim FO, Kiama TN, Bukachi F. Glucose-lowering effects of Momordica charantia (Karela) extract in diabetic rats. AJPT. 2012;1:62–6.
35. Nagy MA, Bastawy MA, Abdel-Hamid NM. Effects of Momordica charantia on Streptozotocin-induced diabetes in rats: role of insulin, oxidative stress and nitric oxide. J Health Sci. 2012;2:8–13.
36. Lanjhiyana S, Garabadu D, Ahirwar D, Bigoniya P, Rana A, Patra K, Lanjhiyana S, Karuppaih MP. Antidiabetic activity of methanolic extract of stem bark of Elaeodendron glaucum Pers. in Alloxanized rat model. Adv Appl Sci Res. 2011;2:47–62.
37. Habibuddin M, Daghriri HA, Humaira T, AlQahtani MS, Hefzi AA. Antidiabetic effect of alcoholic extract of Caralluma sinaica L. on streptozotocin- induced diabetic rabbits. J Ethnopharmacol. 2008;117:215–20.
38. Jain S, Bhatia G, Barik R, Kumar P, Jain A, Dixit VK. Antidiabetic activity of Paspalum scrobiculatum Linn. In alloxan induced diabetic rats. J Ethnopharmacol. 2010;127:325–8.
39. Rotshteyn Y, Zito SW. Application of modified in vitro screening procedure for identifying herbals possessing sulfonylurea-like activity. J Ethnopharmacol. 2004;9:337–44.
40. Kumar DS, Sharathnath KV, Yogeswaran P, Harani A, Sudhakar K, Sudha P, Banji D. A medicinal potency of Momordica charantia. Int J Pharma Sci Rev Res. 2010;1:95–100.
41. Saha SK, Haque E, Islam D, Rahman M, Islam R, Parvin A, Rahman S. Comparative study between the effect of Momordica charantia (wild and hybrid variety) on hypoglycemic and hypolipidemic activity of alloxan induced type 2 diabetic long-evans rats. J Diabetes Mellitus. 2012;2:131–7.
42. Ramos SM, Tovar AR, Torres N. Diet: friend or foe of enteroendocrine cells–how it interacts with enteroendocrine cells. Adv Nutr. 2012;3:8–20.
43. Reimann F, Tolhurst G, Gribble FM. G-protein-coupled receptors in intestinal chemo-sensation. Cell Metabol. 2012;15:421–31.

44. Cicero AF, Tartagni E. Antidiabetic properties of berberine: from cellular pharmacology to clinical effects. Hosp Pract (Minneap). 2012;40:56–63.

45. Habib NC, Honoré SM, Genta SB, Sánchez SS. Hypolipidemic effect of Smallanthus sonchifolius (yacon) roots on diabetic rats. Chem Biol Interact. 2011;194:31–9.

46. Silvas UJE, Cani PD, Delmée E, Neyrinck A, López MG, Delzenne NM. Physiological effects of dietary fructans extracted from *Agave tequilana* Gto. And *Dasylirion spp*.Unidad de Biotecnología e Ingeniería Genética de Plantas, México. Br J Nutr. 2008;99:254–61.

47. Hussein GM, Matsuda H, Nakamura S, Hamao M, Akiyama T, Yoshikawa TK. Mate tea (*Ilex paraguariensis*) promotes satiety and body weight lowering in mice: involvement of glucagon-like peptide-1. Biol Pharm Bull. 2011;34: 1849–55.

48. Hlebowicz J, Hlebowicz A, Lindstedt S, Björgell O, Höglund P, Holst JJ, Darwiche G, Almér LO. Effects of 1 and 3 g cinnamon on gastric emptying, satiety, and postprandial blood glucose, insulin, glucose-dependent insulinotropic polypeptide, glucagon-like peptide 1, and ghrelin concentrations in healthy subjects. Am J Clin Nutr. 2009;89:815–21.

49. Pasman WJ, Heimerikx J, Rubingh CM, Berg R, O'Shea M, Gambelli L, Hendriks HF, Einerhand AW, Scott C, Keizer HG, Mennen LI. The effect of Korean pine nut oil on in vitro CCK release, on appetite sensations and on gut hormones in post-menopausal overweight women. Lipids Health Dis. 2008;20:10.

50. Park S, Ahn IS, Kim JH, Lee MR, Kim JS, Kim HJ. Glyceollins, one of the phytoalexins derived from soybeans under fungal stress, enhance insulin sensitivity and exert insulinotropic actions. J Agric Food Chem. 2010;58:1551–7.

7

Antibacterial mechanism of chelerythrine isolated from root of *Toddalia asiatica* (Linn) Lam

Nan He[†], Peiqing Wang[†], Pengyu Wang[1], Changyang Ma[1,2*] and Wenyi Kang[1,2*] (iD)

Abstract

Background: Antimicrobial resistance was one of serious worldwide problems confused many researchers. To solve this problem, we explored the antibacterial effect of chelerythrine, a natural compound from traditional Chinese medicine and studied its action.

Methods: The contents of chelerythrine from different fractions of *Toddalia asiatica* (Linn) Lam (*T. asiatica*) were determined. The anti-bacterial activities of chelerythrine were tested by disc diffusion method (K-B method). Scanning electron microscopy (SEM), alkaline phosphatase (AKP), bacterial extracellular protein leakage and SDS-PAGE analysis were also used to investigate the antibacterial mechanism of chelerythrine.

Results: Analytic results of High Performance Liquid Chromatography showed that the content of chelerythrine (1.97 mg/g) in the ethyl acetate fraction was the highest, followed by those of methanol fraction and petroleum ether fraction. The in vitro anti-bacterial mechanisms of chelerythrine from *T. asiatica* were assessed. Chelerythrine showed strong antibacterial activities against Gram-positive bacteria, *Staphylococcus aureus* (SA), Methicillin-resistant *S. aureus* (MRSA), and extended spectrum β-lactamase *S. aureus* (ESBLs-SA). The minimum inhibitory concentrations (MICs) of chelerythrine on three bacteria were all 0.156 mg/mL. Furthermore, results suggested that the primary anti-bacterial mechanism of chelerythrine may be attributed to its destruction of the channels across the bacterial cell membranes, causing protein leakage to the outside of the cell, and to its inhibition on protein biosynthesis. Images of scanning electron microscope revealed severe morphological changes in chelerythrine-treated bacteria except control, damage of parts of the cell wall and cell membrane as well as the leakage of some substances.

Conclusions: Chelerythrine isolated from root of *Toddalia asiatica* (Linn) Lam possesses antibacterial activities through destruction of bacterial cell wall and cell membrance and inhibition of protein biosynthesis.

Keywords: Chelerythrine, Antibacterial mechanism, *Toddalia asiatica* (Linn) Lam., HPLC, *Staphylococcus aureus*

Background

With the increasing and widespread use of antibiotics, a large percentage of microorganisms have developed antimicrobial resistance, causing economic loss and even death. Thus, searching new class of effective antimicrobial agents is essential to cope with the continuous emergence of multi-drug-resistance of bacteria, especially resistance to anti-staphylococcal drugs. More and more phytochemicals derived from plants have been considered as a potential

source of promising antibacterial agents [1]. Some components extracted from natural plants showed inhibitory effects against *Staphylococcus aureus* (SA) at low dose. However, the underlying antimicrobial action mechanisms of most natural components are currently unknown [2]. It is quite possible that promising natural compounds can be discovered as the new antibiotic drugs [3].

T. asiatica, belonging to the family Rutaceae, distributes in the dry areas full of hedges and bushes [4]. The root and bark of *T. asiatica* have been used in traditional medicine to treat malaria, diarrhea, cholera and cough [5]. Its leaves have been used to treat lung and skin diseases, and rheumatism [6]. Moreover, the plant also

* Correspondence: macaya1024@sina.com; kangweny@hotmail.com
[†]Nan He and Peiqing Wang contributed equally to this work.
[1]Institute of Chinese Materia Medica, Henan University, Kaifeng 475004, Henan, China
Full list of author information is available at the end of the article

possesses antimicrobial, larvicidal, antidiabetic, anti-oxidant, antinocieptive and anti-inflammatory activities [7–9]. It has been reported that the root and duramen of *T. asiatica* are mainly rich in coumarins, triterpenoids and alkaloids [10–12]. In our previous research, we isolated thirteen compounds from the petroleum fraction and the ethyl acetate fraction of roots of *T. asiatica* and identified them [13, 14]. These compounds were screened out based on anti-bacterial activities. Among them, chelerythrine showed more effective and potent antibacterial activity. Chelerythrine is a kind of benzo [c] phenanthridine alkaloids with many pharmacological activities, such as anti-cancer, anti-bacterial, anti-inflammatory, insecticide, anti-fibrosis activities, etc. [15–19]. In past decades, a majority of studies were focused on its anti-cancer and anti-bacterial activities. It has been suggested by a previous study that chelerythrine may possess antibacterial activities and its antibacterial action mechanisms of chelerythrine against bacterium may be related to its inhibitory effects on DNA synthesis, proteinase synthesis and membrane permeability of bacterium [20]. However, its exact action mechanisms against bacteria are currently unclear and need be further elucidated. Therefore, in this paper, we focused on elucidating its antibacterial mechanisms by detecting the changes in cell wall and cell membrane electrical conductivity,

alkaline phosphatase (AKP), extracellular proteins, electrophoresis protein bands with SEM and TEM.

Methods
Bacterial strains and bacterial culture
Staphylococcus aureus (SA) 25,923 was purchased from Shanghai Tiancheng Bio-information and Technology Co., Ltd., (Shanghai, China). MRSA and ESBLs-SA were provided by Huaihe Hospital (Kaifeng, Henan, China), and identified by Vitek-AMS (Automated Microbic System).

The three *S. aureus*s trains were activated and inoculated into Broth Agar Medium at 37 °C for 24 h in a thermostat, and then bacterial concentration was diluted with sterile broth agar to 10^6 CFU/mL.

Preparation of extracts and drugs
The roots of *T. asiatica* (200801) were collected from Guizhou province, China, in September 2008 and identified by Professor Zhiyou Guo, Qian Nan Normal College for Nationalities, Guizhou, China. The voucher specimen was stored at the Institute of Chinese Materia Medica, Henan University (Kaifeng, Henan, China).

Root powder of *T. asiatica* (1.3 kg) was extracted three times with methanol for 7 days each time. Then the extracts were evaporated and dried under reduced pressure. The concentrated extract was mixed with silica gel, and

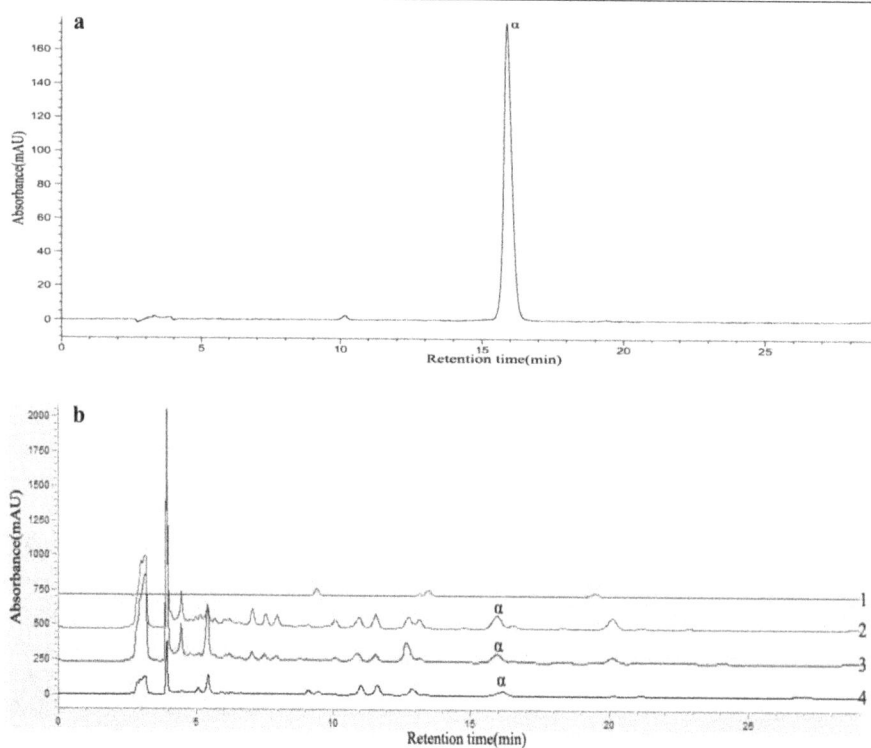

Fig. 1 HPLC chromatograms of (**a**) standard and (**b**) *T. asiatica* fractions (peak α, Chelerythrine). Petroleum ether fraction (1), Ethyl acetate fraction (2), Methanol fraction (3), and Methanol extract (4)

Table 1 Contents (mg/g) of chelerythrine in different fractions extracted from roots of *T. asiatica*

Standard	Petroleum ether fraction	Ethyl acetate fraction	Methanol fraction	Methanol extract
Chelerythrine	ND	1.97	1.19	0.66

ND not detected

eluted successively with petroleum ether, ethyl acetate and methanol to obtain petroleum ether fraction, ethyl acetate fraction and methanol fraction, respectively.

Ethyl acetate fraction was loaded to silica gel column and eluted with CH_2Cl_2: MeOH (v:v = 100:1~ 8:2). Ten sub-fractions were obtained. After the sixth subfraction was repeatly subjected to silica gel column and Sephadex LH-20, chelerythrine (24.5 mg) was obtained. The purity of chelerythrine was higher than 98%. The NMR data of chelerythrine were published on China Pharmacist [14].

Analysis of chelerythrine by HPLC

The HPLC analysis was carried out in an Agilent 1260. Agilent TC-C_{18} column (250 mm × 4.6 mm, 5 μm) with acetonitrile and water containing 0.4% phosphoric acid (30:70) as mobile phase were used. The column temperature was set at 30 °C. The detection wavelength was at 258 nm, the flow rate was 1.0 mL/min and the injection volume was 10 μL.

Antibacterial activity

Antibacterial activity of chelerythrine was tested by disc diffusion test. Sample solution was obtained after dissolving chelerythrine (50 μg) with DMSO (1 mL). Filter paper discs of 6 mm diameter were impregnated with 5 μL of sample solution. A disc prepared with corresponding volume of DMSO was used as negative control and that prepared with berberine was used as the positive control. The plates were incubated at 37 °C for 24 h. Antimicrobial activity was evaluated by measuring the diameter of the inhibition zone (IZ) [21].

According to the results of IZ method, bacteriostatic ring was > 8 mm, then its minimum inhibitory concentration

(MIC) was determined in triplicate by the tube doubling dilution method, and the test sample was serially obtained a series of concentration. MICs were defined as the lowest sample concentration that exhibited IZ.

Inhibitory effects on the bacterial cell wall

Chelerythrine at MIC and 3 × MIC were mixed with bacterial suspension ($5 × 10^6$ CFU). Sterile water was used as negative control group. All the groups were cultured in incubator at 37 °C and time sampling method (0 h, 0.17 h, 0.33 h, 0.5 h, 1 h, 2 h, 3 h, 4 h, 5 h, 7 h, and 9 h) was adopted. Then the testing objects were centrifuged at 3500 rpm for 10 min, the content of AKP in supernatant was measured by the AKP kit assay with time.

Determination of soluble protein

Coomassie brilliant blue method was used to determine the concentration of soluble protein in bacterial suspension treated with chelerythrine (MIC and 3 × MIC) and the control groups, respectively. After resting for 10 min, OD values of all groups were measured with spectrophotometer at 595 nm.

SDS-page

The chelerythrine solution at MIC was added to bacterial suspension and the mixed suspension was cultivated at 37 °C for 24 h. Sterile water was used as negative control. Mixed solution (12 mL) was sampled at 3, 6 and 9 h, respectively. After the samples were diluted and adjusted into the same OD value, the precipitations were obtained by centrifuge, and then 80 μL of sterile water and 20 μL of 5 × SDS sample buffer precipitation were added, mixed thoroughly and boiled in a water bath at 100 °C for 5 min, the solution was centrifuged again and supernatant on standby was collected and used as protein extracts.

The vertical slab gel electrophoresis made from 8% of separating gel and 5% of stacking gel was used to separate proteins. 5 μL of protein maker and 15 μL of each sample were drawn with micro pipette tips. At first, the voltage

Table 2 Inhibition zones of antimicrobial activity of *T. asiatica* fractions and Chelerythrine

Samples	Concentration(mg/mL)	Inhibition zones(mm)		
		SA	MRSA	ESBLs-SA
Petroleum ether fraction	50	8.13 ± 0.18	9.21 ± 0.18	–
Ethyl acetate fraction	50	8.06 ± 0.13	8.00 ± 0.18	–
Methanol fraction	50	7.95 ± 0.28	–	–
Chelerythrine	10	19.07 ± 0.19	18.12 ± 0.14	16.93 ± 0.23
Blank		–	–	–
DMSO		–	–	–
Berberine	2.5	15.04 ± 0.31	15.89 ± 0.24	16.27 ± 0.19

(−) no activity; Berberine-positive control

Table 3 MICs of *T. asiatica* fractions and chelerythrine against SA, MRSA and ESBLs-SA

Tested bacteria	MIC(mg/mL)				
	Pe	Ea	Me	Che	Ber
Staphylococcus aureus	50	50	50	0.156	0.0312
Methicillin-resistant *S.aureus*	25	50	NT	0.156	0.0312
Extended spectrum β-lactamases *S.aureus*	NT	NT	NT	0.156	0.0312

NT not test, *Pe* Petroleum ether fraction, *Ea* Ethyl acetate fraction, *Me* Methanol fraction, *Che* Chelerythrine, and *Ber* Berberine

was set at 60 V and electrophoresis was run, when the bands of samples passed into separating gel, the voltage was adjusted to 120 V and electrophoresis was continuously run until the blue ribbons was one or two centimeters distant from the bottom edge of the gel. The power was turned off and rubber blocks were taken out and stained with Coomassie brilliant blue for 3 h. Thereafter, the stained rubber blocks were de-stained with destainer in a shaking table up to appearing clear bands.

Scanning electron microscope (SEM) and transmission electron microscope (TEM)

Chelerythrine (1 × MIC) was added with bacteria at the concentration of 10^9 CFU/mL for a shaking Table (150 r/min) for 1.5 h and 6 h at 37 °C, respectively. Distilled water was used as control. The depositions were collected by

centrifugation and fixed with 2.5% glutaraldehyde at 4 °C overnight, and washed three times with 0.1 M phosphate buffer solution (PBS, PH 7.2). The samples were dehydrated in a graded series of alcohols (30, 50, 70, 85, 90 and 100%). Tert-butanol was used to replace the ethanol twice before coating onto the metal foil. Eventually, the cells were dried by freeze-drying apparatus (ALPHA1–4, Christ, Germany), and visualized under a scanning electron microscopy (SEM, JSM-5600LV, JEOL, Japan) and a transmission electron microscopy (TEM, JEM-2010, JEOL, Japan), respectively.

Results

Determination of Chelerythrine in *T. asiatica*
The typical chromatograms were showed in Fig. 1. The contents of each sample were presented in Table 1. There content of chelerythrine (1.97 mg/g) in ethyl acetate fraction was the highest among all the samples, while no chelerythrine was detected in petroleum ether fraction.

Antibacterial activity in vitro
In Table 2 and Table 3, petroleum ether fraction and ethyl acetate fraction of roots of *T. asiatica* inhibited the *S. aureus* and the Methicillin-resistant *S. aureus* at the same concentration (50 mg/mL). The IZs of chelerythrine

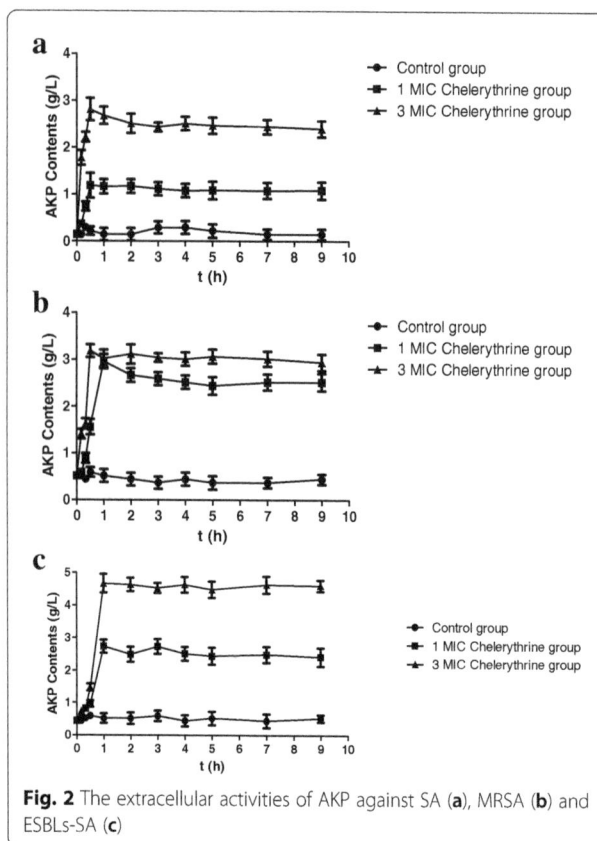

Fig. 2 The extracellular activities of AKP against SA (**a**), MRSA (**b**) and ESBLs-SA (**c**)

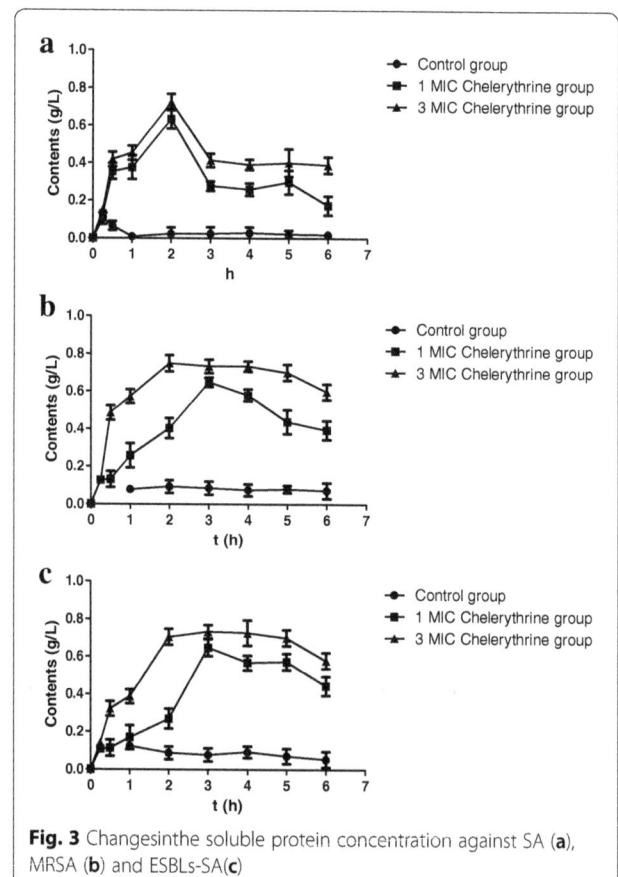

Fig. 3 Changesinthe soluble protein concentration against SA (**a**), MRSA (**b**) and ESBLs-SA(**c**)

Antibacterial mechanism of chelerythrine isolated from root of Toddalia asiatica (Linn) Lam

(10 mg/mL) against SA, MRSA and ESBLs-SA were 19.07 ± 0.19 mm, 18.12 ± 0.14 mm and 16.93 ± 0.23 mm, respectively, and its MICs against three bacteria were 0.156 mg/mL, 0.156 mg/mL and 0.156 mg/mL, respectively.

Antibacterial mechanisms of chelerythrine
Effects on the cell wall of SA, MRSA and ESBLs-SA
Fig. 2 showed that after chelerythrine was added to bacteria, the contents of AKP were increased rapidly and reached the highest level in 1 h as compared to those of the control group. There was a positive correlation between the concentration of chelerythrine and AKP leakage, suggesting that chelerythrine can destroy cell wall of bacteria and lead to the increased AKP leakage for a short period of time.

Effects on the contents of extracellular proteins of SA, MRSA and ESBLs-SA
Fig. 3 showed that concentrations of soluble proteins were increased with increasing the concentrations of

chelerythrine, demonstrating that chelerythrine may cause damage to bacteria and lead to exclusion of soluble proteins, which can, in turn, result in offsetting parts of the proteins consumed by bacteria. The concentrations reached a maximum for SA at 2 h and for MRSA and ESBLs-SA at 2.5 h.

Changes in levels of six bacterial proteins reavealed by SDS-PAGE analysis
In Fig. 4a, six bands (a, b, c, d, e, and f) in map of SA exhibited more obvious changes.

In Fig. 4b, the g-band (72KDa-95KDa) became shallower while h-band (43KDa-55KDa), i-band (34KDa-43KDa) and j-band (34KDa) disappeared at 3 h.

In Fig. 4c, k-band (72KDa-95KDa), l-band (43KDa-55KDa), m-band (43KDa-55KDa), n-band (43KDa) and o-band (34KDa) were becoming shallower or even disappeared as compared with those of the corresponding control groups at 3 h, 6 h and 9 h, respectively, suggesting that

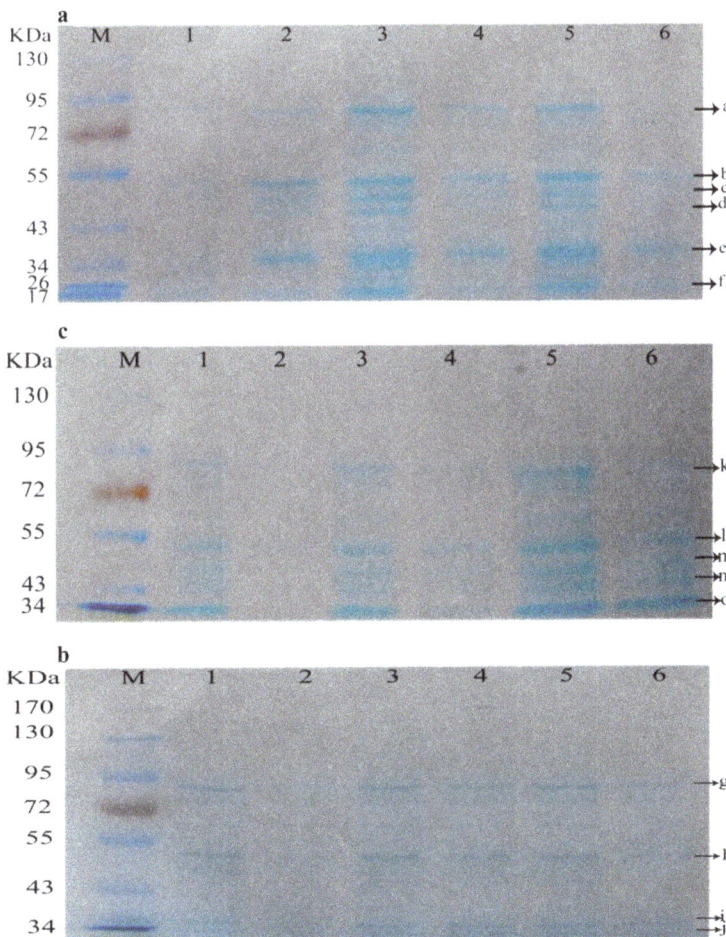

Fig. 4 Changes in SDS-PAGE profiles of SA (**a**), MRSA (**b**) and ESBLs-SA (**c**) affected by chelerythrine. Lanes 1, 3 and 5: Normal electrophoretic bands of SA, MRSA, and ESBLs-SA for 3 h, 6 h, 9 h respectively(control groups); Lanes 2, 4, 6: Electrophoretic bands of SA, MRSA, and ESBLs-SA affected by chelerythrine treatment for 3, 6 and 9 h, respectively

chelerythrine inhibits the expression of these proteins and synthesis of ESBLs-SA.

Ultrastructural changes

The morphology of bacterial cells was examined by transmission electron microscopy (TEM) (Fig. 5). The bacteria of control group (Fig. 5a, d and g) displayed a spherical cell morphology that had a round and plump form without damaged surface. However, the external parts of the bacteria treated with chelerythrine adhered floc and a few cells became smaller or broken.

In Fig. 6, TEM images showed that severe morphological changes were visualized in these chelerythrine-treated bacteria but such changes were not seen in control group (Fig. 6a, d and g), parts of the cell wall and cell membrane were damaged and some substances were leaked.

Discussion

The present study showed that chelerythrine exhibited strong antibacterial effect. Results of HPLC suggested that chelerythrine in ethyl acetate fraction was highest and chelerythrine in petroleum ether fraction was lowest among four samples examined. However, the antibacterial activity of petroleum ether fraction was higher than that of ethyl acetate fraction, which might be due to the reason that other constituent of fractions also contribute to antibacterial functions [22] and the exact reasons need be further studied.

We valued the integrity of the bacterial cell wall by measuring contents of AKP. AKP in bacteria mainly exists between the cell wall and cell membrane of the bacteria. AKP will be leaked into the extracellular by increasing the permeability of bacterial cell wall. The results of AKP can reflect the integrity of the bacterial cell wall indirectly [23, 24]. The results in our study

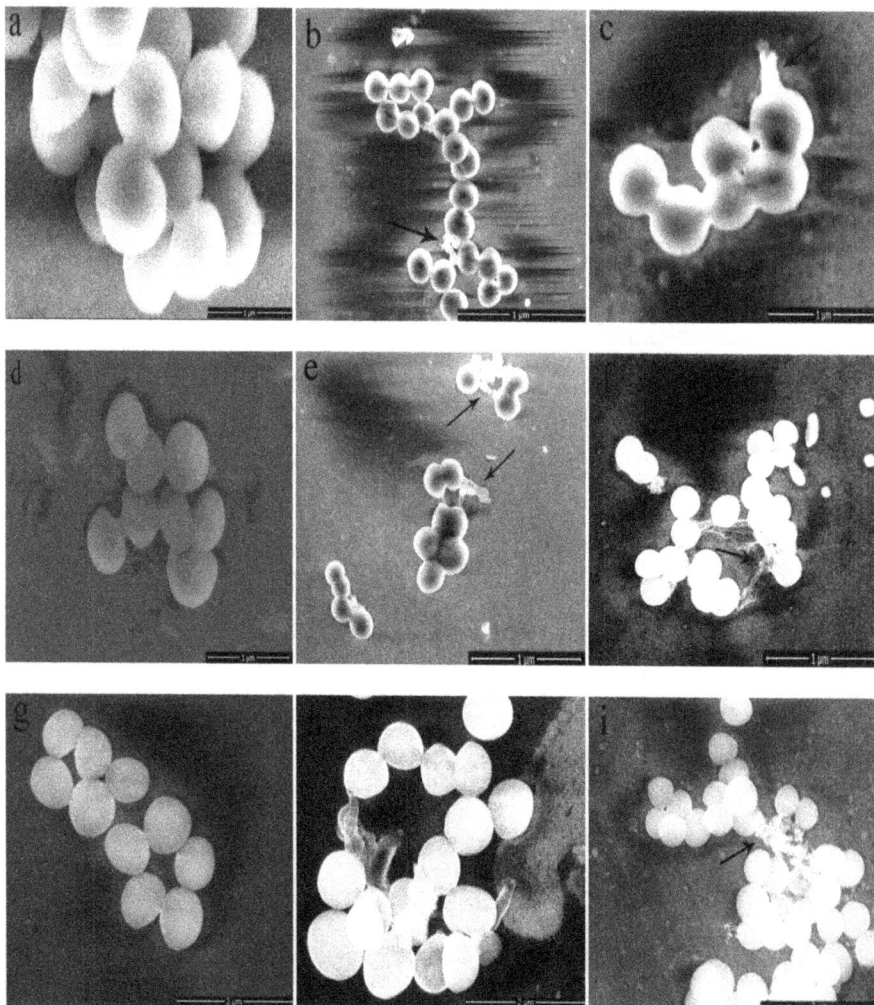

Fig. 5 SEM images of SA (**a**, **b** and **c**), MRSA (**d**, **e** and **f**) and ESBLs-SA (**g**, **h** and **i**) treated by chelerythrine for 1.5 h (**b**, **e** and **h**), 6 h (**c**, **f**, **i**); and control (**a**, **d** and **g**)

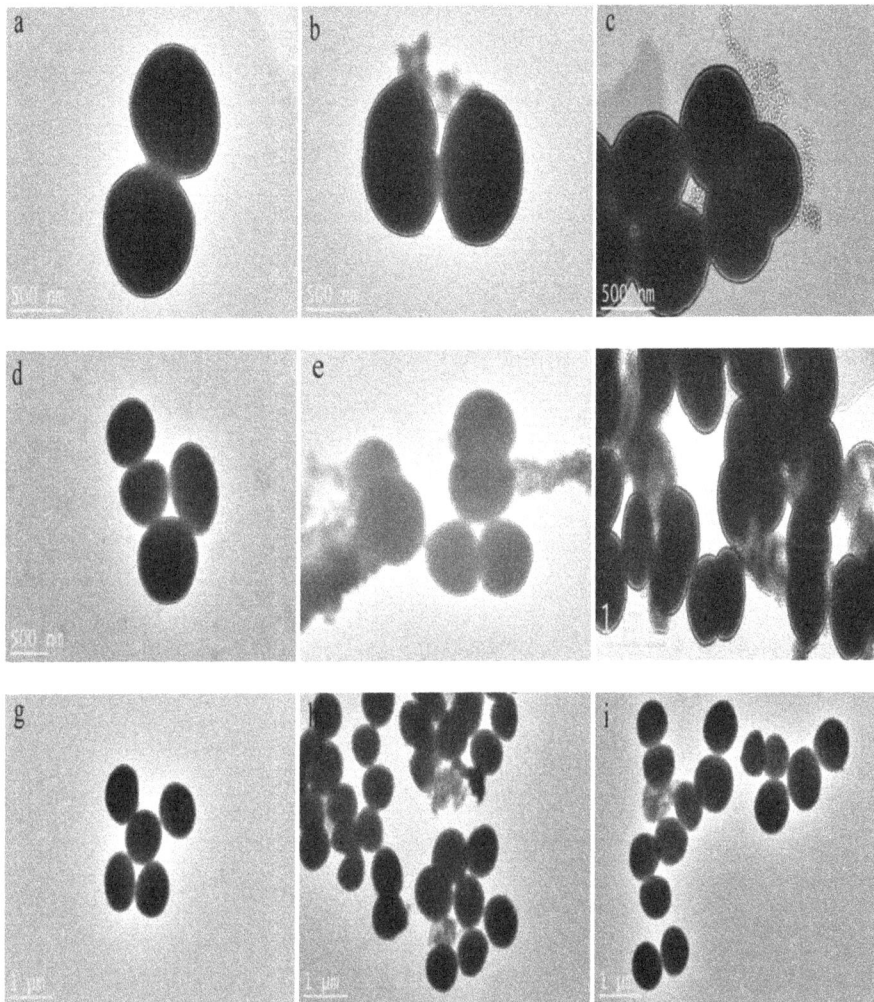

Fig. 6 TEM images of SA (**a**, **b** and **c**), MRSA (**d**, **e** and **f**) and ESBLs-SA (**g**, **h** and **i**) treated by chelerythrine for 1.5 h (**b**, **e** and **h**), 6 h (**c**, **f** and **i**); and control (**a**, **d** and **g**)

showed the permeability of cell walls of three bacterial strains could be increased by chelerythrine in a short-period of time.

Effects on cell membrane were also tested by measuring the leakage of intracellular soluble protein and the electrical conductivity of the bacteria solution [25]. We observed that chelerythrine imposed certain effects on the cell membrane of three strains of bacteria. There are positive correlations between protein leakage of proteins and chelerythrine concentration. It is suggested that the permeability of cell membrane of three bacteria was increased. 2.5 h later the bacterial protein concentrations were decreased gradually. This may be due to the reason that the effect of chelerythrine is decreased with time and the remaining bacteria still grow and consume the soluble proteins in the bacterial fluid. It also may be due to the reason that bacteria have been infringed and activated the self-healing mechanism, which directly caused

a reduction of protein leakage. Therefore, the leaked proteins were not sufficient to offset the consumption of proteins.

SDS-PAGE electrophoresis bands protein were clearly changed when bacteria were treated with Chelerythrine ($1 \times MIC$). In Fig. 4a, the protein bands of treatment groups were darker than the corresponding bands of control groups at 3 h because of the self-repairing mechanism of SA after being treated with chelerythrine and the synthesis of these proteins was accelerated to meet the needs of self-repairing cells. The six bands became shallower or even disappeared as compared with the corresponding bands of the control groups at 6 h and 9 h, which illustrated that there was certain suppression on normal metabolism of proteins. In brief, chelerythrine showed the inhibitory activity on SA by decreasing expression of the bacterial proteins. In Fig. 4b, the disappeared bands [h-band (43KDa-55KDa), i-band (34KDa-43KDa) and j-band (34KDa)] reappeared at 6 h and 9 h but were thinner than those of the control. Results showed that chelerythrine effectively inhibited the expression of such proteins in 3 h, the longer the MRSA were treated, the less effect the chelerythrine caused. On the other hand, the remaining MRSA continued to grow and the synthesis of these proteins was increased, indicating that chelerythrine can hinder protein expression of MRSA.

The morphology of bacterial cells was examined by transmission electron microscopy and results showed that parts but not all of cell membrane and cell wall of bacteria were broken, which this needs further explore.

Conclusions

Chelerythrine is one of the major antibacterial ingredients in *T. asiatica*. The results obtained in this paper indicate that chelerythrine may be capable of destroying the cell wall and membrane of bacterial cells, leading to the increased membrane permeability, thereby causing the cellular contents to leak extracellularly. Meanwhile, chelerythrine could affect and hinder the bacterial protein expression and synthesis, eventually leading to cell death. Together, these results provide additional supporting evidence that chelerythrine can be a natural bactericide.

Funding

This work was supported by Grant (2017YFC1601400) from the Ministry of Science and Technology of the People's Republic of China, Henan Province University Science and Technology Innovation Team (16IRTSTHN019), National Cooperation Project of Henan Province (2015GH12). The materials and analysis were supported by funding.

Authors' contributions

HN, WPQ, WPY, MCY and KWY conceived and designed the experiments. HN, WPQ and MCY performed the experiments. WPY and MCY made substantial contributions to interpretation of data. HN wrote the first draft of the manuscript. MCY and KWY revised the draft and approved the version submitted. All authors read and approved the final manuscript.

Competing interests

The authors declare that they have no competing interests.

Author details

[1]Institute of Chinese Materia Medica, Henan University, Kaifeng 475004, Henan, China. [2]Kaifeng Key Laboratory of Functional Components in Health Food, Kaifeng 475004, Henan, China.

References

1. Gibbons S. Anti-staphylococcal plant natural products. Nat Prod Rep. 2004; 21(2):263–77. [View Article]
2. Sharma A, Gupta S, Sarethy IP, Dang S, Gabrani R. Green tea extract: possible mechanism and antibacterial activity on skin pathogens. Food Chem. 2012;135(2):672–5. [View Article]
3. Wright HT, Reynolds KA. Antibacterial targets in fatty acid biosynthesis. Curr Opin Microb. 2007;10(5):447–53. [View Article]
4. Ramaraj T, Rajarajeswaran J, Murugaiyan P. Analysis of chemical composition and evaluation of antigenotoxic, cytotoxic and antioxidant activities of essential oil of *Toddalia asiatica* (L.) lam. Asian Pac J Trop Biomed. 2012;z3: 1276–S1279. [View Article]
5. Duraipandiyan V, Ignacimuthu S. Antibacterial and antifungal activity of Flindersine isolated from the traditional medicinal plant, *Toddalia asiatica*(L.) lam. J Ethnopharmacol. 2009;123(3):494–8. [View Article]
6. Karunai RM, Balachandran C, Duraipandiyan V, Agastian P, Ignacimuthu S. Antimicrobial activity of Ulopterol isolated from *Toddalia asiatica* (L.) lam.: a traditional medicinal plant. J Ethnopharmacol. 2012;140(1):161–5. [View Article]
7. Liu XC, Dong HW, Zhou L, Du SS, Liu ZL. Essential oil composition and larvicidal activity of Toddalia asiatica roots against the mosquito *Aedes albopictus* (Diptera: Culicidae). Parasit Res. 2013;112(3):1197–203. [View Article]
8. Santiagu SI, Christudas S, Veeramuthu D, Savarimuthu I. Antidiabetic and antioxidant activities of *Toddalia asiatica* (L.) Lam. leaves in Streptozotocin induced diabetic rats. J Ethnopharmacol. 2012;143(2):515–23. [View Article]
9. Kariuki HN, Kanui T, Yenesew A, Patel N, Mbugua PM. Antinocieptive and anti-inflammatory effects of *Toddalia asiatica* (L) Lam. (Rutaceae) root extract in Swiss albino mice. Pan Afr Med J. 2013;14:133. [View Article]
10. Shi L, Li D, Kang WY. Research progress on chemical constituents and pharmacological activities of *Toddalia asiatica* (L.) lam. China Pharm. 2011; 22:666–8.
11. Wang F, Xu Y, Liu JK. New geranyloxy coumarins from *Toddalia asiatica*. J Asian Nat Prod Res. 2009;11(8):752–6. [View Article]
12. Muthumani P, Meera R, Devi P, Mohamed SA, Arabat S, Seshu Kumar Koduri LV, Manavarthi S. Chemical investigation of *Toddalia asiatica* Lin. and *Cardiospermum halicacabum* Lin. Int J Drug Formul Res. 2010;1:224–39. [View Ariticle]
13. Shi L, Wang W, Ji ZQ, Kang WY. Study on chemical constituents in methanol parts of *Toddalia asiatica*. China Pharm. 2014;17:534–7.
14. Shi L, Ji ZQ, Zhang ZW, Li YY. Chemical constituents in ethyl acetate parts of *Toddalia asiatica* (Lin.) lam. China Pharm. 2013;16:1293–5.
15. Chmura SJ, Dolan ME, Cha A, Mauceri HJ, Kufe DW, Weichselbaum RR. In vitro and in vivo activity of protein kinase C inhibitor chelerythrine chloride induces tumorcell toxicity and growth delay in vivo. Clin Cancer Res. 2000; 6(2):737–42. [View Article]
16. Zdařilová A, Malíková J, Dvořák Z, Ulrichováá J, Šimáne kV. Quaternary isoquinoline alkaloids sanguinarine andchelerythrinein vitro and in vivo effects. Chem Listy. 2006;100(1):30.
17. Niu XF, Zhou P, Li WF, Xu HB. Effects of chelerythrine, a specific inhibitor of cyclooxygenase-2, on acute inflammation in mice. Fitoterapia. 2011;82:620–5. [View Article]
18. Miao F, Yang XJ, Ma YN, Zheng F, Song XP, Zhou L. Structural modification of Sanguinarine and Chelerythrine and their in vitro Acaricidal activity against Psoroptescuniculi. Chem Pharm Bull. 2012;60(12):1508–13. [View Article]
19. Szeto CC, Lai KB, Chow KM, CYK S, Wong YK, PKT L. Differential effects of transforming growth factor-beta on the synthesis of connective tissue growth factor and vascular endothelial growth factor by peritoneal mesothelial cell. Nephron Exp Nephrol. 2005;99(4):e95–e104. [View Article]
20. Wang PQ, Yin ZH, Kang WY. Research Progress on Pharmacological Activities of Chelerythrine. China. J Chin Mater Med. 2013;38:2745–9.
21. Wei JF, Zhang Q, Zhao L, Kang WY. Antimicrobial activity of *Musa basjoo* in vitro. Chin J Exp Med Formul. 2010;16(17):69–71. [View Article]
22. Ding W, Wen CF, Chen JH, Huang KX, Dong AW. Primary study on antibacterial activity of extracts from *Toddalia asiatica* (Linn.) lam. Biomass. Chemical. Engineering. 2007;41(5):33–5.
23. Hara S, Yamakawa M. Moricin, a novel type of antibacterial peptide isolated from the silkworm, *Bombyx mori*. J Biol Chem. 1995;270(50):29923–7. [View Article]
24. Lan WQ, Xie J, Hou WF, Li DW. Antimicrobial Activity and mechanism of complex biological fresh-keeping agents against *Staphylococcus sciuri*. Nat Prod Res Dev. 2012;24:741–6. 753.[View Article]
25. Liu SX, Wei HP, Ceng J, Yang JQ. Studies on antibacterial mechanism of the volatile oil from *Eupatorium adenophorum* antibacterial mechanism of *Staphylococcus aureus*. Chin J Hosp Pharm. 2012;32:1742–5. [View Article]

8

Anti-inflammatory effects of *Phyllanthus amarus* Schum. & Thonn. through inhibition of NF-κB, MAPK, and PI3K-Akt signaling pathways in LPS-induced human macrophages

Hemavathy Harikrishnan[1], Ibrahim Jantan[1,2]* 🆔, Md. Areeful Haque[1] and Endang Kumolosasi[1]

Abstract

Background: *Phyllanthus amarus* has been used widely in various traditional medicines to treat swelling, sores, jaundice, inflammatory diseases, kidney disorders, diabetes and viral hepatitis, while its pharmacological and biochemical mechanisms underlying its anti-inflammatory properties have not been well investigated. The present study was carried out to investigate the effects of 80% ethanolic extract of *P. amarus* on pro-inflammatory mediators release in nuclear factor-kappa B (NF-κB), mitogen activated protein kinase (MAPK) and phosphatidylinositol 3-kinase/Akt (PI3K-Akt) signaling activation in lipopolysaccharide (LPS)-induced U937 human macrophages.

Methods: The release of prostaglandin E_2 (PGE$_2$) and pro-inflammatory cytokines, tumor necrosis factor (TNF)-α and interleukin (IL)-1β in a culture supernatant was determined by ELISA. Determination of cyclooxygenase-2 (COX-2) protein and the activation of MAPKs molecules (JNK, ERK and p38 MAPK), NF-κB and Akt in LPS-induced U937 human macrophages were investigated by immunoblot technique. The relative gene expression levels of COX-2 and pro-inflammatory cytokines were measured by using qRT-PCR. The major metabolites of *P. amarus* were qualitatively and quantitatively analyzed in the extract by using validated reversed-phase high performance liquid chromatography (HPLC) methods.

Results: *P. amarus* extract significantly inhibited the production of pro-inflammatory mediators (TNF-α, IL-1β, PGE$_2$) and COX-2 protein expression in LPS-induced U937 human macrophages. *P. amarus*-pretreatment also significantly downregulated the increased mRNA transcription of pro-inflammatory markers (TNF-α, IL-1β, and COX-2) in respective LPS-induced U937 macrophages. It downregulated the phosphorylation of NF-κB (p65), IκBα, and IKKα/β and restored the degradation of IκBα, and attenuated the expression of Akt, JNK, ERK, and p38 MAPKs phosphorylation in a dose-dependent manner. *P. amarus* extract also downregulated the expression of upstream signaling molecules, TLR4 and MyD88, which play major role in activation of NF-κB, MAPK and PI3K-Akt signaling pathways. The quantitative amounts of lignans, phyllanthin, hypophyllahtin and niranthin, and polyphenols, gallic acid, geraniin, corilagin, and ellagic acid in the extract were determined by HPLC analysis.

Conclusion: The study revealed that *P. amarus* targeted the NF-κB, MAPK and PI3K-Akt signaling pathways to exert its anti- inflammatory effects by downregulating the prospective inflammatory signaling mediators.

Keywords: *Phyllanthus amarus*, Macrophages, Inflammation, Cytokines, NF-κB, MAPK, PI3K-Akt

* Correspondence: profibj@gmail.com
[1]Drug and Herbal Research Center, Faculty of Pharmacy, Universiti Kebangsaan Malaysia, Jalan Raja Muda Abdul Aziz, 50300 Kuala Lumpur, Malaysia
[2]School of Pharmacy, Taylor's University, Lakeside Campus, 47500 Subang Jaya, Selangor, Malaysia

Background

Inflammation is an innate immune response occurring in our body to protect against harmful chemicals and invading pathogens. During inflammation, macrophages which reside in tissues and organs of human body are activated by infectious materials or injury. The activated macrophages will produce inflammatory mediators such as nitric oxide (NO), prostaglandin E_2 (PGE_2), interleukin 1 beta (IL-1β) and tumor necrosis factor (TNF-α), to defend against the invading pathogens [1, 2]. The occurrence of prolonged inflammatory response will lead to the development of various chronic diseases such as rheumatoid arthritis, chronic hepatitis, atherosclerosis, cancer, and inflammatory brain diseases [3–5].

Lipopolysaccharide (LPS) is a bacterial endotoxin, which activates the TLR4 receptors on macrophage and stimulates the recruitment of cytoplasmic MyD88 and TRIF adaptor proteins. The binding of the adaptor proteins on TLR4 complex will trigger the activation of nuclear factor-κB (NF-κB) and mitogen activated protein kinase (MAPK) pathways [2]. However, NF-κB is an ubiquitous nuclear transcription factor, regulates the expression of various genes which play pivotal roles in inflammation, autoimmune diseases, apoptosis and carcinogenesis [6]. In a resting cell, the NF-κB which consists of p50/p65 heterodimer bound to the inhibitory protein IκBs and remain inactive in cytoplasm. In response to LPS stimulation, activated IκB kinases (IKKs) will phosphorylate two specific serine residues (Ser32 and Ser36) on IκBs leading to its degradation through the ubiquitination and proteolysis by the 26S proteasome [2, 7, 8]. The resulting free NF-κB in cytoplasm will translocate into nucleus and binds to the specific IκB binding sites in the promoter region of target genes, followed by the transcription of various inflammatory mediators [1, 9, 10]. On the other hand, the MAPKs family consists of three major classes, extracellular signal-regulated kinases 1 and 2 (ERK1/2), c-Jun N-terminal kinase (JNK) and p38. The phosphorylation of the MAPKs in LPS-induced macrophages will trigger the transcriptional activation of NF-κB [2]. Both NF-κB and MAPK pathways will work together to aggravate the inflammatory diseases in LPS-induced inflammation models [11, 12]. The uncontrolled activation of NF-κB and MAPK signaling pathways will cause detrimental effects to the living organisms. Recent studies have found that the phosphatidylinositol 3-kinase/Akt (PI3K-Akt) signaling pathway was responsible for the expression of pro-inflammatory markers through the IκB degradation and NF-κB activation in LPS induced cells. Hence, targeting these signaling pathways will be an attractive therapeutic approach for the development of anti-inflammatory drugs [13].

Currently, non-steroidal anti-inflammatory drugs (NSAIDs) such as aspirin and ibuprofen are available to treat inflammatory diseases by inhibiting cyclooxygenase-2(COX-2) activation. However, they possess adverse effects, which include disturbance in upper gastrointestinal system and heartburn which limit their use [14]. Therefore, many researchers are trying to find a drug with greater efficacy and minimal toxicity to treat the inflammatory related diseases [15]. *Phyllanthus amarus* Schum. & Thonn. (Family: Euphorbiaceae) is a medicinal herb which is widely distributed in tropical and subtropical countries from Africa to Asia, South America and the West Indies [16]. *P. amarus* has been reported to have an array of ethanopharmacological activities such as anti-inflammatory, hepatoprotective, nephroprotective, anti-amnesia, anti-cancer, diuretic, antioxidant, anti-viral, anti-bacterial, anti-hyperglycemic, anti-hypercholesterolemia and so on [17–19]. The plant is a rich source of secondary metabolites such as alkaloids, flavonoids, hydrolysable tannins, lignans, polyphenols, triterpenes, sterols and volatile oils [20–23]. The anti-inflammatory activities of *P. amarus* have been demonstrated in rat models of carrageenan-induced rat paw edema air-pouch inflammation and cotton pellet granuloma [24]. Several lignans isolated from *P. amarus* such as niranthin, nirtetralin and phyltetralin exhibited in vitro and in vivo anti-inflammatory activities [25]. Previously we have reported the in vitro inhibitory effects of *P. amarus* and its isolates on phagocytic activity of human neutrophils and NO production, lymphocyte proliferation and cytokine release from phagocytes [26, 27]. Immunosuppressive effects of the standardized extract of *P. amarus* on cellular and humoral immune responses in Balb/C mice and Wistar-Kyoto rats have also been investigated [28, 29]. Despite its various pharmacological activities, there is no comprehensive investigation on molecular mechanisms underlying the anti-inflammatory effects of *P. amarus* extract in human macrophages. Hence, the present study was conducted to investigate the effects of 80% ethanolic extract of *P. amarus* on the production of pro-inflammatory mediators and the activation of signaling molecules related to NF-κB, MAPK and PI3K-Akt signaling pathways.

Methods

Chemicals and reagents

Roswell Park Memorial Institute (RPMI) 1640 medium, penicillin-streptomycin (Pen Strep), fetal bovine serum (FBS) were purchased from Gibco (Grand Island, NY, USA). Phorbol 12-myristate 13-acetate (PMA), LPS (*Escherichia coli* 055:B5), RIPA buffer, DMSO were purchased from Sigma Chemical Co. (St. Louis, MO, USA). 1× Halt Protease and Phosphatase Inhibitor Cocktail was purchased from Pierce (Rockford, IL, USA). Human

TNF-α and IL-1β enzyme-linked immunosorbent assay (ELISA) kits were purchased from R&D Systems (Minneapolis, MN, USA). Alamar blue reagent for cell viability assay was purchased from Life Technologies (Grand Island, NY, USA). Primary antibodies specific to COX-2, p-p38, p38, p-ERK1/2, ERK1/2, p-JNK1/2, JNK1/2, p-IκBα, IκBα, p-IKKα/β, p-NFκBp65 and β-actin were purchased from Cell Signaling Technology (Beverly, MA) and, in addition, anti-rabbit secondary antibody conjugated to horseradish peroxidase was obtained from Cell Signaling Technology (Beverly, MA). Methanol and acetonitrile of HPLC grade were purchased from Fisher Scientific (Loughborough, UK). Phyllanthin, hypophyllanthin, niranthin gallic acid, ellagic acid, corilagin and geraniin (purity > 98%) were purchased from ChromaDex (CA, USA). Dexamethasone was obtained from CCM Duopharma Biotech Bhd (Selangor, Malaysia).

Preparation of *P. amarus* ethanol extract

The whole plants of *P. amarus* were collected from Marang, Kuala Terengganu, Malaysia, in February 2015. The plant was authenticated by Dr. Abdul Latif Mohamad of Faculty of Science and Technology, Universiti Kebangsaan Malaysia (UKM). A voucher specimen (voucher number UKMB 30075) has been deposited at the Herbarium of UKM, Bangi, Malaysia for future reference. The plant materials were dried at room temperature and powdered. The powdered plant material was macerated with 80% ethanol for 72 h and the crude ethanol extract was filtered through Whatmann No 1 filter paper. The filtrate was solvent-evaporated using rotary evaporator, freeze dried and stored in an airtight container for further investigation.

High performance liquid chromatography analysis

Qualitative and quantitative high performance liquid chromatography (HPLC) analysis of the 80% ethanolic extract of *P. amarus* was carried out according to the method of Jantan et al. with slight modification [27]. These stock solutions (20 mg/mL) were sonicated for 15 min and filtered through 0.45 μm Millipore Millex PTFE membranes (Maidstone, Kent, UK). The solutions for reference standards (phyllanthin, hypophyllanthin, niranthin, gallic acid, ellagic acid, corilagin and geraniin) were prepared at a concentration of 1 mg/mL and further diluted into a series of concentration (1000–125 μg/mL). The HPLC analysis was performed on a Waters 2535 Quaternary Gradient Module equipped with PDA Photodiode Array Detector (Waters 2998) of wavelength ranging from 205 to 270 nm and data were acquired by using Empower 3 software. The chromatographic analysis was performed on an XBridge™ C-18 (250 mm length × 4.6 mm i.d., 5 μm) analytical column (Waters, Milford, MA, USA). Analysis of the extracts and standard solutions of lignans

(phyllanthin, hypophyllanthin, niranthin) followed the following parameter: isocratic elution with solvent A. acetonitrile: solvent B. water (acidified with 0.1% orthophosphoric acid) (55:45) as mobile phase at a flow rate of 1.0 mL/min. The column was maintained at 25 °C and the detection wavelength was 205 nM. The identification and quantification of the polyphenols (geraniin, corilagin, ellagic acid and gallic acid) in the 80% ethanolic extract of *P. amarus* were carried out based on the chromatographic condition as follows: gradient elution with acetonitrile and 0.2% orthophosphoric acid as mobile phase at a flow rate of 1.0 mL/min. Quantification of compounds in the extracts was based on the standard curves equations obtained by plotting calibration curves of five concentrations (1000–125 μg/mL) each of the standard solution of compounds versus the areas under the peaks.

Validation procedures for HPLC analysis

The HPLC method was validated by determining the linearity, precision, limits of quantification (LOQ) and detection (LOD). The precision of the method was determined by studying intra-day and inter-day variations. Separately one concentration of extracts (20 mg/mL) and reference compounds (125, 500, 1000 μg/mL) were injected three times for each concentration in one day and on three different days. The calibration curve was obtained by using phyllanthin, hypophyllanthin and niranthin as external standards. Six concentrations of each standard (31.25–1000 μg/mL) were injected in triplicate, and the curve was constructed by plotting the corresponding peak areas versus the concentration of each standard. The linearity was evaluated by linear calibration analysis while the correlation coefficient (R^2) was calculated from the calibration curves. LOD and LOQ were calculated from RSD and slope (S) of the calibration curves by using following equations: LOD $=3.3 \times$ (RSD/S) and LOQ $=10 \times$ (RSD/S).

LC-MS analysis

LC-MS analysis was performed onThermo Scientific C18 column (AcclaimTM Polar Advantage II, 3 × 150 mm, 3 μm particle size) on an UltiMate 3000 UHPLC system (Dionex). The LC-MS was carried out by using the gradient program at 0.4 mL/min, 40 °C using H_2O + 0.1% Formic Acid (A) and 100% ACN (B) with 22 min total run time with sample injection volume of 1 uL. Gradient started at 5% B (0-3 min); 80% B (3-10 min); 80% B (10-15 min) and 5% B (15–22 min). The positive and negative ionization spectra obtained with MicroTOF QIII Bruker Daltonic with the following settings:- capillary voltage: 4500 V; nebulizer pressure: 1.2 bar; drying gas: 8 L/min at 200 °C. The mass range was at 50–1000 m/z. The accurate mass data of the molecular ions, provided by the TOF analyzer, were processed by Compass Data Analysis software (Bruker Daltonik GmbH). The corresponding peaks of the compounds were identified by comparison with the mass spectral library.

Cell culture and differentiation induction

U937 (ATCC ® CRL-1593.2) cell line was obtained from ATCC (American Type Culture Collection). U937 mononuclear cell line was grown in RPMI 1640 medium supplemented with 10% (v/v) fetal bovine serum (FBS) and 1% (v/v) penicillin G/streptomycin at 37 °C under 5% CO_2. The U937 cells density was maintained between 1×10^5 and 2×10^6 viable cells/mL throughout the experiments. Cells were harvested once the cell confluency reached approximately 80–90%. For all the experiments, the U937 cells were differentiated to obtain macrophage like phenotype by addition of phorbol 12-myristate 13-acetate (PMA) (Sigma-Aldrich) at 200 nM, for 24 h. The following day, cells were washed with complete culture media once and incubated overnight with serum free media for recovery phase [1, 30].

Alamar blue for testing cell viability

The cell viability assay was carried out with Alamar blue reagent according to the manufacturer standard protocol to determine the cytotoxicity effect induced by the 80% ethanolic extract of *P. amarus*. The differentiated macrophages were plated at a density 5×10^5 cells/mL onto 96 well plate. *P. amarus* extract was dissolved in DMSO, and the DMSO concentration did not exceed 1%. The cells were treated with various concentrations of *P. amarus* extract of serial dilutions 60, 30, 15, 7.5, and 3.25 µg/mL and then incubated for 24 h. After 24 h of incubation, 10% *v/v* of 10 x Alamar blue cell viability reagents was added into each well followed by 4 h incubation at 37 °C, 5% CO_2 incubator. Then the reduction of an active compound of Alamar blue, resazurin into resorufin by viable cells was read with Tecan plate reader at 570 nm using 600 nm (normalized to 600 nm value) as a reference wavelength. The results were expressed as percentage of viable cells over control cells [19].

Enzyme-linked immunosorbent assay

To investigate the effect of *P. amarus* extract on cytokines levels from LPS-induced cells, differentiated U937 macrophages (5×10^5 cells/mL) seeded into 24 well plate were pretreated with 60, 30,15,7.5 and 3.75 µg/mL of *P. amarus* extract or with 4, 0.4, 0.04, 0.004 and 0.0004 µg/mL of dexamethasone for 2 h prior to 24 h stimulation with 1 µg/mL LPS. In another experiment, the differentiated cells also pretreated with SB202190 (a p38 inhibitor, 10 µM), U0126 (an ERK inhibitor, 10 µM), SP600125 (a JNK inhibitor, 10 µM), BAY 11–7082 (an NF-κB inhibitor, 10 µM) and LY294002 (an Akt inhibitor,

10 µM) for 2 h and then cultured with LPS of 1 µg/mL for 24 h to study the effect of inhibitors on TNF-α release. The U937 macrophages untreated with LPS which acted as a control was included for comparison. After 24 h, the cell free supernatants were collected and stored at − 20 °C until cytokine analysis. The concentrations of TNF- α and IL-1β in the supernatants of U937 cell cultures were determined using DuoSet® ELISA Development System (R&D Systems, Minneapolis, MN, USA) kit according to the manufacturer protocol [1, 19].

Measurement of PGE₂

The differentiated U937 cells were plated in a 24 well plate and pretreated with concentrations of *P. amarus* (60, 30 and 15 µg/mL) for 2 h and then stimulated with 1 µg/mL of LPS for 24 h. The supernatants were assayed to determine the PGE_2 level. The PGE_2 level was analyzed by using ELISA kit (R&D Systems, Minneapolis, MN, USA) according to manufactures protocol [1, 19].

Quantification of relative gene expression level by qRT-PCR

U937 macrophages (1×10^6 cells/mL) were pre-treated with varying concentrations of *P. amarus* (60, 30, and 15 µg/mL) for 2 h and later cultured with LPS of 1 µg/mL for 1 day. The inhibitory properties of *P. amarus* on the expression of COX-2, TNF-α, and IL-1β were evaluated by qRT-PCR [1, 19]. To determine the gene expression level, total RNA was extracted from LPS treated U937 cells by using innuPREP RNAmini kit (Analytik Jena AG, Germany) and cDNA was synthesized by using SensiFAST™ cDNA Synthesis Kit (Bioline USA Inc., Taunton, MA) following manufacturer protocol. Quantification of mRNA by qRT-PCR was done using CFX96 Touch™ Real-Time PCR Detection System (Biorad, Hercules, California, USA) along with SYBR® Green RT-PCR Master Mix (Bioline USA Inc., Taunton, MA). The cDNA was amplified by using the following primers; COX-2 (Hs_PTGS2_1_SG QuantiTect Primer QT00040586), TNF-α (Hs_TNF_3_SG QuantiTect Primer QT01079561), IL-1β (Hs_IL1B_1_SG QuantiTect Primer QT00021385) and GADPH (Hs_GAPDH_1_SG QuantiTect Primer QT00079247). The PCR reaction mixture consisted of 10 µL of SYBR master mixture, 2 µL of reverse and forward primers, 6 µL of deionized water and 2 µL of cDNA. The reaction was carried out in the following parameter: 95 °C for 2 s, 95 °C for 5 min, 60 °C for 10 min, 72 °C for 20 min (36 cycles). The relative fold difference between samples was determined following the comparative cycle threshold ($2^{-\Delta\Delta Ct}$) method. Glyceraldehyde 3-phosphate dehydrogenase (GADPH) was used as the housekeeping gene for normalizing the data.

Western blotting analysis

Differentiated cells (1×10^6 cells/mL) were plated onto six well plate and pretreated with 60, 30, 15 µg/mL of *P. amarus* extract, SB202190, U0126, SP600125, LY294002 and BAY 11–7082 (10 µM) for 2 h and then stimulated with 1 µg/mL of LPS for 30 min. The cells were harvested by centrifugation at 7000 x *g* for 5 min and washed twice with ice cold PBS. The washed cell pellets were lysed in RIPA buffer and halt protease and phosphatase inhibitor cocktails. The cell lysates were centrifuged at 13,000 x *g* for 10 min and protein concentrations were measured by Bradford assay. Approximately 20 µg of proteins were resolved by 10% SDS-polyacrylamide gel electrophoresis and were electroblotted onto polyvinylidene difluoride (PVDF) membrane. The immunoblot was incubated for 1 h with 5% skim milk powder in TBS-T buffer containing 0.1% Tween 20 to block the nonspecific binding prior to the overnight incubation with specific primary antibodies that recognized COX-2, p-p38 (Thr180/Tyr182), p38, p-ERK1/2 (Thr202/Tyr204), ERK1/2, p-JNK1/2 (Thr183/Tyr185), JNK1/2, p-IκBα (Ser32/36), IκBα, p-IKKα/β (Ser176/180), p-NFκBp65 (Ser536), p-Akt (Ser 473) and β-actin (Cell Signaling Technology Inc., Beverly, MA). The following day, membrane was washed with TBS-T (0.1% Tween 20) 3 times for 10 min each. It was then incubated with anti-rabbit secondary antibody conjugated to horseradish peroxidase for 1 h at room temperature with agitation and washed 3 times with TBST for 10 min each. Each protein band was detected using chemiluminescence detection system according to the manufacturer instruction. The band intensity was quantified using Image Lab™ software [1, 2, 31].

Statistical analysis

Statistical analyses were performed using the GraphPad Prism 6.0 (GraphPad Software, San Diego, CA, USA). For each experiment, three independent experiments were performed and data are expressed as mean ± standard error mean (SEM). Differences between two means were analyzed by one-way analysis of variance (ANOVA) followed by post-hoc Dunnett's test with $P < 0.05$ considered as statistically significant.

Results

Quantitative and qualitative analysis of 80% ethanolic extract of *P. amarus*

To identify and quantify the active components of *P. amarus* we performed HPLC analysis of the ethanol extract and several representative standards as previously reported by Jantan et al. [32]. Peaks with the same retention time as the standard compounds, phyllanthin (11.17 min), hypophyllahtin (11.71 min) and niranthin (14.48 min) were observed in *P. amarus* (Fig. 1a). For the polyphenols, four peaks were identified namely gallic acid (7.89 min), geraniin (23.76 min), corilagin (26.41 min) and ellagic acid (33.42 min) (Fig. 1b). Among the lignans, phyllanthin (660.28 µg/mL) was present at the highest concentration compared to niranthin (575.11 µg/mL) and hypophyllanthin (290.46 µg/mL). Among the identified polyphenols, ellagic acid (601.29 µg/mL) was the most abundant, followed by corilagin (313.41 µg/mL), geraniin (170.49 µg/mL) and gallic acid (163.30 µg/mL). The LC-MS results revealed that *P. amarus* extract consisted of 18 compounds identified via positive ionization mode

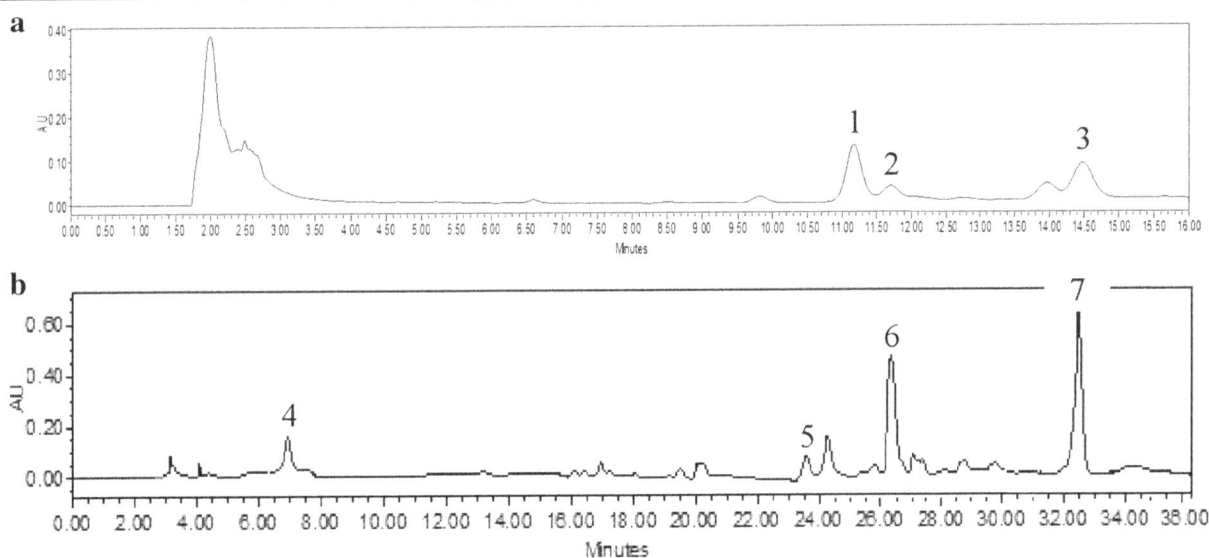

Fig. 1 RP-HPLC chromatogram of the 80% ethanol extracts of *Phyllanthus amarus* **a** for identification and quantification of (1) phyllanthin, (2) hypophyllanthin and (3) niranthin; **b** for identification and quantification of (4) gallic acid, (5) geraniin, (6) corilagin and (7) ellagic acid at the wavelength of 205 nm

while five compounds identified via negative ionization mode (Table 1).

Effects of *P. amarus* on cell viability

U937 macrophages were incubated with the 80% ethanolic extract of *P. amarus* ranging from 0 to 60 μg/mL and cell viability was determined by alamar blue assay after 24 h. The results demonstrated that from 0 to 60 μg/mL of *P. amarus* extract, there was no cytotoxic effect on U937 macrophages (cell viability greater than 90%). These results confirmed that the effects of *P. amarus* on U937 macrophages in this study were not due to cytotoxicity.

Effects of *P. amarus* on pro-inflammatory cytokines production and gene expression

To investigate the anti-inflammatory effects of *P. amarus* extract on LPS-stimulated macrophages, firstly the concentrations of TNF-α and IL-1β in the culture supernatants of U937 macrophages were determined by ELISA kit. The results demonstrated that, the pro- inflammatory cytokines (TNF-α and IL-1β) production was significantly upregulated in LPS induced U937 macrophages while the cells pretreated with *P. amarus* for 2 h prior to LPS stimulation showed suppressive effect on TNF-α and IL-1β production with IC_{50} values of 16.12 and 7.13 μg/mL, respectively (Fig. 2a and b). In addition, the suppressive effect also was observed for sample treated with an standard anti-inflammatory agent, dexamethasone which exhibited inhibitory activity on TNF-α and IL-1β with IC_{50} values of 0.18 μg/mL and 0.002 μg/mL, respectively. Next, we determined the effects of *P. amarus* on pro-inflammatory cytokines expression at pre-translational level by using quantitative Real-Time RT-PCR (qRT-PCR). As shown in Additional file 1: Figure S1, the mRNA expression of TNF-α and IL-1β were significantly ($P < 0.001$) upregulated in U937 macrophages 24 h following LPS stimulation. However, the cells pretreated with *P. amarus* (60, 30 and 15 μg/mL) for 2 h showed a significant inhibition in LPS induced TNF-α (27, 32, and 35 fold, respectively) and IL-1β (12, 32, and 35 fold, respectively) (Fig. 2c and d). These gene expression levels also were comparable with 4 μg/mL dose of dexamethasone pretreated cells prior to LPS induction. Dexamethasone pretreated cells also showed an inhibition of TNF-α and IL-1β expression (8 and 2 fold respectively) (Fig. 2c and d). The consistent inhibition of cytokine expression at protein and mRNA levels suggests that *P. amarus* may exert their anti-inflammatory effects by controlling gene transcription.

Table 1 Tentative compounds detected in 80% ethanol extract of *Phyllanthus amarus* by LCMS analysis

Peak	Retention time (RT)	Molecular ion peak	MS^2 fragment ions	Tentative compounds identified
1	1.7	131 (M-H)$^-$	909, 688, 244, 134	D-glutamine
2	2.0	195 (M-H)$^-$	909, 678, 404, 204	Gluconic acid
3	2.1	228 (M-H)$^-$	897, 709, 405, 238, 129	Naringenin
4	2.1	191 (M-H)$^-$	935, 596, 381, 191	Quinic acid
5	2.6	133 (M-H)$^-$	913, 677, 412, 230, 134	D-(+)-Malic acid
6	2.9	321 (M-H)$^-$	711, 412, 248, 183	Dinitramin
7	3.1	128 (M-H)$^-$	122	4-oxoproline
8	4.2	387 (M-H)$^-$	514, 387, 207	galloyl glucopyroxidase
9	6.5	169 (M-H)$^-$	169	Gallic acid
10	7.0	343 (M-H)$^-$	169	trio-O-methylellagic acid
11	7.9	633 (M-H)$^-$	633, 463, 301	corilagin
12	8.0	331 (M-H)$^-$	169	tuberonic acid hexoside
13	8.5	951 (M-H)$^-$	933, 765, 613, 463, 301	geraniin
14	8.9	965 (M-H)$^-$	933, 765, 609, 300	Rutin
15	9.2	197 (M-H)$^-$	125	Syringic acid
16	9.2	463 (M-H)$^-$	463, 300, 169	Quercetine 3-D-glucoside
17	9.5	206 (M-H)$^-$	873, 704, 558, 226, 147	N-acetyl-D- phenylalanine
18	9.7	247 (M-H)$^-$	247	7-Deshydroxypyrogallin4- carboxylic acid
19	1.6	133 (M-H)$^+$	663, 383, 132	Maleamate
20	1.8	222 (M-H)$^+$	222	Metaxalone
21	1.9	184 (M-H)$^+$	184	4-pyridoxic acid
22	3.6	166 (M-H)$^+$	120	Stachydrine
23	13.9	419 (M-H)$^+$	419, 149	Phyllanthin

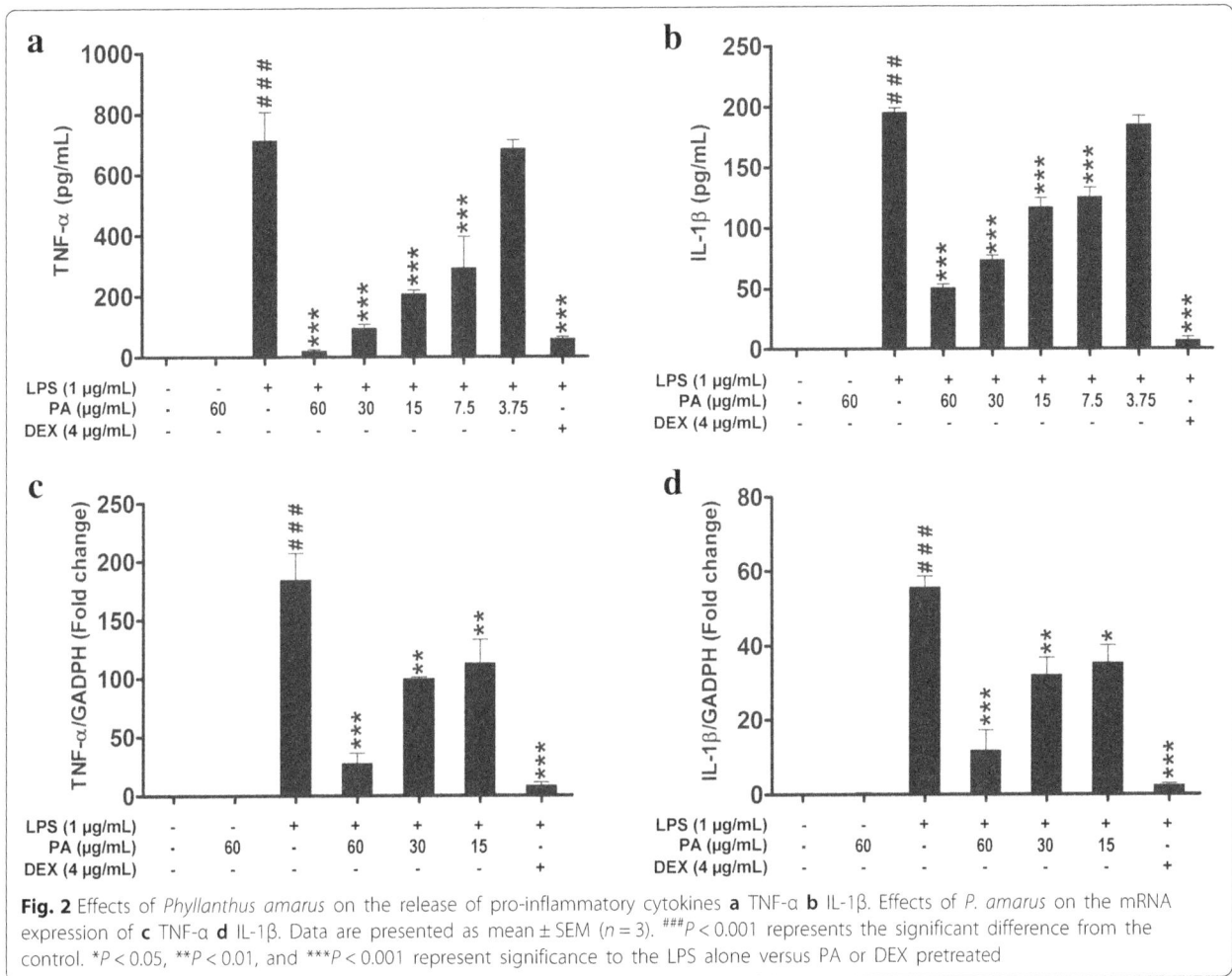

Fig. 2 Effects of *Phyllanthus amarus* on the release of pro-inflammatory cytokines **a** TNF-α **b** IL-1β. Effects of *P. amarus* on the mRNA expression of **c** TNF-α **d** IL-1β. Data are presented as mean ± SEM ($n = 3$). ### $P < 0.001$ represents the significant difference from the control. * $P < 0.05$, ** $P < 0.01$, and *** $P < 0.001$ represent significance to the LPS alone versus PA or DEX pretreated

Effects of *P. amarus* on PGE₂ production and COX-2 expression

To examine the effect of *P. amarus* on PGE_2 release, production of PGE_2 in culture supernatant was measured. PGE_2 production was measured in U937 macrophages induced with LPS for 24 h in the presence and absence of *P. amarus*. As shown in Fig. 3a, LPS (1 µg/mL) induced U937 macrophages produced significant amount of PGE_2 (1128.67 ± 200.07 pg/mL) compared to control (31.33 ± 11.31 pg/mL). However, the production of PGE_2 was significantly attenuated by *P. amarus* pretreatment at 60, 30 and 15 µg/mL in a dose- dependent manner. In order to examine the mechanisms by which *P. amarus* inhibited LPS- induced PGE_2 release, the expression of COX-2 at protein and gene level was measured in U937 macrophages induced with LPS. As shown in Fig. 3b, Western blot analysis showed that 24 h LPS stimulation significantly ($P < 0.001$) upregulated the COX-2 protein expression while 2 h *P. amarus* (60, 30 and 15 µg/mL) pretreatment significantly attenuated the expression in a dose-dependent manner. In addition, we have investigated the effects of *P. amarus* on

gene expression to determine whether *P. amarus* inhibited the LPS induced COX-2 mRNA level in U937 macrophages. As shown in Fig. 3c, the significantly ($P < 0.001$) increased COX-2 mRNA expression (282 fold) in LPS stimulated cells were significantly attenuated in *P. amarus* (60 and 30 µg/mL) pretreated cells (137 and 259 fold, respectively) as compared to control.

Effects of *P. amarus* on NF-κB signaling pathways

To determine the role of IKK/IκB/NF-κB signaling pathway in *P. amarus* mediated inhibition of LPS-induced inflammatory response, we studied the activation of p-NF-κB (p65), NF-κB (p65), p-IκBα, IκBα, p-IKKα/β, and IKKα/β in LPS-induced human macrophages by Western blot. Our results demonstrated that, *P. amarus* altered the NF-κB signaling mechanisms by suppressing the phosphorylation of IKKα/β and IκBα in a dose-dependent manner, which were significantly ($P < 0.001$) upregulated by 30 min LPS treatment. In addition, the 2 h *P. amarus* pretreatment significantly blocked the degradation of

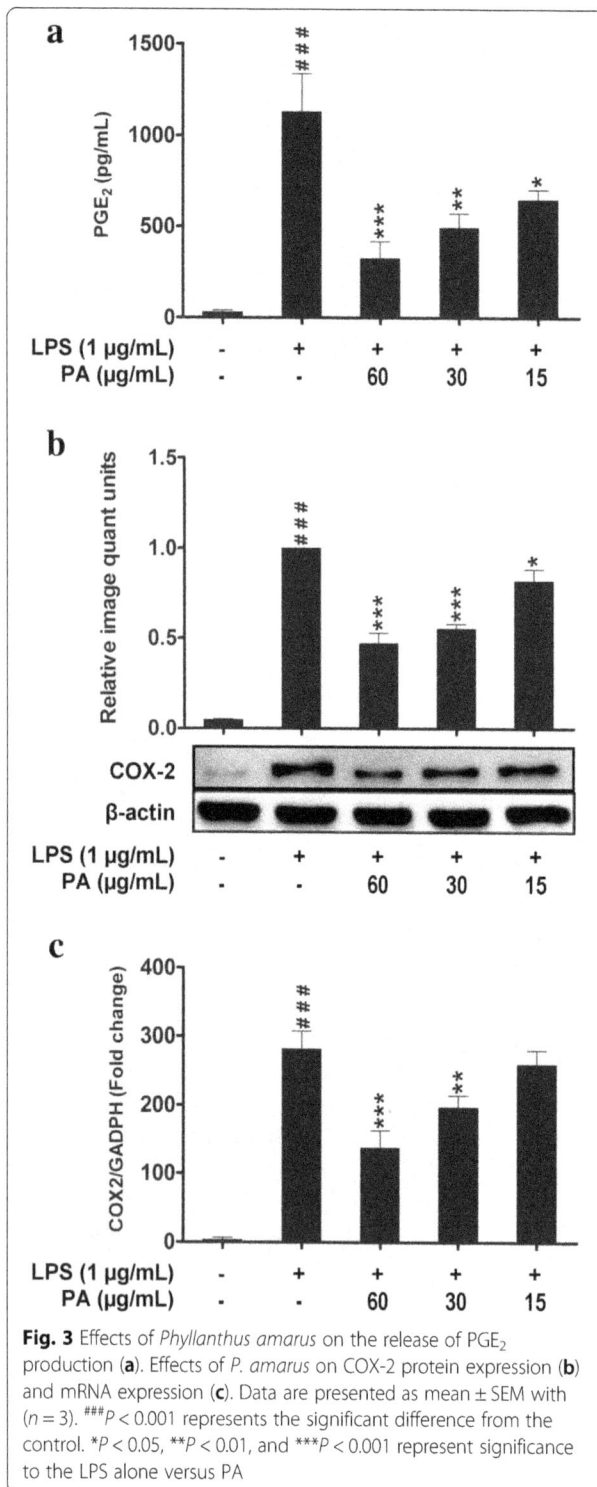

Fig. 3 Effects of *Phyllanthus amarus* on the release of PGE₂ production (**a**). Effects of *P. amarus* on COX-2 protein expression (**b**) and mRNA expression (**c**). Data are presented as mean ± SEM with ($n = 3$). $^{###}P < 0.001$ represents the significant difference from the control. $^*P < 0.05$, $^{**}P < 0.01$, and $^{***}P < 0.001$ represent significance to the LPS alone versus PA

LPS induced IκBα in a concentration-dependent manner (Additional file 2: Figure S2). Furthermore, the 2 h pretreatment with *P. amarus* also significantly attenuated the LPS-induced phospho-p65 without altering the total level of p65 in human U937 macrophages (Fig. 4).

Effects of *P. amarus* on MAPKs and PI3K-Akt activation

Studies have demonstrated that the activation of Akt and MAPKs (JNK1/2, ERK1/2, and p38) signaling molecules is important to initiate and mediate the NF-κB signal transduction pathway. Hence,we investigated the effect of *P. amarus* on phosphorylation of Akt by Western blot analysis. As depicted in Fig. 5, the 30 min LPS induction significantly upregulated Akt phosphorylation while 2 h *P. amarus* pretreatment dose-dependently suppressed the phosphorylation. Furthermore, the effect of PA on phosphorylation activity of three important MAPKs signaling molecules (JNK1/2, ERK1/2, and p38) was also investigated. The LPS induction at 30 min significantly ($P < 0.001$) stimulated the JNK1/2, ERK1/2, and p38 phosphorylation levels in macrophages but the cells pretreated with *P. amarus* (60, 30 and 15 µg/ml) for 2 h significantly suppressed the phosphorylation of JNK1/2, ERK1/2, and p38 protein kinases in a dose-dependent manner without interfering the total level of JNK1/2, ERK1/2, and p38 protein kinases (Fig. 5).

In order to further validate that the suppression of inflammatory mediators by *P. amarus* linked to the NF-κB, MAPKs, and Akt signaling pathway down regulation, we examined the effect of specific NF-κB, MAPKs, and Akt inhibitors on TNF-α production and COX-2 protein expression. The 2 h pretreatment of LPS-induced macrophages with BAY 11–7082 (an NF-κB inhibitor), LY294002 (an Akt inhibitor), SB202190 (a p38 inhibitor), U0126 (an ERK inhibitor) and SP600125 (a JNK inhibitor) showed significant inhibitory effect on TNF-α production and COX-2 expression (Fig. 6). Taken together, our results suggest that *P. amarus* reduced COX-2 expression and TNF-α production by down regulating LPS-activated NF-κB, ERK, JNK, p38MAPKs and Akt signaling pathways.

Effects of *P. amarus* on MyD88 and TLR4 signaling molecules

To further confirm the anti- inflammatory activity of *P. amarus*, the expression of MyD88 and TLR4 were investigated in LPS-induced U937 macrophages. As shown in Fig. 7, 1 h LPS induction significantly ($P < 0.001$) upregulated the expression of MyD88 and TLR4 compared to control cells. However, the cells pretreated with *P. amarus* for 2 h dose- dependently diminished the upregulation of MyD88 and TLR4 protein expression. It was noted that, at the dose of 60 µg/mL, the suppression of *P. amarus* was found highly significant ($P < 0.001$) for the both upstream signaling molecules.

Discussion

P. amarus is a promising herbal resource with therapeutic potential against various diseases due to the presence of numerous active and secondary metabolites [22].

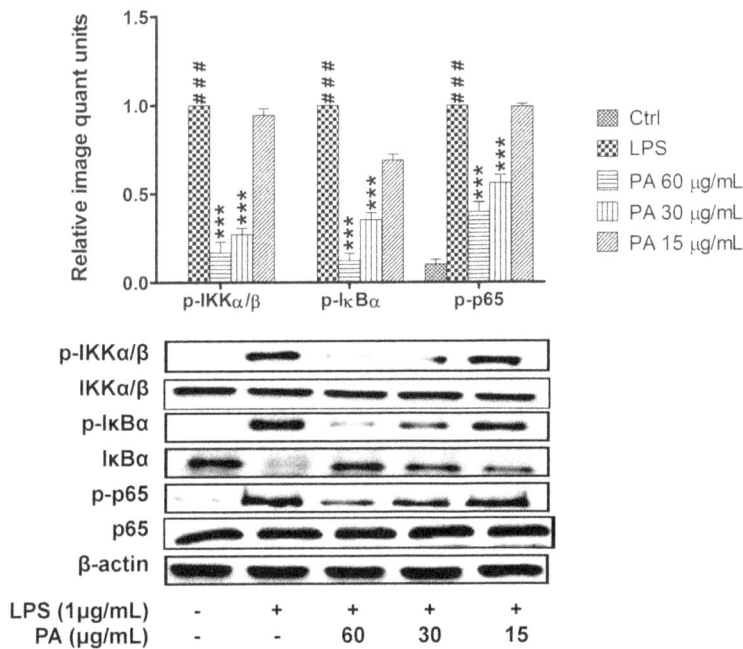

Fig. 4 Effects of *Phyllanthus amarus* on phosphorylation of IKKα/β, IκBα and NF-κB (p65). Data are presented as mean ± SEM with ($n = 3$). ###$P < 0.001$ represents the significant difference from the control. *$P < 0.05$, **$P < 0.01$, and ***$P < 0.001$ represent significance to the LPS alone versus PA

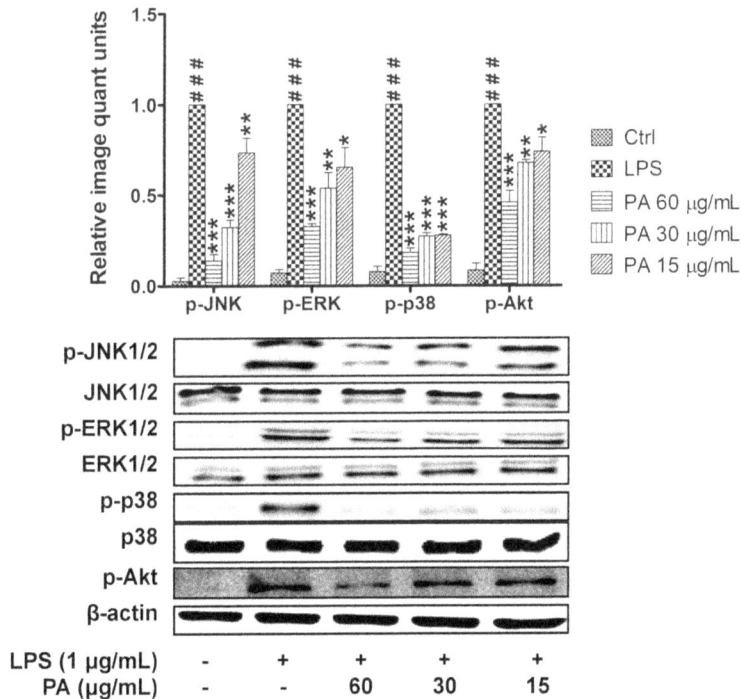

Fig. 5 Effects of *Phyllanthus amarus* on p-JNK, p-ERK, p-p38 and p-Akt expression. Data are presented as mean ± SEM with ($n = 3$). ###$P < 0.001$ represents the significant difference from the control. *$P < 0.05$, **$P < 0.01$, and ***$P < 0.001$ represent significance to the LPS alone versus PA

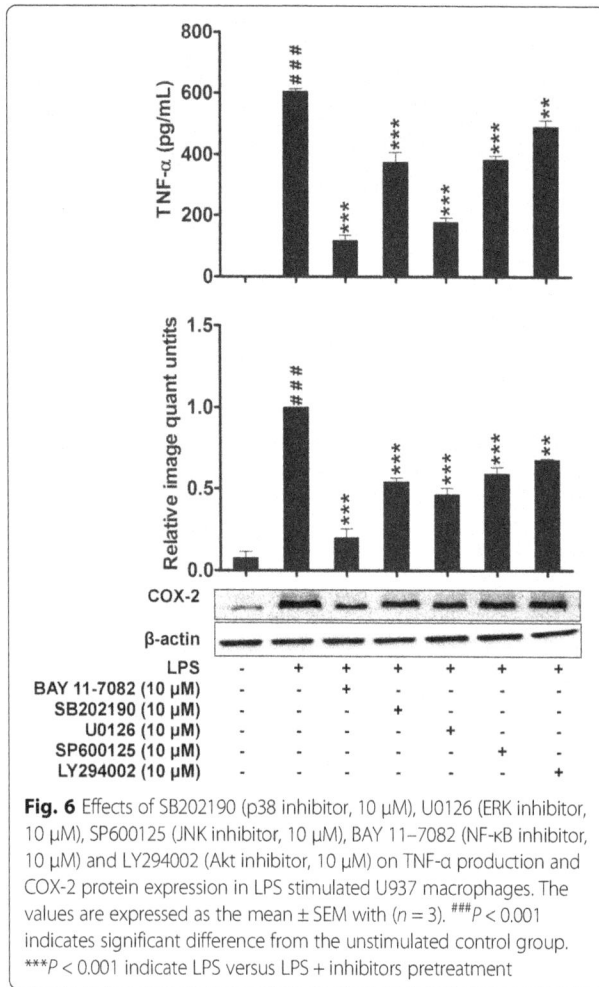

Fig. 6 Effects of SB202190 (p38 inhibitor, 10 μM), U0126 (ERK inhibitor, 10 μM), SP600125 (JNK inhibitor, 10 μM), BAY 11–7082 (NF-κB inhibitor, 10 μM) and LY294002 (Akt inhibitor, 10 μM) on TNF-α production and COX-2 protein expression in LPS stimulated U937 macrophages. The values are expressed as the mean ± SEM with ($n = 3$). $^{\#\#\#}P < 0.001$ indicates significant difference from the unstimulated control group. $^{***}P < 0.001$ indicate LPS versus LPS + inhibitors pretreatment

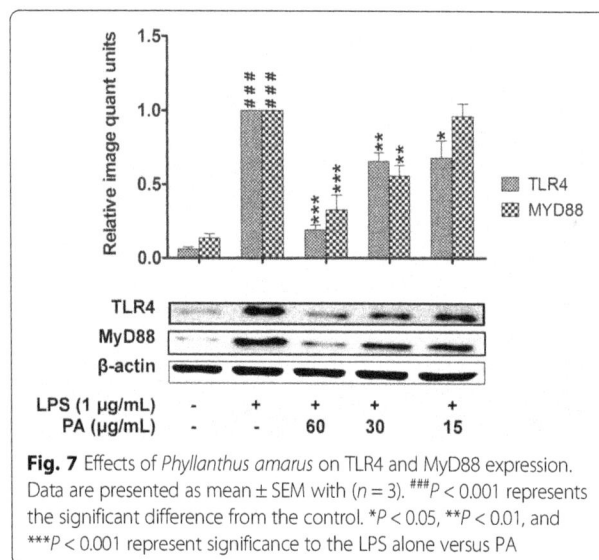

Fig. 7 Effects of *Phyllanthus amarus* on TLR4 and MyD88 expression. Data are presented as mean ± SEM with ($n = 3$). $^{\#\#\#}P < 0.001$ represents the significant difference from the control. $^*P < 0.05$, $^{**}P < 0.01$, and $^{***}P < 0.001$ represent significance to the LPS alone versus PA

Although *P. amarus* extracts have been previously shown to possess immunosuppressive activity on immune cells but the mechanism underlying the anti-inflammatory activity of the plant remain unknown [27, 32–34]. Therefore, in the present study we investigated the in vitro effects of *P. amarus* by using LPS-activated U937 human macrophage, which mimics the inflammatory model [1]. Macrophages can be activated by LPS to produce pro-inflammatory molecules such as IL-6, TNF-α, IL-1β, PGE$_2$ and NO by triggering intracellular signaling pathways including NF-κB and MAPKs [1, 2, 35].

COX is known as an enzyme which aid in the process converting the arachidonic acid to prostaglandins and it exists as COX-1 and COX-2 isomers. COX-1 is responsible for the homeostatic function of PGE$_2$ while COX-2 triggers the excess release of PGE$_2$ at the region of inflammation which is known to play critical role during pathogenesis of chronic diseases [31, 36, 37]. Besides, it is also reported that overexpression of COX-2 leads to the upregulation of several angiogenic mediators [38]. Therefore, potent inhibitory effects of anti-inflammatory drugs on COX-2 expression have been revealed by several researches to be valuable in preventing and curing these disorders [39]. In current study, we found that *P. amarus* extract suppressed the PGE$_2$ production in LPS stimulated U937 macrophages by down regulating the COX-2 protein and gene expression. These finding suggest that the suppression of PGE$_2$ release by *P. amarus* extract might be due to the inhibition of COX-2 elevation upon the LPS induction of macrophages. Furthermore, Kiemer et al. also reported the inhibitory effect of *P. amarus* extract on PGE$_2$ production in rat Kupffer cells and RAW264.7 macrophages, whick were in consistent with our present finding. Like COX-2, iNOS is also one of the enzyme that is involved in the production of excess NO during chronic inflammatory disorders to alleviate the pathogenesis of disease state [38]. It is to be noted that from our experiment NO could not be detected at measurable quantity in the LPS induced U937 macrophages which is in agreement with the previous report [40]. The probable reason for this occurrence may linked to the statement that, U937 cells lack of BH4 (tetrahydrobiopterin) which is the crucial cofactor for NO production [19, 41]. TNF-α and IL-1β are known as a key pro-inflammatory cytokines that are secreted during the development of chronic inflammatory diseases [42]. In this study we found that the extract of *P. amarus* and positive control, dexamethasone showed a significant inhibition of pro-inflammatory cytokines in a concentration-dependent manner in LPS-stimulated human macrophages. The outcome was found in line with the previous study where the inhibitory effect of *P. amarus* on pro-inflammatory cytokines such as TNF-α, IL-1β and IFN-γ in LPS induced immune cells has also been observed [32].

NF-κB signaling plays a major role in macrophages to regulate the cell survival genes and induces transcription and translation of other mediators that are involved in inflammatory response [43]. Thus, the inhibition of these signaling pathways may highlight the potential of *P. amarus* as a suppressor of inflammatory cytokines. Consistent with previous report, *P. amarus* ethanolic extract inhibited the production of LPS-induced TNF-α and IL-1β that are known to regulate by NF-κB signaling pathway. Interestingly, our present findings revealed that *P. amarus* extracts dose –dependently diminished the phosphorylation of IKKα/β and IκBα in response to LPS. Furthermore, LPS-induced IκBα degradation in U937 cells also inhibited by *P. amarus* in a dose dependent manner. These findings indicate that the downregulation of LPS-induced inflammatory cytokines production by *P. amarus* results from the blockade of IKK/IκB/NF-κB signaling pathway. A study has reported that *P. amarus* inhibited the DNA binding activity of NF-κB binding factors and also iNOS and COX-2 expression in LPS-induced murine macrophages [32]. This is in agreement with our findings which showed that *P. amarus* was able to downregulate the NF-κB activation by suppressing the release of pro- inflammatory mediators.

Apart from NF-κB, LPS-induced macrophages also activate MAPKs signaling pathway, which regulate the expression of inflammatory mediators by controlling NF-κB activity [44]. Our study demonstrated that pretreatment of cell with *P. amarus* inhibited the early activation of cell by LPS in a dose-dependent manner. Thus, our study strongly indicates that the MAPKs (JNK, ERK, and p38) were involved in inhibitory activity of *P. amarus* on the expression of pro-inflammatory mediators. Apart from NF-κB and MAPKs, phosphatidylinositol 3-kinase/Akt (PI3K-Akt) is another signaling pathway which is activated in LPS induced macrophages to control the expression of inflammatory markers by activating the NF-κB signal transduction pathway [45]. Hence, blocking the phosphorylation activity of Akt in response to LPS induction is known to be an important target to control inflammatory disorders. Supportingly, our study revealed that, *P. amarus* pretreatment significantly attenuated the LPS induced Akt phosphorylation in LPS induced human macrophages. Furthermore, in this study we proved that the suppression of TNF-α production and COX-2 protein expression by *P. amarus* were due to the blockage of NF-κB, MAPKs, and Akt pathways through the use of NF-κB, MAPKs, and Akt inhibitors.

TLR4 is known to specifically bind with LPS and trigger inflammatory response by activating NF-κB, MAPKs, and PI3K-Akt signaling pathways which lead to the production of inflammatory mediators [1, 46, 47]. The activated TLR4 sequentially transmit the inflammatory signals through the adaptor protein, Myd88 [48].

This suggests that, TLR4 and MyD88 act as a specific molecular target to inititate inflammatory responses [47, 49]. Our investigation demonstrates that *P. amarus* significantly inhibited LPS-induced TLR4 and MyD88 expression in U937 macrophages. These findings propose that TLR4 and MyD88 participated in the inhibitory action of *P. amarus* on the LPS-induced production of PGE$_2$ and pro-inflammatory cytokines.

Conclusions

In conclusion, the present study demonstrated that *P. amarus* potently suppressed the inflammatory responses in LPS-induced U937 macrophages via inhibition of MyD88-dependent signaling pathway, which may be linked to the inhibitory effects exerted by *P. amarus* on pro-inflammatory mediators. Therefore, the ethanol extract of *P. amarus* have promising anti-inflammatory activity which acts through the suppression of NF-κB, MAPKs, and PI3K-Akt signaling pathways and may have beneficial therapeutic applications for treating inflammatory disorders.

Abbreviation

ATCC: American type culture collection; COX2: Cyclooxygenase 2; ELISA: Enzyme-linked immunosorbant assay; ERK: Extracellular signal-regulated kinase; FBS: Fetal bovine serum; HPLC: High performance liquid chromatography; IL-1β: Interleukin 1 beta; iNOS: Inducible nitric oxide synthase; IκB: I-kappa B kinase; JNK: c-Jun N-terminal kinase; LPS: Lipopolysaccharide; MAPK: Mitogen activated protein kinase; MyD88: Myeloid differentiation primary response gene 88; NF-κB: Nuclear factor-kappa B; NO: Nitric oxide; NSAID: Non-steroidal anti-inflammatory drug; PA: *Phyllanthus amarus*; PGE$_2$: Prostaglandin E2; PMA: Phorbol 12-myristate 13-acetate; RPMI: Roswell park memorial institute; TLR4: Toll like receptor 4; TNF-α: Tumor necrosis factor-alpha

Acknowledgements

This work was supported by the Ministry of Agriculture and Agro-based Industry, Malaysia, under the NKEA Research Grant Scheme (NRGS) (Grant no. NH1014D020).

Funding

This study was funded by the Ministry of Agriculture Malaysia under the NKEA Research Grant Scheme (NRGS) (no. NH0811D003).

Authors' contributions

HK carried out the experiments, analyzed and interpreted the data, and drafted the manuscript. IJ and EK designed the study and participated in analysis and interpretation of data. IJ coordinated the study, revised the manuscript and approved the final version to be submitted for publication. MAH helped in the analysis and interpretation of data. All authors read and approved the final manuscript.

Competing interests

The authors declare that they have no competing interest.

References

1. Haque MA, Jantan I, Harikrishnan H. Zerumbone suppresses the activation of inflammatory mediators in LPS-stimulated U937 macrophages through MyD88-dependent NF-κB/MAPK/PI3K-Akt signaling pathways. Int Immunopharmacol. 2018;55:312–22.

2. Haque MA, Jantan I, Harikrishnan H, Abdul Wahab SM. Magnoflorine enhances LPS-activated pro-inflammatory responses via MyD88-dependent pathways in U937 macrophages. Planta Med. 2018; https://doi.org/10.1055/a-0637-9936.

3. Chen GY, Nunez G. Sterile inflammation: sensing and reacting to damage. Nat Rev Immunol. 2010;10(12):826–37.

4. Shacter E, Weitzman SA. Chronic inflammation and cancer. Oncology. 2002; 16(2):217–226, 229. discussion 230-212

5. Killeen MJ, Linder M, Pontoniere P, Crea R. NF-kappabeta signaling and chronic inflammatory diseases: exploring the potential of natural products to drive new therapeutic opportunities. Drug Discov Today. 2014;19(4):373–8.

6. Aggarwal BB. Nuclear factor-kappaB: the enemy within. Cancer Cell. 2004; 6(3):203–8.

7. Karin M, Ben-Neriah Y. Phosphorylation meets ubiquitination: the control of NF-[kappa]B activity. Annu Rev Immunol. 2000;18:621–63.

8. Pasparakis M. Regulation of tissue homeostasis by NF-kappaB signalling: implications for inflammatory diseases. Nat Rev Immunol. 2009;9(11):778–88.

9. Guha M, Mackman N. LPS induction of gene expression in human monocytes. Cell Signal. 2001;13(2):85–94.

10. Lawrence T, Fong C. The resolution of inflammation: anti-inflammatory roles for NF-kappaB. Int J Biochem Cell Biol. 2010;42(4):519–23.

11. Thalhamer T, McGrath MA, Harnett MM. MAPKs and their relevance to arthritis and inflammation. Rheumatol. 2008;47(4):409–14.

12. Vanden Berghe W, Plaisance S, Boone E, De Bosscher K, Schmitz ML, Fiers W, Haegeman G. p38 and extracellular signal-regulated kinase mitogen-activated protein kinase pathways are required for nuclear factor-kappaB p65 transactivation mediated by tumor necrosis factor. J Biol Chem. 1998; 273(6):3285–90.

13. Hwang PA, Chien SY, Chan YL, Lu MK, Wu CH, Kong ZL, Wu CJ. Inhibition of lipopolysaccharide (LPS)-induced inflammatory responses by Sargassum hemiphyllum sulfated polysaccharide extract in RAW 264.7 macrophage cells. J Agric Food Chem. 2011;59(5):2062–8.

14. Paccani SR, Boncristiano M, Ulivieri C, D'Elios MM, Del Prete G, Baldari CT. Nonsteroidal anti-inflammatory drugs suppress T-cell activation by inhibiting p38 MAPK induction. J Biol Chem. 2002;277(2):1509–13.

15. Patil VV, Bhangale SC, Patil VR. Studies on immunomodulatory activity of Ficus carica. Int J Pharm Pharm Sci. 2010;2(4):97–9.

16. Jayathirtha MG, Mishra SH. Preliminary immunomodulatory activities of methanol extracts of Eclipta alba and Centella asiatica. Phytomedicine. 2004; 11(4):361–5.

17. Patel JR, Tripathi P, Sharma V, Chauhan NS, Dixit VK. Phyllanthus amarus: ethnomedicinal uses, phytochemistry and pharmacology: a review. J Ethnopharmacol. 2011;138(2):286–313.

18. Calixto JB, Santos AR, Cechinel Filho V, Yunes RA. A review of the plants of the genus Phyllanthus: their chemistry, pharmacology, and therapeutic potential. Med Res Rev. 1998;18(4):225–58.

19. Harikrishnan H, Jantan I, Haque MA, Kumolosasi E. Anti-inflammatory effects of hypophyllanthin and niranthin through downregulation of NF-κB/MAPKs/PI3K-Akt signaling pathways. Inflammation. 2018;41(3):984–95.

20. Foo LY. Amariin, a di-dehydrohexahydroxydiphenoyl hydrolysable tannin from Phyllanthus amarus. Phytochemistry. 1993;33(2):487–91.

21. Sharma A, Singh RT, Handa SS. Estimation of phyllanthin and hypophyllanthin by high performance liquid chromatography in Phyllanthus amarus. Phytochem Anal. 1993;4(5):226–9.

22. Houghton PJ, Woldemariam TZ, O'Shea S, Thyagarajan S. Two securinega-type alkaloids from Phyllanthus amarus. Phytochemistry. 1996;43(3):715–7.

23. Moronkola DO, Ogunwande IA, Oyewole IO, Başer KHC, Ozek T, Ozek G. Studies on the volatile oils of Momordica charantia L. (Cucurbitaceae) and Phyllanthus amarus Sch. Et Thonn (Euphorbiaceae). J Essent Oil Res. 2009;21(5):393–9.

24. Mahat M, Patil B. Evaluation of antiinflammatory activity of methanol extract of Phyllanthus amarus in experimental animal models. Indian J Pharm Sci. 2007;69(1):33.

25. Kassuya CA, Silvestre A, Menezes-de-Lima O, Marotta DM, Rehder VLG, Calixto JB. Antiinflammatory and antiallodynic actions of the lignan niranthin isolated from Phyllanthus amarus: evidence for interaction with platelet activating factor receptor. Eur J Pharmacol. 2006;546(1):182–8.

26. Yuandani IM, Jantan I, Mohamad HF, Husain K, Abdul Razak AF. Inhibitory effects of standardized extracts of Phyllanthus amarus and Phyllanthus urinaria and their marker compounds on phagocytic activity of human neutrophils. Evid Based Complement Alternat Med. 2013;2013:603634.

27. Jantan I, Ilangkovan M, Mohamad HF. Correlation between the major components of Phyllanthus amarus and Phyllanthus urinaria and their inhibitory effects on phagocytic activity of human neutrophils. BMC Complement Altern Med. 2014;14(1):429.

28. Ilangkovan M, Jantan I, Mesaik MA, Bukhari SNA. Immunosuppressive effects of the standardized extract of Phyllanthus amarus on cellular immune responses in Wistar-Kyoto rats. Drug Des Dev Ther. 2015;9:4917.

29. Ilangkovan M, Jantan I, Mesaik MA, Bukhari SNA. Inhibitory effects of the standardized extract of Phyllanthus amarus on cellular and humoral immune responses in Balb/C mice. Phytother Res. 2016;30(8):1330–8.

30. Sock-Jin L, Kumolosasi E, Azmi N, Bukhari SNA, Jasamai M, Fauzi NM. Effects of synthetic chalcone derivatives on oxidised palmitoyl arachidonoyl phosphorylcholine-induced proinflammatory chemokines production. RSC Adv. 2015;5(84):68773–80.

31. Aluwi MFFM, Rullah K, Haque MA, Yamin BM, Ahmad W, Amjad MW, Leong SW, Fahmizar NA, Jalil J, Abas F. Suppression of PGE2 production via disruption of MAPK phosphorylation by unsymmetrical dicarbonyl curcumin derivatives. Med Chem Res. 2017;26(12):3323–35.

32. Kiemer AK, Hartung T, Huber C, Vollmar AM. Phyllanthus amarus has anti-inflammatory potential by inhibition of iNOS, COX-2, and cytokines via the NF-κB pathway. J Hepatol. 2003;38(3):289–97.

33. Ilangkovan M, Jantan I, Mohamad HF, Husain K, Abdul Razak AF. Inhibitory effects of standardized extracts of Phyllanthus amarus and Phyllanthus urinaria and their marker compounds on phagocytic activity of human neutrophils. Evid Based Complement Alternat Med. 2013;2013, Art. ID. 603634. p. 9.

34. Yuandani IJ, Ilangkovan M, Husain K, Chan KM. Inhibitory effects of compounds from Phyllanthus amarus on nitric oxide production, lymphocyte proliferation, and cytokine release from phagocytes. Drug Des Dev Ther. 2016;10:1935.

35. Roh K-B, Kim H, Shin S, Kim Y-S, Lee J-A, Kim MO, Jung E, Lee J, Park D. Anti-inflammatory effects of Zea mays L. husk extracts. BMC Complement Altern Med. 2016;16(1):298.

36. Lee SH, Soyoola E, Chanmugam P, Hart S, Sun W, Zhong H, Liou S, Simmons D, Hwang D. Selective expression of mitogen-inducible cyclooxygenase in macrophages stimulated with lipopolysaccharide. J Biol Chem. 1992;267(36):25934–8.

37. Xie W, Chipman JG, Robertson DL, Erikson R, Simmons DL. Expression of a mitogen-responsive gene encoding prostaglandin synthase is regulated by mRNA splicing. Proc Natl Acad Sci. 1991;88(7):2692–6.

38. Mohamed SIA, Jantan I, Haque MA. Naturally occurring immunomodulators with antitumor activity: an insight on their mechanisms of action. Int Immunopharmacol. 2017;50:291–304.

39. Baraf HS. Efficacy of the newest COX-2 selective inhibitors in rheumatic disease. Curr Pharm Des. 2007;13(22):2228–36.

40. Tham CL, Liew CY, Lam KW, Mohamad A-S, Kim MK, Cheah YK, Zakaria Z-A, Sulaiman M-R, Lajis NH, Israf DA. A synthetic curcuminoid derivative inhibits nitric oxide and proinflammatory cytokine synthesis. Eur J Pharmacol. 2010; 628(1–3):247–54.

41. Bertholet S, Tzeng E, Felley-Bosco E, Mauel J. Expression of the inducible NO synthase in human monocytic U937 cells allows high output nitric oxide production. J Leukoc Biol. 1999;65(1):50–8.

42. Jung H-W, Seo U-K, Kim J-H, Leem K-H, Park Y-K. Flower extract of Panax notoginseng attenuates lipopolysaccharide-induced inflammatory response via blocking of NF-κB signaling pathway in murine macrophages. J Ethnopharmacol. 2009;122(2):313–9.

43. Oeckinghaus A, Ghosh S. The NF-κB family of transcription factors and its regulation. Cold Spring Harb Perspect Biol. 2009;1(4):a000034.

44. Kaminska B. MAPK signalling pathways as molecular targets for anti-inflammatory therapy-from molecular mechanisms to therapeutic benefits. Biochim Biophys Acta. 2005;1754(1–2):253–62.

45. Laird MH, Rhee SH, Perkins DJ, Medvedev AE, Piao W, Fenton MJ, Vogel SN. TLR4/MyD88/PI3K interactions regulate TLR4 signaling. J Leukoc Biol. 2009; 85(6):966–77.

Antioxidant and skin-whitening effects of aerial part of *Euphorbia supina* Raf. Extract

Sa-Haeng Kang[1], Yong-Deok Jeon[2]ⓘ, Ji-Yoon Cha[1], Sung-Woo Hwang[1], Hoon-Yeon Lee[1], Min Park[1], Bo-Ri Lee[1], Min-Kyoung Shin[2], Su-Jeong Kim[3], Sang-Min Shin[3], Dae-Ki Kim[4], Jong-Sik Jin[2*] and Young-Mi Lee[1*]

Abstract

Background: *Euphorbia supina* (ES) has been widely used in folk medicine owing to its antibacterial, hemostatic, and anti-inflammatory properties. The aim of this study was to evaluate the antioxidant and skin-whitening effects of a 70% ethanol extract of ES.

Methods: The aerial parts of ES plant were extracted with 70% ethanol. The viability of B16F10 cells was evaluated by MTT assay to determine the non-toxic doses for further experiments. The tyrosinase and cellular tyrosinase activities were then measured using an enzyme-substrate assay. In addition, the expression of whitening-related proteins was measured using western blot.

Results: The antioxidant activity of the ES samples increased in a dose-dependent manner, as confirmed by their radical scavenging activities in the 2,2-diphenyl-1-1-picrylhydrazyl and 2,2-azino-bis-(3-ethylbenzthiazoline-6-sulfonic acid) assays. The ES extract significantly reduced tyrosinase activity and melanin content in a dose-dependent manner. Furthermore, it decreased α-melanocyte stimulating hormone (MSH)-induced protein expression of tyrosinase and microphthalmia-associated transcription factor (MITF).

Conclusions: Our results indicate that the ES extract attenuated α-MSH-stimulated melanin synthesis by modulating tyrosinase and MITF expression. Therefore, the ES extract could be a promising therapeutic agent to treat hyperpigmentation and as an ingredient for skin-whitening cosmetics.

Keywords: *Euphorbia supina* (ES), DPPH, Melanogenesis, Tyrosinase, MITF, α-MSH

Background

Melanin is a major pigment that controls skin and hair color. It is a high-molecular-weight compound widely distributed in animals and plants [1]. Melanin protects the skin from ultraviolet radiation. However, when produced in excess, the pigment accumulates in the skin to form spots and freckles, and these lesions may cause skin cancer [2]. Therefore, to prevent an excess of skin pigmentation, it is necessary to inhibit the production of melanin [3]. Melanocytes, located in the basal layer of the epidermis and controlled by tyrosinase, produce melanin via melanogenesis, and contain enzymes such as tyrosinase-related protein-1 (TRP-1) and dopachrome tautomerase (DCT) [4]. Tyrosinase catalyzes 3,4-dihydroxyphenylalanine (DOPA) quinone formation from DOPA, and melanin formation from DOPA quinone via autoxidation and enzymatic reactions [5]. Therefore, melanin production is related to tyrosinase expression and TRP-1 activation. Thus, we investigated whether *Euphorbia supina* (ES) could influence the relationship between tyrosinase and melanin.

Tyrosinase activity is important in skin-whitening studies [6]. Various chemicals and plant extracts, such as kojic acid, arbutin, vitamin C, and hydroquinone, are used in skin-whitening cosmetics. However, their use has been limited due to their side effects such as coloration, odor, and cytotoxicity [7]. Therefore, recent studies are focused on the development of skin-whitening agents from skin-safe natural products.

* Correspondence: jongsik.jin@jbnu.ac.kr; ymlee@wku.ac.kr
[2]Department of Oriental Medicine Resources, Chonbuk National University, 79 Gobongro, Iksan, Jeollabuk-do 54596, South Korea
[1]Department of Oriental Pharmacy, College of Pharmacy, Wonkwang-Oriental Medicines Research Institute, Wonkwang University, Iksan, Jeollabuk-do 54538, South Korea
Full list of author information is available at the end of the article

In this study, ES was used to develop a safe compound with antioxidant and skin-whitening effects. ES is an annual herbaceous plant, and is widely used in traditional herbal formulations. It is widely distributed in temperate and tropical regions such as Korea, China, and Japan. It is used in folk medicine against various inflammatory disorders [8, 9]. Studies focused on the components of ES such as tannins [10, 11], phenolic substances and flavonoids [12, 13], and terpenoids [14, 15] have been reported. In addition, the in vitro anticancer effect in breast cancer metastasis [16], and the antioxidant activity of phenolic mixtures of ES have been reported [17]. However, the in vitro antioxidant activities in 2,2-diphenyl-1-1-picrylhydrazyl (DPPH) and 2,2′-azino-bis-3-ethylbenzthiazoline-6-sulfonic acid (ABTS) assays, and skin-whitening effects of ES extracts on melanoma cells have not been understood. Therefore, the aim of this study was to determine the antioxidant and skin-whitening effects of ES in vitro and confirm its efficacy as a novel skin-whitening agent.

Methods
Preparation of the ES extract
ES was provided by Wonkwang pharmaceutical company (Iksan, Jeonbuk, Korea). The aerial parts (stem and leaf) of ES (250 g) were boiled with 70% ethanol at 70 °C for 2 h. After filtration, the residue was again boiled twice as described above. The combined filtrates were evaporated at 45 °C and lyophilized to obtain the crude extract at a yield of 60 g (24%). The extract was stored at 4 °C before experiments. A voucher specimen (JUHES-1660) has been deposited at the Department of Oriental Medicine Resources, Chonbuk National University (Iksan, Korea).

Cell culture
The B16F10 murine melanoma cells (CRL-6475) were purchased from the American Type Culture Collection (ATCC; Manassas, VA, USA). The cells were cultured in Dulbecco's Modified Eagle's Medium (DMEM) containing 2 mM glutamine, supplemented with 10% fetal bovine serum (FBS), 100 units/mL of penicillin, and 100 μg/mL of streptomycin in culture flasks in a CO_2 incubator with a humidified atmosphere of 5% CO_2 in air at 37 °C. All the experiments were performed in triplicate, and were repeated thrice to ensure reproducibility.

Cell viability assay
To evaluate the safety of the ES extract, an MTT assay was performed to determine the viability of the cells after treatment with the extract. This method was based on the reduction of 3-(4,5-dimethylthiazol-2-yl)-2,5-diphenyl tetrazolium bromide (MTT) to formazan by mitochondrial enzymes (NAD(P)H-dependent cellular

oxidoreductase) in viable cells [18]. Briefly, B16F10 cells (1×10^4 cells/well) were incubated with various concentrations of ES extract (8, 40, 200 μg/mL) in a 96-well microplate for 24 h. Then, the MTT solution (500 μg/mL) was added to each well and the plate was incubated at 37 °C for 8 h. The formazan crystals produced by living cells were dissolved in 600 μL of DMSO. The absorbance of each well was measured at 540 nm on a VersaMax microplate reader (Molecular Devices, Sunnyvale, CA, USA).

Antioxidant activities
The DPPH radical scavenging activity was evaluated according to the method described in [19] with minor modifications. The various concentration (8, 40, 200 μg/mL) of ES extract or 20 μg/mL of ascorbic acid (used as positive control) at 500 μL were added to 1 mL of 0.1 mM DPPH solution. The reaction was allowed to proceed for 30 min in the dark at room temperature (RT) after vortexing. The absorbance was measured at 517 nm on a VersaMax microplate reader. We conducted an experiment to confirm the extent to which radicals were reduced by the electron-donating effect with respect to the ABTS radical scavenging activity [20]. After radical formation, a solution of 7.4 mM ABTS and 2.6 mM potassium persulfate was added and the resulting mixture was allowed to react for 12 h at RT; ABTS solution was measured and showed an absorbance of 0.70 ± 0.03 (mean ± S.D.) measured using a microplate reader. The ES extract (100 μL) was added to 900 μL of ABTS solution, and was allowed to react for 10 min at RT. The absorbance of 200 μL solution mixture was measured at 732 nm using a microplate reader.

Measurement of melanin content
Melanin content was measured after adding minor modifications to the previously described protocol [21]. The B16F10 melanoma cells were seeded at 1×10^5 cells/well in 3 mL of medium in 6-well culture plates and incubated overnight to allow cells to adhere. The cells were exposed to various concentrations (8, 40, 200 μg/mL) of the ES extract or 10 mM arbutin for 72 h in the presence or absence of 100 nM of α-melanocyte-stimulating hormone (α-MSH; Sigma-Aldrich, St. Louis, MO, USA). At the end of the treatment, the cells were washed with PBS (pH 7.2) and lysed with 300 μL of 1 M NaOH containing 10% DMSO for 2 h at 80 °C. The absorbance of 200 μL mixture was measured at 400 nm using a microplate reader.

Determination of cellular tyrosinase activity
Cellular tyrosinase activity was measured according to a method previously described by Lee et al. [22] with some modifications. Six-well plates containing 2 mL of DMEM

were seeded with B16F10 melanoma cells at a density of 1×10^5 cells/well. Each well was separated into 6 different groups as follows; Vehicle: non-treatment, Control: 100 nM of α-MSH, ESEE 8: α-MSH and ES extract (8 μg/mL), ESEE 40: α-MSH and ES extract (40 μg/mL), ESEE 200: α-MSH and ES extract (200 μg/mL), Arbutin: α-MSH and arbutin (10 mM). Plates were incubated overnight in a humidified incubator at 37 °C with 5% CO_2 atmosphere to allow cells to adhere. Cells were then exposed to 100 nM of α-MSH for 48 h and then treated with increasing doses of the ES extract or arbutin for 24 h. The cells were washed with PBS (pH 6.8) and re-suspended in lysis buffer. Next, the cells were ruptured by freezing and thawing, and the lysate was clarified by centrifugation at 16,000 g for 20 min. The protein content of the lysate was determined using a BCA Protein Assay Kit (Thermo Scientific, Vantaa, Finland). After quantifying the protein levels, the concentrations were adjusted such that all the samples contained the same amount of protein (20 μg). These lysates were then added to the wells of a 96-well plate containing 2.5 mM L-DOPA in 0.1 M phosphate buffer (pH 6.8). Following incubation at 37 °C for 1 h, the absorbance of the different lysates was measured at 475 nm using a spectrophotometer. Tyrosinase activity in the protein was calculated by the following formula:

$$\text{Tyrosinase activity } (\%) = (OD_s - OD_b)/\text{Control} \times 100$$
$$OD_s : \text{sample absorbance value}$$
$$OD_b : \text{vehicle absorbance value}$$

Mushroom tyrosinase activity
L-DOPA was used as the substrate for the measurement of mushroom tyrosinase activity. The reaction buffer (total 3 mL) used in the experiment contained 2.8 mL of 0.5 mM L-DOPA in 50 mM Na_2HPO_4-NaH_2PO_4 buffer (pH 6.8) and 100 μL of different concentrations of ES. An aqueous solution of mushroom tyrosinase (100 μL) was added to the mixed buffer. The solution (200 μL) was immediately evaluated for the linear increase in optical absorbance at 475 nm using a microplate reader.

Western blot analysis
The B16F10 melanoma cells (1×10^6 cells/well) were cultured in 60-mm² dishes. Then, cells were treated with various concentrations (8, 40, 200 μg/mL) of ES extract and 10 mM of arbutin for 24 h. The cells were then lysed in a buffer containing 50 mM Tris-HCl with pH 7.4, 2 mM EGTA, 1 mM phenylmethyl-sulfonyl fluoride, 10 mM β-glycerophosphate, 10 mM β-mercaptoethanol, 1 mM sodium orthovanadate, and 0.1% deoxycholic acid sodium salt. The lysates (25 μg) were resolved by 10% SDS-polyacrylamide gel electrophoresis and transferred electrophoretically to polyvinylidene difluoride

membranes and blocked overnight with 5% skim milk in TBST buffer (20 mM Tris-HCl pH 7.4, 100 mM NaCl, and 0.1% Tween 20) at 4 °C. After the membranes were washed in TBST buffer, they were incubated for 3 h with a primary antibody of tyrosinase, MITF, and β-actin (ratio 1:1000). After incubation with a secondary antibody (ratio 1:1000) for 1 h at RT, the protein-antibody complexes were visualized with ECL Western blotting Luminol Reagent (Santa Cruz Biotech, CA, USA), and detected using the Fluorchem E image analyzer (Cell Biosciences, CA, USA).

GC-MS analysis
The ethanol extract sample was dried with a speed vacuum and derivatized with N,O-bis(trimethylsilyl)trifluoroacetamide (BSTFA) (Sigma Aldrich, St. Louis, MO, USA). GC-MS analysis was performed using a QP2010 gas chromatograph coupled with a mass spectrometer (Shimadzu) at an ionization voltage of 70 eV. GC analysis was performed in a temperature-programming mode with a Restek column (0.25 mm, 30 m; XTI-5). The initial column temperature was set at 70 °C for 3 min, increased linearly at 10 °C/min to 300 °C, and then held for 5 min. The temperature of the injection port was 280 °C, and the GC/MS interface was maintained at 290 °C. The helium carrier gas flow rate was 1.0 mL/min.

Statistical analysis
The data for melanin synthesis, cytotoxicity, and tyrosinase activity assay were statistically evaluated by ANOVA, followed by Dunnett's test. The data are presented as mean ± SD. A P value < 0.05 indicated statistical significance.

Results
Effect of the ES extract on B16F10 cell viability
The MTT assay was used to assess the effect of the ES 70% ethanol extract on the viability of B16F10 melanoma cells. The cells were treated with various concentrations of the extract (8, 40, 200 μg /mL) for 24 h, and then the MTT assay was performed. The results are expressed as percent of viability relative to control. The ES extract had a non-cytotoxic effect on B16F10 cell proliferation (Fig. 1). However, at a concentration of 1000 μg/mL, clear cytotoxicity was observed in B16F10 cells (data not shown).

Antioxidant capacities of the ES extract
The DPPH and ABTS assays were used to measure the antioxidant activity of the ES extract. To measure the DPPH radical scavenging activity of the ES extract, various concentrations of the ES extract (8, 40, 200 μg/mL) were used. The DPPH radical scavenging activity of the

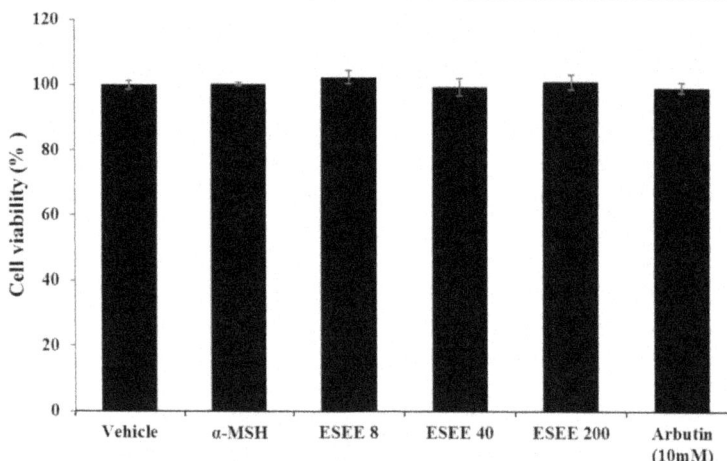

Fig. 1 Cell viability of the ES extract on the B16F10 cells. B16F10 cells were treated with various concentration of ES extract (8, 40, 200 μg/ml) for 24 h and the cell viability was measured by MTT assay. The absorbance was measured at 540 nm on a VersaMax microplate reader. Values represent the mean ± S.D. of triplicate experiments

ES extract increased in a dose-dependent manner. Ascorbic acid used as a positive control and showed over 50% DPPH radical scavenging activity (Fig. 2a). The ABTS+ radical scavenging activity of 8 and 40 μg/mL of ES extract was also significantly high, presenting a result similar to the positive control group. The ES extract showed $93.05 \pm 0.6\%$ activity at 200 μg/mL, which was almost the same as that of ascorbic acid (Fig. 2b).

Effect of the ES extract on mushroom tyrosinase activity, B16F10 melanin content, and intracellular tyrosinase activity

To measure the inhibitory effect of the ES extract on mushroom tyrosinase activity, the tyrosinase inhibition assay was performed. The results indicated that the mushroom tyrosinase activity was inhibited by the ES extract at high concentrations. Tyrosinase activity was $88.35 \pm 1.28\%$, $70.81 \pm 2.52\%$, and $45.43 \pm 0.48\%$ after treatment with 8, 40, and 200 μg/mL of the ES extract,

respectively (Fig. 3a). To examine the antimelanogenic activity of the ES extract, the inhibitory effect of the ES extract on melanin was evaluated in B16F10 cells. The B16F10 cells were treated with the ES extract at 8, 40, and 200 μg/mL or with arbutin at 10 mM, and stimulated with α-MSH (10 nM) for 48 h. The ES extract presented a significant dose-dependent inhibitory effect on melanin synthesis. The melanin content was represented as percentage of the vehicle. The melanin content was $146.17 \pm 0.07\%$, $110 \pm 0.1\%$, and $76.95 \pm 0.39\%$ after treatment with 8, 40, and 200 μg/mL of the ES extract, respectively (Fig. 3b). When the B16F10 cells were treated with the positive control arbutin (10 mM), the intracellular melanin content was $84.82 \pm 1.28\%$. To determine the mechanism underlying the inhibitory effect of the ES extract on melanogenesis, we assessed the intracellular tyrosinase activity in B16F10 melanoma cells. Therefore, another group of B16F10 cells was treated with various concentrations of the ES extract (8, 40, 200 μg/mL) or

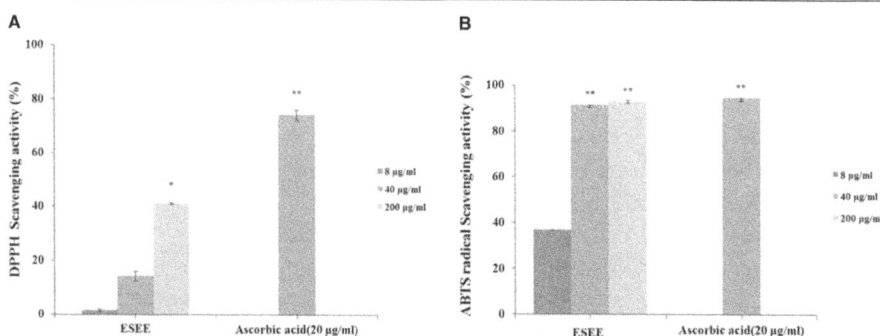

Fig. 2 Antioxidant activities of ES extract. **a** Scavenging effect of ES on DPPH radical (**b**) ABTS+ radical scavenging activity of the extract. The ES ethanol extract (ESEE) (8, 40, 200 μg/ml), ascorbic acid (20 μg/ml) were incubated with DPPH, ABTS+ solution, respectively. Results are represented as percentages of control, and the data represent mean ± S.D. for three separate experiments. Values are significantly different by comparison with control. *: $p < 0.05$, **: $p < 0.01$

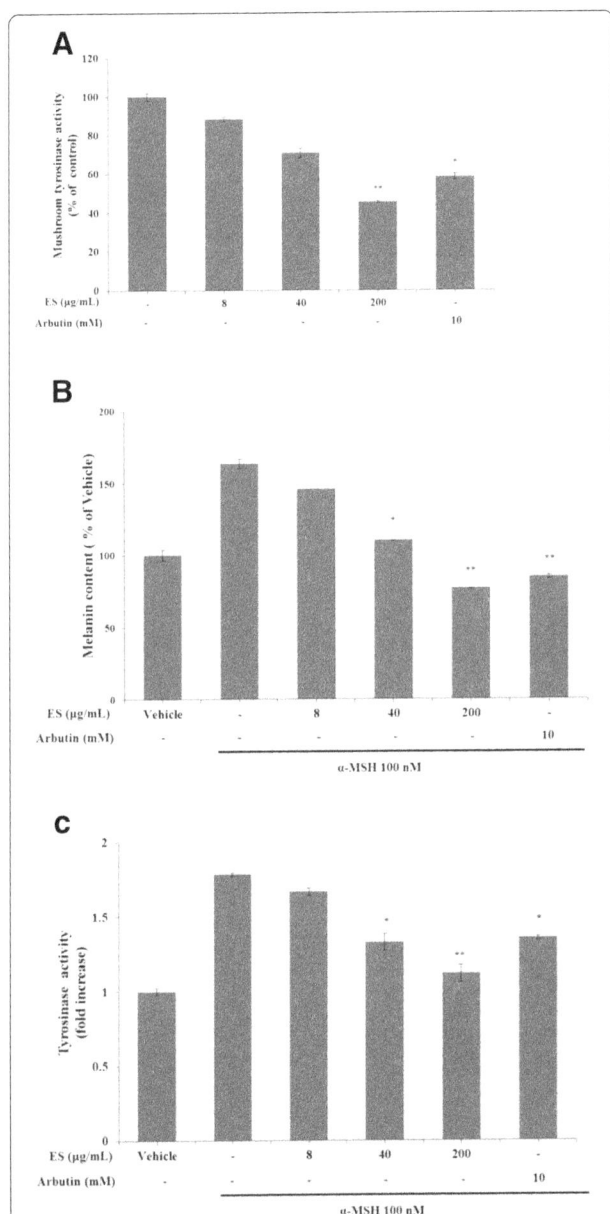

Fig. 3 Inhibitory effect of ES extract on mushroom tyrosinase activity, B16F10 melanin content and intracellular tyrosinase activity. **a** Different concentrations of the ES extract (8, 40, 200 μg/ml) or arbutin (10 mM) was incubated with the same units of mushroom tyrosinase. Following incubation, the amount of dopachrome produced was determined at 490 nm. **b** and **c** B16F10 melanoma cells were stimulated with α-MSH (100 nM) for 48 h, and then the melanin content or intracellular tyrosinase activity were measured after treatment with various concentrations of the ES extract (8, 40,200 μg/ml) or arbutin (10 mM) for another 24 h. Results are represented as percentages of control, and data are presented as mean ± S.D. for three separate experiments. Values are significantly different by comparison with control. *: $p < 0.05$, **: $p < 0.01$ α-MSH treatment alone

arbutin (10 mM) and stimulated with α-MSH (10 nM) for 48 h. The ES extract significantly inhibited α-MSH-induced tyrosinase activity in a dose-dependent manner (Fig. 3c).

Inhibitory effect of the ES extract on proteins related to melanogenesis in B16F10 cells

To investigate whether ES could influence melanogenic protein expression, western blotting was performed using the lysate of B16F10 melanoma cells treated with ES and stimulated with α-MSH (10 mM). Tyrosinase and MITF expression levels were evaluated by western blot (Fig. 4). We confirmed that tyrosinase and MITF expression significantly increased when cells were stimulated with α-MSH. The ES extract was able to suppress tyrosinase and MITF expression stimulated by α-MSH in a dose-dependent manner.

Chemical composition of ES

The chemical composition of the ES extract was analyzed by GC-MS (Fig. 5). The retention times of gallic and protocatechuic acids, two of the major components of the ES extract, were 19.810 and 18.290 min, respectively. The two compounds were successfully detected in the ES extract.

Discussion

In this study, we evaluated whether the ES extract exhibited a skin-whitening effect by suppressing melanin production in B16F10 melanoma cells. The ES extract inhibited tyrosinase enzyme activity, decreased melanin content, and showed an antioxidant effect. Melanin production may be stimulated by UV or α-MSH. The α-MSH binds MC1R and activates the signaling protein adenylate cyclase to increase cyclic AMP (cAMP) production [23]. cAMP responsive element binding protein (CREB) is activated continuously by protein kinase A (PKA), and activation by CREB increases the expression of MITF protein and promotes the expression of tyrosinase [24]. After stimulating B16F10 cells with α-MSH to induce melanogenesis, the whitening effect of ES was confirmed by melanin quantification. Melanin content was found to be suppressed in a dose-dependent manner, and at the highest concentration (200 μg/mL) used in the experiment, more than 50% suppression of the melanin content was observed in comparison with the α-MSH only treatment group.

ES has been used in traditional herbal formulations. It belongs to the Euphorbiaceae family, and is traditionally used in eastern Asia for medicinal purposes. ES contains numerous biologically active substances including tannins, terpenoids, and polyphenols [25]. DPPH is a relatively stable free radical. The DPPH

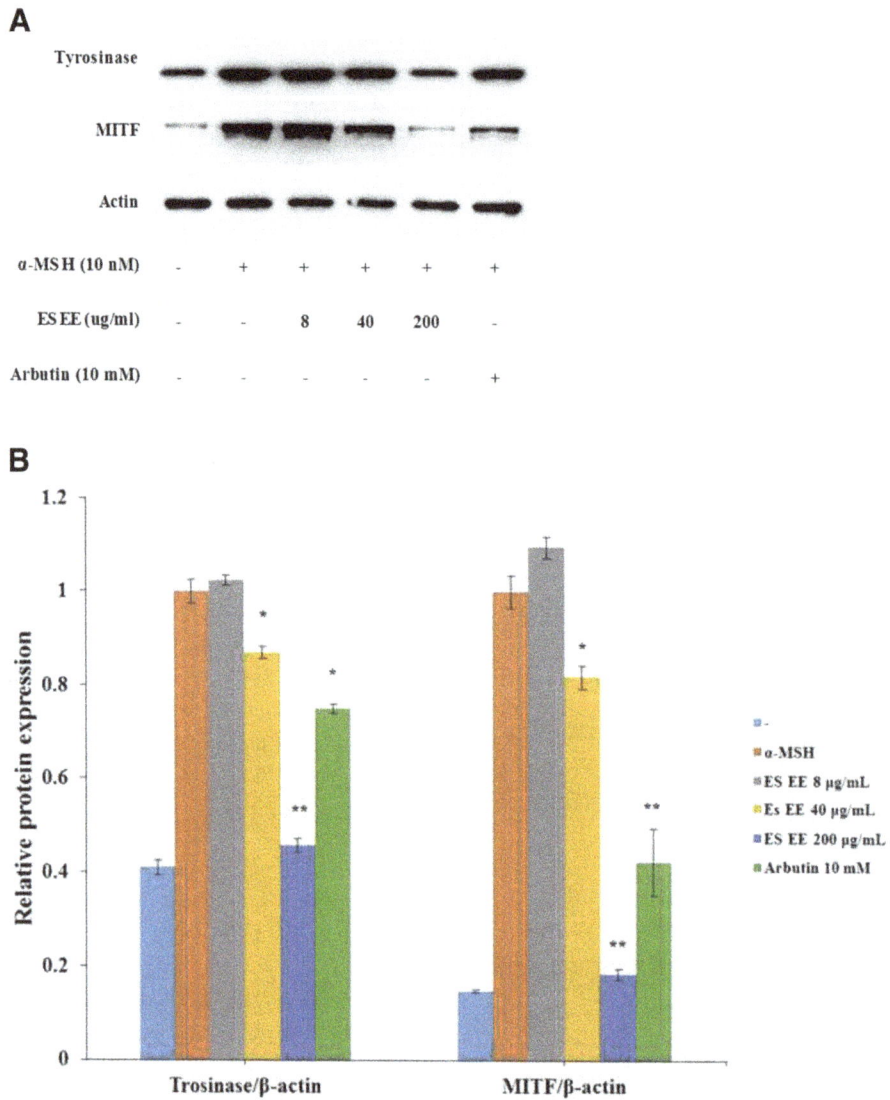

Fig. 4 Effect of ES extract on melanogenesis-related proteins expression. **a** B16F10 cells were cultured with α-MSH (100 nM) for 24 h and then treated with various concentration of the ES extract (8, 40, 200 µg/ml) or arbutin (10 mM) for another 24 h. Then the content of cellular MITF, tyrosinase proteins were analyzed by western blotting assay. **b** Densitometry was normalized to the α-MSH group. Values are mean ± S.D. Data were analyzed by Student's t-test. *: $p < 0.05$, **: $p < 0.01$ versus α-MSH treatment alone

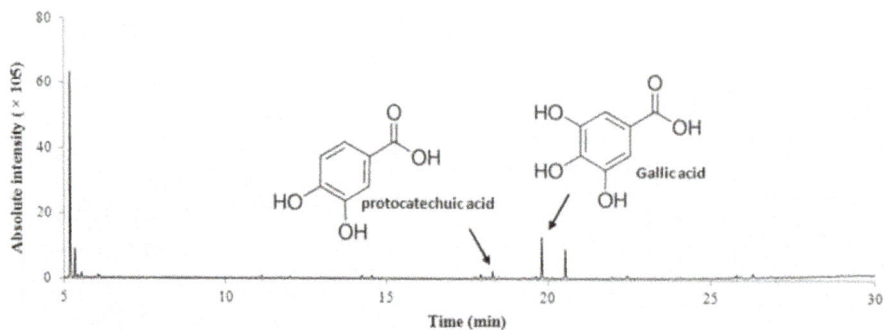

Fig. 5 GC-MS Chromatograms of the methanol extract ES

assay is widely used to measure the antioxidant activity of plants, indicated by a decrease in the deep purple color of the solution by reducing agents such as ascorbic acid, tocopherol, polyhydroxy aromatic compounds, and aromatic amines [26]. In addition, ABTS radical scavenging activity is more useful than DPPH radical scavenging activity with respect to measurement of hydrogen-donating antioxidants, chain-breaking antioxidants, and antioxidant ability of hydrophilic and hydrophobic substances [27]. Studies have reported the antioxidant activity of ES. However, its skin-whitening effect has not been evaluated thus far. Therefore, in this study, we confirmed the skin-whitening effect of ES (Fig. 2). We verified its influence on tyrosinase activity, which determines the initial rate of melanogenesis (Fig. 3). As an enzyme that promotes the production of melanin, tyrosinase is widely used as a target compound to identify new inhibitors that can suppress melanin formation [28]. To investigate the mechanism by which ES inhibits melanogenesis, we determined whether the ES extract could inhibit tyrosinase activity directly [29]. For this assay, arbutin was used as the positive control. We observed a skin-whitening effect, which was remarkably higher than that of arbutin (10 mM). The ES extract significantly decreased the mushroom tyrosinase activity after 24 h of treatment and inhibited cellular tyrosinase activity. Thus, we confirmed that the ES extract exhibits an excellent antioxidant effect as well as skin-whitening activity.

Tyrosinase is the main enzyme involved in melanogenesis [30]. The MITF transcription factors are important regulators in the development and differentiation of melanocytes [31]. The suppression of tyrosinase and MITF expression by the ES extract increased in a dose-dependent manner. These results suggest that ES suppresses the transcription factor MITF, and thus inhibits tyrosinase expression.

There has been an increase in the interest in various natural products with skin-whitening and wrinkle-improvement effects as base materials for food and cosmetics. The use of products containing ingredients with various skin-protecting properties, such an anti-wrinkle, moisturizing, whitening, and anti-inflammation, has increased in the global beauty market [32]. In this study, we found that the ES extract had strong antioxidant effects, inhibited tyrosinase, and regulated whitening-related protein expression. The activities might be attributed to gallic acid and protocatechuic acid detected in ES extract [33, 34]. Therefore, ES appears to have the potential to be used for the development of natural cosmetics for skin whitening for effective reduction or prevention of excessive melanin pigmentation in the skin.

Conclusions
In conclusion, ES extract regulated tyrosinase activities and MITF protein expression in B16F10 cells. The ES extract showed antioxidant activities in DPPH and ABTS assays. This study provides experimental evidence that ES could be a useful therapeutic agent for the treatment of skin diseases.

Abbreviations
ABTS: 2,2'-azino-bis-3-ethylbenzthiazoline-6-sulfonic acid; cAMP: Cyclic AMP; CREB: cAMP responsive element binding protein; DCT: Dopachrome tautomerase; DMEM: Dulbecco's Modified Eagle's Medium; DPPH: 2,2-Diphenyl-1-1-picrylhydrazyl; ES: *Euphorbia supina*; FBS: Fetal bovine serum; MITF: Microphthalmia-associated transcription factor; MTT: 3-(4,5-dimethylthiazol-2-yl)-2,5-diphenyl tetrazolium bromide; PKA: Protein kinase A; RT: Room temperature; TRP-1: Tyrosinase-related protein-1; α-MSH: α-melanocyte-stimulating hormone

Funding
This research was supported by the Ministry of Trade, Industry & Energy (MOTIE), Korea Institute for Advancement of Technology (KIAT) through the Encouragement Program for The Industries of Economic Cooperation Region (R0004536).

Authors' contributions
SHK, JYC and MP performed the in vitro experiments and analyzed the data. SWH, HYL, BRL contributed design the all experiments also acquisition of experimental data. SJK and SMS provided technical support and gave the material support of ES. MKS performed analysis of extract constituent. SWH, HYL, BRL and YDJ interpreted results of data. SHK, YDJ and DKK collected the data, undertook the statistical analyses, and wrote the manuscript. JSJ and YML designed and supervised the study, including editing of the manuscript. All authors shared the raw data of this experimental study. Also, all authors contributed to and have approved the final manuscript.

Competing interests
The authors declare that they have no competing interests.

Author details
[1]Department of Oriental Pharmacy, College of Pharmacy, Wonkwang-Oriental Medicines Research Institute, Wonkwang University, Iksan, Jeollabuk-do 54538, South Korea. [2]Department of Oriental Medicine Resources, Chonbuk National University, 79 Gobongro, Iksan, Jeollabuk-do 54596, South Korea. [3]Laboratory of YOUCEL, YOUCEL, INC, 78 Iksandaero, Iksan, Jeollabuk-do 54526, South Korea. [4]Department of Immunology and Institute of Medical Science, Jeonbuk National University Medical School, Jeonju, Jeollabuk-do 54896, South Korea.

References
1. Baumann L. Cosmetic dermatology. New York: McGraw-Hill; 2001. p. 98.
2. Iwata M, Corn T, Iwata S, et al. The relationship between tyrosinase activity and skin color in human foreskins. J Invest Dermatol. 1990;95:9–15.
3. Cabanes J, Chazarra S, Garcia-Carmona F. Kojic acid, a cosmetic skin whitening agent, is a slow-binding inhibitor of catecholase activity of tyrosinase. J Pharm Pharmacol. 1994;46:982–5.
4. Kim YJ, Uyama H. Tyrosinase inhibitors from natural and synthetic sources: structure, inhibition mechanism and perspective for the future. Cell Mol Life Sci. 2005;62:1707–23.
5. Jimenez Cervantes C, Garcia Borron JC, Valverde P, et al. Tyrosinase isoenzymes in mammalian melanocytes. 1. Biochemical characterization of two melanosomal tyrosinases from B16 mouse melanoma. Eur J Biochem. 1993;271:549 56.

6. Ye Y, Chou GX, Wang H, et al. Flavonoids, apigenin and icariin exert potent melanogenic activities in murine B16 melanoma cells. Phytomedicine. 2010;18:32–5.

7. Yamakoshi J, Otsuka F, Sano A, et al. Lightening effect on ultraviolet-induced pigmentation of Guinea pig skin by oral administration of a proanthocyanidin-rich extract from grape seeds. Pigment Cell Res. 2003;16:629–38.

8. Choi JG. The medicine of grasses, flowers and trees. Hanmunhwa, Seoul, Korea; 2004. p. 193–201.

9. National China Medical Administration. China medical herbs. Shanghai science technology publisher, Shanghai, China; 1999. p. 789–792.

10. Lee SH, Tanaka T, Nonaka G, et al. Tannins and related compounds. CV. Monomeric and dimeric hydrolysable tannins having a dehydrohexahydroxydiphenoyl group, supinanin, euphorscopin, euphorhelin and jolkianin, from Euphorbia species. Chem Pharm Bull. 1991;39:630–8.

11. Agata I, Hatano T, Nakaya Y, et al. Tannins and related polyphenols of euphorbiaceous plants. VII. Eumaculin a and eusupinin a, and accompanying polyphenols from Euphorbia maculate L. and E. supina Rafin. Chem Pharm Bull. 1991;39:881–3.

12. Fang Z, Zeng X, Zhang Y, et al. Chemical constituents of spottedleaf euphorbia (Euphorbia supina). Zhongcayao. 1993;24:230–3.

13. An RB, Kwon JW, Kwon TO, et al. Chemical constituents from the whole plants of Euphorbia supina Rafin. Kor J Pharmacogn. 2007;38:291–5.

14. Tanaka R, Matsunaga S. Terpenoids and steroids from several Euphorbiaceae and Pinaceae plants. Yakugaku Zasshi. 1999;119:319–39.

15. Chung BS, Kim HG. Studies on the terpenoid constituents of Euphorbia supina Rafin. Kor J Pharmacogn. 1985;16:155–9.

16. Ko YS, Lee WS, Joo YN, et al. Polyphenol mixture of Euphorbia supine the inhibit invasion and metastasis of highly metastatic breast cancer MDA-MB-231 cells. Oncol Rep. 2015;34:3035–42.

17. Hong HK, Kwak JH, Kang SC, et al. Antioxidative constituents from whole plants of Euphorbia supina. Kor J Pharmacogn. 2008;39:260–4.

18. Mosmann T. Rapid colorimetric assay for cellular growth and survival: application to proliferation and cytotoxicity assays. J Immunol Methods. 1983;65:55–63.

19. Blois ML. Antioxidant determination by the use of a stable free radical. Nature. 1958;181:1199–200.

20. Re R, Pellegrini N, Proteggente A, et al. Antioxidant activity applying an improved ABTS radical cation decolorization assay. Free Radic Biol Med. 1999;26:1231–7.

21. Hosoi J, Abe E, Suda T, et al. Regulation of melanin synthesis of B16 mouse melanoma cells by 1 alpha, 25-dihydroxyvitamin D3 and retinoic acid. Cancer Res. 1985;45:1474–8.

22. Lee MH, Lin YP, Hsu FL, et al. Bioactive constituents of Spatholobus suberectus in regulating tyrosinase-related proteins and mRNA in HEMn cells. Phytochemistry. 2006;67:1262–70.

23. Yamaguchi Y, Hearing VJ. Physiological factors that regulate skin pigmentation. Biofactors. 2009;35:193–9.

24. Hearing VJ, Jimenez M. Mammalian tyrosinase-the critical regulatory control point in melanocyte pigmentation. Int J BioChemiPhysics. 1987;19:1141–7.

25. Song Y, Jeong SW, Lee WS, et al. Determination of polyphenol components of Korean prostrate spurge (Euphorbia supina) by using liquid chromatography—tandem mass spectrometry: overall contribution to antioxidant activity. J Anal Methods Chem. 2014. https://doi.org/10.1155/2014/418690.

26. Choi CH, Song ES, Kim JS, et al. Antioxidative activities of Castanea crenata Flos. Methanol extracts. Korean J Food Sci Technol. 2003;35:1216–20.

27. Busca R, Ballotti R. Cyclic AMP a key messenger in the regulation of skin pigmentation. Pigment Cell Res. 2000;13:60–9.

28. Hwang JH, Lee BM. Inhibitory effects of plant extracts on tyrosinase, L-DOPA oxidation, and melanin synthesis. J Toxicol Environ Health A. 2007;70: 393–407.

29. Tayarani NZ, Akaberi M, Vatani M, et al. Evaluation of antioxidant and antimelanogenic activities of different extracts from aerial parts of Nepeta binaludensis Jamzad in murine melanoma B16F10 cells. Iran J Basic Med Sci. 2016;19:662–9.

30. Kim DS, Kim SY, Park SH, et al. Inhibitory effects of 4-n-Butylresorcinol on Tyrosinase activity and melanin synthesis. Biol Pharm Bull. 2005;28:2216–9.

31. Goding CR. Melanocytes: the new black. Int J Biochem Cell Biol. 2007;39: 275–9.

32. Jeong SC, Park JH, Kim JH. The development trend of skin beauty food with skin protection effects from natural source. Kor J Aesthet Cosmetol. 2013;11:203–12.

33. Truong XT, Park SH, Lee YG, et al. Protocatechuic acid from pear inhibits Melanogenesis in melanoma cells. Int J Mol Sci. 2017;21, 18(8).

34. Su TR, Lin JJ, Tsai CC, et al. Inhibition of melanogenesis by gallic acid: possible involvement of the PI3K/Akt, MEK/ERK and Wnt/β-catenin signaling pathways in B16F10 cells. Int J Mol Sci. 2013;14(10):20443–2058.

Water/ethanol extract of *Cucumis sativus* L. fruit attenuates lipopolysaccharide-induced inflammatory response in endothelial cells

Chiara Bernardini* ⓘ, Augusta Zannoni, Martina Bertocchi, Irvin Tubon, Mercedes Fernandez and Monica Forni

Abstract

Background: It is widely accepted the key role of endothelium in the onset of many chronic and acute vascular and cardiovascular diseases.

In the last decade, traditional compounds utilized in "folk medicine" were considered with increasing interest to discover new bioactive molecules potentially effective in a wide range of diseases including cardiovascular ones. Since ancient times different parts of the *Cucumis sativus* L. plant were utilized in Ayurvedic medicine, among these, fruits were traditionally used to alleviate skin problem such as sunburn irritation and inflammation. The main purpose of the present research was, in a well-defined in vitro model of endothelial cells, to investigate whether a water/ethanol extract of *Cucumis sativus* L. (CSE) fruit can attenuate the damaging effect of pro-inflammatory lipopolysaccharide (LPS).

Methods: Cell viability, gene expression of endothelial cell markers, cytokines secretion and in vitro angiogenesis assay were performed on porcine Aortic Endothelial Cells exposed to increasing doses (0.02; 02; 2 mg/ml) of CSE in the presence of pro-inflammatory lipopolysaccharide (LPS 10 μg/ml).

Results: CSE reduced LPS-induced cytotoxicity and decreased the cellular detachment, restoring the expression of tight junction ZO-1. The increase of TLR4 expression induced by LPS was counterbalanced by the presence of CSE, while the protective gene Hemeoxygenase (HO)-1 was increased. *Cucumis sativus* L. inhibited the early robust secretion of inflammatory IL-8 and GM-CSFs, furthermore inhibition of inflammatory IL-6 and IL-1α occurred late at 7 and 24 h respectively. On the contrary, the secretion of anti-inflammatory IL-10, together with IL-18 and IFN-γ was increased. Moreover, the in vitro angiogenesis induced by inflammatory LPS was prevented by the presence of *Cucunis sativus* L. extract, at any doses tested.

Conclusions: Our results have clearly demonstrated that *Cucumis sativus* L. extract has attenuated lipopolysaccharide-induced inflammatory response in endothelial cells.

Keywords: Endothelium, *Cucumis sativus* L., Inflammation, Hemeoxygenase-1, Cytokines, Angiogenesis

Background

Vascular integrity contributes to the maintenance of the homeostasis of the whole organism [1]. The break of the vascular balance causes many pathological alterations, including cardiovascular diseases (CDVs), that represent the principle cause of death globally [2].

Among vascular cellular components, endothelial cells (EC) establish the inner lining of blood vessels and perform a pivotal role in the maintenance of the vascular integrity [1, 3–5]. Moreover endothelial cells have a key position in the beginning, progression, control and resolution of the vascular dysfunction [6–9]. Several endogenous and exogenous pro-inflammatory stimuli, such as lipopolysaccharide (LPS), induce "EC activation". The phenotype of activated endothelial cells promotes phenomena of vasoconstriction, leukocyte adhesion, coagulation and thrombosis. This change involves the up-regulation of pro-inflammatory genes, including secretion of inflammatory cytokines and chemokines. If the pro-inflammatory

* Correspondence: chiara.bernardini5@unibo.it
Department of Veterinary Medical Sciences – DIMEVET, University of Bologna, Via Tolara di Sopra 50, Ozzano Emilia, 40064 Bologna, Italy

status is not counterbalanced by the synthesis of pro-tective molecules, the endothelial activation converts into the endothelial dysfunction and then in the vas-cular disease [10, 11].

In full accordance with the principle of "Replacement", one of the commonly-accepted 3Rs rules (Replacement, Reduction and Refinement) for more ethical use of ani-mals in experimental testing, primary culture of porcine Aortic Endothelial Cells (pAECs) were successfully used in many different in vitro models, preceding the in vivo, confirming swine as a relevant animal model for transla-tional medicine [12–17].

In the last decade, traditional compounds utilized in "folk medicine" have been considered with increasing interest to discover new bioactive molecules potentially ef-fective in a wide range of diseases including cardiovascular ones. Nevertheless, to support the traditional medicine use of these compounds, scientific informations regarding the phytochemical or biological activity are needed. [18, 19].

Cucumber (Cucumis sativus L.) is a popular vegetable crop member of the Cucurbitaceae family commonly cultivated for its edible fruits. Since ancient times, differ-ent parts of the cucumber plant have been employed in Ayurvedic medicine, among these, fruits are traditionally used to alleviate skin problem such as sunburn's irrita-tion and inflammation [20, 21]. Recently in vitro evi-dences [22] suggested that a Cucumis sativus extract show strong anti-oxidant capacity and ability to stability the membrane of human red blood. Moreover, Patil [23] demonstrated that aqueous extracts of Cucumis sativus is efficacious on inflammatory model of ulcerative colitis in in vivo model of Wister rats.

Nowadays no studies have investigated the effect of Cucumis sativus L. on vascular endothelial cells. There-fore, to provide new scientific evidence to support trad-itional medicine use of Cucumis sativus L., the main purpose of the present research was to investigate whether a water/ethanol extract of Cucumis sativus L. fruit (CSE) can attenuate the deleterious effects of LPS in in vitro model of endothelial cells.

Methods
Chemicals and reagents
Human endothelial SFM medium, heat inactivated FBS (Fetal Bovine Serum), antibiotic-antimycotic and Dulbec-co's phosphate buffered saline (DPBS) were purchased from Gibco-Life technologies (Carlsbad CA, USA).

RNA isolation was performed with NucleoSpin RNA kit (Macherey-Nagel GmbH & Co. KG, Düren Germany), iScript cDNA synthesis kit and iTaq Universal SYBR Green Supermix were used for cDNA synthesis and qPCR analysis (Bio-Rad Laboratories Inc., Hercules, CA, USA). All plastic supports were purchased from Falcon, Beckton-Dickinson.

A water/ethanol extract of Cucumis sativus L. fruit (CSE), titrated for total iminosugar acids content by HPLC-MS (2 g/100g), was kindly provided by Naturalea (Naturalea SA, Lugano, CH - Cuvrex batch number CE1501).

Cell culture
Porcine Aortic Endothelial Cells (pAECs) were isolated and maintained as previously described by Bernardini and colleagues [12]. Briefly thoracic aortic traits were collected in a local slaughterhouse from adult pigs. After collection, thoracic aortic traits were washed with DPBS, ligated at the ends, and transferred to the laboratory within 1 h on ice. After ligation of all arterial side branches, aortas were cannulated with modified syringe cones and silicone tubes to set up a closed system. The vessels were repeatedly flushed with DPBS and then filled with a collagenase solution and incubated for 20 min at 37 °C. The cellular sospension were then cen-trifuged at 800 x g for 10 min. The cellular pellet was re-suspended in 1 mL human endothelial basal growth medium (Gibco-Invitrogen, Paisley, UK) supplemented with 5% fetal bovine serum (Gibco-Invitrogen) and 1% antibiotics-antimicotics (Gibco-Invitrogen). Cell number and viability (85–90%) were determined using a Burker chamber under a phase-contrast microscope after vital staining with trypan blue dye. Cells were maintained in a logarithmic growth phase by routine passages every 2–3 days at a 1:3 split ratio. To confirm their endothelial origin, cultured cells were checked by immunocitochem-istry for endothelial cell markers: CD31 and Caderine. Then cells were expanded till 20th passages. All experi-ments were performed with cells from the third to the eighth passage. The first seeding after thawing was al-ways performed in T-25 tissue culture flasks (3×10^5 cells/flask) and successive experiments were conducted in 24-well plates (qPCR and western blot analysis), in 96-well assay plates (cytotoxicity) and 8-well slide cham-ber for in vitro angiogenesis assay. Cells were cultured in Human endothelial SFM medium, added with FBS (5%) and antimicrobial/antimycotic solution (1×) in a 5% CO_2 atmosphere at 38.5 °C.

Cytotoxicity
Since the non-toxicity of the extract is a fundamental pre-requisite, we first tested the cytotoxicity of the CSE in a concentration range of 0.0002–2 mg / ml. No tox-icity was showed at any doses tested.

pAECs were seeded in a 96 wells plate (approximately 3×10^3 cells/well) and exposed to increasing doses of Cucumis sativus L. (CSE) (0.02; 0.2; 2 mg/ml) in pres-ence of lipopolysaccharide (LPS) (10 μg/ml) (E. coli 055:B5, Sigma-Aldrich Co, St Louis, MO, USA) for 24 h. Cytotoxicity was evaluated by trypan Blue exclusion dye

Quantitative real time PCR for ZO-1, TLR4, HO-1

pAECs were seeded in a 24 wells plate (approximately 4×10^4 cells/well) and exposed to increasing doses (0.02; 0.2; 2 mg/ml) of CSE in presence of LPS (10 μg/ml) for 1, 7 and 24 h. At the end of experimental times, treated or control cells were collected and stored until gene expression analysis.

Total RNA was isolated using the NucleoSpin®RNA Kit, and high quality RNA, with A260/A280 ratio above 2.0 was used for cDNA synthesis. Total RNA (500 ng) was reverse-transcribed to cDNA using the iScript cDNA Synthesis Kit in a final volume of 20 μL. Swine primers were designed using Beacon Designer 2.07 (Premier Biosoft International, Palo Alto, CA, USA). Primer sequences, expected PCR product lengths and accession numbers in the NCBI database are shown in Table 1.

Quantitative real-time PCR was performed to evaluate gene expression profiles in CFX96 (Bio-Rad) thermal cycler using SYBR green detection system. A master mix of the following reaction components was prepared in nuclease free water to the final concentrations indicated: 0.2 μM forward primer, 0.2 μM reverse primer, 1X iTaq Universal SYBR Green Supermix. One μl of cDNA was added to 19 μl of the master mix. All samples were analyzed in duplicate. The qPCR protocol used was: 10 min at 95 °C, 40 cycles at 95 °C for 15 s and at 61 °C for 30 s, followed by a melting step from 55 °C to 95 °C (80 cycle of 0.5 °C increase/cycle).

The expression level of interest genes was calculated as fold of change using the $2^{-\Delta\Delta CT}$ method [24].

Western blot for TLR4 and HO-1

pAECs were seeded in a 24 wells plate (approximately 4×10^4 cells/well) and exposed to increasing doses (0.02; 0.2; 2 mg/ml) of CSE for 24 h. At the end of experimental time, cells were harvested and lysed in SDS solution (Tris–HCl 50 mM pH 6.8; SDS 2%; glycerol 5%). Protein Assay Kit (TP0300, Sigma) was used to determine the protein content of cellular lysates. Aliquots containing 20 μg of proteins were separated on NuPage 4–12% bis-Tris Gel (Gibco-Life-Technologies) for 50 min at 200 V. The proteins were then electrophoretically transferred onto a nitrocellulose membrane by Turbo Blot System (Bio-Rad). The blots were washed in PBS and protein transfer was checked by staining the nitro-cellulose membranes with 0.2% Ponceau Red. Non-specific binding on nitrocellulose membranes was blocked with 5% milk powder in PBS-T20 (Phosphate Buffer Saline-0.1% Tween-20) for 1 h at room temperature. The membranes were then incubated over-night at 4 °C with a 1:500 dilution of anti-HO-1 rabbit polyclonal antibody (SPA 896 StressGen Biotecnologies Corp, Victoria BC, Canada) and 1:1000 anti TLR4 mouse monoclonal antibody (NB100–56566 Novus Biologicals, Littleton, CO, USA). After several washings with PBS-T20, the membranes were incubated with the secondary biotin-conjugate antibody and then with a 1:1000 dilution of an anti-biotin horseradish peroxidase (HRP)-linked antibody.

The western blots were developed using chemiluminescent substrate (Super Signal West Pico Chemiluminescent Substrate, Pierce Biotechnology, Inc., Rockford, IL, USA) according to the manufacturer's instructions. Chemidoc instrument using Quantity One Software (Bio-Rad) acquired the intensity of the luminescent signal of the resultant bands.

In order to normalize the HO-1 and TLR4 data on the housekeeping protein, membranes were stripped (briefly: the membranes were washed 5 min in water, then 5 min in 0.2 M NaOH and then washed again in water) and re-probed for housekeeping α-tubulin (1:500 of anti α-tubulin MA1–19162, Thermo Fisher Scientific, Rockford, IL, USA).

The relative protein content (HO-1 or TLR4/α-tubulin) was expressed as arbitrary units (AUs).

Multiparametric enzyme-linked immunosorbent assay (ELISA) for cytokines and chemokines

Concentration of 13 cytokines and chemokines (GM-CSF, IFN-γ, IL-1α, IL-1β, IL-1ra, IL-2, IL-4, IL-6, IL-8, IL-10, IL-12, IL-18, TNF-α) was measured by quantitative multiparametric ELISA (Enzyme-linked immunosorbent assay). (Porcine Cytokine/Chemokine Magnetic Bead Panel kit, Milliplex Map Kit, EMD Millipore Corporation, Billerica MA USA), following the manufacturer's instructions. The Luminex xMAP bead-based multiplexed immunoassay technology and MAGPIX instrument provided with xPONENT 4.2 software were used.

Table 1 Primer sequence used for quantitative Real Time PCR analysis

Genes	Forward (5'-3')	Reverse (5'-3')	Product size (bp)	Accession Number
HPRT	GGACAGGACTGAACGGCTTG	GTAATCCAGCAGGTCAGCAAAG	115	AF143818
HO-1	CGCTCCCGAATGAACAC	GCTCCTGCACCTCCTC	112	NM_001004027
TLR4	CAGATACAGAGGGTCATGCTTTC	GGGGATGTTGTCAGGGATTTG	215	NM_001113039.1
ZO-1	AGTGCCGCCTCCTGAGTTTG	CATCCTCATCTTCATCATCTTCTACAG	147	AJ318101

Capillary-like tube formation assay

The experiments were carried out using 8-well slide chamber (BD Falcon Bedford, MA USA) coated with un-diluted Geltrex™ LDEV-Free Reduced Growth Factor Basement Membrane Matrix. Extracellular matrix coating was carried out for 3 h in a humidified incubator, at 38.5 °C, 5% CO_2. pAECs (8×10^4 cells/well) were exposed to increasing doses (0.02; 0.2; 2 mg/ml) of (CSE) in the presence of LPS (10 µg/ml) for 24 h.

At the end of experimental time, images were acquired using a digital camera installed on a Nikon epifluorescence microscope (Nikon, Yokohama, Japan) and analyzed by open software Image J 64.

Statistical analysis

Each treatment was replicated three times or six times (cytotoxicity) in three independent experiments. The data were analysed by a one-way analysis of variance (ANOVA) followed by the Tukey post hoc comparison Test. Differences of at least $p < 0.05$ were considered significant. Statistical analysis was carried out by using R software (http://www.R-project.org) [25].

Results

CSE prevented LPS-induced cell death and ZO-1 reduction

The protective effect of *Cucumis sativus* L. extract on LPS-induced toxicity was evaluated in pAECs. LPS treatment provoked an increased number of round and detached cells after 24 h (Fig. 1a), while CSE reduced the cellular detachment in a dose dependent manner (Fig. 1b-d). Cytotoxicity assay confirmed the ability of CSE to protect cells against LPS-induced cellular death (Fig. 1e). Moreover, we studied the expression of ZO-1, a critical component of tight junction scaffold; LPS induced the downregulation of ZO-1 gene expression, while CSE restored ZO-1 expression to control level at the intermediate and higher doses (Fig. 1f).

Effect of CSE on TLR-4 and HO-1 expression

We studied the effect of CSE on the expression of the Toll-like receptor 4 (TLR4) that is the main receptor for LPS recognition. LPS induced a significant increase of TLR4 mRNA after 1 and 7 h of treatment, while CSE inhibited its expression at all doses studied (Fig. 2a). This inhibitory effect was confirmed at protein level by western blot analysis as shown in Fig. 2b and c. Moreover, we studied the effect of CSE on the vascular protective molecule HO-1. LPS induced HO-1 expression in pAECs, additionally CSE increased HO-1 induction at both mRNA (Fig. 3a) and protein level (Fig. 3b and c).

Effect of CSE on cytokine/chemokines secretion

To assess whether CSE could influence the LPS-induced secretion of inflammatory mediators we evaluated the

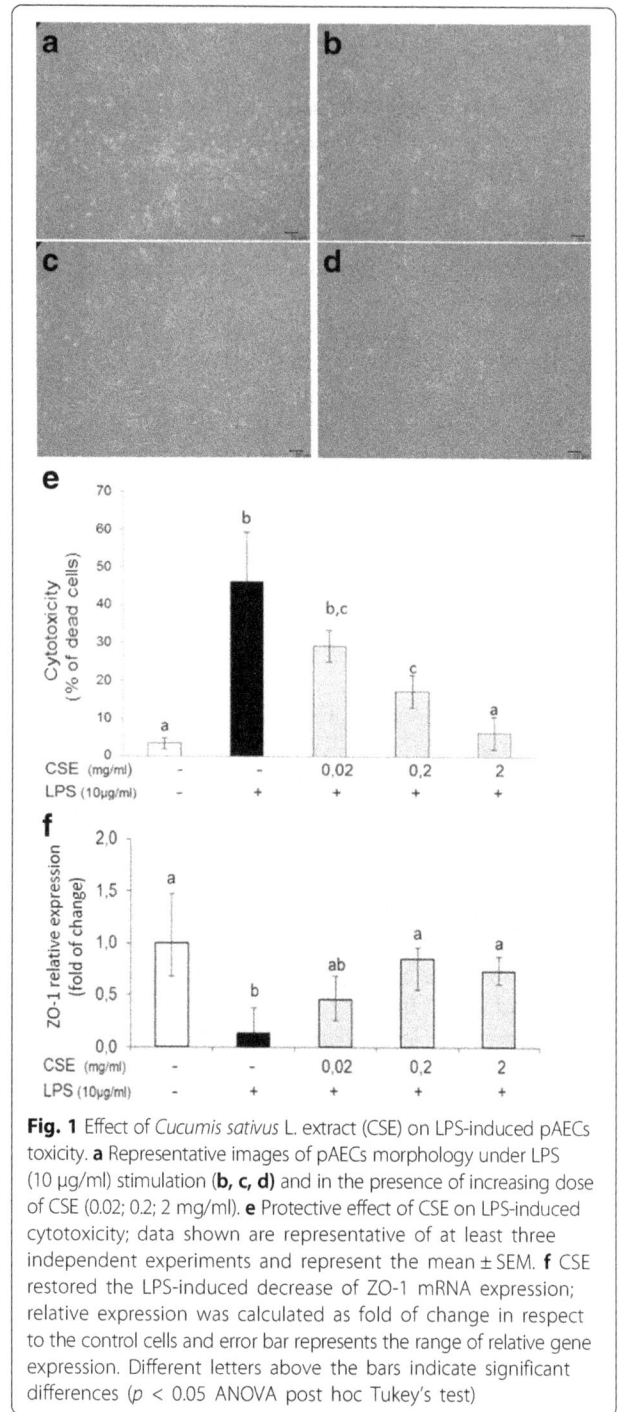

Fig. 1 Effect of *Cucumis sativus* L. extract (CSE) on LPS-induced pAECs toxicity. a Representative images of pAECs morphology under LPS (10 µg/ml) stimulation (b, c, d) and in the presence of increasing dose of CSE (0.02; 0.2; 2 mg/ml). e Protective effect of CSE on LPS-induced cytotoxicity; data shown are representative of at least three independent experiments and represent the mean ± SEM. f CSE restored the LPS-induced decrease of ZO-1 mRNA expression; relative expression was calculated as fold of change in respect to the control cells and error bar represents the range of relative gene expression. Different letters above the bars indicate significant differences ($p < 0.05$ ANOVA post hoc Tukey's test)

presence of 13 cytokines/chemokines in the culture medium of pAECs treated with LPS in the presence or absence of CSE (2 mg/ml). LPS-treated endothelial cells released significant level of Il-6, Il-8, IL-10, IL-18, GM-CSF and IFN-γ. CSE significantly influenced these cytokines setting; in particular, the presence of the extract decreased the concentration of GM-CSF, IL-8 and IL-1α with a different kinetic, whereas the concentration

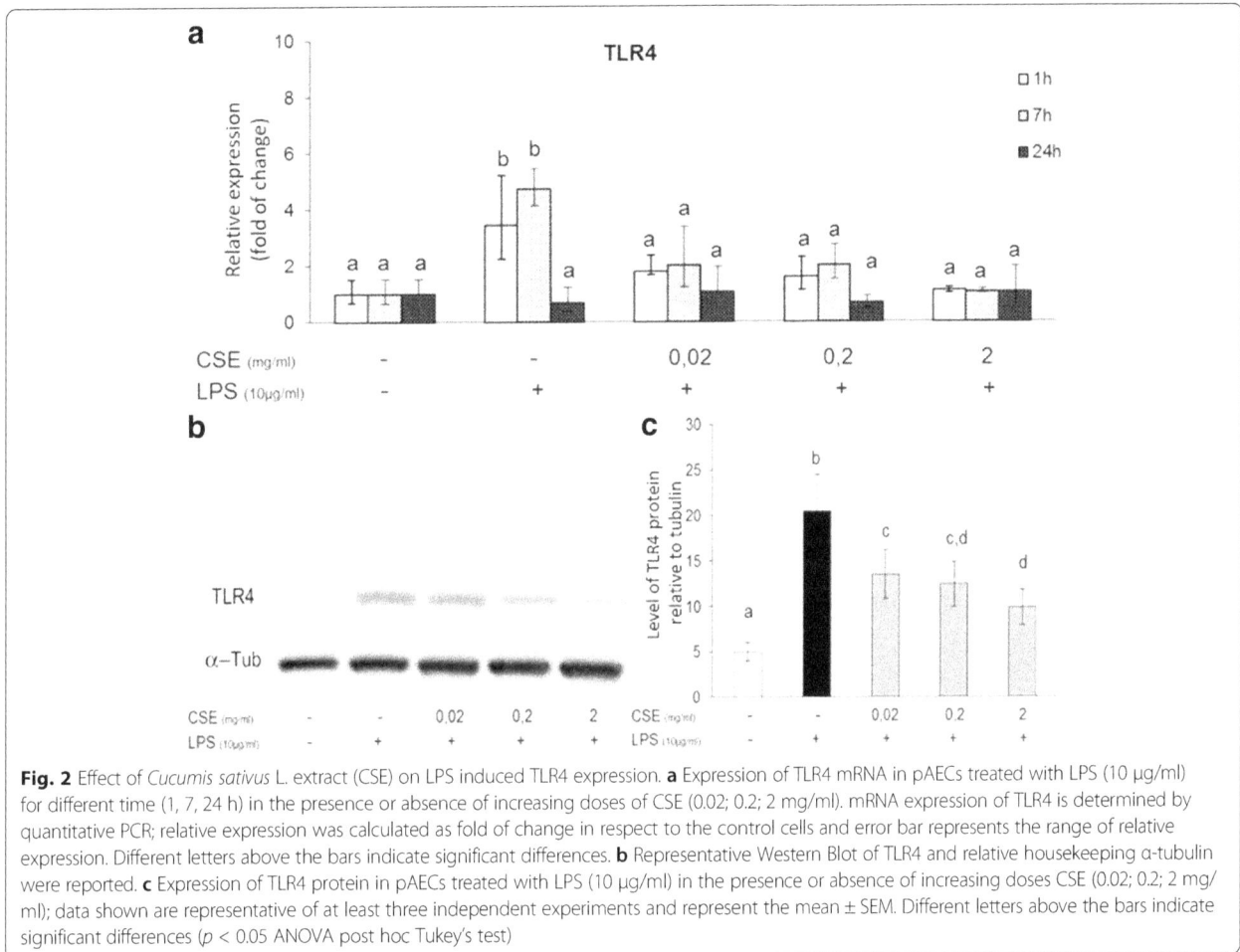

Fig. 2 Effect of *Cucumis sativus* L. extract (CSE) on LPS induced TLR4 expression. **a** Expression of TLR4 mRNA in pAECs treated with LPS (10 µg/ml) for different time (1, 7, 24 h) in the presence or absence of increasing doses of CSE (0.02; 0.2; 2 mg/ml). mRNA expression of TLR4 is determined by quantitative PCR; relative expression was calculated as fold of change in respect to the control cells and error bar represents the range of relative expression. Different letters above the bars indicate significant differences. **b** Representative Western Blot of TLR4 and relative housekeeping α-tubulin were reported. **c** Expression of TLR4 protein in pAECs treated with LPS (10 µg/ml) in the presence or absence of increasing doses CSE (0.02; 0.2; 2 mg/ml); data shown are representative of at least three independent experiments and represent the mean ± SEM. Different letters above the bars indicate significant differences ($p < 0.05$ ANOVA post hoc Tukey's test)

of IL-10, IL-18 and IFN-γ was increased at each experimental point, as shown in Table 2. The level of IL-6 showed a precocious increase (1 h) in presence of CSE but after 7 and 24 h, cells treated with plant extract produced less IL-6 than cells only treated with LPS. IL-1β, IL-1ra, IL-2, IL-4, IL-12 and TNF-α were never detected in cell culture medium (data not shown).

Effect of CSE on LPS-induced angiogenesis

We examined the effect of CSE on in vitro LPS-induced pAECs angiogenesis in an extracellular matrix-based assay. Cells cultured on extracellular matrix in the presence of pro-inflammatory LPS assembled in a complete tube and network formation (Fig. 4a and e), while the in vitro angiogenesis induced by inflammatory LPS was prevented by the presence of *Cucunis sativus* L. extract, at any doses tested (Fig. 4b-e).

Discussion

It is widely accepted the key role of endothelium in the onset of many chronic and acute vascular and cardiovascular diseases. The shift from the healthy endothelium to the endothelial dysfunction is a complex process involving many different factors that starts with "the activation of endothelial cells".

Recently, great effort is attempted to translate the potential activity of traditional compounds into the modern therapy, in a broad range of pathologies including cardiovascular disease [18]. *Cucumis sativus* L. is a very popular vegetable, native of India but nowadays commercially cultivated all over the world. Furthermore, since ancient time, Ayurvedic medicine has always used its fruits and seeds for their refrigerant, haemostatic tonic properties. It is now evident that fruits contain many interesting phyto-complex [20, 26] that makes it an interesting candidate for anti oxidant [27] and anti-inflammatory action [28] but the study of their effect still requires scientific supports.

The present study demonstrates that the protective effects reported for *Cucumis sativus* L., might be also mediated by its protective activity on the vascular endothelium.

Being the pig an excellent model for translational researches [29], in vitro approaches based on primary cell culture are required to better define the subsequent eventual in vivo activities to respect the 3Rs rules. We used in vitro cultures of porcine Aortic Endothelial Cells

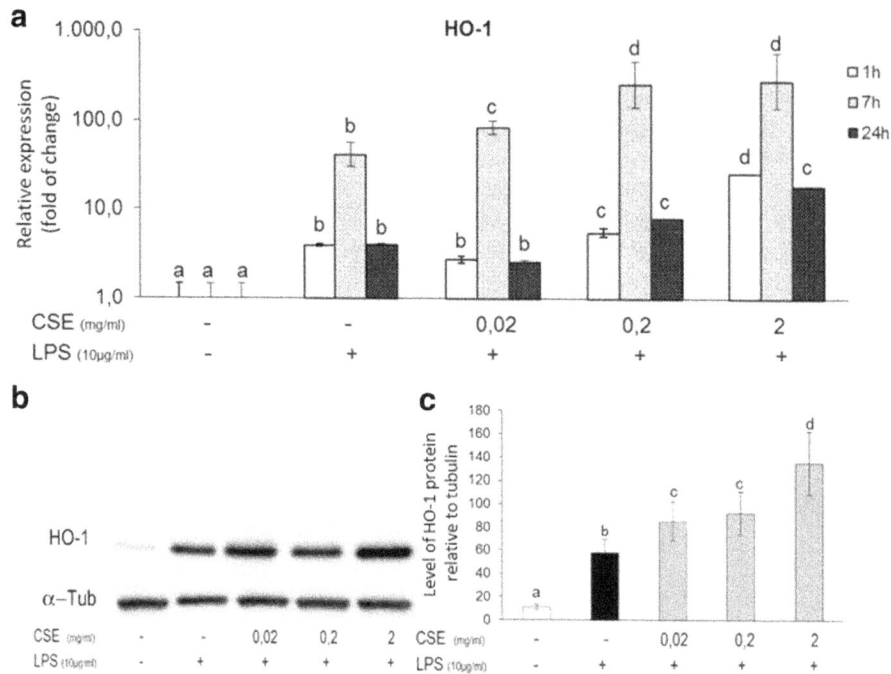

Fig. 3 Effect of *Cucumis sativus* L. extract (CSE) on LPS induced HO-1 expression. **a** Expression of HO-1 mRNA in pAECs treated with LPS (10 μg/ml) in the presence or absence of increasing doses of *Cucumis sativus* L. extract (0.02, 0.2, 2 mg/ml). mRNA expression of HO-1 as determined by quantitative PCR. Relative expression was calculated as fold of change in respect to the control cells and error bar represents the range of relative gene expression. Different letters above the bars indicate significant differences. **b** Representative Western Blot of HO-1 and relative housekeeping α-tubulin were reported. **c** Expression of HO-1 protein in pAECs treated with LPS (10 μg/ml) in the presence or absence of increasing doses CSE (0.02; 0.2; 2 mg/ml); data shown are representative of at least three independent experiments and represent the mean ± SEM. (AU = Arbitrary Units) Different letters above the bars indicate significant differences (p < 0.05 ANOVA post hoc Tukey's test)

(pAECs), previously isolated and cultured by us to study vascular endothelial response to different shock, including LPS [12, 13, 30].

In the present research, LPS-induced effects on pAECs is contrasted by the contemporary administration of *Cucumis sativus* L. extract; in fact CSE protected endothelial cells against LPS-induced toxicity, in a dose dependent manner. Furthermore LPS reduced the expression of the tight junction molecule ZO-1, increasing the number of round and detached cells. Instead,

Cucumis sativus L. extract, restored the ZO-1 expression, contributing to maintain the integrity of cellular tight junction, as confirmed by the reduction of cellular detachment.

It is well demonstrated that the exposure to LPS induces endothelial cell activation through the binding of a receptor complex that includes TLR4 [31–34]. In our model TLR4 expression is increased by LPS making cells more responsive to the stimulation, according to what seen by other researchers [35, 36]. In contrast, the

Table 2 Levels of cytokines/chemokines in culture medium of pAECs stimulated with LPS (10 μg/ml) in the presence or absence of *Cucumis sativus* L. extract (CSE 2 mg/ml). Data shown are representative of at least three independent experiments and represent the mean ± SEM. Significant differences are indicated by (p < 0.05) *, and (p < 0.001) by ** nd not detectable

ng/ml	1 h		7 h		24 h	
	CSE-/LPS+	CSE+/LPS+	CSE-/LPS+	CSE+/LPS+	CSE-/LPS+	CSE+/LPS+
IL-1α	nd	nd	nd	nd	0.0592 ± 0.0019	0.0140 ± 00002**
IL-6	nd	0.1574 ± 0.0064	4.3163 ± 0.0893	3.3889 ± 0.0835*	8.0129 ± 0.3067	3.9270 ± 0.0335**
IL-8	6.3445 ± 0.4821	2.3809 ± 0.0434**	> 50	24.2300 ± 2.2100	31.5600 ± 3.8210*	25.1500 ± 2.7210
IL-10	0.0077 ± 0.0023	0.0355 ± 0.0010**	0.0187 ± 0.0025	0.0395 ± 0.0034*	0.0209 ± 00017	0.0400 ± 0.0056**
IL-18	0.0319 ± 0.0021	0.1796 ± 0.0049**	0.0572 ± 0.0011	0.1897 ± 0.0033**	0.0606 ± 0.0034	0.1913 ± 0.0056**
GM-CSF	0.1083 ± 0.0071	nd	0.1895 ± 0.0221	nd	0.2061 ± 0.0094	0.0021 ± 0.0037**
IFN-γ	0.0501 ± 0.0436	1.5529 ± 0.0292**	0.2654 ± 0.0889	0.5230 ± 0.0725*	0.0725 ± 0.0378	0.3522 ± 0.0340**

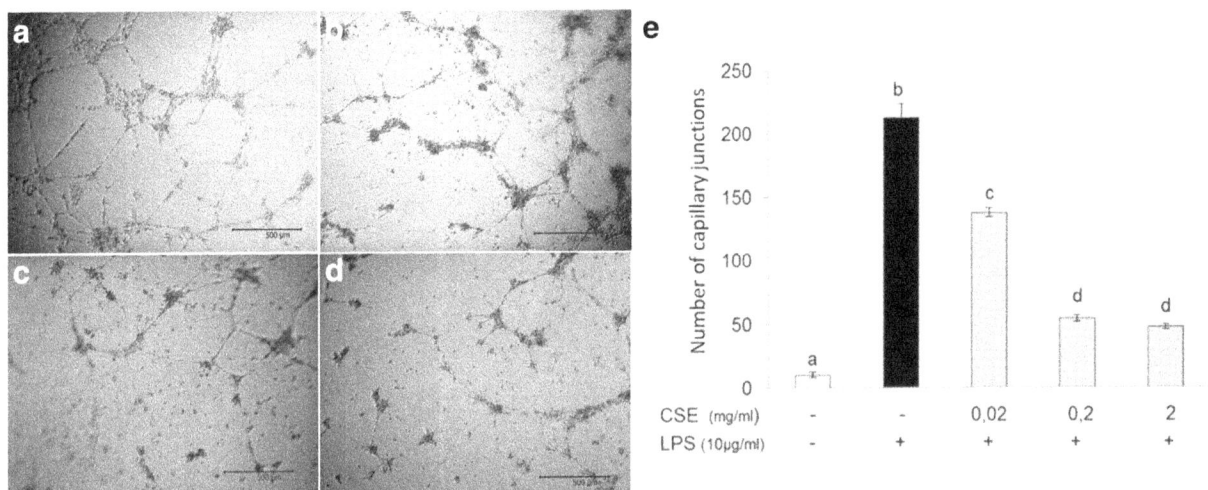

Fig. 4 Effect of *Cucumis sativus* L. extract on LPS-induced angiogenesis. pAECs were cultured on a extracellular matrix with LPS (10 μg/ml) in the absence (**a**) or presence of increasing doses (0.02; 0.2; 2 mg/ml) of *Cucumis sativus* L. extract (**b, c, d** respectively) for 18 h. LPS induced a capillary like network (**a, e**) while CSE reduced LPS-induced angiogenesis at any doses tested (**b-e**). Data shown are representative of at least three independent experiments and represent the mean ± SEM. Different letters above the bars indicate significant differences (p < 0.05 ANOVA post hoc Tukey's test)

presence of *Cucumis sativus* L. extract, inhibited the LPS-induced expression of TLR4.

The inflammatory signalling driven by TLR4 in endothelial cells goes through the activation of NF-κB and the consequently induction or shutdown of several genes including those for cytokines/chemokines synthesis [37].

The presence of CSE in the culture medium contrasted early the robust secretion of inflammatory IL-8 and GM-CSFs; while inhibition of inflammatory IL-6 and IL-1α occurred late at 7 and 24 h respectively. On the contrary, the anti-inflammatory IL-10 is increased together with IL-18 and IFN-γ.

Since the production and function of cytokines overlaps, what is the meaning of our results? Considering that in vivo endothelial cells mainly produce IL-6 and IL-8 and being, among the major functions of these cytokines, the induction of angiogenesis [11], the anti-angiogenic effect of CSE, evidenced by the in vitro-angiogenesis assay, is in agreement with the inhibition of these cytokines. Moreover interleukin 18 (IL-18), firstly described as a novel cytokine that stimulates interferon-γ (IFN-γ) production, possessed potent antitumor effects achieved by the inhibition of angiogenesis in vivo [38], so the increase of IL-18 in our model, could also contribute to a reduction in inflammatory angiogenesis.

Overall, our results demonstrate that the extract of *Cucumis sativus* L. influenced the secretion of cytokines/chemokines trough the reduction of TLR4 expression; moreover, the effect of this modulation inhibited the inflammation-induced angiogenesis. Overall, these important results suggest that *Cucumis sativus* L. extract could be a very interesting candidate in counteracting

inflammatory pathologies in which TLR play a crucial modulatory role.

Furthermore, to avoid that the endothelial cell activation results in dysfunction, the induction of protective genes must be strictly regulated. Among protective genes, Hemeoxygenase (HO)-1, the rate-limiting enzyme in the heme catabolism, has been demonstrated to present important beneficial roles in the vasculature [39]; in particular HO-1 exerts antiapoptotic, antioxidants, antithrombotic and anti-atherogenic effects [39]. Our previous reports showed the LPS ability to induce HO-1 expression [12]; in the present research we demonstrated that *Cucumis sativus* L. extract increased the expression of vascular protective HO-1. Moreover, the role of HO-1 in angiogenesis is intriguing in fact HO-1 activity is necessary for VEGF-induced angiogenesis, whereas HO-1 has the opposite effect in the pathological angiogenesis [39]. Therefore, in our model, the increase of HO-1 could exert protective effect including the inhibition of LPS-induced inflammatory angiogenesis.

Conclusions

Our results demonstrate the efficacy of a water/ethanol extract of *Cucumis sativus* L. fruit to protect vascular endothelial cells against LPS-challenge: decreasing LPS-induced TLR4 expression, influencing cytokines secretion, increasing the expression of protective HO-1. Moreover, the presence of *Cucumis sativus* L. extract inhibited the LPS-induced cellular toxicity and inflammation-induced angiogenesis. These impressive and robust results propose the *Cucumis sativus* L. extract as a promising natural compound in vascular endothelium protection.

Abbreviations
CDVs: Cardiovascular diseases; CSE: *Cucumis sativus* L extract; EC: Endothelial cells; GM-CSF: Granulocyte-macrophage colony-stimulating factor; HO-1: Heme oxygenase 1; IFN-γ: Interferon γ; IL-10: Interleukin 10; IL-12: Interleukin 12; IL-18: Interleukin 18; IL-1ra: Interleukin-1 receptor antagonist; IL-1α: Interleukin 1α; IL-1β: Interleukin1β; IL-2: Interleukin 2; IL-4: Interleukin 4; IL-6: Interleukin 6; IL-8: Interleukin 8; LPS: Lipopolysaccharide; pAECs: Porcine aortic endothelail cells; TLR4: Toll-like receptor 4; TNF-α: Tumor necrosis factor α; ZO-1: Zona occludens-1

Funding
This work was supported by: "Programma di Ricerca Fondamentale Orientata 2015 (RFO-MIUR ex 60%)". The funding source was not involved in study design, collection of samples, analysis of data, interpretation of data, writing of the report and decision to publish.

Authors' contributions
CB and MFo conceived and designed the research; CB, AZ, MB, IT and MFe made substantial contribution to perform experiments, analyse data and contributed to write the manuscript. MFo supervised the work and revised critically the manuscript. All authors read and approved the final version of the manuscript.

Competing interests
The authors declare that they have no competing interests.

References
1. Aird WC. Endothelium and haemostasis. Hamostaseologie. 2015;35:11–6.
2. WHO | Cardiovascular diseases (CVDs). WHO. World Health Organization; 2016. http://www.who.int/cardiovascular_diseases/en/.
3. Bazzoni G, Dejana E. Endothelial cell-to-cell junctions: molecular organization and role in vascular homeostasis. Physiol Rev Am Physiol Soc. 2004;84:869–901.
4. Aird WC. Phenotypic heterogeneity of the endothelium: I. Structure, function, and mechanisms. Circ Res Lippincott Williams & Wilkins. 2007;100:158–73.
5. Burger D, Touyz RM. Cellular biomarkers of endothelial health: microparticles, endothelial progenitor cells, and circulating endothelial cells. J Am Soc Hypertens. 2012;6:85–99.
6. Aird WC. Endothelium in health and disease. Pharmacol Rep. 2008;60:139–43.
7. Cahill PA, Redmond EM. Vascular endothelium – gatekeeper of vessel health. Atherosclerosis. 2016;248:97–109.
8. Chistiakov DA, Orekhov AN, Bobryshev YV. Endothelial barrier and its abnormalities in cardiovascular disease. Front Physiol. 2015;6:365.
9. Regina C, Panatta E, Candi E, Melino G, Amelio I, Balistreri CR, et al. Vascular ageing and endothelial cell senescence: molecular mechanisms of physiology and diseases. Mech Ageing Dev. 2016;159:14–21.
10. Sprague AH, Khalil RA. Inflammatory cytokines in vascular dysfunction and vascular disease. Biochem Pharmacol. 2009;78:539–52.
11. Akdis M, Aab A, Altunbulakli C, Azkur K, Costa RA, Crameri R, et al. Interleukins (from IL-1 to IL-38), interferons, transforming growth factor β, and TNF-α: receptors, functions, and roles in diseases. J Allergy Clin Immunol. 2016;138:984–1010.
12. Bernardini C, Zannoni A, Turba ME, Fantinati P, Tamanini C, Bacci ML, et al. Heat shock protein 70, heat shock protein 32, and vascular endothelial growth factor production and their effects on lipopolysaccharide-induced apoptosis in porcine aortic endothelial cells. Cell Stress Chaperones Springer; 2005;10:340–348.
13. Bernardini C, Gaibani P, Zannoni A, Vocale C, Bacci ML, Piana G, et al. Treponema denticola alters cell vitality and induces HO-1 and Hsp70 expression in porcine aortic endothelial cells. Cell Stress Chaperones. 2010;15:509–16.
14. Botelho G, Bernardini C, Zannoni A, Ventrella V, Bacci ML, Biochemistry FMC, Physiology PC. Effect of tributyltin on mammalian endothelial cell integrity. Comp Biochem Physiol Part C Elsevier Inc. 2015;177:79–86.

15. Dao VT-V, Medini S, Bisha M, Balz V, Suvorava T, Bas M, et al. Nitric oxide up-regulates endothelial expression of angiotensin II type 2 receptors. Biochem. Pharmacol. 2016;112:24–36.
16. Dushpanova A, Agostini S, Ciofini E, Cabiati M, Casieri V, Matteucci M, et al. Gene silencing of endothelial von Willebrand factor attenuates angiotensin II-induced endothelin-1 expression in porcine aortic endothelial cells. Sci Rep. 2016;6:30048.
17. Grossini E, Farruggio S, Qoqaiche F, Raina G, Camillo L, Sigaudo L, et al. Monomeric adiponectin increases cell viability in porcine aortic endothelial cells cultured in normal and high glucose conditions: data on kinases activation. Data Br. 2016;8:1381–6.
18. Pan S-Y, Zhou S-F, Gao S-H, Yu Z-L, Zhang S-F, Tang M-K, et al. New perspectives on how to discover drugs from herbal medicines: CAM's outstanding contribution to modern therapeutics. Evidence-Based Complement Altern Med. 2013;2013:1–25.
19. Accardi G, Aiello A, Gambino CM, Virruso C, Caruso C, Candore G. Mediterranean nutraceutical foods: strategy to improve vascular ageing. Mech Ageing Dev. 2016;159:63–70.
20. Mukherjee PK, Nema NK, Maity N, Sarkar BK. Phytochemical and therapeutic potential of cucumber. Fitoterapia. 2013;84:227–36.
21. Park SY, Kim YH, Park G. Cucurbitacins attenuate microglial activation and protect from neuroinflammatory injury through Nrf2/ARE activation and STAT/NF-κB inhibition. Neurosci Lett. 2015;609:129–36.
22. Muruganantham N, Solomon S, Senthamilselvi MM. Anti-oxidant and anti-inflammatory activity of Cucumis sativas (cucumber) flowers. Int J Pharm Sci Res. 2016;7:1740–5.
23. Patil VM, Kandhare AD, Bhise SD. Effect of aqueous extract of Cucumis sativus Linn. Fruit in ulcerative colitis in laboratory animals. Asian Pac J Trop Biomed. 2012;2(5962-9):39–11.
24. Livak KJ, Schmittgen TD. Analysis of relative gene expression data using real-time quantitative PCR and the 2−ΔΔCT method. Methods Academic Press. 2001;25:402–8.
25. R Core Team. R: a language and environment for statistical computing [Internet]. R Found. Stat. Comput. Vienna, Austria. 2015. Available from: https://www.r-project.org/
26. Chu Y-F, Sun J, Wu X, Liu RH. Antioxidant and antiproliferative activities of common vegetables. J Agric Food Chem. 2002;50:6910–6.
27. Nema NK, Maity N, Sarkar B, Mukherjee PK. Cucumis sativus fruit-potential antioxidant, anti-hyaluronidase, and anti-elastase agent. Arch Dermatol Res Springer-Verlag. 2011;303:247–52.
28. Qiao J, Xu L, He J, Ouyang D, He X. Cucurbitacin E exhibits anti-inflammatory effect in RAW 264.7 cells via suppression of NF-κB nuclear translocation. Inflamm Res SP Birkhäuser Verlag Basel; 2013;62:461–469.
29. Prather RS, Lorson M, Ross JW, Whyte JJ, Walters E. Genetically engineered pig models for human diseases. Annu Rev Anim Biosci Annual Reviews. 2013;1:203–19.
30. Bernardini C, Greco F, Zannoni A, Bacci ML, Seren E, Forni M. Differential expression of nitric oxide synthases in porcine aortic endothelial cells during LPS-induced apoptosis. J Inflamm. 2012;9:47.
31. Dauphinee SM, Karsan A. Lipopolysaccharide signaling in endothelial cells. Lab Investig. 2006;86:9–22.
32. Zeuke S, Ulmer AJ, Kusumoto S, Katus HA, Heine H. TLR4-mediated inflammatory activation of human coronary artery endothelial cells by LPS. Cardiovasc Res. 2002;56:126–34.
33. Andonegui G, Bonder CS, Green F, Mullaly SC, Zbytnuik L, Raharjo E, et al. Endothelium-derived toll-like receptor-4 is the key molecule in LPS-induced neutrophil sequestration into lungs. J Clin Invest. 2003;111:1011–20.
34. Mai CW, Kang YB, Pichika MR. Should a toll-like receptor 4 (TLR-4) agonist or antagonist be designed to treat cancer? TLR-4: its expression and effects in the ten most common cancers. Onco Targets Ther. 2013;6:1573–87.
35. Heo S-K, Yun H-J, Noh E-K, Park W-H, Park S-D. LPS induces inflammatory responses in human aortic vascular smooth muscle cells via toll-like receptor 4 expression and nitric oxide production. Immunol Lett. 2008;120:57–64.
36. Wang Y, Zhang MX, Meng X, Liu FQ, Yu GS, Zhang C, et al. Atorvastatin suppresses LPS-induced rapid upregulation of toll-like receptor 4 and its signaling pathway in endothelial cells. Am J Physiol Heart Circ Physiol American Physiological Society. 2011;300:H1743–52.

37. Sun R, Zhu Z, Su Q, Li T, Song Q. Toll-like receptor 4 is involved in bacterial endotoxin-induced endothelial cell injury and SOC-mediated calcium regulation. Cell Biol Int. 2012;36:475–81.
38. Zheng J-N, Pei D-S, Mao L-J, Liu X-Y, Sun F-H, Zhang B-F, et al. Oncolytic adenovirus expressing interleukin-18 induces significant antitumor effects against melanoma in mice through inhibition of angiogenesis. Cancer Gene Ther. 2010;17:28–36.
39. Calay D, Mason JC. The multifunctional role and therapeutic potential of HO-1 in the vascular endothelium. Antioxid Redox Signal. 2014;20:1789–809.

Phenolics from *Barleria cristata* var. Alba as carcinogenesis blockers against menadione cytotoxicity through induction and protection of quinone reductase

Ali M. El-Halawany[1,2], Hossam M. Abdallah[1,2*], Ahmed R. Hamed[3], Hany Ezzat Khalil[4,5] and Ameen M. Almohammadi[6]

Abstract

Background: There are increasing interests in natural compounds for cancer chemoprevention. Blocking agents represent an important class of chemopreventive compounds. They prevent carcinogens from undergoing metabolic activation and thereby suppressing their interaction with cellular macromolecular targets.

Methods: The effect of phenolic compounds isolated from *Barleria cristata* var. alba as chemopreventive agent was evaluated. The ethyl acetate fraction of *B. cristata* was subjected to different chromatographic techniques for isolation of its major phenolic compounds. The isolated compounds were evaluated for their potential to induce the cancer chemopreventive enzyme marker NAD(P)H quinonereductase 1 (NQO1) in murine Hepa-1c1c7 cell model.

Results: The ethyl acetate fraction of *B. cristata* var. alba yielded five known compounds identified as verbascoside (**1**), isoverbascoside (**2**), dimethoxyverbascoside (**3**), *p*-hydroxy benzoic acid (**4**), and apigenin-7-O-glucoside (**5**). Among the tested compounds, isoverbascoside (**2**) was shown to potently induce the activity of the enzyme in a dose –dependent manner. As a functional assay for detoxification, compound **2** was the strongest to protect Hepa-1c1c7 against the toxicity of menadione, a quinone substrate for NQO1.

Conclusion: This effect seemed to be attributed to the compound's potential to induce both the catalytic activity and protein expression of NQO1 as revealed by enzyme assay and Western blotting, respectively.

Keywords: Chemoprevention, Quinonereductase 1, Menadione, Phenolic compounds

Background

Cancer is a condition in which a cell divides and grows in an uncontrolled manner forming a neoplastic tumor which may spread to other tissues and becomes malignant. Cancer incidence is neither rare anywhere in the world, nor restricted to rich countries. However, deaths from cancer in developing countries are higher than in developed countries [1]. Therefore it is becoming highly recognized that the strategies for cancer prevention are forming the logic and cost effective approach to control this global problem of cancer mortalities as alternative to the high costs of the chemotherapy or radiotherapeutic programs and this should reflect positively on the local and global economies. There are increasing interests in natural compounds for chemoprevention against cancer. These great interests are mainly due to a high number of population studies that showed reduced cancer risk in people consuming dietary phytochemicals compared to people who consume less dietary phytochemicals [2]. Based on the classified stages of carcinogenesis process, the term 'cancer chemoprevention' has been defined as the use of relatively non-toxic chemical agent (natural or synthetic) to inhibit, arrest or reverse the carcinogenesis

* Correspondence: hmafifi2013@gmail.com
[1]Department of Natural Products, Faculty of Pharmacy, King Abdulaziz University, Jeddah 21589, Saudi Arabia
[2]Department of Pharmacognosy, Faculty of Pharmacy, Cairo University, Cairo 11562, Egypt
Full list of author information is available at the end of the article

at early stages [3, 4]. Blocking agents is one important class of compounds in chemoprevention. They prevent carcinogens from undergoing metabolic activation and thereby suppressing their interaction with cellular macromolecular targets such as DNA, RNA and proteins. Blocking agents elicit chemopreventive actions through the induction of a set of phase II detoxifying and antioxidant enzymes such as the chemopreventive marker NAD(P)H quinonereductase 1 (NQO1 or QR1), glutathione-s-transferase (GST), UDP-glucuronosyltransferase (UGT), γ-glutamate cysteine ligase (γ -GCL), glutathione reductase (GR), catalase and Mn superoxide dismutase which act in the detoxification and elimination of harmful reactive intermediates and oxidative stress [5]. There have been accumulating evidences for the promising value of natural products in chemoprevention against cancer. The reason for this is largely due to their low toxicity and high diversity of their chemical structures [6].

Genus *Barleria* is belonging to family Acanthaceae. Ten species from this genus are growing in Saudi flora. Plants belonging to this genus are widely used as an ethnomedicines for variety of illnesses [7, 8]. *Barleria cristata* L. as an example of this genus is an ornamental plant with two varieties named on the basis of their flower color including var. alba and var. purpurea for the white and purple flowers, respectively. *B. cristata* var. purpurea is also known as Philippine Violet or Blue Bell Barleria. Leaves and stems of the plant are used as anti-inflammatory, anemia treatment, antiplasmodial, anti-oxidant and analgesic for toothache. The plant was reported to contain alkaloids, flavonoids, iridoids and to be rich in phenolic contents [8].

The phenolic content of the plant encouraged its use as a chemopreventive and cytoprotective agent. In addition, there is no published chemical or biological data on the other variety (alba) of the plant, which encouraged us to investigate its possible chemopreventive effect, based on expected similarity in active constituents' classes to that of the variety purpurea. Therefore, in continuation to our interest in isolating bioactive chemopreventive agent from plants [5] and based on the chemopreventive activity of phenolics [9], which represent a major constituent in, *B.cristata* var. alba, the current study was performed.

Methods

General experimental procedures

UV spectra were recorded in MeOH using a UV IKON940 spectrophotometer.1D and 2D NMR spectra (chemical shifts in ppm and coupling constants in Hz) were recorded on a Bruker DRX-600 MHz Ultrashield spectrometer (Bruker BioSpin, Billerica, MA, USA) using DMSO-d6 as solvent, with TMS as the internal reference. Column

chromatographic separations were performed on silica gel 60 (70–230 mesh, Merck, Darmstadt, Germany), Silica gel $100C_{18}$-Reversed phase (0.04–0.063 mm, Merck, Darmstadt, Germany) and Sephadex LH-20(Pharmacia Fine Chemicals Inc., Uppsala, Sweden). TLC analysis was performed on pre-coated TLC plates with silica gel 60 F_{254}(Merck, Darmstadt, Germany). Purification of the isolated compounds was performed on a preparative HPLC Agilent1200 equipped with a multi-wavelength detector and ZorbaxSB-C18 column (9.4 × 250 mm).

Plant material

Aerial parts of *B. cristata* L. var. alba were collected from El-Orman Public Garden, Giza, Egypt during April and June 2010. Authentication of plant material was established by Agricultural Engineer Traiz Labib, taxonomy specialist in El-Orman public garden, Giza, Egypt. Voucher specimen (Reg. No. BS1110) is kept in the Herbarium of the Department of Natural Products and Alternative Medicine, Faculty of Pharmacy, King Abdulaziz University, KSA.

Materials for the biology

All chemicals and reagents for cell culture and bioassays were purchased from Lonza (Verviers, Belgium) or Sigma-Aldrich (Steinheim, Germany). Plastic ware for cell culture and assays were prom Griener Bio One (Frickenhausen, Germany). Murine hepatoma cells (Hepa1c1c7, ATCC, USA).

Extraction and isolation of main active constituents

The air dried powdered aerial parts (3 Kg) were exhaustively extracted at room temperature (14 days) using 25 L 70% methyl alcohol, applying cold maceration method to avoid damage of active principals. The solvent mixtures were distilled off under reduced pressure using rotary evaporator and then freeze-dried to yield the total dry extract (210 g), which was stored in deep freezer for further analysis. The total extract was suspended in water (500 mL) and fractionated with chloroform (3 × 1 L) followed by EtOAc (3 × 1 L) and finally *n*-butanol saturated with water. The EtOAc fraction (10 g) was fractionated using RP-18 VLC (5 × 20 cm) using MeOH: H_2O (0–70% *v*/v, 5% increment) and four major fractions were collected. Fraction 1 (2.3 g) was placed on silica gel column (2 × 50 cm) using $CHCl_3$:MeOH (9.5:0. 5 *v*/v) as mobile phase. Subfraction 1–5 was further purified using Sephadex LH-20 (2 × 50 cm) using MeOH as an eluent to give 50 mg of **1**. Fraction 2 was rechromatographed on silica gel column (2 × 50 cm) using Hexane:EtOAc (1:1) to give 20 mg of compound **2**.Subfraction3 was purified on RP-18 HPLC using the following mobile phase system acetonitrile: water (2:8) to yield two pure compounds **3** (3 mg) and **4** (5 mg). Fraction 4 was purified on RP-18 HPLC using the following mobile phase system acetonitrile: water (3:7) to yield compound **5** (2 mg).

Hepa-1c1c7 cell culture

Murine hepatoma cell line Hepa-1c1c7 was maintained as monolayer culture in α- modified Minimum Essential Medium Eagle (α-MEME) supplemented with 10% (v/v) heat-and charcoal–inactivated fetal bovine serum, 2 mM L-glutamine, 100 U/ml penicillin, 100 μg/ml streptomycin sulphate in humidified incubator (Sartorius CMAT, Germany, 5% CO_2/95% air). At about 80% confluence, cells were routinely sub-cultured with Trypsin EDTA solution.

Assessment of the induction of NQO1 in Hepa-1c1c7 cells

The induction of NQO1 in Hepa-1C1C7 cells was assessed. Briefly, cells (1.5×10^5 cells/ml) were seeded onto 6-well plates and left overnight to adhere and form semi-confluent monolayers. Monolayers were treated with either vehicle (final concentration 0.5% v/v DMSO) or test compounds for additional 48 h. Media were then aspirated and monolayers were washed with ice-cold Dulbecco's PBS (1 ml/well). Cells were then scrapped in ice-cold lysis buffer (25 mMTris-Cl, pH 7.4, 250 mM sucrose and 5 μM FAD) and transferred to microcentrifuge tubes. Cell suspensions were then sonicated on ice for 5 s (20% amplitude). Sonicates were then centrifuged (15,000×g for 10 min) and the supernatant (cytosolic fraction) was aliquoted and stored at – 80 °C until assayed.

NQO1 assay

The dicoumarol-sensitive NQO1 activity was measured in cell lysate according to [10] as optimized in our laboratory for spectrophotometer measurement in 500 μl cuvettes. Briefly, the reaction mixture contained in a final volume of 500 μl: 25 mM Tris buffer (pH 7.4), 0. 7 mg/ml bovine serum albumin, 5 μM FAD, 0.2 mM β-NADH as electron donor, 20 μM 2,6-dichlorophenolindophenol (DCPIP) as electron acceptor in the absence (total reductase activity) or the presence of 20 μM dicoumarol (inhibited non-NQO-1 activity). The reaction was started by the addition of 10 μl of supernatant of cell lysates to 490 μl of the reaction mixture in disposable cuvettes. The kinetic determination of enzyme activity was carried out using UV-visible spectrophotometer monitoring the decrease in absorbance of DCPIP at 600 nm for 1 min. The instrument software was used to calculate the average reaction rate per minute (ΔA/minute). Total proteins were determined using Bradford assay [11]. The enzyme activity was

normalised to 1 mg of total proteins and expressed as ΔA/minute/mg protein.

Effect of compounds on menadione-induced cytotoxicity in Hepa-1c1c7 cells

First, The cytotoxic effect of menadione (MD), a quinone substrate for NQO1, on Hepa-1c1c7 cells was determined using a modified sulforhodamin B assay for cellular protein content which is essentially based on method mentioned by [12]. Briefly, Hepa-1c1c7 cells (100,000 cells/ml) were seeded onto 96-well plates and incubated to adhere overnight at 5% CO_2/95% air incubator. At the next day, cells were treated with either vehicle (0.1% DMSO) or increasing concentrations of menadione (1.5–100 μM) and incubated for further 24 h. Culture medium was then aspirated and monolayers were fixed with 10% TCA for 1 h at 4 °C after which all wells were washed with deionized water (4 washes). Air-dried plates were then stained with 0.4% SRB in 1% acetic acid for 30 min at room temperature. Excess dye was removed with washing with 1% acetic acid (4 washes). Bound SRB in air-dried plates were then quantified by solubilisation in 10 mM unbuffered Tris base. The absorbance (OD) was read at 540 nm on a microplate reader (FLUOstar Optima, BMG LAB-TECH GmbH, Ortenberg, Germany). Percentage viability to vehicle control (100%) was calculated from the mean values of the OD of test concentrations. Dose response curves were plotted on Graphpad Prism V6.0 and analysed using non-linear regression to calculate the concentration of MD causing 50% cytotoxicity (IC_{50}).

To test the potential of compounds **1**, **2**, **4** and **5** to protect Hepa-1c1c7 cells against MD cytotoxicity, cells were pre-treated with either DMSO or 3.125 μM from compounds for 24 h before being intoxicated with 20 μM of menadione (MD) for a further 24 h. The Plate was then air-dried and processed for SRB cytotoxicity assay as mentioned above.

NQO1 western blotting

Cells were cultured and treated as mentioned above. NQO1 protein expression was assessed in cell sonicates by Western blotting. Samples, including vehicle control, positive control (sulforaphane at 5 μM) and compound **2**-treated lysates (15 μg total proteins/lane) were resolved by electrophoresis on 10% acrylamide/bis acrylamide gel (200 Volts for 1 h). Resolved proteins were then transferred to nitrocellulose membrane at 100 V for 90 min. Membranes were blocked in 5% non-fat milk in Tris-buffered saline with 0.1% Tween 20 (TBST) for 1 h at 25 °C and then probed overnight (4 °C) with primary antibodies against NQO1 and β-actin (abcam, UK). After three washes in TBST (10 min each), membranes were probed with appropriate secondary antibodies for 1 h at 25 °C, washed three times in TBST and then developed using enzyme chemiluminescence (ECL). Protein bands were visualized on developed membranes using x-ray film. Protein band intensities were determined and normalized to β-actin using Image Studio Lite software v 5.2 (Li-COR® Biosciences, USA).

Results

The ethyl acetate fraction of *B. cristata* var. alba yielded five known compounds. The isolated compounds (Fig. 1) were identified based on their NMR data (Additional file 1: Figures S1–10) and by comparison with the reported data as; verbascoside (**1**) [13], isoverbascoside (**2**) [13], dimethoxyverbascoside (**3**), p-hydroxybenzoic acid (**4**) [14] and apigenin-7-O-glucoside (**5**) [15].

Induction of NQO1 activity by B.Cristata var. alba phenolic constituents

In the present study, we evaluated compounds (**1**, **2**, **4** & **5**) isolated from *B. cristata* for their potential to induce the cancer chemopreventive marker enzyme NQO1 in murine Hepa-1c1c7 cells. A shown in Fig. 2, tested compounds caused differential potencies as inducers for the activity of NQO1 following a 48 h treatment period. The most active compound was shown to be compound **2** (isoverbascoside) causing 8.8-fold induction of NQO1

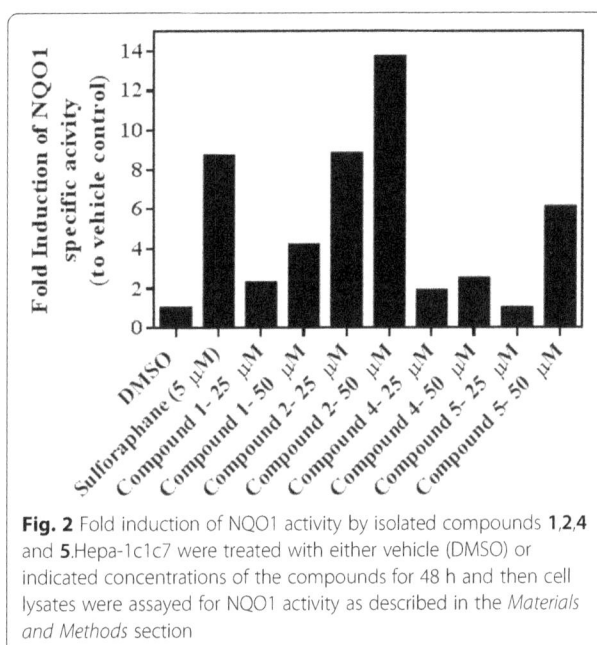

Fig. 2 Fold induction of NQO1 activity by isolated compounds **1**,**2**,**4** and **5**.Hepa-1c1c7 were treated with either vehicle (DMSO) or indicated concentrations of the compounds for 48 h and then cell lysates were assayed for NQO1 activity as described in the *Materials and Methods* section

activity at 25 μM over vehicle control activity level. Higher inducer potency (13.9-fold over control) was recorded with 50 μM of compound 2. Lower inducer activities were shown by compounds **1**, **4** and **5** as displayed in Fig. 2.

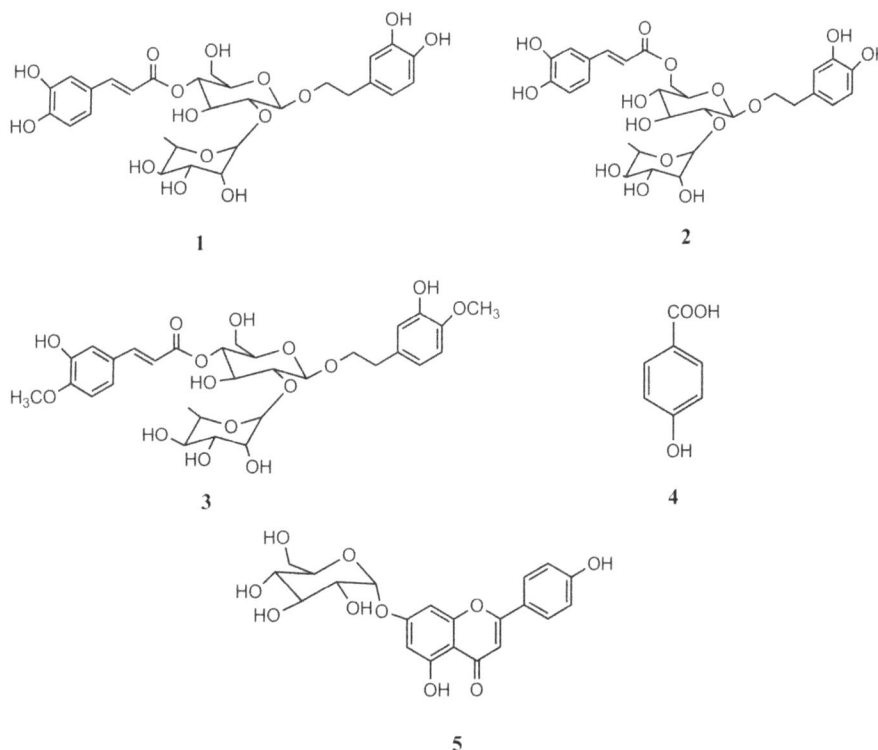

Fig. 1 Chemical structure of isolated phenolic constituents from *B. cristata*varalba

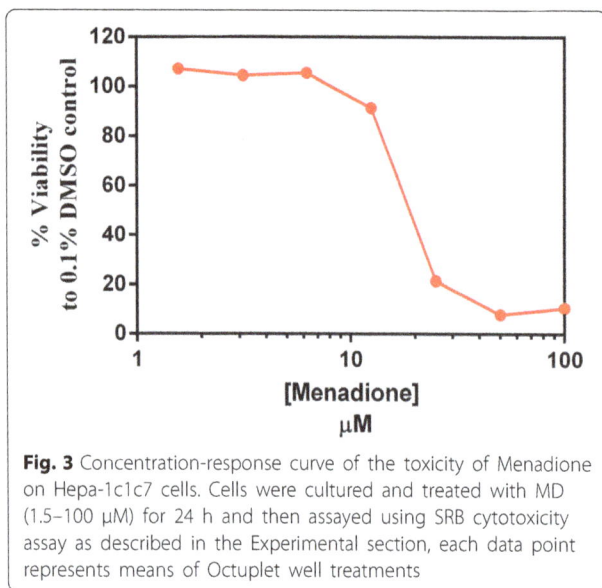

Fig. 3 Concentration-response curve of the toxicity of Menadione on Hepa-1c1c7 cells. Cells were cultured and treated with MD (1.5–100 μM) for 24 h and then assayed using SRB cytotoxicity assay as described in the Experimental section, each data point represents means of Octuplet well treatments

Effect of compounds from *B. cristata* on menadione-induced toxicity (functional assay of NQO1)

Among the tested compounds (Fig. 3), compound **2** (isoverbascoside) was the most active one to protect Hepa-1c1c7 cells against MD cytotoxicity. This is matched with the potency of this compound as NQO1 inducer (Fig. 2). The induction of NQO1 by isoverbascoside helped to detoxify MD through 2-electron reduction to the hydroquinone form menadiol. Menadiol is easily excreted and this prevents the phase I single electron reduction of MD to the toxic semiquinone. Lower protection was produced by the other compounds which

can be ordered from high to low activity as Compound 5 > Compound 1 > Compound 4 as displayed in Fig. 4.

Compound **2** was also shown to cause a concentration-dependent upregulation of the protein expression level of NQO1 using Western blotting analysis as displayed in Fig. 5a and b.

Taken together, the present study shed some light on the mechanism-based potential of the phenolic constituents of the ornamental plant *B. cristata* var. alba as chemopreventive agents. As shown, this activity is through the induction of the cytoprotective enzyme NQO1 at the activity and protein expression levels.

Discussion

Many experimental evidences exist to support the protective roles of NQO1 in the prevention against the toxicity and neoplastic effects of quinones, quinoneimenes and azo dyes in vitro as well as in experimental animals. For example, Wu et al., [16] investigated the protective role of indole-3-carbinol (I3C), a known cruciferous NQO1 inducer, to reduce the incidence of prostate cancer in mice model of transgenic adenocarcinoma of mouse prostate (TRAMP mice). Feeding TRAMP mice with 1% I3C diet has significantly abolished the number of palable tumors, compared with the untreated TRAMP group. This effect was found to occur via the induction

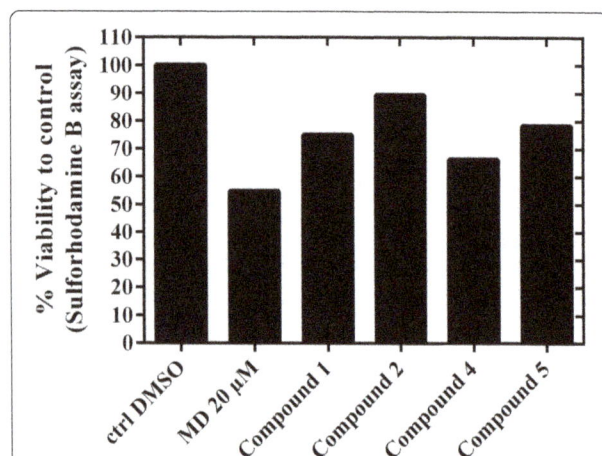

Fig. 4 Protection of Hepa-1c1c7 cells against menadione-induced cytotoxicity. Hepa-1c1c7 cells were pretreated with either DMSO or 3.125 μM from indicated compounds for 24 h before being intoxicated with 20 μM of menadione (MD) for a further 24 h. Cell monolayers were then fixed with TCA for 1 h and processed for SRB cytotoxicity assay. Data are means of at least quadrate treatments for each concentration

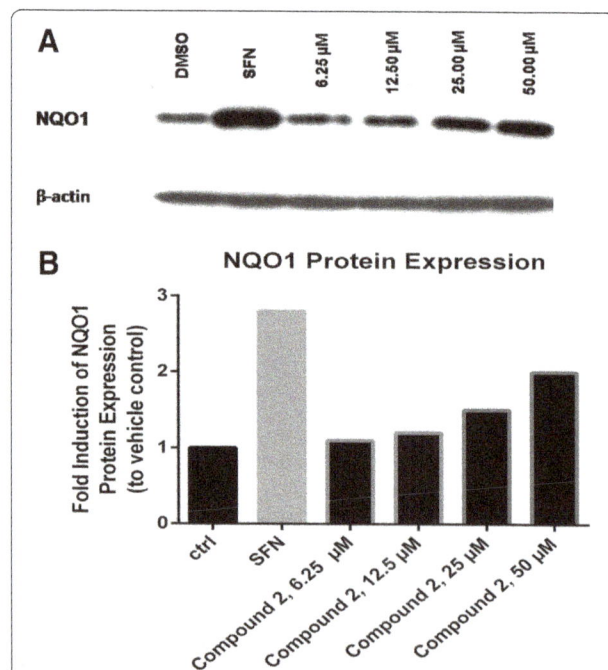

Fig. 5 Concentration -dependent upregulation of NQO1 protein expression by Compound 2 in Hepa1c1c7 cells. Cells were cultured and assayed using Western blotting (**a**) as described in the Experimental section. Densitometric determination (**b**) of the fold of NQO1 induction over DMSO control (ctrl) was performed using Image Studio Lite

of the Nrf2-target gene NQO1 expression. The induction of Nrf2-target genes NQO1 and Glutathione S Transferase (GST) by ursolic acid inhibited the development of lung cancer in nude mice injected with the lung cancer cells A549 [17]. Moreover, inducers of NQO1 in vitro in the Hepa-1c1c7 model were also able to suppress the carcinogenic effects of diverse cancer promoting agents related to different types of cancers, with sulforaphane being the prototype NQO1 inducer [18, 19]. Phenolic phytochemicals were found to be potent inducers of NQO1 by many investigators. For example, (+)-tephropurpurin, a chalcone isolated from *Tephrosia purpurea* induced NQO1 activity in the murine hepatoma hepa-1c1c7 model [20]. Protection against azoxymethane-induced intestinal adenocarcinoma was accomplished in F344 rats administered with the flavonoid morin via significant increase in the activity of GST and NQO1 enzymes over those of untreated control [21]. Morin was also shown to protect against 4-nitroquinone 1-oxide-induced tongue carcinogenesis in F344 rat through induction of GST and NQO1 enzymatic activities [22].

In present study; to further elucidate the potency of tested compounds as inducers of the cancer chemopreventive marker NQO1 at the functional level, we used an assay system at which the NQO1 substrate menadione (MD), a toxic quinone which is known to cause redox cycling and oxidative damage through 1-electron reduction catalyzed by NADH Cytochrome P450 reductase and this results in the formation of unstable toxic semiquinone [23]. NQO1 is known to detoxify quinones through direct 2-electron-reduction into the more water soluble, more stable, easily conjugated hydroquinone and therefore minimizing the formation of the toxic semiquinone metabolite of MD [13, 24].

Treatment of Hepa-1c1c7 cells with 20 μM MD alone caused a dramatic loss of cell viability near to 50% compared to DMSO control (calculated MD IC$_{50}$ from dose response curve = 19.7 μM, Fig. 3). Pretreatment of Hepa-1c1c7 cells with 3.125 μM from tested compounds inhibited the cytotoxic effect caused by MD treatment, displaying higher cell viability % of cells compared to the 20 μM MD only treated cells. Therefore, the protection of Hepa-1c1c7 cells pretreated by compounds **1**, **2**, **4** or **5**, seems to be largely attributed to their NQO1 inducer activities (Fig. 2) that resulted in detoxification of MD compared to MD treated cells.

Conclusion

The present study shed light on the mechanism-based potential of the phenolic constituents of the ornamental plant *B. cristata* var. alba as chemopreventive agents. As shown, this activity is through the induction of the cytoprotective enzyme NQO1 at the activity and protein expression levels.

Acknowledgments

This work was funded by the Deanship of Scientific Research (DSR), King Abdulaziz University, Jeddah, under grant No. (166-929-D1435). The authors, therefore, acknowledge with thanks DSR technical and financial support.

Funding

This work was funded by the Deanship of Scientific Research (DSR), King Abdulaziz University, Jeddah, under grant No. (166–929-D1435).

Authors' contributions

AME, HMA, HEK performed extraction, isolation and identification of pure compounds and shared in writing the manuscript. ARH carried out the biological study and shared in writing the manuscript. AMA suggested the idea of the manuscript, shared in fund raising and edited the manuscript. All authors read and approved the final manuscript.

Competing interests

The authors declare that they have no competing interest.

Author details

[1]Department of Natural Products, Faculty of Pharmacy, King Abdulaziz University, Jeddah 21589, Saudi Arabia. [2]Department of Pharmacognosy, Faculty of Pharmacy, Cairo University, Cairo 11562, Egypt. [3]Phytochemistry Department and Biology Unit lab 610, Central Laboratory for the Pharmaceutical and Dug Industries Research Division, National Research Centre, Giza, Dokki 12622, Egypt. [4]Department of Pharmacognosy, Faculty of Pharmacy, Minia University, Minia 61519, Egypt. [5]Department of Pharmaceutical Sciences, College of Clinical Pharmacy, King Faisal University, Al-Ahsa, Saudi Arabia. [6]Department of Clinical Pharmacy, Faculty of Pharmacy, King Abdulaziz University, Jeddah 21589, Saudi Arabia.

References

1. Ali NS, Khalil HZ. Cancer prevention and early detection among Egyptians. *Cancer nursing.* 1996;**19**(2):104–11.
2. Surh Y-J. Cancer chemoprevention with dietary phytochemicals. Nat Rev Cancer. 2003;3(10):768–80.
3. Manson MM, Gescher A, Hudson EA, Plummer SM, Squires MS, Prigent SA. Blocking and suppressing mechanisms of chemoprevention by dietary constituents. Toxicol Lett. 2000;112:499–505.
4. Zhao CR, Gao ZH, Qu XJ. Nrf2-ARE signaling pathway and natural products for cancer chemoprevention. Cancer Epidemiol. 2010;34(5):523–33.
5. Hamed AR, Hegazy M-EF, Higgins M, Mohamed TA, Abdel-Azim NS, Pare PW, Dinkova-Kostova AT: Potency of extracts from selected Egyptian plants as inducers of the Nrf2-dependent chemopreventive enzyme NQO1. J Nat Med. 2016;70(3):683–8.
6. Crowell JA. The chemopreventive agent development research program in the division of Cancer prevention of the US National Cancer Institute: an overview. Eur J Cancer. 2005;41(13):1889–910.

7. Harraz FM, El-Halawany AM, El Gayed SH, Abdel-Sattar E. Iridoid glycosides from Barleria trispinosa. Nat Prod Res. 2009;23(10):903–8.
8. Hemalatha K. Chemical constituents isolated from leaves of *Barleria cristata* Linn. Int J Pharm Bio Sci. 2012;3(1):609–15.
9. Swanson H: Mechanisms by which flavonoids exert their beneficial anti-cancer effects. In: *Flavonoids, Inflammation and Cancer.* edn. Singapore: World Scientific; 2016; 25–58.
10. Benson AM, Hunkeler MJ, Talalay P. Increase of NAD(P)H:quinone reductase by dietary antioxidants: possible role in protection against carcinogenesis and toxicity. Proc Natl Acad Sci U S A. 1980;77(9):5216–20.
11. Bradford MM. A rapid and sensitive method for the quantitation of microgram quantities of protein utilizing the principle of protein-dye binding. Anal Biochem. 1976;72(1–2):248–54.
12. Vichai V, Kirtikara K. Sulforhodamine B colorimetric assay for cytotoxicity screening. Nat Protoc. 2006;1(3):1112–6.
13. Dietz BM, Kang Y-H, Liu G, Eggler AL, Yao P, Chadwick LR, Pauli GF, Farnsworth NR, Mesecar AD, Van Breemen RB. Xanthohumol isolated from *Humulus lupulus* inhibits menadione-induced DNA damage through induction of quinone reductase. Chem Res Toxicol. 2005;18(8):1296–305.
14. Abdallah HM, Mohamed MA, Abdou AM, Hamed MM, Abdel-Naim AB, Ashour OM. Protective effect of *Centaurea pallescens* Del. Against CCl$_4$-induced injury on a human hepatoma cell line (Huh7). Med Chem Res. 2013;22(12):5700–6.
15. Shabana MM, El-Sherei MM, Moussa MY, Sleem AA, Abdallah HM. Investigation of phenolic constituents of *Carduncellus eriocephalus* Boiss. Var. albiflora Gauba and their biological activities. Nat Prod Commun. 2007;2(8):823–8.
16. Wu TY, Saw CL, Khor TO, Pung D, Boyanapalli SS, Kong AN. In vivo pharmacodynamics of indole-3-carbinol in the inhibition of prostate cancer in transgenic adenocarcinoma of mouse prostate (TRAMP) mice: involvement of Nrf2 and cell cycle/apoptosis signaling pathways. Mol Carcinog. 2012;51(10):761–70.
17. Liu W, Tan X, Shu L, Sun H, Song J, Jin P, Yu S, Sun M, Jia X. Ursolic acid inhibits cigarette smoke extract-induced human bronchial epithelial cell injury and prevents development of lung cancer. Molecules. 2012;17(8):9104–15.
18. Zhang Y, Talalay P, Cho CG, Posner GH. A major inducer of anticarcinogenic protective enzymes from broccoli: isolation and elucidation of structure. Proc Natl Acad Sci U S A. 1992;89(6):2399–403.
19. Radjendirane V, Joseph P, Lee YH, Kimura S, Klein-Szanto AJ, Gonzalez FJ, Jaiswal AK. Disruption of the DT diaphorase (NQO1) gene in mice leads to increased menadione toxicity. J Biol Chem. 1998;273(13):7382–9.
20. Chang LC, Gerhauser C, Song L, Farnsworth NR, Pezzuto JM, Kinghorn AD. Activity-guided isolation of constituents of Tephrosia purpurea with the potential to induce the phase II enzyme, quinone reductase. J Nat Prod. 1997;60(9):869–73.
21. Tanaka T, Kawabata K, Kakumoto M, Makita H, Ushida J, Honjo S, Hara A, Tsuda H, Mori H. Modifying effects of a flavonoid morin on azoxymethane-induced large bowel tumorigenesis in rats. Carcinogenesis. 1999;20(8):1477–84.
22. Kawabata K, Tanaka T, Honjo S, Kakumoto M, Hara A, Makita H, Tatematsu N, Ushida J, Tsuda H, Mori H. Chemopreventive effect of dietary flavonoid morin on chemically induced rat tongue carcinogenesis. Int J Cancer. 1999; 83(3):381–6.
23. Burdette JE, Chen SN, Lu ZZ, Xu H, White BE, Fabricant DS, Liu J, Fong HH, Farnsworth NR, Constantinou AI. black cohosh (*Cimicifuga racemosa* L.) protects against menadione-induced DNA damage through scavenging of reactive oxygen species: bioassay-directed isolation and characterization of active principles. J Agric Food Chem. 2002;50(24):7022–8.
24. Dinkova-Kostova AT, Fahey JW, Talalay P. Chemical structures of inducers of nicotinamide quinone oxidoreductase 1 (NQO1). Methods Enzymol. 2004; 382:423–48.

Antidiabetic activity, glucose uptake stimulation and α-glucosidase inhibitory effect of *Chrysophyllum cainito* L. stem bark extract

Hau Van Doan, Siriporn Riyajan, Roongtip Iyara and Nuannoi Chudapongse[*]

Abstract

Background: *Chrysophyllum cainito* L., a tropical fruit tree, has been used as an alternative medicine for the treatment of diabetic patients in many countries. However, there is very limited scientific rationale for this medical use. The present study aimed to evaluate the antidiabetic activity of the extract from *C. cainito* stem bark and the possible mechanisms underlying this activity.

Methods: Phytochemistry and in vitro antioxidant capacity of the extract were studied. Hypoglycemic activity of the extract was examined in normal and alloxan-induced diabetic mice. The effect of *C. cainito* extract on glucose absorption and glucose uptake were conducted using mouse isolated jejunum and abdominal muscle, respectively. Finally, an in vitro effect of *C. cainito* extract on α-glucosidase activity was evaluated.

Results: *C. cainito* extract possessed a strong antioxidant activity comparable to the ascorbic acid and butylated hydroxytoluene. The extract at 500 mg/kg significantly reduced the area under curve of blood glucose level in oral glucose tolerance test in normal mice. In alloxan-induced diabetic model, similar to glibenclamide, a single dose of the extract significantly decreased fasting blood glucose level from 387.17 ± 29.84 mg/dl to 125.67 ± 62.09 mg/dl after 6 h of administration. From the isolated jejunum experiment, the extract at any doses used did not inhibit glucose absorption. However, the extract at 50 μg/ml significantly increased the amount of glucose uptake by abdominal muscles in the presence of insulin ($P < 0.05$). Lastly, it was found that the extract produced stronger inhibition of α-glucosidase activity ($IC_{50} = 1.20 \pm 0.09$ μg/ml) than acarbose ($IC_{50} = 198.17 \pm 4.74$ μg/ml).

Conclusion: Direct evidence of antidiabetic activity of *C. cainito* stem bark with possible modes of action, glucose uptake stimulation and α-glucosidase inhibitory effect, was reported for the first time herein. These data support the potential use of this plant for the treatment of diabetic patients.

Keywords: *Chrysophyllum cainito*, Antidiabetic activity, Glucose uptake, α-glucosidase, Alloxan

Background

Diabetes mellitus, one of the most common metabolic disorders, has been reported to affect approximately 415 million people worldwide in 2015 and the number of cases has been estimated to increase to 642 millions in 2040 [1]. Chronic hyperglycemic patients have been living with a high risk of macrovascular complications (e.g., coronary artery disease, peripheral arterial disease, and/or stroke) and microvascular complications (e.g., retinopathy, nephropathy, and neuropathy) [2]. Being supplied with high blood glucose, cells can generate the formation of free radicals and reactive oxygen species. In turn, an overload of free radicals can damage cellular macromolecules including lipid, protein and nucleic acids leading to the progression of diabetes and the development of its complications. Therefore, the antioxidant therapy is one of the important therapeutic strategy in diabetes management [3]. Plants have been widely accepted that they provide natural antioxidant compounds

* Correspondence: nuannoi@sut.ac.th
School of Preclinical Sciences, Institute of Science, Suranaree University of Technology, Nakhon Ratchasima 30000, Thailand

[4, 5]. In addition, plant products and their derivatives also possess many other pharmacological activities, such as anti-inflammatory, antimicrobial, anticancer and anti-diabetic activity. Thus, traditional medicines have been proved to be a vital source of future drugs to counteract many diseases including diabetes mellitus [6].

Chrysophyllum cainito L. (commonly known as Star Apple) is a tropical fruit tree of which many biological activities have been demonstrated. The documented benefits of *C. cainito* include antihypertensive, anti-inflammatory [7], antioxidant and wound healing [8], antibacterial [9] and antidiabetic activity [10, 11]. The stem bark decoction has been traditionally used as tonic, stimulant, antidiarrheals [12] and antidiabetics [13]. Although several parts of *C. cainito*, such as fruit, leaf and stem, have been used as alternative medicines for the treatment of diabetic patients in many countries, there is limited pharmacological basis for this therapeutic application. The present study was carried out to evaluate the antidiabetic activity of the aqueous extract of *C. cainito* stem bark in animal models. In addition, the effects on glucose absorption, glucose uptake and α-glucosidase activity were also examined as the possible mechanisms underlying antidiabetic property of the extract.

Methods
Chemicals
2,2-Diphenyl-1-picrylhydrazyl (DPPH), 2,2′-Azino-bis (3-ethylbenzothiazoline-6-sulfonic acid) diammonium salt (ABTS), 2,4,6-tripyridyl-s-triazine (TPTZ), Peroxidase-glucose oxidase (PGO) enzyme, α-glucosidase, alloxan monohydrate were purchased from Sigma-Aldrich (MO, USA). Folin–Ciocalteu reagent was purchased from Carlo-Erba (Val de Reuil Cedex, France). Blood glucose test strips were purchased from Terumo (Tokyo, Japan).

Plant extraction
The stem bark of *C. cainito* was collected from Mo Cay Nam district, Ben Tre, Vietnam. Plant verification was performed by Dr. Santi Watthana, a plant taxonomist, School of Biology, Institute of Science, Suranaree University of Technology, Thailand. Voucher specimens of leaf, fruit, flowers, and stem was stored at Suranaree University of Technology Botanical Garden under collected number H.DOAN-1. The bark was dried under the shade for a week before ground. In this study, water was chosen as an extraction solvent because water formulations are safe for human consumption compared to other organic solvents. It also increases bioavailability of active compounds. Furthermore, water maceration and decoction of this plant have been used by Vietnamese for treatment of diabetic patients. We have chosen simple maceration rather than decoction to prevent chemical degradation from high temperature. Briefly, 50 g of

ground material were shaken with 200 ml of deionized water at room temperature for 2 h. The process was repeated four times. The combined extract was centrifuged at 5000 rpm for 15 min to remove solid residue. The supernatant was evaporated and dried by lyophilizer. The extract of *C. cainito* stem bark (CE) was kept at -20 °C until used for the experiments.

Phytochemical screening and total phenolic content determination
Phytochemical screening for tannin, phenols, alkaloids, flavonoids, saponin, steroids and glycosides were conducted as previously described [14]. The presence of terpenoids was also examined [15].

Total phenolic content was determined by Folin–Ciocalteu reagent using gallic acid as a standard. Briefly, after incubation at room temperature for 30 min, the absorbance of the mixture of CE and Folin–Ciocalteu reagent was measured at 750 nm by spectrophotometer. Total phenolic content of CE was expressed as mg of gallic acid equivalents (GAE) per gram of dried extract [16].

In vitro antioxidant activity
DPPH radical scavenging activity
To perform DPPH assay, one milliliter of various concentrations of CE (0–25 µg/ml) was mixed with 2 ml of 0.1 mM DPPH in methanol and left standing for 1 h at room temperature in the dark. The absorbance was measured at 515 nm. Percentage of inhibition was calculated using the equation below. The antioxidant activity was expressed by the concentration required for 50% of scavenging of free radical (IC_{50}) [17].

$$\% \text{ inhibition} = [(\text{Absorbance}_{control} - \text{Absorbance}_{sample})/$$
$$\text{Absorbance}_{control}] \times 100$$

ABTS radical scavenging activity
The scavenging activity of CE against ABTS• was measured as previously described with minor modifications [16]. ABTS radical cation (ABTS•) was produced by adding 14 mM ABTS solution to 4.9 mM potassium persulfate solution (1:1; v/v) for 16 h in the dark at room temperature. The 150 µl of CE at various concentrations (0–25 µg/ml), ascorbic acid or butylated hydroxytoluene (BHT) was added to 2850 µl of diluted ABTS• solution, mixed and then incubated in the dark for 6 min. Finally, the absorbance of the reaction mixture was measured at 734 nm. The radical scavenging activity of CE was expressed by IC_{50} value.

Ferric reducing antioxidant power (FRAP) assay

FRAP assay was performed to investigate the reducing power of CE [18]. The absorbance of the resulting mixture was measured at 593 nm. The standard calibration curve was created using $FeSO_4 \cdot 7H_2O$. The FRAP capacity of the extract was expressed as mM Fe^{2+} per gram extract.

Experimental animals

Male Jcl:ICR mice of 6-week old (28–34 g), obtained from Nomura Siam International Co., Ltd., Bangkok, Thailand, were used in this study. Mice were housed in stainless steel cages lined with wood shavings at Laboratory Animal Facility, Suranaree University of Technology, under standard condition of 25 ± 2 °C, 45–50% relative humidity and 12-h light/dark cycle. Normal food and water were given ad libitum. The experiments were performed after 7 days of acclimatization. The extract was dissolved in distilled water and was administered to animal using oral gavage method. All mice were sacrificed by CO_2 inhalation at the end of experiment and for tissue collection. All procedures were approved and conducted following the guidelines of the Institutional Animal Care and Use Committee, Suranaree University of Technology, Thailand (Approval number No. 1/2561).

Oral glucose tolerance test in normal mice

The effect of CE on blood glucose level was first evaluated via oral glucose challenge. Six-hour fasted normal mice were randomly divided into 3 different groups ($n = 6$) as the following.

Group 1: normal mice + deionized water
Group 2: normal mice + 500 mg/kg CE
Group 3: normal mice + 10 mg/kg glibenclamide (Daonil®, Jakarta, Indonesia)

All mice were pretreated with drugs prior to the oral glucose administration at the dose 2 g/kg (2 h for CE and deionized water; 30 min for glibenclamide based on the onset of action from our preliminary study). Blood glucose level was monitored at 0, 30, 60 and 120 min from small incision of tail tip using Medisafe® EX glucose meter. The area under the curve was calculated using the same formula in the previous report [19].

Hypoglycemic test in alloxan-induced diabetic mice

Overnight fasted mice were received an intraperitoneal injection of 130 mg/kg of alloxan monohydrate dissolved in cold 0.85% saline solution to induce type 2 diabetes [20]. Diabetic induction was checked after 3 days of alloxan injection. Mice showed glucose level greater than 200 mg/dl (survived without insulin) was considered as type 2 diabetic mice [21] and used for the experiment. Mice were randomly divided into 4 groups as follow.

Group 1: normal mice + deionized water ($n = 6$)

Group 2: diabetic mice + deionized water ($n = 6$)
Group 3: diabetic mice + 500 mg/kg CE ($n = 6$)
Group 4: diabetic mice + 10 mg/kg glibenclamide ($n = 5$)

After the single dose of drug administration, blood glucose levels were determined at 0, 1, 2, 4 and 6 h to evaluate acute hypoglycemic effect of the extract as described in the previous study [22].

Effect of the extract on glucose absorption

The inhibitory effect of CE on glucose absorption was investigated using isolated mouse jejunum. The jejunum was isolated from normal mouse and placed in oxygenated Kreb-Henseleit solution (composition in g/l; NaCl 6.92, KCl 0.35, $MgSO_4.7H_2O$ 0.29, $CaCl_2$ 0.28, KH_2PO_4 0.16, $NaHCO_3$ 2.1, and D-glucose 1.4), pH 7.4. The jejunum was cut into 6 cm long segments, tied edges, everted and filled with Kreb-Henseleit solution. The sacs were incubated in 10 ml of Kreb-Henseleit solution containing each of the following substances CE (25 and 50 µg/ml) or acarbose (1 mg/ml) for 1 h in the presence of carbogen at 37 °C. Glucose concentrations inside the sacs were determined using PGO enzyme. Ten µl of diluted buffer was interacted with 190 µl of PGO enzyme solution in a microtiter plate. The reaction mixture was incubated at 37 °C in the dark for 30 min. The intensity of the brown color was measured at 450 nm using spectrophotometer. The concentration of glucose was calculated using standard curve of D-glucose. The amount of glucose absorption was calculated using the following formula [23].

$$\text{Amount of glucose absorbed} = (\text{amount of glucose after} \\ - \text{amount of glucose before}) \\ /\text{g of jejunum}$$

Effect of the extract on glucose uptake

Glucose uptake by mouse abdominal muscle was measured as previously described [24]. Briefly, after animals were sacrificed, abdominal muscles were removed and soaked in the Kreb's-Ringer bicarbonate (KRB) buffer, pH 7.4 with continuously supply of carbogen for 10 min. The muscle was then incubated with KRB buffer containing 200 mg/dl of D-glucose, CE 25 or 50 µg/ml with or without insulin (100 mU/ml) for 30 min. Then, buffer was collected and analyzed for the remaining glucose using PGO enzyme as described in the previous section. The amount of glucose uptake was calculated by the formula below.

$$\text{Amount of glucose uptake} = (\text{amount of glucose before} \\ - \text{amount glucose after}) \\ /\text{g of muscle}$$

Examination of the effect on α-glucosidase activity

The α-glucosidase inhibitory activity was measured as described previously [16]. Briefly, a mixture of 10 µl of

0.25 U/ml α-glucosidase (Sigma–Aldrich, USA), 50 µl of 0.1 M potassium phosphate buffer (pH 6.8) and 20 µl of various concentrations of the extract or the α-glucosidase inhibitor acarbose (Fluka, USA) was incubated at 37 °C for 10 min. Then, 10 µl of 5 mM p-nitrophenyl-α-D-glucopyranoside (PNPG) was added and further incubated for 30 min. To terminate the reaction, 50 µl of 0.1 M Na_2CO_3 was added. The absorbance was measured at 405 nm optically by using a spectrophotometer. Results were expressed as the concentration where the activity of α-glucosidase is inhibited by 50% (IC_{50}).

Statistical analysis

Each experiment was repeated at least 3 times and the result values were expressed as mean ± SEM. The comparisons between means were done using One way- or Two way-ANOVA followed by Student-Newman-Keuls. A value of $P < 0.05$ was considered as statistically significant differences.

Results

Phytochemistry and total phenolic content

The results of extract yield and phytochemicals screening were presented in Table 1. In this study, extract yield of *C. cainito* stem bark prepared by maceration method using water was $11.22 \pm 0.54\%$. The phytochemical screening revealed the presence of phenols, tannin, glycosides, terpenoids, and saponin but the absence of flavonoids, alkaloids, and steroids. Total phenolic compounds found in the extract was 871.75 ± 10.41 mg GAE/g extract (Table 2).

Antioxidant activity

To access the antioxidant activity of the extract, DPPH, ABTS free radical scavenging and FRAP assay were performed. The concentrations of CE were varied from 0 to 25 µg/ml. The extract showed the maximum radical scavenging activity in the highest experimental concentration by 92% in DPPH assay and 99% in ABTS assay (Fig. 1). The IC_{50} values found for CE, ascorbic acid, and BHT from DPPH and ABTS assays were presented in Table 2. The reducing potential of CE was determined using $FeSO_4$ standard curve. The FRAP value of CE was 291.56 ± 3.25 mM Fe^{2+} equivalent per gram of dried extract (Table 2).

Oral glucose tolerance test in normal mice

The results of the oral glucose tolerance test in normal mice are shown in Fig. 2. As seen in Fig. 2a, the initial blood glucose levels of all groups prior to drug administration were no difference. The blood glucose levels after glucose loading reached a peak at 30 min and decreased subsequently over time, in all groups. It was found that CE or glibenclamide had significantly improved glucose tolerance in normal mice. Mice received CE (500 mg/kg) and glibenclamide (10 mg/kg) noticeably suppressed the elevation of glucose after 30 min of glucose load compared to control group ($P < 0.05$). In addition, the area under the curve (AUC) was significantly reduced in both treated groups when compared to control mice (Fig. 2b).

Antidiabetic effect of *C. cainito* extract in alloxan-diabetic mice

Fig. 3 shows kinetics of blood glucose observed during the period of experiment. In this study, alloxan injection destroyed pancreatic β cells and reduced insulin secretion leading to an elevated blood glucose level compared to normal control mice. The extract and glibenclamide started to suppress the rise of blood glucose in diabetic mice after 2 h of treatment, but not statistically significant. However, after 4 h and longer blood glucose levels of the CE and glibenclamide groups declined significantly more than the diabetic control group ($P < 0.05$).

Effect of *C. cainito* extract on glucose absorption

The everted sacs of the small intestines from mice were used for investigating the inhibitory effect of CE on glucose absorption ex vivo. The results shown in Fig. 4 indicated that the extract at the experimental concentrations (25 and 50 µg/ml) did not inhibit glucose absorption when compared to control. In contrast, acarbose at 1 mg/ml profoundly suppressed glucose absorption by everted sacs ($P < 0.05$).

Effect of *C. cainito* extract on glucose uptake

The effect of CE on glucose uptake is presented in Fig. 5. In normal group, low glucose uptake was found in the absence of insulin. Addition of insulin to the KRB buffer increased the glucose uptake significantly ($P < 0.05$). This

Table 1 Phytochemical screening and yield of the aqueous extract of *C. cainito* stem bark

Test for	Results
Phytochemistry	
Phenols	+
Tannins	+
Glycosides	+
Terpenoids	+
Saponin	+
Flavonoids	−
Steroids	−
Alkaloids	−
Yield (%)	11.22 ± 0.54^a

+ present; − absent
[a]Value is expressed as mean ± SEM ($n = 3$)

Table 2 Total phenolic content and antioxidant activities of *C. cainito* stem bark extract

	DPPH IC$_{50}$ (µg/ml)	ABTS IC$_{50}$ (µg/ml)	FRAP (mM Fe^{2+} /g extract)	Phenolic Content (mg GAE/g CE)
CE	4.66 ± 0.14*	2.10 ± 0.06#	291.56 ± 3.25	871.75 ± 10.41
AA	3.49 ± 0.12	1.86 ± 0.03	–	–
BHT	4.68 ± 0.03	5.07 ± 0.19	–	–

The values are expressed as mean ± SEM, *n* = 3. CE, AA, BHT were abbreviations of *C. cainito* extract, ascorbic acid and butylated hydroxytoluene, respectively
*$P < 0.05$ compared with AA; #$P < 0.05$ compared with BHT by one-way ANOVA followed by Student-Newman-Keuls as post hoc test

effect was also observed in all experiments when compared to the non-insulin treated groups. The results showed that treatment of CE at 50 µg/ml with insulin significantly increased glucose uptake from 7.86 ± 0.52 (control) to 9.45 ± 0.82 mg/g tissue. However, without insulin, CE at the doses used had no significant effect on glucose uptake.

α-Glucosidase inhibitory effect of *C. cainito* extract

α-Glucosidase enzyme is one of the medication targets in diabetic management. The enzyme is involved in digestion of polysaccharide into monosaccharide that can be absorbed by the intestine. In this study, α-glucosidase isolated from *Saccharomyces cerevisiae* was chosen as the target enzyme. The aqueous extract from *C. cainito*

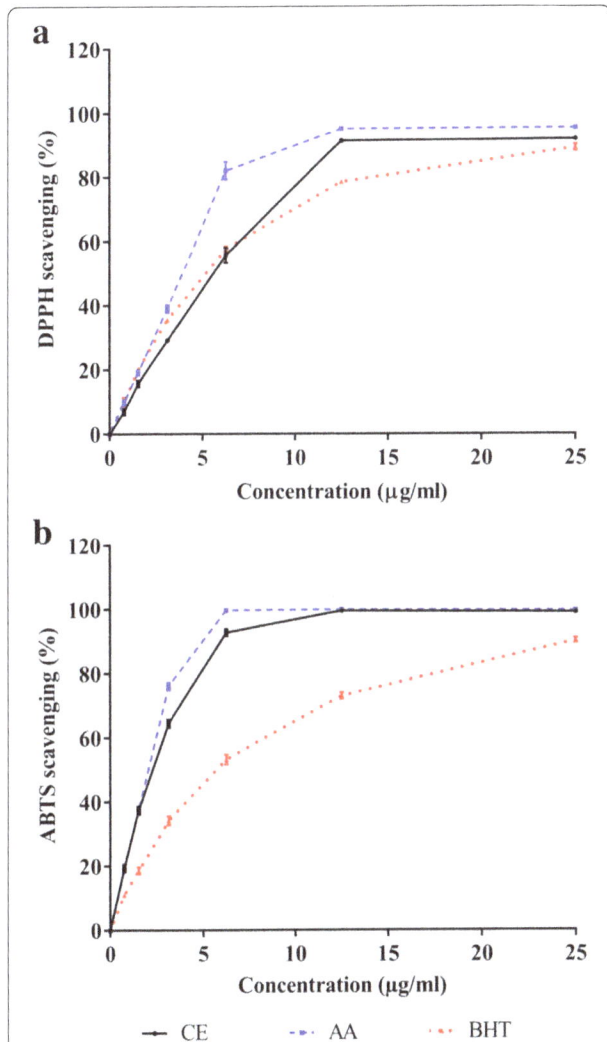

Fig. 1 Antioxidant activity of *C. cainito* extract. Panel **a** and **b** are the results from DPPH and ABTS) radical scavenging methods, respectively. The values are expressed as mean ± SEM, *n* = 3. AA: ascorbic acid; BHT: butylated hydroxytoluene; CE: *C. cainito* extract

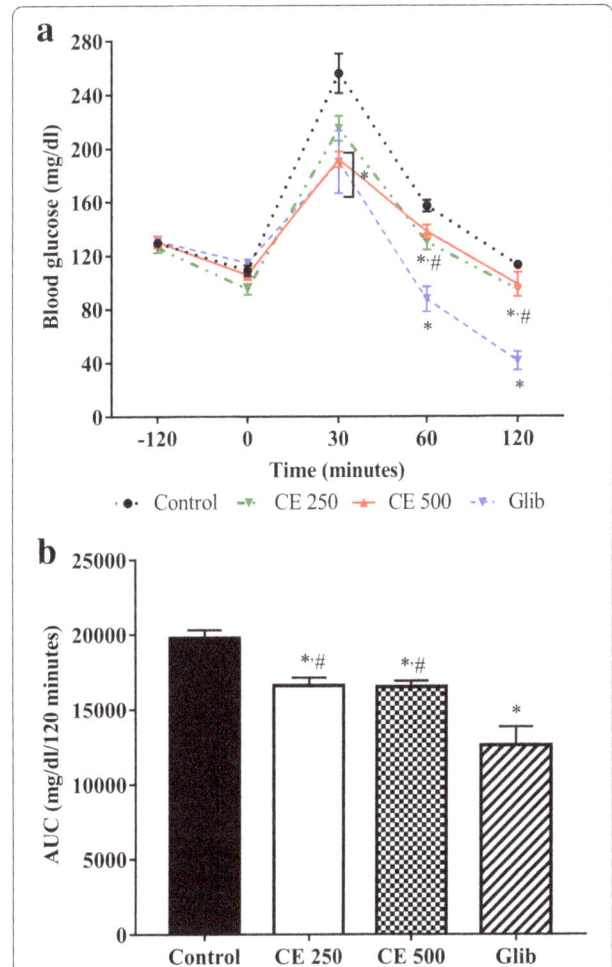

Fig. 2 Effect of *C. cainito* extract on OGTT in normal mice. Panel **a** is blood glucose level during oral glucose challenge whereas Panel **b** is the area under the curve (AUC) of the blood glucose level over time. *$P < 0.05$ compared with control mice; #$P < 0.05$ compared with glibenclamide treated mice by one-way ANOVA followed by Student-Newman-Keuls as post hoc test. The values are expressed as mean ± SEM, *n* = 6. Glib: glibenclamide; CE: *C. cainito* extract

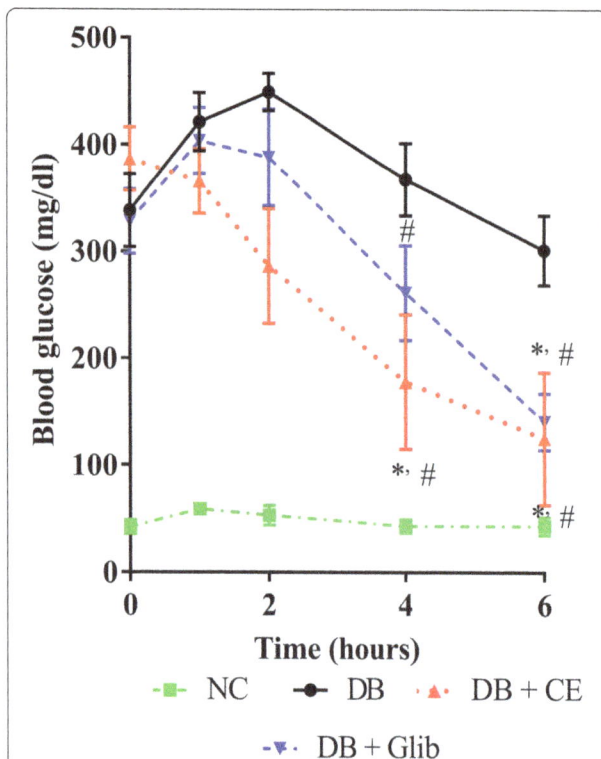

Fig. 3 Acute effect of *C. cainito* extract on alloxan-induced diabetic mice. NC: normal control; DB: diabetic control; DB + CE: diabetes + CE 500 mg/kg; DB + Glib: diabetes + glibenclamide 10 mg/kg. *P < 0.05 compared with diabetic control mice at the same time of experiment, #P < 0.05 compared to the initial level in the same treatment by one-way ANOVA followed by Student-Newman-Keuls as post hoc test. The values are expressed as mean ± SEM, n = 5–6

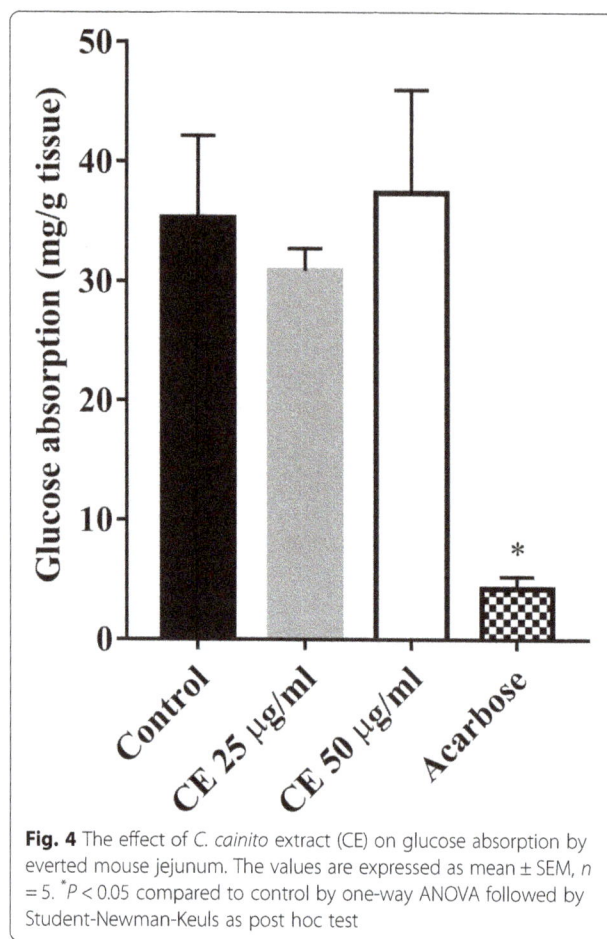

Fig. 4 The effect of *C. cainito* extract (CE) on glucose absorption by everted mouse jejunum. The values are expressed as mean ± SEM, n = 5. *P < 0.05 compared to control by one-way ANOVA followed by Student-Newman-Keuls as post hoc test

exhibited much greater inhibition on α-glucosidase activity compared to acarbose. The IC_{50} of CE was 1.20 ± 0.09 μg/ml whereas that of acarbose was 198.17 ± 4.74 μg/ml (Fig. 6).

Discussion

It is widely accepted that the rapidly increasing incidence of diabetes mellitus has become a major health problem worldwide. The modern oral hypoglycemic agents such as sulphonylureas, biguanides, thiozolidinediones and α-glucosidase inhibitors are commonly used for the treatment of type 2 diabetes. However, it is well known that they can produce side effects associated with their applications [25]. Moreover, a progressive decline in their effectiveness, termed secondary failure have been reported [26]. During the past decade, there is a growing interest in alternative herbal medicine due to their efficacy, less side effects in clinical practice and relatively low costs. It has been estimated that about 800 plants have antidiabetic potentials [27]. Most of them have been used as folk medicines in many countries around the world. *C. cainito*, commonly called Star Apple in English and Vú Sữa (literally: milky breast) in

Vietnamese, is one of medicinal plants which has long been prescribed by local practitioners for traditional treatment of diabetes mellitus. However, there is a paucity of scientific evidence that confirms its antidiabetic activity. Herein, we first evaluated the antidiabetic effect of the extract from *C. cainito* stem bark to confirm its benefits according to the use of this plant in Vietnam.

In this study, antidiabetic effect of the *C. cainito* extract was conducted in healthy and alloxan-diabetic mice. In normal mice, the hypoglycemic effect of the extract was investigated through an oral glucose tolerance test (OGTT). A 6-h fasting is considered as a best fasting duration for establishing an OGTT in mice [28]. The rise in blood glucose after 30 min confirmed successful oral glucose loading in every group (Fig. 2). The antidiabetic drug glibenclamide used in this study as a positive control reduces the postprandial hyperglycemia by increasing insulin secretion from β cell. Based on our preliminary experiment, the dose at 500 mg/kg was chosen for oral administration. As shown in Fig. 2a and b, the extract and glibenclamide improved glucose tolerance compared to vehicle control.

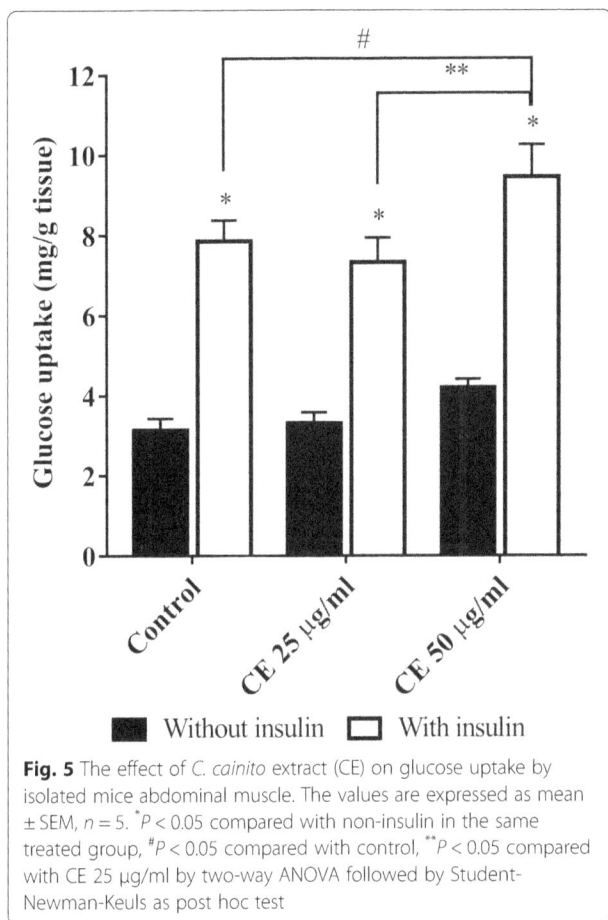

Fig. 5 The effect of *C. cainito* extract (CE) on glucose uptake by isolated mice abdominal muscle. The values are expressed as mean ± SEM, $n = 5$. $^*P < 0.05$ compared with non-insulin in the same treated group, $^{\#}P < 0.05$ compared with control, $^{**}P < 0.05$ compared with CE 25 µg/ml by two-way ANOVA followed by Student-Newman-Keuls as post hoc test

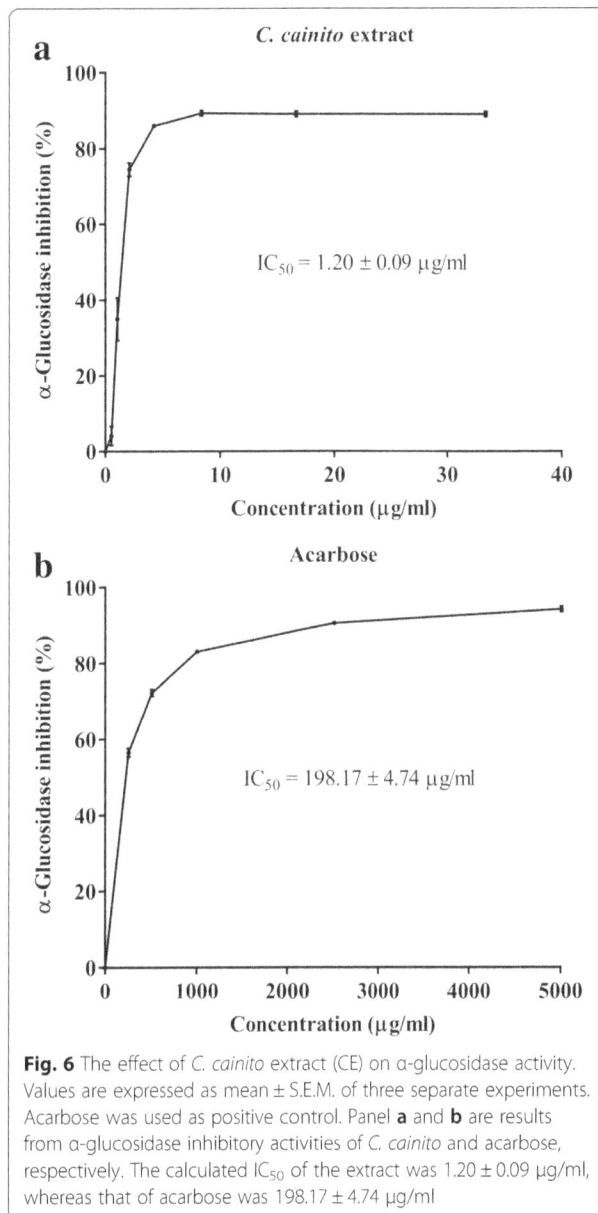

Fig. 6 The effect of *C. cainito* extract (CE) on α-glucosidase activity. Values are expressed as mean ± S.E.M. of three separate experiments. Acarbose was used as positive control. Panel **a** and **b** are results from α-glucosidase inhibitory activities of *C. cainito* and acarbose, respectively. The calculated IC$_{50}$ of the extract was 1.20 ± 0.09 µg/ml, whereas that of acarbose was 198.17 ± 4.74 µg/ml

Alloxan, a toxic glucose analogue, enters pancreatic β-cell via GLUT2 glucose transporter. This chemical plays an important role in hyperglycemic animal model through its specific inhibition of glucokinase and stimulation of reactive oxygen species production, consequently causing necrosis and destruction of β-cells [29]. The data from Fig. 3 clearly showed that the administration of CE reduced blood glucose level in alloxan-induced diabetic mice similar to that of glibenclamide. These in vivo experiments provide the first scientific evidence supporting an anti-hyperglycemic activity of *C. cainito* stem bark.

Numerous mechanisms of action have been proposed for medicinal plants used in the treatment of diabetes mellitus. However, none has been postulated for antidiabetic activity of *C. cainito*. In this study, two possible mechanisms underlying its acute antidiabetic activity, an inhibition of glucose absorption and a stimulation of glucose uptake were examined. The glucose absorption was performed using everted jejunal sacs of mice. Acarbose, a well-known α-glucosidase inhibitor currently used for the treatment of diabetic patients, was used as a positive control because it has been shown to additionally inhibit the absorption of D-glucose from the intestinal lumen into the blood stream [23, 30]. The data

in Fig. 4 showed that unlike acarbose, CE did not inhibit the glucose absorption.

Isolated skeletal muscle such as epitrochlearis muscle [31, 32] and abdominal muscle [24, 33, 34] have been exploited in the glucose uptake study. In the current study, we isolated the abdominal muscle from mice and incubated in a bicarbonate buffer with carbogen supplied constantly. The effect of CE on glucose uptake was evaluated in the absence and presence of insulin. The data in Fig. 5 shows that in the presence of insulin CE at 50 µg/ml significantly enhanced glucose uptake by the muscle (9.45 ± 0.82 mg/g tissue) compared to control (7.86 ± 0.52 mg/g tissue). Without insulin, CE treatment also showed an increase of glucose uptake, but not statistical significant. These in vitro experiments revealed that the extract promoted glucose transport in the skeletal muscle, especially in the presence of insulin, but no effect on glucose absorption. It is likely that the enhancement on glucose uptake contributes to the antidiabetic effect of CE.

In this study, the in vivo experiments were done only in the acute treatment mainly to provide scientific evidence to support the hypoglycemic activity of the extract. One may argue that the postulated action on glucose uptake in this study could not explain the acute anti-hyperglycemic effect of the extract. Skeletal muscle is recognized as the major site of insulin-mediated glucose uptake after carbohydrate consumption in human [35]. Insulin resistance is a hallmark of non-insulin dependent diabetic mellitus. Peroxisome proliferator-activated receptor gamma (PPARγ) is a key factor in insulin sensitivity. The activation of PPARγ by insulin sensitizers (e.g. thiazolidinediones) markedly improve the sensitivity to insulin, however, it requires long-term effect to cause gene expression change [36]. Moreover, PPARγ is prominently present in adipose tissue and nearly absent in muscle [37]. The enhancement of insulin action in skeletal muscle by CE found in this study tend to be mediated via other mechanism(s).

It is well established that glucose uptake by skeletal muscle is mostly via glucose transporter 4 (GLUT4). It has been shown that GLUT4 recruitment from cytosol to the cell surfaces of muscle can be acutely stimulated by both insulin and exercise independent of transcription or translation [38, 39]. The translocation of GLUT4 from intracellular vesicles to accumulate in the plasma membrane in the response to insulin was demonstrated to depend on the activation of the insulin receptor substrate 1, PI3K, PDK1 and Akt2 [40]. In addition, the data from a previous study suggested that an acute stimulation effect on insulin-mediated glucose uptake in skeletal muscle was related to the elevation of the phosphorylation and activation of key proteins involving in the translocation of GLUT4 such as Rac1, AS160 and Akt [41]. Other studies suggested that the rising in glucose uptake was due to the increase of AMPK phosphorylation [31, 42]. This pathway supports the acute anti-hyperglycemic effect of the CE by increasing glucose uptake in the muscle.

α-Glucosidase is a digestive enzyme which catalyzes the breakdown of polysaccharides into monosaccharide, the form of carbohydrate that the intestine can only be able to transport into the blood circulation. Therefore, the inhibition of α-glucosidase is one of the important approaches in oral antidiabetic medication. Reducing postprandial glucose level by delay glucose absorption after meal is the prominent benefit from α-glucosidase inhibitor [43]. In addition to the glucose uptake stimulation which is proposed as a mechanism underlying the

acute hypoglycemic effect of C. cainito extract in this study, α-glucosidase inhibitory effect was also investigated. The IC$_{50}$ value of the extract was found at 1.20 ± 0.09 µg/ml, approximately 200 times lower than that of acarbose which is used clinically as antidiabetic drug. Although this action could not be attributed to the anti-hyperglycemic mechanism in this study, it could be anticipated to contribute to the blood lowering effect when used as alternative medicine in diabetic patients. Moreover, this plant could be a potential candidate for a search of a new α-glucosidase inhibitory drug for diabetic care.

Free radicals are found to be associated with many diseases, including diabetes. In diabetes mellitus, the supplement of antioxidant agents show promising effect on the reverse of the oxidative stress biomarkers and diabetic complications [3]. Major antioxidant ability can be classified into two groups, hydrogen atom transfer and single electron transfer based assays. For in vitro antioxidant measurement, a single assay may not provide sufficient evidence for antioxidant potential of a compound. Therefore, in this study, the antioxidant activity of CE was assessed by different methods including DPPH, ABTS, and FRAP assays. DPPH, a stable organic nitrogen radical, is used to perform a simple technique assay. DPPH assay has been considered as a valid accurate and easy method to determine radical scavenging activity of antioxidants. However, the disadvantages of this method are (1) the cross interaction between DPPH radical and other radicals and (2) the time response curve to reach the final stable state is not linear with different ratios of antioxidant and DPPH [44]. In ABTS assay, the oxidant was generated by the reaction between ABTS ammonium and potassium persulfate. This assay has been used commonly in many laboratories although it costs time to prepare the radical. The FRAP assay is an electron transfer based assay. The oxidant involves many Fe (III) species and many metal chelators in food extract. The redox potential of Fe (III) salt in FRAP assay is comparable to ABTS$^{·}$ in ABTS assay [45]. As shown in Table 2, the results from all methods used in this study were in agreement that the extract had quite strong antioxidant activity.

Phytochemical analysis of CE obtained from this study showed the presence of phenols, tannin, glycosides, terpenoids, and saponin of which the antidiabetic effects have been established [46–49]. The extract contains great amounts of phenolic compounds (871.75 ± 10.41 mg GAE/g extract) and had high antioxidant potential comparable to antioxidant power of the standard antioxidant ascorbic acid and butylated hydroxytoluene (Table 2). These results agree with previous report that high phenolic content was correlated with strong antioxidant activity [48]. It can be anticipated that the antioxidant activity of CE may be beneficial in the long-term treatment of diabetic patients. Nine polyphenolic compounds, (+)-catechin, (+)-gallocatechin, (−)-epigallocatechin, quercetin, quercitrin, isoquercitrin, myricitrin, gallic acid and (−)-epicatechin were isolated from fruit of *C. cainito* [49]. Others including ursolic acid, β-sitosterol, lupeol and gallic acid were extracted from the leaves [50]. It has been demonstrated that these compounds possess antidiabetic activity [51–54]. In terms of the compositions of *C. cainito* stem bark, there is lack of information. Phytochemical verification and identification of the active ingredients responsible for its antidiabetic activity need further investigation.

Conclusion

In conclusion, the aqueous extract from *C. cainito* stem bark possesses a strong in vitro antioxidant activity and in vivo antidiabetic effects. It is postulated that the mechanism of action contributing the acute anti-hyperglycemic effect of the extract is the enhancement of glucose uptake by the muscles. Moreover, the extract was also found to possess strong α-glucosidase inhibitory effect which may contribute to its anti-hyperglycemic action when used in diabetic patients. The results obtained in the present study provide scientific rationale to corroborate the use of *C. cainito* stem bark for its traditional diabetic treatment.

Acknowledgements
The authors would like to extend their appreciation to the Office of the Higher Education Commission under NRU Project of Thailand and Suranaree University of Technology (SUT) for partial financial support (salary for researcher assistant, RI). We are thankful to Dr. Santi Watthana for plant verification.

Funding
Suranaree University of Technology for its funding of this research under the SUT-PhD Scholarship program for ASEAN.

Authors' contributions
HVD conceived the study and performed the experiments. He contributed to the interpretation, analysis of the data and drafted the manuscript. SR and RI participated in the performing of the animal experiments and in vitro studies. NC supervised the experimental design and data analysis. She revised the manuscript for submission. All authors read and approved the final manuscripts.

Competing interests
The authors declared that they have no competing interests.

References
1. Ogurtsova K, da Rocha Fernandes JD, Huang Y, Linnenkamp U, Guariguata L, Cho NH, et al. IDF diabetes atlas: global estimates for the prevalence of diabetes for 2015 and 2040. Diabetes Res Clin Pract. 2017;128:40–50.
2. Fowler MJ. Microvascular and macrovascular complications of diabetes. Clin Diabetes. 2008;26:77–82.
3. Johansen JS, Harris AK, Rychly DJ, Ergul A. Oxidative stress and the use of antioxidants in diabetes: linking basic science to clinical practice. Cardiovasc Diabetol. 2005;4:5.
4. Pietta P, Simonetti P, Mauri P. Antioxidant activity of selected medicinal plants. J Agric Food Chem. 1998;46:4487–90.
5. Krishnaiah D, Sarbatly R, Nithyanandam R. A review of the antioxidant potential of medicinal plant species. Food Bioprod Process. 2011;89:217–33.
6. Yashwant Kumar A, Nandakumar K, Handral M, Talwar S, Dhayabaran D. Hypoglycaemic and anti-diabetic activity of stem bark extracts *Erythrina indica* in normal and alloxan-induced diabetic rats. Saudi Pharm J. 2011;19:35–42.
7. Meira NA, Klein LCJ, Rocha LW, Quintal ZM, Monache FD, Cechinel Filho V, et al. Anti-inflammatory and anti-hypersensitive effects of the crude extract, fractions and triterpenes obtained from *Chrysophyllum cainito* leaves in mice. J Ethnopharmacol. 2014;151:975–83.
8. Shailajan S, Gurjar D. Wound healing activity of *Chrysophyllum cainito* L. leaves: evaluation in rats using excision wound model. J Young Pharm. 2016;8:96–103.
9. Oranusi SU, Braide W, Umeze RU. Antimicrobial activities and chemical compositions of *Chrysophyllum cainito* (star apple) fruit. Ambit J. 2015;1:8–24.
10. Koffi N, Ernest AK, Marie-Solange T, Beugre K, Noeuml ZG. L. Effect of aqueous extract of *Chrysophyllum cainito* leaves on the glycaemia of diabetic rabbits. African J Pharm Pharmacol. 2009;3:501–6.
11. Hegde K, Arathi A, Mathew A. Evaluation of antidiabetic activity of hydro alcoholic extract of *Chrysophyllum cainito* fruits. Int J Pharm Sci Res. 2016;7:4422–8.
12. Morton JF. The star apple. In: Fruits of Warm Climates. Miami: Julia F. Morton; 1987. p. 408–10.
13. Koffi N, Konan Édouard K, Kouassi K. Ethnobotanical study of plants used to treat diabetes, in traditional medicine, by Abbey and Krobou people of Agboville (Côte-d'Ivoire). Am J Sci Res. 2009;2009:45–58.
14. Yadav RNS, Agarwala M. Phytochemical analysis of some medicinal plants. J Phytol. 2011;3:10–4.
15. Sharma V, Paliwal R. Preliminary phytochemical investigation and thin layer chromatography profiling of sequential extracts of Moringa oleifera pods. Int J Green Pharm. 2013;7:41–5.
16. Kumkrai P, Weeranantanapan O, Chudapongse N. Antioxidant, α-glucosidase inhibitory activity and sub-chronic toxicity of *Derris reticulata* extract: its antidiabetic potential. BMC Complement Altern Med. 2015;15:35.
17. Abdennacer B, Karim M, Yassine M, Nesrine R, Mouna D, Mohamed B. Determination of phytochemicals and antioxidant activity of methanol extracts obtained from the fruit and leaves of Tunisian *Lycium intricatum* Boiss. Food Chem. 2015;174:577–84.
18. Sudan R, Bhagat M, Gupta S, Singh J, Koul A. Iron (FeII) chelation, ferric reducing antioxidant power, and immune modulating potential of *Arisaema jacquemontii* (Himalayan cobra lily). Biomed Res Int. 2014;2014:179865.
19. Ibrahim MA, Islam MS. Butanol fraction of Khaya senegalensis root modulates beta-cell function and ameliorates diabetes-related biochemical parameters in a type 2 diabetes rat model. J Ethnopharmacol. 2014;154:832–8.
20. Alam MM, Meerza D, Naseem I. Protective effect of quercetin on hyperglycemia, oxidative stress and DNA damage in alloxan induced type 2 diabetic mice. Life Sci. 2014;109:8–14.
21. Shahid S, Bukhari I, Abbasi MH, Ahmad MK. Dose optimization of alloxan for diabetes in albino mice. Biologica. 2015;61:301–5.
22. Parra-Naranjo A, Delgado-Montemayor C, Fraga-López A, Castañeda-Corral G, Salazar-Aranda R, Acevedo-Fernández JJ, et al. Acute hypoglycemic and antidiabetic effect of teuhetenone a isolated from *Turnera diffusa*. Molecules. 2017;22:559.
23. Widyawati T, Yusoff AN, Asmawi ZM, Ahmad M. Antihyperglycemic effect of methanol extract of *Syzygium polyanthum* (Wight.) leaf in streptozotocin-induced diabetic rats. Nutrients. 2015;7(9):7764–80.
24. Hassan Z, Yam MF, Ahmad M, Yusof APM. Antidiabetic properties and mechanism of action of *Gynura procumbens* water extract in streptozotocin-induced diabetic rats. Molecules. 2010;15:9008–23.
25. Fowler MJ. Diabetes treatment, part 2: Oral agents for glycemic management. Clin Diabetes. 2007;25:131–4.
26. Groop LC, Pelkonen R, Koskimies S, Bottazzo GF, Doniach D. Secondary failure to treatment with oral antidiabetic agents in non-insulin-dependent diabetes. Diabetes Care. 1986;9:129–33.
27. Grover JK, Yadav S, Vats V. Medicinal plants of India with anti-diabetic potential. J Ethnopharmacol. 2002;81:81–100.
28. Andrikopoulos S, Blair AR, Deluca N, Fam BC, Proietto J. Evaluating the glucose tolerance test in mice. Am J Physiol Endocrinol Metab. 2008;295:E1323–32.
29. Lenzen S. The mechanisms of alloxan- and streptozotocin-induced diabetes. Diabetologia. 2008;51:216–26.
30. Hirsh AJ, Yao SY, Young JD, Cheeseman CI. Inhibition of glucose absorption in the rat jejunum: a novel action of alpha-D-glucosidase inhibitors. Gastroenterology. 1997;113:205–11.
31. Ma X, Iwanaka N, Masuda S, Karaike K, Egawa T, Hamada T, et al. *Morus alba* leaf extract stimulates 5′-AMP-activated protein kinase in isolated rat skeletal muscle. J Ethnopharmacol. 2009;122:54–9.

32. Kleinert M, Liao Y-H, Nelson JL, Bernard JR, Wang W, Ivy JL. An amino acid mixture enhances insulin-stimulated glucose uptake in isolated rat epitrochlearis muscle. J Appl Physiol. 2011;111:163–9.

33. O'Harte FP, Gray AM, Flatt PR. Gastric inhibitory polypeptide and effects of glycation on glucose transport and metabolism in isolated mouse abdominal muscle. J Endocrinol. 1998;156:237–43.

34. Boyd AC, Abdel-Wahab YH, McKillop AM, McNulty H, Barnett CR, O'Harte FP, et al. Impaired ability of glycated insulin to regulate plasma glucose and stimulate glucose transport and metabolism in mouse abdominal muscle. Biochim Biophys Acta. 2000;1523:128–34.

35. DeFronzo RA, Tripathy D. Skeletal muscle insulin resistance is the primary defect in type 2 diabetes. Diabetes Care. 2009;32:S157–63.

36. Olefsky JM. Treatment of insulin resistance with peroxisome proliferator-activated receptor γ agonists. J Clin Invest. 2000;106:467–72.

37. Ferré P. The biology of peroxisome proliferator-activated receptors. Diabetes. 2004;53:S43–50.

38. Herman MA, Kahn BB. Glucose transport and sensing in the maintenance of glucose homeostasis and metabolic harmony. J Clin Invest. 2006;116:1767–75.

39. Rose AJ, Richter EA. Skeletal muscle glucose uptake during exercise: how is it regulated? Physiology. 2005;20:260–70.

40. Satoh T. Molecular mechanisms for the regulation of insulin-stimulated glucose uptake by small guanosine triphosphatases in skeletal muscle and adipocytes. Int J Mol Sci. 2014;15:18677–92.

41. Röhling M, Herder C, Stemper T, Müssig K. Influence of acute and chronic exercise on glucose uptake. J Diabetes Res. 2016;2016:2868652.

42. Vlavcheski F, Naimi M, Murphy B, Hudlicky T, Tsiani E. Rosmarinic acid, a rosemary extract polyphenol, increases skeletal muscle cell glucose uptake and activates AMPK. Molecules. 2017;22:E1669.

43. Mohamed EAH, Siddiqui MJA, Ang LF, Sadikun A, Chan SH, Tan SC, et al. Potent α-glucosidase and α-amylase inhibitory activities of standardized 50% ethanolic extracts and sinensetin from Orthosiphon stamineus Benth as anti-diabetic mechanism. BMC Complement Altern Med. 2012;12:176.

44. Kedare SB, Singh RP. Genesis and development of DPPH method of antioxidant assay. J Food Sci Technol. 2011;48:412–22.

45. Huang D, Ou B, Prior RL. The chemistry behind antioxidant capacity assays. J Agric Food Chem. 2005;53:1841–56.

46. Abdallah HM, Salama MM, Abd-elrahman EH, El-Maraghy SA. Antidiabetic activity of phenolic compounds from pecan bark in streptozotocin-induced diabetic rats. Phytochem Lett. 2011;4:337–41.

47. Nazaruk J, Borzym-Kluczyk M. The role of triterpenes in the management of diabetes mellitus and its complications. Phytochem Rev. 2015;14:675–90.

48. Piluzza G, Bullitta S. Correlations between phenolic content and antioxidant properties in twenty-four plant species of traditional ethnoveterinary use in the Mediterranean area. Pharm Biol. 2011;49:240–7.

49. Luo XD, Basile MJ, Kennelly EJ. Polyphenolic antioxidants from the fruits of Chrysophyllum cainito L. (star apple). J Agric Food Chem. 2002;50:1379–82.

50. Shailajan S, Gurjar D. Pharmacognostic and phytochemical evaluation of Chrysophyllum cainito Linn. leaves. Int J Pharm Sci Rev Res. 2014;26:106–11.

51. Castro AJG, Frederico MJS, Cazarolli LH, Mendes CP, Bretanha LC, Schmidt ÉC, et al. The mechanism of action of ursolic acid as insulin secretagogue and insulinomimetic is mediated by cross-talk between calcium and kinases to regulate glucose balance. Biochim Biophys Acta. 2015;1850:51–61.

52. Gupta R, Sharma AK, Dobhal MP, Sharma MC, Gupta RS. Antidiabetic and antioxidant potential of beta-sitosterol in streptozotocin-induced experimental hyperglycemia. J Diabetes. 2011;3:29–37.

53. Gupta R, Sharma AK, Sharma MC, Dobhal MP, Gupta RS. Evaluation of antidiabetic and antioxidant potential of lupeol in experimental hyperglycaemia. Nat Prod Res. 2012;26:1125–9.

54. Oboh G, Ogunsuyi OB, Ogunbadejo MD, Adefegha SA. Influence of gallic acid on α-amylase and α-glucosidase inhibitory properties of acarbose. J Food Drug Anal. 2016;24:627–34.

Ipomoea batatas L. Lam. ameliorates acute and chronic inflammations by suppressing inflammatory mediators, a comprehensive exploration using in vitro and in vivo models

Muhammad Majid[1], Bakht Nasir[1], Syeda Saniya Zahra[1], Muhammad Rashid Khan[2], Bushra Mirza[2] and Ihsan-ul Haq[1*]

Abstract

Background: *Ipomoea batatas* L. Lam. is a functional food and belongs to family Convolvulaceae. It is used as an antiinflammatory, aphrodisiac, antiasthmatic, anticonvalescent, antitumor, antanemic and antidiabetic agent by local communities. This study has been planned to evaluate its antiinflammatory and antiarthritic potentials.

Methods: Dry powder of *I. batatas* tuber and roots were extracted with ethyl acetate (IPT-EA, IPR-EA) and methanol (IPT-M, IPR-M), respectively. These extracts were tested for total phenolic and flavonoid contents (TPC and TFC), HPLC finger printing, multidimensional in vitro and in vivo antioxidant potential and albumin denaturation inhibition. Carrageenan-induced paw edema, croton oil-induced ear and anal edema inhibition and Complete Freund's Adjuvant (CFA)-induced antiarthritic assays were executed at a dose of 300 mg/kg body weight on Sprague-Dawley rats. Serum levels of interleukins IL-1β and IL-6 and nitric oxide (NO) were assessed to measure the inhibition of inflammation.

Results: Maximal TPC (319.81 ± 14.20 µg GAE/mg dry extract) and TFC (208.77 ± 9.09 µg QE/mg DE) were estimated in IPR-EA extract. IPT-EA and IPR-EA yielded the maximum amounts of rutin (7.3 ± 1.12 and 4.5 ± 0.55), caffeic acid (1.60 ± 0.25 and 2.17 ± 0.26) and myricetin (2.7 ± 0.14 and 1.01 ± 0.08 µg/mg DE), respectively in HPLC-DAD analysis. All extracts showed dose dependent response in in vitro antioxidant assays. Best inhibition (76.92 ± 3.07%) of albumin denaturation was shown by IPT-EA in comparison to ibuprofen (79.48 ± 4.71%). IPR-EA exhibited highest edema inhibition in models of carrageenan-induced paw edema (79.11 ± 5.47%) and croton oil-induced ear and anal edema (72.01 ± 7.80% and 70.80 ± 4.94%, respectively). Significant inhibition of CFA-induced arthritic edema and arthritic score were observed by IPR-EA as compared to ibuprofen. Suppression of pro-inflammatory cytokines (IL-1β, IL-6) and NO levels was shown by IPR-EA and IPT-EA, respectively.

Conclusion: These results depict that richness of polyphenols and phytoconstituents in *I. batatas* ameliorates oxidative stress and inflammation of acute and chronic nature. Dose dependent antioxidant potential and inhibition of inflammatory edema, pro-inflammatory cytokines and hematological, biochemical and histological changes prove *I. batatas* therapeutic potential as an antiinflammatory and antiarthritic agent.

Keywords: Inflammation, Arthritis, Sweet potato, *Ipomoea*, CFA, Antioxidant, Interleukin

* Correspondence: ihsn99@yahoo.com
[1]Department of Pharmacy, Faculty of Biological Sciences, Quaid-i-Azam University, Islamabad 45320, Pakistan
Full list of author information is available at the end of the article

Background

Inflammation is considered to be an important causative agent of morbidity and mortality associated with a range of diseases. Inflammation involves several metabolic and cellular events coordinated by mediators like cytokines, interleukins (IL), prostaglandins (PGs) and thromboxanes. A number of inflammatory disorders such as rheumatoid arthritis (RA), several carcinomas, atherosclerosis and asthma have high prevalence worldwide [1]. Rheumatoid arthritis, a chronic inflammatory problem, is an auto-immune disorder responsible for series of erratic articular cartilage and subcondral bone damages [2]. It involves several cellular and metabolic events involving profuse amount of mediators like interleukins, cytokines, thromboxanes and prostaglandins [3]. Although, it is a protective effort of immune system of the organism to eradicate the invading pathogens and initiate the process of healing in stressed tissues [4]; however; unrestrained inflammation may lead to the beginning of several diseases like rheumatoid arthritis, atherosclerosis and vasomotor rhinorrhea [1]. Though several molecules like tumor necrosis factor (TNF), IL and PGs are the causative agents of RA pathology [5] but reactive oxygen species (ROS) are much notorious for stimulating inflammatory pathways via their harmful attitude towards macromolecules of the cells [6].

Reactive nitrogen species (RNS) and ROS are continuously produced as byproducts during the routine metabolic processes [7, 8]. According to the circumstances and situations, free radicals act as dual-edged sword either friend or foe. When friendly, they carry important jobs in neurotransmission, defense against microbes and cytotoxicity [9] but in excess, these lead to oxidative stress, which is the root cause of many chronic inflammatory disorders such as rheumatism, diabetes, cancer, aging and circulatory disorders [10]. ROS invades and damages endothelial cells with increase in the permeability of the microvasculature facilitating the migration of neutrophils to the foci of inflammation [11]. Extensive experimental investigations concerning assays of nitro-tyrosine residues in synovial fluids of RA patients or in vitro exposure of chondrocytes to peroxynitrite concluded that conversion of superoxide anions to NO leads to cartilage abrasion. Several endogenous detoxifying enzymes and metabolites provide first line of defense inside the living system to eliminate the deleterious effects of free radicals [12]. Catalase (CAT), peroxidase (POD), and superoxide dismutase (SOD) are the notable and significant detoxifying enzymes.

Diseases of cartilage abrasions such as rheumatoid and osteoarthritis (OA) involve unstable phenotype of differentiated chondrocytes, localize inflammation, progressive cartilage abrasion, aching and joints tenderness [13–15]. Assessment of cytokines, chemokines and NO [16–18] levels are helpful in finding degrees of arthritic progression. Most commonly practiced therapy for these inflammatory disorders are non-steroidal antiinflammatory drugs (NSAIDs), as they are good at reducing pain, redness, edema and fever. But these drugs are accompanied with numeral adverse effects of supreme severity in case of multi-dose treatment [19]. Hence, the use of natural substances including food plants with medicinal virtues is getting more attention for arthritis management.

Efficient food products are intended to introduce human dietary constituents that aid specific physiological functions in addition to being nutritive. Sweet potato (*Ipomoea batatas* L. Lam.), the 7th most important food crop in the world (FAO 1997) [20] and a member of family Convolvulaceae, is an imperative root vegetable with large size, high starch content and sweet taste [21]. It is used in folk medicine as aphrodisiac, antiinflammatory, astringent, demulcent, energizer, laxative, bactericidal and antifungal agent. It's also helpful in treating mouth and throat tumors, asthma, bug bites, burns, catarrh, diarrhea, fever, nausea, splenosis, stomach distress [22], anemia, hypertension, diabetes and prostatitis [23]. Several phytochemical studies of *I. batatas* have detected numerous potential compounds with profound medicinal worth like vitamins such as pantothenic acid (vitamin B5), pyridoxine (vitamin B6), and thiamin (vitamin B1), as well as niacin, riboflavin [21], β-carotene, iron, calcium, zinc, protein [24], polyphenols like anthocyanin and phenolic acids such as caffeic, monocafeoyl quinic, dicaffeoylquinic, and tricaffeoylquinic acids [25, 26]. The tubers are packed with many essential vitamins.

Functional food likeness, non-toxic attitude and antiinflammatory potential of *I. batatas* make it a strong candidate to be assessed as a natural remedy to prevent and control inflammatory diseases. Literature review demonstrates its antiinflammatory potential but the studies performed were not comprehensive and no antiarthritic study on any part of the plant has been conducted. Therefore, multi-mode validation of the potency in terms of antiinflammatory prospective was needed. Scientists have been using tubers and veins of *I. batatas* for the investigation of several biological and phytochemical inquiries. We, for the first time, have used *I. batatas* roots along with tuber to inquire its phytochemical and biological aptitude. A detailed in vitro and in vivo study was conducted to prove antirheumatoid arthritis abilities of roots and tubers of *I. batatas*.

Methods

Chemicals and reagents

Complete Freund's Adjuvant (CFA), carrageenan, ibuprofen, tween 80, ascorbic acid, 2,2- diphenyl-1-picrylhydrazyl (DPPH), thiobarbituric acid, ferric chloride, aluminum chloride, 2,2-azino-bis-(3-ethylbenzothiazoline-6-sulphonic acid) diammonium salt, potassium persulphate, trichloroacetic acid, phenazine methosulphate, and Folin–Ciocalteu reagent were purchased from Sigma (Chemicals Co. St. Louis, USA). Disodium hydrogen phosphate, sodium dihydrogen phosphate, hydrogen peroxide, sodium hydroxide, sodium carbonate, sodium nitrite, potassium ferricyanide, sulphuric acid, deoxyribose, ferrous chloride were purchased from Merck KGaA Darmstadt Germany. All other chemicals were obtained from Sigma (Chemicals Co. St. Louis, USA). All the chemicals were of analytical grade.

Preparation of extract

Plant was recognized by its local name and collected from the District Sargodha in January 2016. The plant sample was identified and authenticated by Prof. Dr. Rizwana Aleem Qureshi, Department of Plant Sciences, Faculty of Biological Sciences, Quaid-i-Azam University, Islamabad, Pakistan. It was then deposited (Accession No. PHM-501) at the Herbarium of Pakistan, Quaid-i-Azam University. Tubers and roots of I. batatas were washed with fresh water and air dried with no exposure to direct sunlight. Fully shade dried parts of the plant were first powdered followed by successive extraction with n-hexane, ethyl acetate, methanol and distilled water. These extracts were dried under vacuum in a rotary evaporator at 40 °C and evaluated for several bench top assays. On the bases of high phenolic and flavonoid contents and significant antioxidant activity ethyl acetate (IPT-EA) and methanol extracts (IPT-M) from tubers while ethyl acetate (IPR-EA) and methanol extracts (IPR-M) from roots were selected for further in vitro and in vivo experiments.

Phytochemical and antioxidant profiling
Reckoning the total phenolic content (TPC)

The total phenolic contents were estimated according to slightly modified procedure as described previously using Folin–Ciocalteu reagent [27]. An aliquot of 20 µl from 4 mg/ml DMSO stock solution of each test sample was transferred in respective well of 96-well plate followed by addition of 90 µl of Folin–Ciocalteu reagent. The plate was incubated for 5 min after which 90 µl of sodium carbonate was added to the reaction mixture. Gallic acid was used as standard and absorbance of each reaction mixture was taken at 630 nm using microplate reader (Biotech USA, microplate reader Elx 800) in triplicate. Gallic acid (6.25–50 µg/ml) was used as a positive control and the results are expressed as µg gallic acid equivalent per mg dry extract (µg GAE/mg DE).

Estimation of total flavonoid content (TFC)

For total flavonoid content determination, aluminum chloride colorimetric method was employed with slight modifications according to system suitability [28]. The crude extracts (20 µl of 4.0 mg/ml in DMSO) were transferred to each well of 96-well plate. Subsequently, 10 µl of each 10% aluminum chloride and 1.0 M potassium acetate

was added followed by the addition of 160 µl of distilled water. The resulting mixture was kept at room temperature for 30 min. Then absorbance of the plate was measured at 415 nm using microplate reader. The calibration curve was drawn by using quercetin as standard at final concentrations of 0, 2.5, 5, 10, 20, 40 µg/ml. The resultant flavonoid contents were calculated as quercetin equivalent per mg dry extract (µg QE/mg DE).

High performance liquid chromatography (HPLC) exploration

For the detection and quantification of polyphenols, HPLC-DAD analysis was conducted following the methodology of Sahreen et al. [29] with little modifications. HPLC analysis of IPT-EA, IPT-M, IPR-EA and IPR-M was carried out by using HPLC-DAD (Agilent Germany) equipment using Zorbax RX-C8 (4.6 × 250 mm, 5 µm particle size, Agilent, USA). Mobile phase consisted of eluent A, (acetonitrile:methanol:water:acetic acid/ 5:10:85:1) and eluent B (acetonitrile:methanol:acetic acid/ 40:60:1). Following gradient (A:B) was utilized: 0–20 min (0 to 50% B), 20–25 min (50 to 100% B), and isocratic 100% B (25–40 min) at flow rate of 1 ml/min. The injection volume of the sample was 20 µl. Before the injection, samples were filtered through 0.45 µm membrane filter. Among the standards, rutin was analyzed at 257 nm, gallic acid and catechin at 279 nm, caffeic acid and apigenin at 325 nm while quercetin, myricetin and kaempferol were analyzed at 368 nm. Each time the column was reconditioned for 10 min before the next analysis. All samples were assayed in triplicates. Quantification was carried out by the integration of the peak using the external standard method. All chromatographic operations were carried out at an ambient temperature.

Determination of in vitro antioxidant activity

The different concentrations of sample ranging from 0 to 500 µg/ml were used in all in vitro antioxidant tests. The stock solution of the sample was prepared by mixing 4 mg in 1 ml of DMSO and dilutions were made for each in vitro antioxidant assay. Standard compounds were used for the comparisons of antioxidant potential of the sample.

The antioxidant potential of IPT-EA, IPR-EA, IPT-M and IPR-M extracts against DPPH, nitric oxide, hydroxyl radical and iron chelation capacity was determined following the previous protocols [29]. The scavenging activity was calculated using the following equation:

$$\% \text{scavenging activity} = 1 - (\text{OD of sample})/(\text{OD of control}) \times 100$$

Reducing power (TRP) and total antioxidant capacity (TAC) was determined by the methodology illustrated by

Phull et al. [30]. The results were expressed as μg QE/mg DE.

Animal ethical statement

The experiment was conducted by strictly following the guidelines approved by the ethical committee of Quaid-i-Azam University, Islamabad, Pakistan (Letter No. QAU-PHM-017/2016 for the animal care and Letter No. QAU-PHM-023/2016 dated 24/10/2016 for experiments). Blood sampling from healthy volunteers was also approved by Institutional Review board of Quaid-i-Azam University (Letter No. IRB-QAU-116 dated 4/11/2016). The study followed ethical guidelines of minimal distress, discomfort and pain to the subject animals ensuring that experiments provided new knowledge or lead for human/animals wellbeing. Appropriate sedation, analgesia and anesthesia techniques were used where necessary as well as informed consent was obtained from human subject. Euthanasia was done by cervical dislocation under chloroform anesthesia.

Experimental animals

Male Sprague-Dawley rats having weight of ~ 150–200 g were used for this study and were kept in cages (made up of aluminum) under controlled conditions (12 h light/dark cycle, 25 ± 1 °C temperature). All the animals were supplied with standard feed along with water ad libitum prior to use in experiments. Animals were divided into seven groups and each group comprised of 6 male Sprague-Dawley rats for each treatment. Specified doses of *I. batatas*, positive and negative controls were orally administered to each group as follows;

Group-I: IPT- EA (300 mg/Kg)
Group-II: IPT-M (300 mg/Kg)
Group-III: IPR- EA (300 mg/Kg)
Group-IV: IPR-M (300 mg/Kg)
Group-V: Positive (ibuprofen 10 mg/Kg)
Group-VI: Disease control
Group-VII: Normal

Toxicity assessment
Isolation and monolayer culture of rabbit articular chondrocytes

Three weeks old local strain of rabbits of either sex at Primate Facility of Faculty of Biological Sciences, Quaid-i-Azam University, Islamabad were sacrificed and articular cartilage pieces were collected. Thereafter, chondrocytes were isolated from cartilage slices using collagenase type II (381 units/ml) for 12 h at 37 °C in CO_2 incubator. The cells were cultured in DMEM medium supplemented with 10% bovine calf serum, streptomycin (50 μg/ml), and penicillin (50 unit/ml). The chondrocytes were seeded at density of 1×10^4 cells per well in 96-well plate for toxicity and viability assay. Culture media was replaced every 2 days and cells at 75% confluence were used for further study [30].

Isolation of lymphocytes from blood

Lymphocytes were isolated from human blood using previously described protocol with some modifications [31, 32]. A volume of 3 ml of blood was obtained from a healthy donor by venipuncture and diluted (1,1) with PBS. It was layered over 2 ml Histopaque-1077 and centrifuged at 800 X g for 20 min. The buffy coat was aspirated into 5 ml of PBS and centrifuged at 350 rpm for 4 min to pellet the lymphocytes. The pellet was suspended in 1 ml of RPMI-1640 and cell density was adjusted to get 1×10^5 cells/ml.

In vitro toxicity assessment on rabbit articular chondrocytes

The methylthiazole tetrazolium (MTT) assay and microscopic observation were performed to evaluate the cytotoxic effects of *I. batatas* on rabbit articular chondrocytes following previously described protocol [13]. Initially, 1×10^4 chondrocytes were seeded in each well (three wells for each dose) and incubated in a CO_2 incubator overnight for attachment. Thereafter, cells were exposed to various concentrations (0 to 1000 μg/ml) of test sample for 24 h. Then, 10 μl of reagent 1 (methyl tetrazolium, 1%) was added in each well and kept in a CO_2 incubator for 4 h until purple formazan crystals developed. Followed by the addition of 100 μl of reagent 2 (solubilization buffer, 10% SDS with 0.01 N HCl and DMSO) the plate was incubated in a CO_2 incubator for 12 h after which absorbance was measured at 590 nm using a Versa-Max microplate reader (Molecular Devices Co., Sunnyvale, CA, USA). The experiment was performed in triplicate.

In vitro toxicity assessment on blood lymphocytes

To assess genotoxicity, comet assay was performed with little modifications in the previously described protocol [33]. Briefly, 20 μl of samples (100 μg/ml) or ethyl methane sulfonate (20 μg/ml) or 1% DMSO in PBS and 180 μl of lymphocyte suspension were incubated in 96-well plate at 37 °C for 3 h in humidified 5% carbon dioxide incubator (Panasonic, Japan MCO-18 AC-PE). After 3 h, the cells were centrifuged to pellet, washed with PBS and 0.5% LMA at 37 °C was added in cells. Then 75 μl of this suspension containing approximately 1000 cells was plated on frozen slides pre-coated with 1% NMA and a cover slip was gently placed over it. The slide was placed on icepacks for about 8–10 min. Cover slip was detached and again LMA was added and placed on ice packs for solidification. After three coatings with low melting point agarose, electrophoresis was performed and 1% ethidium bromide was used to stain. The slides were visualized under fluorescent microscope and CASP 1.2.3.b image analysis software was used to evaluate the extent of DNA damage. In each sample, 50–100 cells were analyzed for comet length, head length, tail length, tail moment, DNA content in head and tail of lymphocytes.

In vivo acute toxicity assessment in rats

For the acute toxicity assay, rats were randomly divided into control and test groups ($n = 6$). The test groups were treated with increasing doses of 300, 500, 1000, 2000, and 4000 mg/kg of test samples. The toxic symptoms, mortality rates and behavioral pattern such as lethargy, salivation, lacrimation, nasal secretions, balance, mood and aggression, piloerection, frequency of urination and defecation, sleep, symptomatic observation for any injury and pain were observed on daily basis for two weeks after intragastric administration of the sample. Control group was administered with saline (10 ml/kg of animals) and toxicity assessment was executed by following the Organization for Economic Cooperation and Development (OECD) guidelines 425.

Antiinflammatory and antiarthritic evaluation
In vitro antiinflammatory activity

The antiinflammatory efficacy was gauged by inhibition of albumin denaturation procedure with minor amendments in methodology of Leelaprakash et al. [34]. The test extracts were incubated with 1% aqueous solution of bovine albumin fraction at 37 °C for 20 min having pH 7.4. After incubation, samples were heated to to 51 °C for 20 min, cooled and turbidity was measured at 660 nm. Experiment was repeated thrice and the % inhibition of protein denaturation was calculated as follows:

$$\text{Percentage inhibition} = (\text{Abs Control} - \text{Abs Sample}) \times 100/\text{Abs control}$$

Test sample and standard drug for in vivo analysis

Solutions of samples were prepared by dissolving in 10% DMSO at dose of 300 mg/kg body weight (BW) per rat and standard drug ibuprofen was prepared at dose of 10 mg/kg BW. Test sample and positive control were orally administered. Four extracts of *I. batatas* (IPT-EA, IPT-M, IPR-EA and IPR-M) were used in the present study.

Carrageenan-induced inflammation impediment in rats

The antiinflammatory competence of *I. batatas* was appraised with the help of carrageenan-induced rat paw edema model [10]. Among seven groups of experimental animals (Sprague-Dawley rats) as described above, Group I-IV were test groups, i.e., IPT-EA, IPT-M, IPR-EA and IPR-M extracts at the dose of 300 mg/kg BW, Group V was positive control ibuprofen at the dose of 10 mg/kg BW, Group VI was carrageenan control and Group VII was saline control, which received 0.1 ml normal saline.

The drugs were administered an hour before injection of 150 µl of carrageenan suspension (0.9% *w/v* in saline) in left hind paw of each rat for the duration of one day. The paw volume was measured at different time periods (1, 3, 6, 12, 24 h) by using Plethysmometer (Ugo Basile 7140, Italy). Results were calculated as.

$$\text{Edema volume} = \text{PVt–PVc}$$

where PVt is paw volume (ml) at specific time after carrageenan administration while PVc is paw volume (ml) before carrageenan administration.

$$\text{Percent inhibition} = \text{EVc–EVt/EVc} \times 100$$

where EVc is edema volume of control group. EVt is edema volume of treated group.

Croton oil-induced ear edema constraint

Method described by Reanmongkol et al. was used with minor modifications [35]. Cutaneous inflammation was induced by applying 100 µl of acetone solution containing the irritant (5% croton oil) to the inner surface of the right ear of the mice. Acetone was applied to the left ear as vehicle. IPT-EA, IPT-M, IPR-EA and IPR-M (5.0 mg/ear each) were applied topically to the right ear 1 h before application of croton oil. Ibuprofen (1 mg/ear) served as a reference antiinflammatory drug. A plug (7-mm diameter) was removed from both the treated and untreated ears after sacrificing the rats four hours later. The % inhibition of edema was calculated as the difference of weight in two plugs.

Croton oil-induced anus edema inhibition

Croton oil-induced edematous response of anus was evaluated by modifying the methodology of Reanmongkol et al. [35]. A cotton swab soaked with the inducer (0.2 ml of 6% croton oil in diethyl ether) was introduced into the anus of rats for 10 s. One hour later, vehicle control, IPT-EA, IPT-M, IPR-EA and IPR-M (300 mg/kg each), and ibuprofen (10 mg/kg) were orally given OD for 3 days to respective groups. On the fourth day, size of each anaesthetized rat's anus (mm) was scaled with the help of a vernier caliper.

Complete Freund's adjuvant-induced arthritis in rats

Arthritic rat model was prepared by using Complete Freund's adjuvant (heated-killed Mycobacterium tuberculosis in 1 ml of liquid paraffin at 10 mg/kg). Briefly, 200 µl of CFA emulsion was injected subcutaneously at the base of the tail of rat under anesthesia [36]. Study plan was sub-divided in following two schemes.

Treatment mode

In this study mode, arthritis was induced till 11–13 days and IPT-EA, IPT-M, IPR-EA, IPR-M (300 mg/kg each) and ibuprofen (10 mg/kg) were given through oral route on alternate days to respective groups. Reversal of maximum arthritic symptoms was assessed.

Preventive mode

In this study mode, single dose CFA was injected and IPT-EA, IPT-M, IPR-EA, IPR-M (300 mg/kg each) and ibuprofen (10 mg/kg) were given concurrently through oral route on alternate days and evaluation of prevention from arthritis was done in test groups with comparison to the controls.

Adjuvant-induced arthritic scoring

Experimental animals were investigated on a daily basis for the signs of arthritic severity through well-established scoring system [36]. Severity of the inflammation in paws was graded on the basis of swelling, induration and erythema using 5-point scale scoring system. In this scale, no sign of diseases (non-toxic), signs involving the wrist/ankle, signs involving the ankle plus tarsal of the hind paw and/or wrist plus carpals of the fore paw, signs extending to the metatarsals or metacarpals and severe disease involving the entire hind or fore paw were assigned as 0 to 4 scores [37]. Paw volume was measured on alternate days using Plethysmometer (Ugo Basile 7140, Italy). Paw edema was monitored from the total paw volumes of 4 paws.

Histological investigation

On the last day (25th day) of experiment, the arthritic rats were sacrificed. The dissected tissue of arthritic joint was fixed by buffered formaldehyde (10%, pH 7.4) at room temperature for 12 h. The water and infiltrated wax of fixed tissue was removed by repeated washing with ethanol. The tissue was cut into small pieces of 5 μm thickness with rotary microtome. The sections were stained with Eosin and Haematoxylin. Histological investigation was carried out under Nikon Microscope (Eclipse 80i, Japan).

Determination of body weight and relative organ weight of rats

Rats and their major organs such as liver, kidney, spleen and thymus were weighed in grams and index of the organ or relative weight was calculated as

$$ROW = AOW/(BW)^* 100$$

ROW = relative organ weight, AOW = absolute organ weight (g), BW = body weight on final day (g).

Collection of blood sample and biochemical analysis

On the last day, experimental rats were anaesthetized by chloroform inhalation and euthanized by cervical dislocation. The blood samples were collected under anesthesia via the abdominal aorta in specific tubes (BD vacutainer) for hematological, biochemical and serological investigations. Serum was separated by centrifuging blood samples at 6000 rpm for 15 min at 4 °C that was either analyzed or stored at – 20 °C. Afterwards, the animals were dissected via a ventral longitudinal abdominal incision. Major organs, i.e., liver, spleen, thymus, and kidney were identified and dissected out for relative organ weight analysis.

Hematological studies

The white blood cells (WBCs), red blood cells (RBC) and platelets were counted by using neubauer hemocytometer (Feinoptik, Germany). The hemoglobin (Hb) content was estimated by Sahli's hemoglobin meter. Erythrocyte sedimentation rate was measured through the modified Westergren method [38].

Determination of biochemical parameters

Different parameters such as urea, creatinine, alkaline phosphatase (ALP), alanine transaminase (ALT), aspartate transaminase (AST) and testosterone were determined from the sera of experimental rats using standard AMP diagnostic kits (Stattogger Strasse 31b 8045 Graz, Austria). The protein concentration was determined by the Bradford method [39].

Determination of endogenous antioxidant enzymes of rats

Activities of serum catalase (CAT) were evaluated by monitoring the rate of H_2O_2 hydrolysis at 240 nm [40]. The superoxide dismutase (SOD) activity in serum was measured by quercetin autoxidation inhibition method [41]. Peroxidases (POD) were determined by following the slightly modified method as described previously [40].

Measurement of cytokines and NO levels in serum

The levels of cytokines (IL-1β and IL-6) from serum were measured by enzyme-linked immunosorbent assay (ELISA), according to the manufacturer's protocol (BD Biosciences, USA) while NO levels were determined by mixing serum (30 μl) with 0.3 M NaOH and 5% ZnSO4. After centrifugation for 15–20 min at 6400×g, an aliquot of 10 μl of the supernatant was mixed with 200 μl of Griess reagent in 96-well plate. The absorbance was recorded at 540 nm. Sodium nitrite curve was used to quantify nitrite amount in serum [42].

Statistical analysis

Data obtained in this study was presented as mean ± SD. One way analysis of variance was performed to determine the variability among groups by Statistix 8.1. GraphPad Prim 5 was used to determine the correlation of IC_{50} values of antioxidant assays with TPC and TFC by Pearson's correlation coefficient. Significant differences among groups were calculated by Tukey's multiple comparison and Kruskal-Wallis tests. Statistical significance was set at $p < 0.05$, $p < 0.01$ and $p < 0.001$.

Results

Phytochemical investigation

Total phenolic and flavonoid contents

Considering the standard regression lines for gallic acid ($y = 0.0083x + 0.0182$; $R^2 = 0.9766$) and quercetin ($y = 0.0088x + 0.0151$; $R^2 = 0.9922$), the equivalents of TPC and TFC were calculated (Table 1). IPR-EA showed maximum quantity of TPC (319.81 ± 14.20 µg GAE/mg DE) followed by IPT-EA (286.68 ± 4.90 µg GAE/mg DE), IPR-M (262.59 ± 5.70 µg GAE/mg DE) and IPT-M (229.45 ± 5.01 µg GAE/mg DE). Flavonoids were found to be rich in IPR-EA (208.77 ± 9.09 µg QE/mg DE) followed by IPT-EA (188.89 ± 2.40 µg QE/mg DE), IPR-M (177.81 ± 2.50 µg QE/mg DE) and IPT-M (146.27 ± 2.80 µg QE/mg DE).

HPLC-DAD quantification

Reverse phase HPLC based qualitative and quantitative sketching of *I. batatas* phenolics was done by comparing the retention time and UV spectra of reference compounds with those of the test sample, shown in Fig. 1. Rutin, gallic acid, catechin, caffeic acid, apigenin, myricetin, quercetin and kaempferol were identified and quantified in different extracts of IPT-EA, IPT-M, IPR-EA and IPR-M. Maximum amount of rutin was detected in IPT-EA (7.3 ± 1.12 µg/mg dry extract) while minimum quantity of apigenin (0.13 ± 0.020 µg/mg dry extract) was quantified in IPR-EA. The results are summarized in Table 2.

In vitro antioxidant activities

I. batatas demonstrated dose dependent antioxidant activity in various in vitro antioxidant assays, including scavenging of DPPH, nitric oxide and hydroxyl (•OH) radicals as well as iron chelating competency. It also exhibited significant total reducing potential and total antioxidant

capacity. *I. batatas* displayed antioxidant capacity in different assays in the subsequent order; nitric oxide scavenging > iron chelating ability > DPPH free radical scavenging > hydroxyl radical (•OH) scavenging (Additional file 1: Figure S1b). Furthermore, the total antioxidant capacity was found to be greater than its total reducing power potential as shown in Table 1. All the antioxidant assays were significantly correlated to TPC and TFC (Table 3).

In vitro and in vivo toxicity investigation

In vitro results showed non-toxic nature of *I. batatas* on rabbit articular chondrocytes as evaluated by microscopic observations and MTT viability assay at various doses (0–1000 µg/ml) and the results are presented in Fig. 2 and Additional file 2: Figure S2b. Non-toxic nature of the *I. batatas* extracts was also confirmed by neutrophil genotoxicity assessment via comet assay as shown in Fig. 3 and Table 4. Further, results of acute toxicity showed that *I. batatas* did not exhibit any significant variation in behavioral pattern and signs of toxicity or death during the observation period of 2 weeks. The investigation was performed at the doses of 300–4000 mg/kg of rats. The IPT-EA, IPT-M, IPR-EA and IPR-M extracts were found safe up to the highest dose of 4000 mg/kg. So, *I. batatas* extracts were rendered non-toxic and safe for additional pharmacological testing within described range.

In vitro antiinflammatory proficiency

For the evaluation of in vitro antiinflammatory potential of *I. batatas* extracts, inhibition of heat induced albumin denaturation assay was conducted. Maximum inhibition was exhibited by IPT-EA ($76.92 \pm 3.07\%$) followed by IPR-EA ($71.79 \pm 4.87\%$), IPR-M ($66.66 \pm 3.61\%$) and IPT-M ($66.66 \pm 2.76\%$) in comparison to the standard, ibuprofen ($79.48 \pm 4.71\%$) at the concentration of 500 µg/ml. The results are summarized in Fig. 4.

Effect on carrageenan-induced inflammation in rats

Carrageenan-induced rat paw edema model (inflammatory model) was used to assess the antiinflammatory activity of the sample. The results showed that *I. batatas* have significant antiinflammatory activity compared to the

Table 1 Total phenolic content, total flavonoid content, total antioxidant capacity and total reducing power of *I. batatas* extracts

Samples	TPC(µg GAE/mg DE)	TFC(µg QE/mg DE)	TAC(µg QE/mg DE)	TRP(µg QE/mg DE)
IPT-EA	286.68 ± 4.90^b	188.89 ± 2.40^b	442.48 ± 4.85^b	332.48 ± 4.06^b
IPT-M	229.45 ± 5.01^d	146.27 ± 2.80^d	361.65 ± 3.35^d	256.09 ± 4.56^d
IPR-EA	319.81 ± 14.20^a	208.77 ± 9.09^a	485.71 ± 4.26^a	370.67 ± 5.28^a
IPR-M	262.59 ± 5.70^c	177.81 ± 2.50^c	416.15 ± 5.95^c	304.71 ± 4.42^c

Data values shown represent mean ± SD ($n = 3$). Means with different superscript (a-d) letters in the column sare significantly ($p < 0.05$) different from one another
TPC total phenolic content, *TFC* total flavonoid content, *TAC* total antioxidant capacity, *TRP* total reducing power, *GAE* gallic acid equivalent, *QE* quercetin equivalent, *DE* dry extract

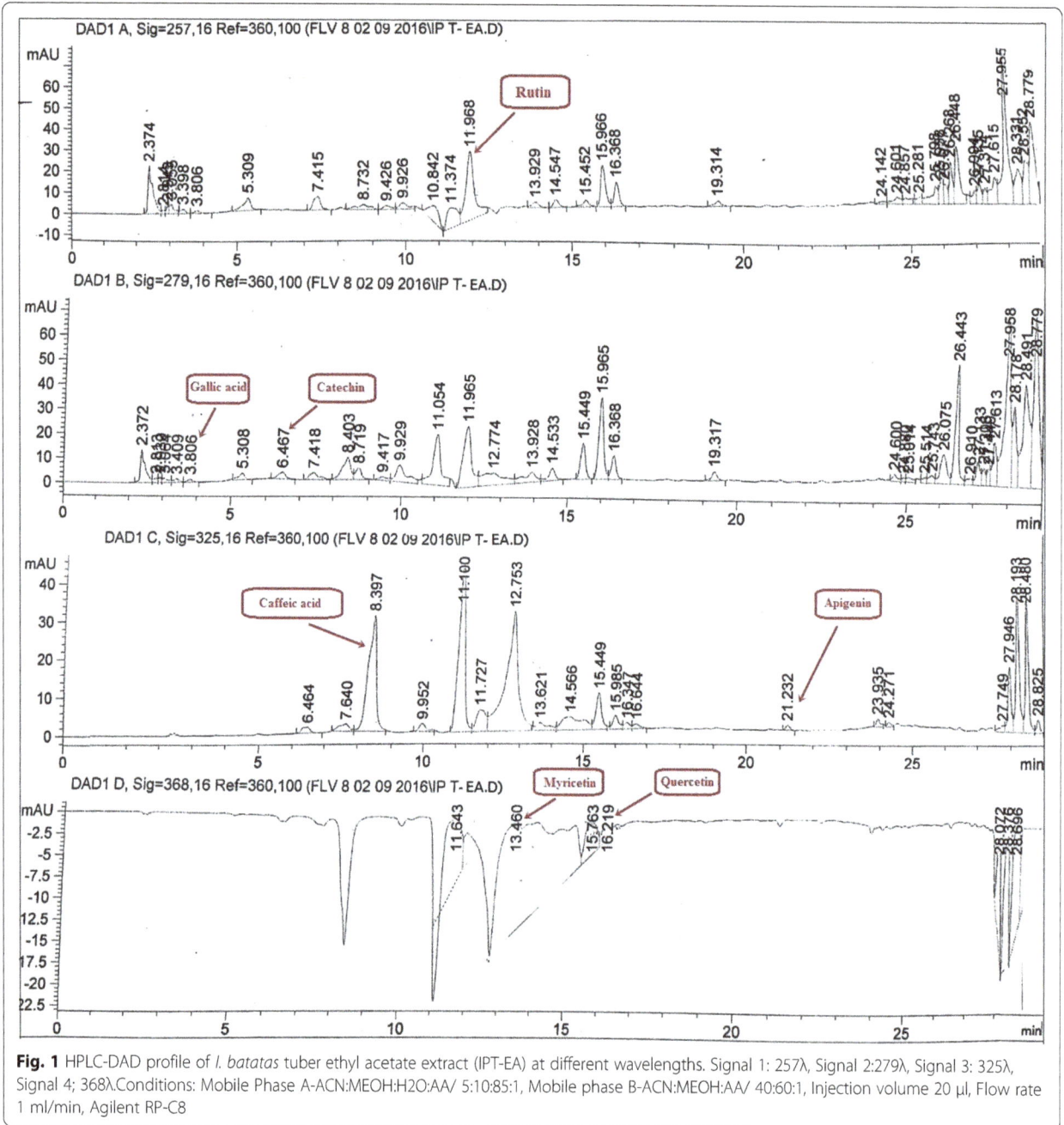

Fig. 1 HPLC-DAD profile of *I. batatas* tuber ethyl acetate extract (IPT-EA) at different wavelengths. Signal 1: 257λ, Signal 2:279λ, Signal 3: 325λ, Signal 4; 368λ.Conditions: Mobile Phase A-ACN:MEOH:H2O:AA/ 5:10:85:1, Mobile phase B-ACN:MEOH:AA/ 40:60:1, Injection volume 20 µl, Flow rate 1 ml/min, Agilent RP-C8

control model. IPR-EA showed maximum inhibition of inflammation ($79.11 \pm 5.47\%$) at 6 h. It was followed by IPT-EA ($74.20 \pm 5.14\%$), IPR-M ($68.67 \pm 5.32\%$) and IPT-M ($63.02 \pm 4.21\%$) in comparison to ibuprofen ($85.25 \pm 6.98\%$). Experimental results are presented in Table 5.

Croton oil-induced inflammation inhibition

Croton oil-induced ear edema and anal edema model (inflammatory model) were used to further assess the anti-inflammatory activity of the *I. batatas*. The results showed that *I. batatas* extracts have significant antiinflammatory activity compared to the control model. IPR-EA showed maximum inhibition of ear inflammation ($72.01 \pm 7.80\%$) followed by IPT-EA ($62.94 \pm 4.12\%$), IPR-M ($60.03 \pm 4.22\%$) and IPT-M ($52.58 \pm 3.45\%$) in comparison to ibuprofen ($80.58 \pm 5.03\%$). Moreover, IPR-EA showed maximal inhibition of anal inflammation ($70.80 \pm 4.94\%$) followed by IPT-EA ($63.04 \pm 4.17\%$), IPR-M ($54.53 \pm 3.80\%$) and IPT-M ($51.75 \pm 3.79\%$) in comparison to ibuprofen ($82.50 \pm 6.21\%$). Experimental results are presented in Table 6.

Table 2 Correlation of IC_{50} values of different antioxidant activities of *I. batatas* with total phenolic and total flavonoid contents

Antioxidant Activity	Correlation R^2	
	TFC	TPC
DPPH radical scavenging activity	0.9382^*	0.9732^*
Nitric Oxide radical scavenging Activity	0.90455^*	0.9754^*
Hydroxyl radical scavenging activity	0.8487^{ns}	0.9654^*
Iron chelating assay	0.8139^{ns}	0.7012^{ns}
Phosphomolybdenum assay (TAC)	0.9837^{**}	0.9975^{**}
Reducing power assay (TRP)	0.9805^{**}	0.9995^{***}

Column with different superscripts are significantly correlated where $^* = p < 0.05$, $^{**} = p < 0.01$, $^{***} = p < 0.001$ and $^{ns} = p > 0.05$ (non-significant), total flavonoid content (TFC), total phenolic content (TPC)

In vivo antiarthritic activity on CFA-induced arthritic rats

Effect on paw volume in treatment mode

Antiarthritic efficacy of *I. batatas* was evaluated by measuring the paw volume. Swelling of paw is the most critical contributing factor in the evaluation of inflammation severity and also shows the curative efficacy of the antiarthritic drugs. Treatment with IPT-EA, IPT-M, IPR-EA and IPR-M extracts (300 mg/kg) and ibuprofen (10 mg/kg) have exhibited significant reduction in paw edema from the 15th to 25th day ($p < 0.05$) as compared to arthritic control group (Fig. 5a).

Effect on paw volume in preventive mode

After injecting CFA to induce arthritis, rat groups were given IPT-EA, IPT-M, IPR-EA and IPR-M extracts (300 mg/kg) and ibuprofen (10 mg/kg) straightaway from day 1st and the prevention of arthritis has been assessed by measuring the hind paw volume. *I. batatas* and -ibuprofen exhibited maximal prevention from arthritic inflammation of paw (Fig. 5b). Arthritic scoring was also done according to the said procedure and maximum recovery from disease was observed in ibuprofen, which lowered the swelling from 17th day of dosing and onward followed by IPR-EA, IPT-EA, IPR-M and IPT-M (Fig. 5c).

Effect on arthritis-induced physical changes

In the current study, we have studied the in vivo efficacy of *I. batatas* on CFA-induced arthritic physical changes. At the final day of experiment, arthritic rats (-5.00 ± 1.28 g, $p < 0.05$) were found to have significantly lower body weight change compared to the normal rats (55.5 ± 3.7 g) as presented in the Fig. 6a. *I. batatas* treated rats exhibited an increase in the body weight as IPR-EA (31.5 ± 2.06 g) followed by IPT-EA (29.67 ± 1.98 g), IPR-M (27.51 ± 2.7 g) and IPT-M (25.01 ± 2.7 g) while ibuprofen treated rats showed an increase in body weight of 40.66 ± 2.7 g (Fig. 6a). Furthermore, relative organ weights were measured, which are presented as an index of the organ. As arthritis affects the key organs of an organism; therefore, in the present study arthritic-induced effects on major organs such as liver, kidney, thymus and spleen were also determined. After the completion of treatment, arthritic rats were found to have a significantly higher liver index, a decreased thymus and spleen index while the effect on the kidney was statistically insignificant compared to the normal rats as shown in the Fig. 6b. Administration of IPR-EA restored the liver (12.96%), thymus (26.20%) and spleen (17.54%) followed by IPT-M (8.43, 18.19 and 11.58%, respectively), IPT-EA (9.25, 21.39 and 16.88%, respectively) and IPR-M (5.34, 13.91 and 9.62%, respectively) at the dose of 300 mg/kg compared to the arthritic control. On the other hand, ibuprofen exposed animals showed 10.3, 17.7 and 21.68% recovery in same organs, respectively.

Effect on histology of normal and inflamed joint

The histological evaluation revealed that arthritic rats have severe edema, inflammatory cells infiltration and

Table 3 HPLC-DAD analysis of *I. batatas* extracts

Flavonoid/Phenolics	Signal wavelength	Quantity (µg/mg dry extract)			
		IPT-EA	IPT-M	IPR-EA	IPR-M
Rutin	257	7.3 ± 1.12^c	0.75 ± 0.08^a	4.5 ± 0.55^c	3.7 ± 0.13^c
Gallic acid	279	0.24 ± 0.080	nd	nd	Nd
Catechin	279	0.74 ± 0.04^a	nd	nd	0.87 ± 0.09^a
Caffeic acid	325	1.60 ± 0.25^a	0.52 ± 0.07^a	2.17 ± 0.26^b	0.78 ± 0.11^a
Apigenin	325	0.21 ± 0.040	0.18 ± 0.04	0.13 ± 0.020	0.31 ± 0.05
Myricetin	368	2.7 ± 0.14^b	nd	$01.01 \pm .08^a$	0.26 ± 0.03
Quercetin	368	0.45 ± 0.05	nd	1.39 ± 0.12^a	0.29 ± 0.06
Kaempferol	368	nd	nd	0.31 ± 0.040	Nd

Each value is presented as mean $\pm$ SD ($n = 3$)

IPT-EA I. batatas tuber-ethyl acetate extracts, *IPT-M I. batatas* tuber-methanol extract, *IPR-EA I. batatas* root-ethyl acetate extract, *IPR-M I. batatas* root-methanol extract

[a, b, c] represents the significance of flavonoid/phenolics quantified and [nd] stands for not detected

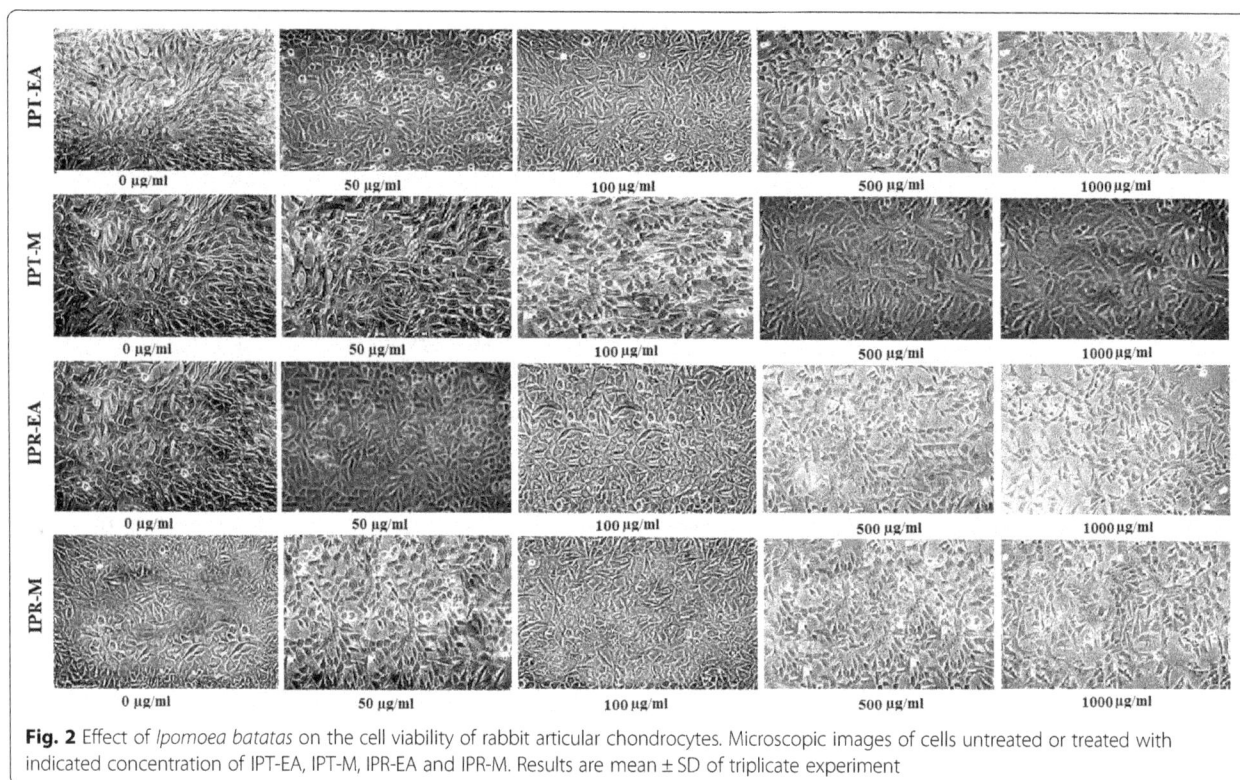

Fig. 2 Effect of *Ipomoea batatas* on the cell viability of rabbit articular chondrocytes. Microscopic images of cells untreated or treated with indicated concentration of IPT-EA, IPT-M, IPR-EA and IPR-M. Results are mean ± SD of triplicate experiment

abnormal joint architecture with increased erosion, cartilage destruction and decreased joint space. However, IPR-EA, IPT-M, IPR-EA, IPR-M extracts and standard drug treated groups exhibited protective effects on the altered histology and joint architecture (Fig. 7).

Arthritis-induced hematological variations

The results of the arthritis-induced hematological variations are presented in Table 7. It was observed from the results that arthritis progression altered the hematological parameters such as decrease in hemoglobin RBCs, platelets, whereas augmented levels of ESR and WBCs in arthritic animals. Administration of the *I. batatas* extracts significantly restored these altered hematological parameters as shown in the Table 7.

Enzymatic and biochemical regulation

Results showed that *I. batatas* extracts were effective in restoring the stress induced altered enzyme levels and biochemical parameters such as ALT, AST, ALP, urea, creatinine, albumin, and decreased levels of testosterone, bilirubin in arthritic rats. Administration of the *I. batatas* extracts significantly recovered the biochemical and enzymatic profile and detailed results are presented in Table 8.

Effect on antioxidant enzymes

Arthritic condition causes the induction of oxidative stress and endogenous antioxidant enzymes are critical

system to counteract such oxidative damages. A significant reduction in expression of antioxidant enzymes such as CAT, POD, and SOD was observed in the arthritic group by 57.02, 51.88 and 47.01%, respectively in comparison to normal control. Compared to arthritic group, ibuprofen treated animals established a reduction in expression of 10.17, 8.74 and 7.49%, respectively. In case of *I. batatas*, IPR-EA altered the levels of CAT, POD and SOD by 12.11, 14.43 and 10.86%, respectively while IPT-M altered maximally by 16.32, 18.11 and 16.85%, respectively. Results are presented in the Fig. 8.

Effect on interleukins and NO levels

Levels of interleukins and NO are supposed to increase in arthritic condition, as these macromolecules have been shown to modulate extracellular matrix turnover, accelerate the degradation of cartilage and induce chondrocyte apoptosis in the development of OA. Highest levels of IL-1β (7.23 ± 0.43 pg/ml), IL-6 (27.16 ± 1.22 pg/ml) and NO (62.56 ± 3.23 μM/ml) were shown by arthritic control in comparison to IPR-EA (4.28 ± 0.55 pg/ml, 21.28 ± 1.56 pg/ml and 38.73 ± 2.11 μM/ml) and ibuprofen (4.11 ± 0.44 pg/ml, 20.72 ± 1.14 pg/ml and 36.22 ± 1.78 μM/ml). Results are presented in the Fig. 8.

Discussion

Immune system is both a blessing as well as a curse in certain situations. It may bring about certain incurable

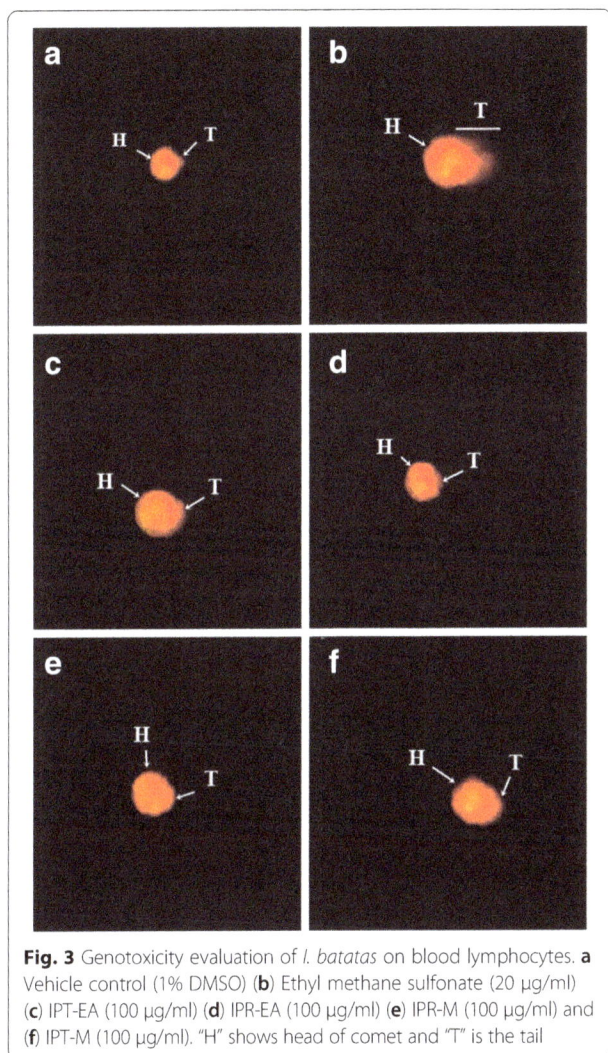

Fig. 3 Genotoxicity evaluation of *I. batatas* on blood lymphocytes. **a** Vehicle control (1% DMSO) (**b**) Ethyl methane sulfonate (20 μg/ml) (**c**) IPT-EA (100 μg/ml) (**d**) IPR-EA (100 μg/ml) (**e**) IPR-M (100 μg/ml) and (**f**) IPT-M (100 μg/ml). "H" shows head of comet and "T" is the tail

engrossment [44]. Cytokines are the key factors with job to regulate a variety of inflammations, which are involved in the onset and pathogenesis of rheumatoid arthritis. Tendered joints with degrees of arthritic swellings, definitely creates a situation of imbalance between pro and antiinflammatory cytokines, which is an open invitation to autoimmune reaction ultimately commencing chronic inflammation and joint injury [45]. Cartilage abrasion, tissue destruction and hyperalgesic situations due to inflammation are mainly due to cyclooxygenase, arachidonic acid and lipooxygenase triggered local inflammatory mediators like prostaglandins, leukotrienes, thromboxane A_2 and prostacyclin [46]. In early acute phase, arthritis comprises pain of severe degrees, lack of mobility, cessation of body weight gain and inflammation and swelling of hind and fore paw joints while in late acute phase (12+ days) rats are unable to move because of high level joint inflammations [2]. Cartilage can bear a high degree of stress and load due to its extracellular matrix constituting proteoglycan (PG) and collagen helix fibers [47]. Cartilage tissues exclusively lack vascularization, have least number of stem cells and measured turnover of collagen, which clearly depict its limited interior repair extent and ability. Yet extrinsic mechanism of mesenchymal stromal cells of connective tissues play some role in cartilage repairing. When ROS level exceeds the biological concentrations, it plays role in amplification and aggressing RA [48]. Histological slides clearly depict these worst conditions in disease controls. The characteristic ability of medicinal plants to cure a number of diseases due to existence of versatile compounds of therapeutic worth has heightened their reputation and is aiding physicians to fight confidently against the upcoming disorders [49].

In the present study, phytochemical screening of IPT-EA, IPT-M, IPR-EA and IPR-M yielded TPC and TFC, justifying the medicinal inference of the food plant. HPLC-DAD quantified significant amounts of rutin, gallic acid, caffeic acid, catechin, apigenin, myricetin and quercetin that is additional clue for the medicinal propensity of the plant. Rutin, gallic acid and quercetin are acknowledged and well alleged secondary metabolites of

diseases due to some serious hypersensitive or allergic reactions causing various complications of intense severity like serum sickness, myasthenia gravis, pernicious anemia and reactive arthritis with unknown etiology [43]. RA is one of the most common autoimmune inflammatory conditions of indefinite etiology well-appointed with symmetric erosive synovitis and in fewer cases extra-articular

Table 4 Cytotoxicity assessment on blood lymphocytes by comet parameters

Sample	Comet length(μm)	Head length(μm)	Tail length(μm)	% DNA in head	% DNA in tail	Tail moment(μm)
IPT-EA	51.56 ± 3.01	44.32 ± 2.56	7.24 ± 0.32[b]	85.95 ± 3.7[ab]	14.04 ± 1.48[b]	0.15 ± 0.03[b]
IPT-M	56.63 ± 4.21	47.12 ± 1.98	9.51 ± 0.25[b]	83.20 ± 4.17[b]	16.79 ± 1.32[b]	0.21 ± 0.04[b]
IPR-EA	49.21 ± 3.65	43.21 ± 2.78	5.99 ± 0.22[a]	87.82 ± 3.52[a]	12.17 ± 0.89[a]	0.11 ± 0.02[a]
IPR-M	53.87 ± 2.89	44.94 ± 2.43	8.93 ± 0.45[b]	83.42 ± 3.30[b]	16.57 ± 1.69[b]	0.18 ± 0.04[b]
EMS	60.31 ± 3.91	43.12 ± 3.21	17.21 ± 1.5[c]	71.67 ± 4.31[c]	28.33 ± 1.91[c]	1.68 ± 0.32[c]
Vehicle Control	46.11 ± 3.14	40.32 ± 2.78	5.79 ± 0.34[a]	88.44 ± 4.67[a]	11.56 ± 3.01[a]	0.12 ± 0.02[a]

IPT-EA, IPT-M, IPR-EA and IPR-M were dosed at 100 μg/ml whereas EMS (Ethyl methane sulfonate) was given in 20 μg/ml concentration. Vehicle = 1% DMSO. Values are expressed as mean ± SD (*n* = 6). Means with letter "b" indicate significant difference from normal control, "a" and "c" from Ethyl methane sulfonate treated group according to Kruskal-Wallis test at *p* < 0.05

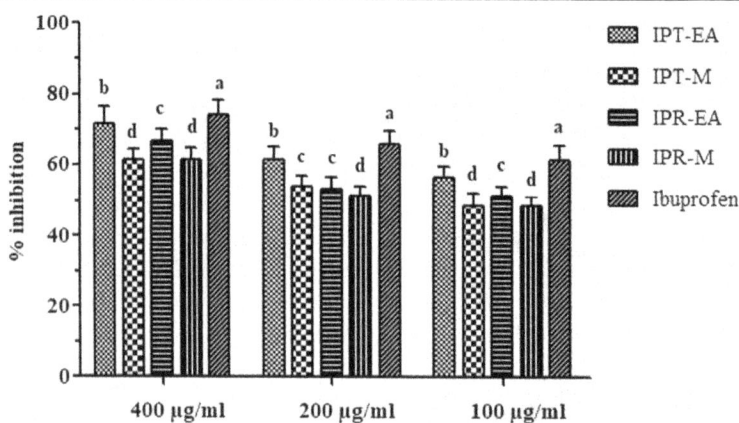

Fig. 4 In vitro antiinflammatory assessment of *I. batatas* extracts via albumin denaturation. Each value is represented as mean ± SD ($n = 3$). Means with different superscript (a-d) letters in the column are significantly ($p < 0.05$) different from one another

plants with admirable role in hepato-protection, neurological disorders and apoptosis as well as have antiinflammatory and antioxidant potential [10]. Similarly, complementary antioxidant results in the plant extracts are due to these proficient polyphenols. These polyphenols added massive abilities to *I. batatas* extracts to scavenge high counts of oxidants.

I. batatas extracts were evaluated for the chondrocyte toxicity and viability testing and genotoxicity via lymphocytic electrophoresis. Most of the exposed chondrocytes remained viable at various increasing doses of *I. batatas* extracts. For the evaluation of safety parameters at molecular level, assessment of lymphocyte genotoxicity via comet assay has been conducted. Size of comet head and concentration of the DNA in that region was proof of geno-protective aptitude of food plant. Comet tail was much smaller than that of standard geno-toxic drug ethyl methane sulfonate proving DNA protecting aptitude of

the extracts. The non-toxic nature of plant sanctioned its safety and suitability for in vivo usage. Outcomes of acute toxicity added to the safety of extracts as high doses up to 4000 mg/kg body weight had no deleterious effects in rats.

A physical or chemical stress like use of heat, strong acid or base, an organic solvent or concentrated inorganic salt that cause loss of tertiary and secondary structure of protein is termed as protein denaturation. This denaturation of protein is the leading cause of inflammation [50]. To evaluate mechanistic antiinflammatory activity, competence of the plant extract to inhibit protein denaturation was appraised. It was effective in inhibiting heat induced albumin denaturation. Maximum inhibition of 76.92 ± 3.07% was observed at the concentration of 500 µg/ml in comparison to the standard drug ibuprofen (79.48 ± 4.71%). Administration of *I. batatas* did not exhibit any physiological and behavioral adverse

Table 5 Effect of *I. batatas* on carrageenan-induced paw edema in rat

Groups	Edema volume (ml) Percent edema inhibition				
	1st h	3rd h	6th h	12th h	24th h
IPT-EA(300 mg/kg)	0.28	0.39	0.21	0.285	0.386
	24.52 ± 2.81[c]	38.58 ± 2.67[bc]	74.20 ± 5.14[c]	70.97 ± 5.75[c]	66.49 ± 4.30[c]
IPT-M (300 mg/kg)	0.315	0.487	0.301	0.39	0.542
	15.09 ± 1.43[e]	23.30 ± 1.70[d]	63.02 ± 4.21[e]	60.28 ± 5.13[e]	52.95 ± 4.13[e]
IPR-EA (300 mg/kg)	0.26	0.364	0.17	0.24	0.34
	29.91 ± 2.91[b]	42.67 ± 3.71[b]	79.11 ± 5.47[b]	75.56 ± 6.06[b]	70.48 ± 4.61[b]
IPR-M (300 mg/kg)	0.3	0.41	0.255	0.335	0.463
	19.13 ± 1.72[d]	35.43 ± 3.07[c]	68.67 ± 5.32[d]	65.88 ± 5.94[d]	59.80 ± 3.90[d]
Ibuprofen (10 mg/kg)	0.22	0.26	0.12	0.17	0.26
	40.70 ± 3.08[a]	59.05 ± 4.51[a]	85.25 ± 6.98[a]	82.68 ± 6.39[a]	77.43 ± 6.05[a]
Carrageenan Control	0.371	0.635	0.814	0.982	1.152
Saline Control	0.256 ± 0.05	0.301 ± 0.04	0.2 ± 0.03	0.14 ± 0.03	0.11 ± 0.04

Data values shown represent mean ± SD ($n = 6$). Means with different superscript ([a-e]) letters in the column are significantly ($p < 0.05$) different from one another

Table 6 Effect of *I. batatas* on croton oil-induced ear and anal edema in rat

Groups	Weight of left ear (mg)	Weight of right ear (mg)	Edema (Δ mg)	% reduction of inflammation	Anus size (mm)	Edema (mm)	% reduction of inflammation
IPT-EA	91.44 ± 1.7	93.73 ± 1.5	2.29 ± 0.20	62.94 ± 4.1[c]	39.13 ± 1.65	4.52 ± 0.21	63.04 ± 4.17[c]
IPT-M	87.3 ± 1.30	90.23 ± 1.2	2.93 ± 0.25	52.58 ± 3.4[d]	40.81 ± 1.87	5.90 ± 0.32	51.75 ± 3.79[d]
IPR-EA	86.34 ± 2.1	88.07 ± 1.8	1.73 ± 0.15	72.01 ± 7.8[b]	38.18 ± 1.43	3.57 ± 0.29	70.80 ± 4.94[b]
IPR-M	83.8 ± 1.02	86.27 ± 1.2	2.47 ± 0.11	60.03 ± 4.2[c]	40.17 ± 1.87	5.56 ± 0.38	54.53 ± 3.80[d]
Ibuprofen	84.7 ± 1.67	85.9 ± 2.01	1.20 ± 0.10	80.5 ± 5.03[a]	36.75 ± 1.01	2.14 ± 0.12	82.50 ± 6.21[a]
Croton oil	93.4 ± 1.10	99.58 ± 2.1	6.18 ± 0.74		46.84 ± 1.21	12.23 ± 0.8	
Normal	80.04 ± 1.4	80.0 ± 2.02			34.61 ± 0.90		

Data values shown represent mean ± SD ($n = 6$). Means with different superscript ([a-d]) letters in the column are significantly ($p < 0.05$) different from one another

effect or mortality in rat model; hence, recommended safer for further investigation in test animals. Among the various models of antiinflammatory activity assessment, carrageenan-induced inflammatory model is a typical model used to investigate the activity of trial drugs [30]. Development of edema with carrageenan is a biphasic model, which involves the contribution of vascular and inflammatory mediators. Initial phase (0–1 h) of edema is attributed by the release of histamine, 5-hydroxytryptamine and bradykinin and is not repressed by the use of NSAIDs such as ibuprofen or aspirin. During the 2nd phase (1–6 h) of edema development, elevated levels of prostaglandins and inducible cyclooxygenase (COX-2) have been demonstrated in hind paw edema of rat. The inhibition of

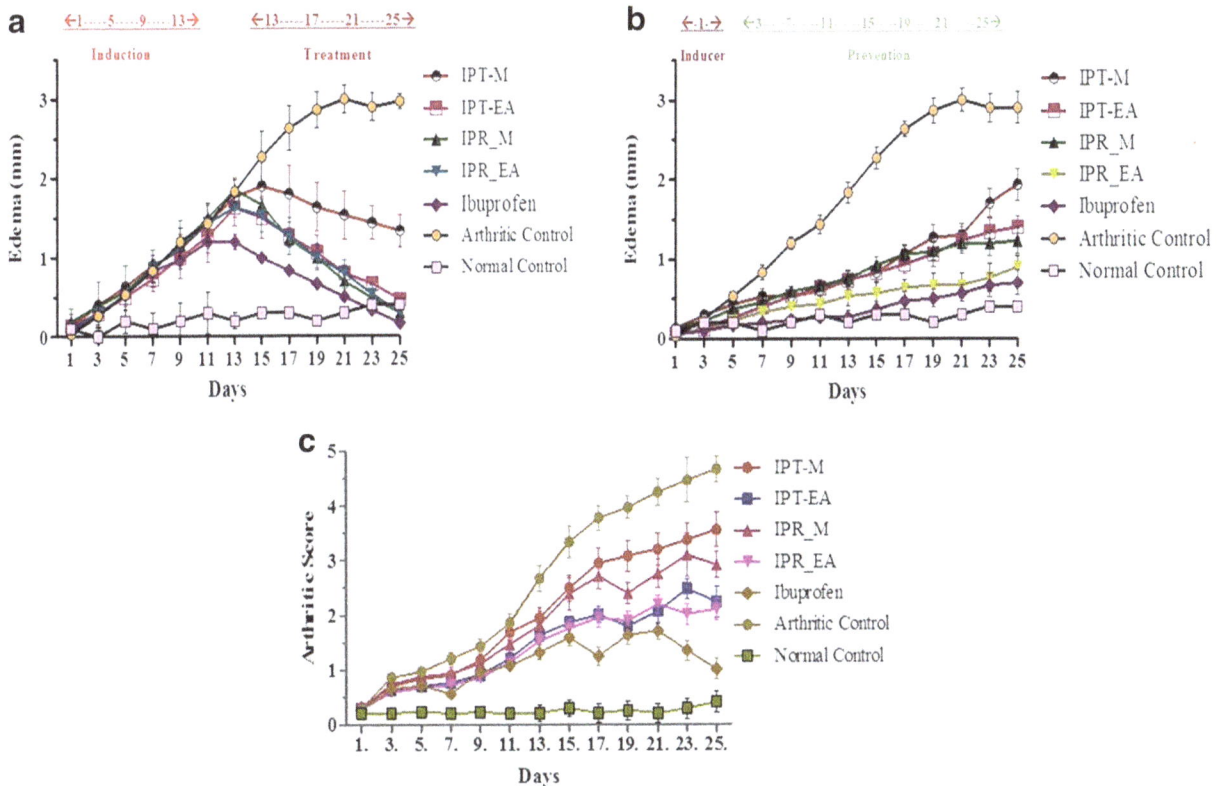

Fig. 5 Assessment of arthritic edema and arthritic score. Data is presented as the mean arthritic score ± SEM ($n = 6$/group). **a** Treatment mode of studies where the induction was done till day 13 and then dose was started. Edema in arthritic control group increased with the passage of time. IPR-EA and IPR-M have significantly decreased arthritic edema after 15th day in comparison to ibuprofen. **b** Preventive mode of study where dose was given after inducer at day 1. Arthritic control group has not prevented the induction of the disease while IPR-EA and IPR-M have significantly prevented arthritic edema in comparison to ibuprofen. **c** Arthritic score where arthritic control group has higher arthritic score compared to normal and other groups. The ibuprofen treated animals showed significant decrease in arthritic score after first week onwards during the experiment

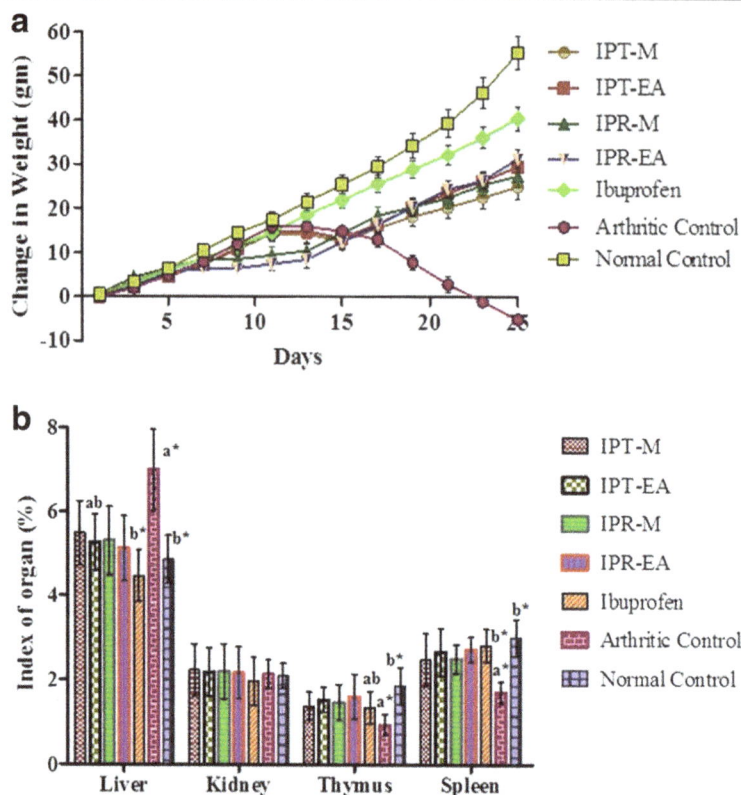

Fig. 6 Assessment of the change in body weight and organ index in experimental animals. **a** Variation in mean body weight over indicated period of time. **b** Normal and arthritic altered organs index. Each value represents the mean ± SD ($n = 6$/group). Differences were considered significant at the level of * $p < 0.05$

inflammation during the early and the late phase of edema with *I. batatas* extracts suggest that they have reduced the antiinflammatory activity by constraining the release of mediators of inflammation. Presence of polyphenols in the extracts has contributed towards the antiinflammatory activity by inhibiting the infiltration of neutrophils, suppression of IL-1β, IL-6 and NO [51].

Histamine is released in response to allergic reactions and causes skin, nose, throat and lung irritation. During inflammation, it plays its role through vasodilation, edema, increased vascular permeability and recruitment of eosinophil. It regulates the leukocyte function and migration, proliferation of T cells, B cell differentiation and release of lysosomal enzymes in neutrophils [52]. The antiinflammatory activity of any extract/compound can be assessed by the croton oil-induced ear and anus edema. Endothelial nitric oxide synthase (eNOS) plays a pivotal role during the histamine-induced paw edema. Thus, lowering down the levels of NO may aid in the reduction of inflammation as NO is directly accounted for the macromolecular gush induced by histamine inflammation [53]. In this study, *I. batatas* extracts appreciably inhibited the croton oil-induced inflammation in rat ear and anus suggesting that the antiinflammatory efficacy

observed is because of the stabilization of mast cell membranes, lowering down the levels of NO synthesis and histamine inhibition. Earlier Sajid et al. [50] has narrated the similar histamine based inflammatory findings.

Adjuvant-induced arthritic rat model has extensively been used as classical animal model sharing several characteristic features of human rheumatoid arthritis patients, such as immunology and histology [54]. Adjuvant-induction results in activation of the cell-mediated immune response and stimulates immunoglobulin production in organisms, which results in the induction of primary and secondary chronic arthritis [55]. A large amount of pro-inflammatory cytokines are produced in adjuvant arthritis that may cause inflammation at different sites, also known as polyarthritis. Pro-inflammatory cytokines and interleukins are involved in osteoclast differentiation, inflammation and bone erosion [50]. The scheme of CFA-induced arthritis has been summarized in Fig. 9 [56].

In the present study, extracts of *I. batatas* tuber and root have significantly reduced the extent and level of inflammation in the late phase (fourth week) of the disease in comparison to the arthritic control with progressive inflammation and lesions. Inhibition of TNF-α and IL-1β, IL-2, IL-6 and NO mainly contributes in the

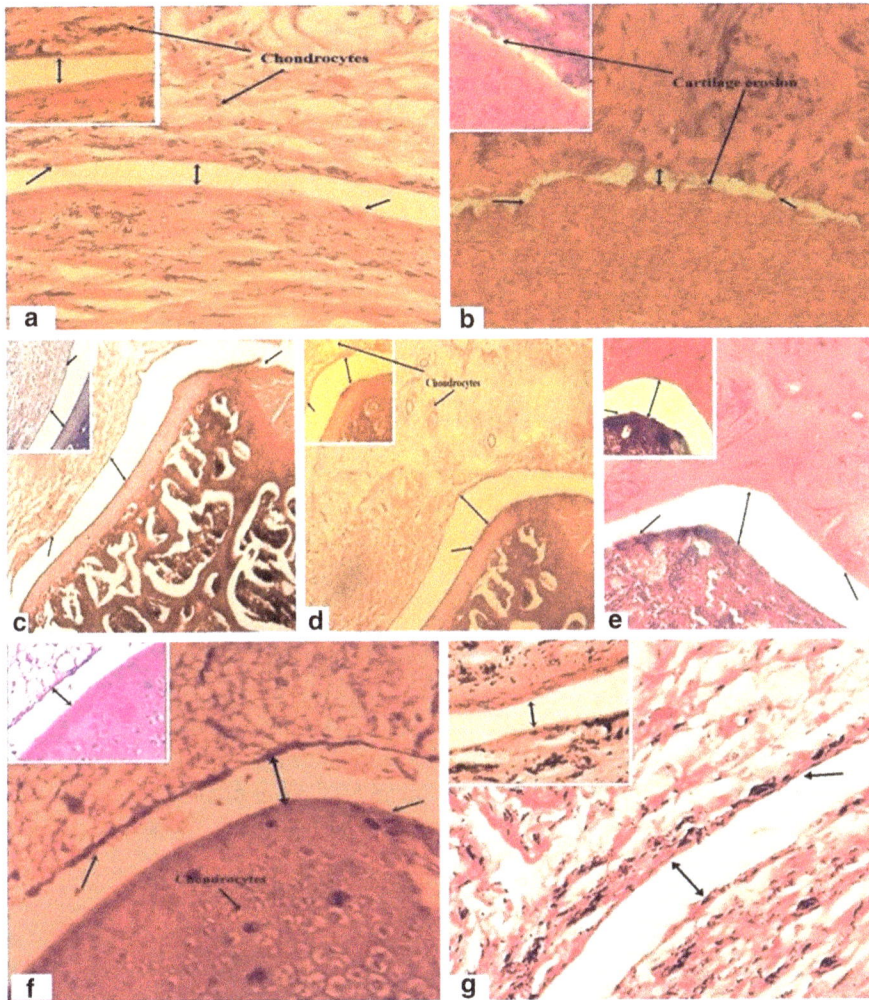

Fig. 7 Investigation of histological architecture (**a**) normal rat; (**b**) arthritic rat; (**c**) IPR-EA 300 mg/kg; (**d**) IPT-EA 300 mg/kg; (**e**) IPR-M 300 mg/kg; (**f**) IPT-M 300 mg/kg; (**g**) ibuprofen 10 mg/kg. The black double arrow shows variation in joint spaces among different groups, while single arrows represent the chondrocytes or cartilage erosion

eradication of inflammations as these macromolecules are purely responsible for the synthesis of metallo-proteinases and proliferation of synovial cells resulting in cartilage degradation [57]. The inhibition of IL-1β, IL-6 and NO proves *I. batatas* as an antiarthritic agent as not only levels of inflammation have been reduced as obvious in arthritic score, but cartilage erosion is also minimized (histology). Significant inhibition of inflammation in treatment mode of the study is possibly due to the suppression of these over expressing cytokines causing damages to the joint cartilage and synovial cell proliferation. Similarly, the plant extracts exhibited significant inhibition of the onset

Table 7 The haematological investigation of normal control and arthritic rats

Groups	RBCs (× 10⁶)/µl	WBCs (×10³) /µl	Platelets (×10³) /µl	Hb (g/dl)	ESR (mm/h)
IPT-EA	5.81 ± 0.019^b	3.89 ± 0.011^{ab}	558 ± 02.811^{ab}	8.03 ± 0.47^b	4.98 ± 0.053^b
IPT-M	5.40 ± 0.013^b	4.67 ± 0.012^b	498 ± 03.2120^c	7.81 ± 0.54^c	5.49 ± 0.089^c
IPR-EA	6.01 ± 0.012^{ab}	3.72 ± 0.014^{ab}	571 ± 02.710^{ab}	8.26 ± 0.71^b	4.83 ± 0.072^b
IPR-M	5.62 ± 0.071^b	4.15 ± 0.017^b	535.10 ± 1.91^b	7.72 ± 0.25^c	5.13 ± 0.10^{bc}
Ibuprofen	5.44 ± 0.032^b	6.31 ± 0.020^c	394.5 ± 02.29^d	7.84 ± 0.70^c	4.96 ± 0.023^b
Arthritic Control	4.14 ± 0.025^c	7.02 ± 0.035^d	346.67 ± 2.51^e	6.31 ± 0.12^d	9.44 ± 0.061^d
Normal	6.78 ± 0.078^a	3.51 ± 0.045^a	594.81 ± 4.58^a	10.33 ± 0.9^a	4.35 ± 0.045^a

Results are presented as mean ± SD ($n = 6$). Means with different superscript ($^{a-e}$) letters in the column are significantly ($p < 0.05$) different from one another

Table 8 Enzymatic and biochemical investigation of control and arthritic rats

Groups	ALT (U/L)	AST (U/L)	ALP (U/L)	Urea (mg/dl)	Creatinine(mg/dl)	Bilirubin (mg/ml)	Albumin (mg/dl)	Testosterone (ng/ml)
IPT-EA	60.21 ± 2.7^c	56.3 ± 2.4^c	156.4 ± 3.8^d	61.12 ± 2.8^c	1.63 ± 0.1^d	6.03 ± 0.1^d	5.58 ± 0.19^c	5.87 ± 0.4^b
IPT-M	73.16 ± 2.9^b	67.2 ± 2.1^b	184.3 ± 5.8^b	66.71 ± 2.3^b	1.8 ± 0.21^b	5.8 ± 0.12^f	5.21 ± 0.30^b	5.46 ± 0.3^d
IPR-EA	54.77 ± 2.8^d	47.2 ± 2.5^d	141.3 ± 4.3^e	57.07 ± 1.8^d	1.56 ± 0.12^e	6.1 ± 0.07^c	5.8 ± 0.12^{cd}	6.37 ± 0.8^a
IPR-M	69.2 ± 2.4^{bc}	64.3 ± 2.9^{bc}	172.8 ± 5.4^c	63.3 ± 2.4^{bc}	1.76 ± 0.11^c	5.9 ± 0.11^e	5.3 ± 0.24^{bc}	5.7 ± 0.45^c
Ibuprofen	45.44 ± 2.1^e	39.9 ± 1.3^e	123.3 ± 2.9^f	54.1 ± 1.9^{de}	1.48 ± 0.11^f	6.2 ± 0.08^b	5.91 ± 0.23^d	5.9 ± 0.38^b
Arthritic Control	93.37 ± 2.4^a	103.9 ± 2.1^a	334.1 ± 7.1^a	71.3 ± 2.34^a	2.54 ± 0.22^a	5.6 ± 0.21^g	2.71 ± 0.14^a	4.37 ± 0.4^e
Normal	39.00 ± 0.5^e	26.7 ± 0.6^f	115.2 ± 2.1^g	51.3 ± 1.89^e	1.34 ± 0.12^g	6.4 ± 0.23^a	6.11 ± 0.28^e	6.6 ± 0.67^a

Data is mean $\pm$ SD ($n = 6$). Means with different superscript ($^{a-g}$) letters in the column are significantly ($p < 0.05$) different from one another

of disease in preventive mode of study, which justifies its antiarthritic capabilities as they subdued the levels of pro-inflammatory cytokines. Previous studies reported that polyphenols like caffeic acid [58], rutin and quercetin [59], gallic acid [60], kaempferol [61], catechin [62] and apigenin [63] are good antiinflammatory compounds that decrease the inflammatory reaction by blocking neutrophil transfer associated with the reduction in TNF-α, IL-1β levels and oxidative stress [51]. Additionally our study is in good correlation with the phenolic contents quantified. The extracts with high TPC and TFC showed best results in multiple experiments; hence, authenticating the antiinflammatory role of polyphenols. Our findings are in consensus with the outcomes of Younis et al. [1].

In the current investigation, histopathological examinations were also performed that clearly depict the restoration of joint cartilage, integrity of leukocytes in synovial fluid and expansion of joint spaces by *I. batatas* extracts. On the other hand, extensive cartilage destruction, narrowing of joint spaces and infiltration of leukocytes in synovial region were observed in arthritic control. The extracts possibly enhanced the expression of extracellular matrix like collagen helix fibers and proteoglycan (PrG), which play extensive role in cartilage restoration.

Reduction of total body weight is an important parameter to find the extent and progression of disease. Altered weight of vital organs like liver, kidney, thymus and spleen is helpful in assessment of various ailments. In

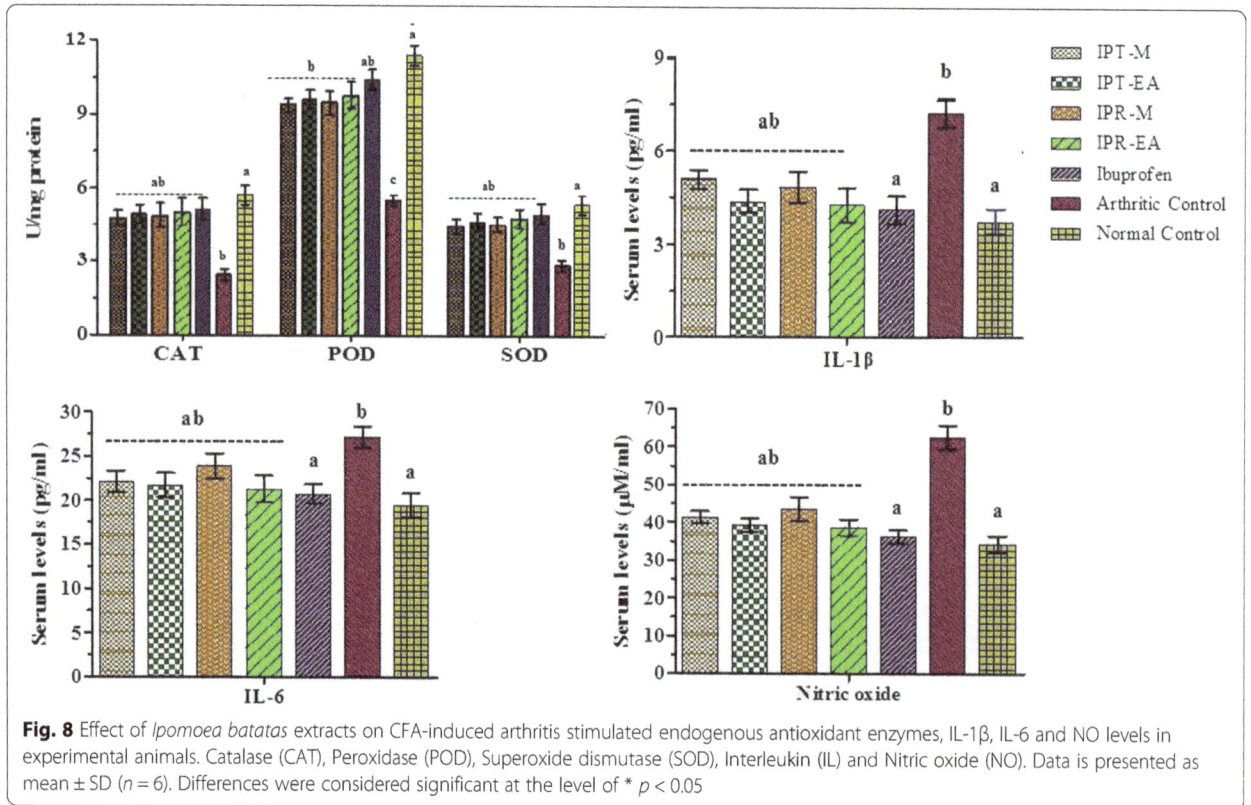

Fig. 8 Effect of *Ipomoea batatas* extracts on CFA-induced arthritis stimulated endogenous antioxidant enzymes, IL-1β, IL-6 and NO levels in experimental animals. Catalase (CAT), Peroxidase (POD), Superoxide dismutase (SOD), Interleukin (IL) and Nitric oxide (NO). Data is presented as mean $\pm$ SD ($n = 6$). Differences were considered significant at the level of * $p < 0.05$

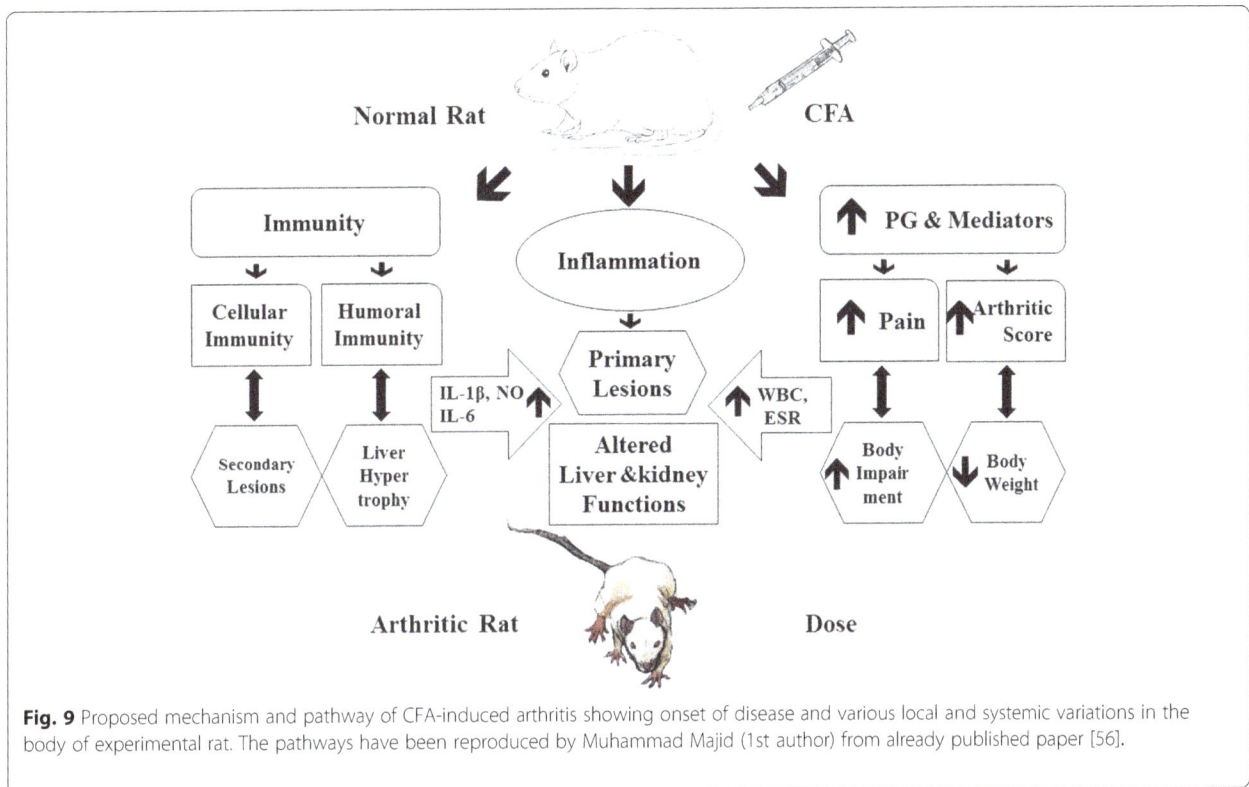

Fig. 9 Proposed mechanism and pathway of CFA-induced arthritis showing onset of disease and various local and systemic variations in the body of experimental rat. The pathways have been reproduced by Muhammad Majid (1st author) from already published paper [56].

the current study, total body weight and indices of the vital organs were measured. The normal and sample treated rats showed a gain of weight, while arthritic animals were found to significantly loose body weight. Likewise, altered organ indices were observed in diseased and test groups in comparison to the normal rats (Fig. 6a, b). Body weight and organ indices based study was also done by Jiang et al. [64] who found positive correlation between body weight variation and arthritis. Atrophy of the liver and thymus in ibuprofen group in the current study clearly suggests its toxicity in multi-dose treatment while the *I. batatas* extracts showed no such deleterious effects. This strengthens our claim of *I. batatas* a better alternative antiarthritic candidate with less or no side effects.

An increased number of the WBCs and ESR in arthritic animals might be due the immune response of pathogenic microorganisms. The decreased RBCs and Hb levels show the anemic condition of arthritic rats (Table 7). ESR is an important hematological tool to index diagnostic or prognostic assessment of inflammatory diseases. Nutritious components like vitamin B, β-carotene, iron, calcium, zinc, and protein are abundantly present in *I. batatas* [23]. The plant is a rich source of anthocyanin and polyphenols responsible for potentiating its ability as antineoplastic, vasotonic, vasoprotective and antiinflammatory agent [25]. The current results are in complete agreement to the abilities reported

as they have completely regulated the blood profile of test group in comparison to the arthritic group. *I. batatas* treatment reversed the altered blood parameters in arthritic animals via inhibition of cytokines such as cyclooxygenase and suppression of pro-inflammatory immune response as reported earlier by Hasan et al. [65].

Elevated levels of different serum enzymes, including ALP, ALT, AST and biochemical parameters such as bilirubin indicate abnormality of liver function [66]. These enzymes were monitored to ascertain the normal function of the liver. The significantly elevated serum enzyme shows the toxic response of arthritis in experimental rats (Table 8). High levels of AST, ALT and ALP as well as creatinine and low level of albumin in arthritic rat clearly denote hepatic injuries that were restored in test groups. Hepatic damage is associated with enhanced generation of ROS in hepatocytes that cause cellular death due to DNA damage, protein oxidation and lipid peroxidation. Polyphenole abundance imparts *I. batatas* an ability to scavenge free radicals, which ultimately reduces ROS and hepatocellular death. Batool et al. [42] also mentioned that polyphenols imparts hepatoprotective potential to the plants.

Endogenous antioxidant enzymes, including CAT, POD and SOD protect the oxidation induced cartilage destruction in inflammatory conditions such as rheumatoid arthritis. Inconsistency of the oxidative system in arthritis promotes and intensifies cellular response and increase the destruction of cartilage and bone [33]. When ROS establishes a stress condition, endogenous antioxidants provide protection against the invading free radicals to cope the stressed situation. Administration of an exogenous antioxidant source like *I. batatas* not only scavenges abundant free radicals by oxidizing them but also restore the amount of natural antioxidants. In this study, the enormous production of free radicals with the help of CFA generated an oxidative stress that extensively damaged the liver. This reduced the expression of antioxidative enzymes in arthritic control. On the other hand, polyphenol rich *I. batatas* extracts provided a fine line of defense to the rat liver against ROS. The current study is in agreement to the findings of Khan et al. [67] and Kazmi et al. [68]. Moreover, *I. batatas* extracts provided significant inhibition of free radicals in vitro, which fortifies their capabilities to provide a better line of defense in in vivo. *I. batatas* extracts are rich in antioxidant compounds that are the major factors of its ability to scavenge the blend of free radicals continuously produced in disease condition like arthritis and provide a real time protection.

All the phytochemical, in vitro and in vivo results clearly depict the therapeutic worth of *I. batatas* extracts against inflammatory disorder like arthritis. It strongly lessened the inflammation, increased thresholds of pain, enhanced the levels of endogenous enzymes, maintained normal blood profile and upheld the levels of liver and kidney enzymes.

Conclusion

Multi-mode phytochemical and pharmacological evaluation of *I. batatas* L. Lam. justifies its medicinal worth as a potential agent for curing acute and chronic inflammatory arthritis. High quantity of potent polyphenols along with massive quantity of dietary components makes this food plant a safe and effective candidate in therapeutic rivalry of finding newer potential agents. The histological restoration, body weight and organ weight index stabilization, hematological and biochemical repair as well as endogenous enzymes revitalization clearly defend the benefit of *I. batatas* in arthritis condition. High percentage of inflammation inhibition by the roots of *I. batatas* clearly suggests detailed evaluation of the plant at molecular level. The plant already in use as an antiinflammatory agent in folk medicine is for the first time investigated and presented as an effective antiarthritic agent with good recovery from acute and chronic stages of the disease.

Additional files

Additional file 1: Figure S1b. Chondrocytes exposed to different concentrations of the IPT-EA, IPT-M, IPR-EA and IPR-M for 24 h and cell viability/toxicity was investigated through MTT assay. Results are mean of triplicate experiment ±SD.

Additional file 2: Figure S2b. In vitro antioxidant activities assessment (A) DPPH radical scavenging activity (B) Nitric oxide scavenging activity (C) Hydroxyl radical scavenging activity (D) iron chelating % inhibition. Each value represents mean ± SD ($n = 3$).

Abbreviations
ALP: Alkaline phosphatase; ALT: Alanine aminotransferase; AST: Aspartate Aminotransferase; CFA: Complete Freund's Adjuvant; IPR-EA: *Ipomea batatas* root ethyle acetate extract; IPR-M: *Ipomea batatas* root methanol extract; IPT-EA: *Ipomea batatas* tuber ethyle acetate extract; IPT-M: *Ipomea batatas* tuber methanol extract; MTT: methylthiazole tetrazolium; OECD: Organization for Economic Cooperation and Development; POD: Peroxidase; PrG: Proteoglycan; SOD: Superoxide dismutase

Funding
The project was funded by Department of Pharmacy, Quaid-i-Azam University Islamabad Pakistan.

Authors' contributions
All authors have made considerable contribution to the work and approved the final version of publication. MM has significant contribution to experimentation, acquisition and drafting of the manuscript. SSZ and BN helped in experimental work. IH and MRK has made substantial contribution in designing, analyzing and drafting of the manuscript. BM provided HPLC facility and acquisition of the data. All authors read and approved the final manuscript.

Ethics approval and consent to participate
We confirm that any aspect of the work covered in this manuscript that has involved either experimental animals or human subjects has been conducted by strictly following the guidelines as approved by the ethical committee of Quaid-i-Azam University, Islamabad, Pakistan (Letter No. QAU-PHM-017/2016 for the animal care and Letter No. QAU-PHM-023/2016 for experimentation dated 24/10/2016). Blood sampling from healthy volunteer was also approved by Institutional Review board of Quaid-i-Azam University (Letter No. IRB-QAU-116 dated 4/11/2016). Blood sampling was done under duly signed consent by the healthy volunteer with no known infection.

Competing interests
The authors declare that they have no competing interests.

Author details
[1]Department of Pharmacy, Faculty of Biological Sciences, Quaid-i-Azam University, Islamabad 45320, Pakistan. [2]Department of Biochemistry, Faculty of Biological Sciences, Quaid-i-Azam University, Islamabad 45320, Pakistan.

References
1. Younis T, Khan MR, Sajid M, Majid M, Zahra Z, Shah NA. *Fraxinus xanthoxyloides* leaves reduced the level of inflammatory mediators during in vitro and in vivo studies. BMC Complement Altern Med. 2016;16(1):230.
2. Amresh G, Singh P, Rao CV. Antinociceptive and antiarthritic activity of *Cissampelos pareira* roots. J Ethnopharmacol. 2007;111(3):531–6.
3. Mueller M, Hobiger S, Jungbauer A. Anti-inflammatory activity of extracts from fruits, herbs and spices. Food Chem. 2010;122(4):987–96.
4. Gambhire M, Wankhede S, Juvekar A. Antiinflammatory activity of aqueous extract of *Barleria cristata* leaves. J Young Pharm. 2009;1(3):220.
5. Blake DR, Allen R. Inflammation: basic principles and clinical correlates. Ann Rheum Dis. 1988;47(9):792.
6. Delaporte RH, Sánchez GMN, Cuellar AC, Giuliani A, de Mello JCP. Antiinflammatory activity and lipid peroxidation inhibition of iridoid lamiide isolated from *Bouchea fluminensis* (Vell.) mold.(Verbenaceae). J Ethnopharmacol. 2002;82(2):127–30.
7. Tahir I, Khan MR, Shah NA, Aftab M. Evaluation of phytochemicals, antioxidant activity and amelioration of pulmonary fibrosis with *Phyllanthus emblica* leaves. BMC Complement Altern Med. 2016;16(1):406.
8. Ali S, Khan M, Sajid M. Protective potential of *Parrotiopsis jacquemontiana* (Decne) Rehder on carbon tetrachloride induced hepatotoxicity in experimental rats. Biomed Pharmacother. 2017;95:1853.

9. Bokhari J, Khan MR, Haq IU. Assessment of phytochemicals, antioxidant, and anti-inflammatory potential of *Boerhavia procumbens* Banks ex Roxb. Toxicol Ind Health. 2016;32(8):1456–66.

10. Majid M, Khan MR, Shah NA, Haq IU, Farooq MA, Ullah S, Sharif A, Zahra Z, Younis T, Sajid M. Studies on phytochemical, antioxidant, anti-inflammatory and analgesic activities of *Euphorbia dracunculoides*. BMC Complement Altern Med. 2015;15(1):349.

11. Haddad JJ. Antioxidant and prooxidant mechanisms in the regulation of redox (y)-sensitive transcription factors. Cell Signal. 2002;14(11):879–97.

12. Afonso V, Champy R, Mitrovic D, Collin P, Lomri A. Reactive oxygen species and superoxide dismutases: role in joint diseases. Joint Bone Spine. 2007;74(4):324–9.

13. Phull A-R, Eo S-H, Abbas Q, Ahmed M, Kim SJ. Applications of chondrocyte-based cartilage engineering: an overview. Biomed Res Int. 2016;2016:1879837.

14. Blanco FJ, Guitian R, Vázquez-Martul E, de Toro FJ, Galdo F. Osteoarthritis chondrocytes die by apoptosis: a possible pathway for osteoarthritis pathology. Arthritis Rheum. 1998;41(2):284–9.

15. Ma B, Leijten J, Wu L, Kip M, van Blitterswijk C, Post J, Karperien M. Gene expression profiling of dedifferentiated human articular chondrocytes in monolayer culture. Osteoarthr Cartil. 2013;21(4):599–603.

16. Tinker AC, Wallace AV. Selective inhibitors of inducible nitric oxide synthase: potential agents for the treatment of inflammatory diseases? Curr Top Med Chem. 2006;6(2):77–92.

17. Feldmann M, Maini SRN. Role of cytokines in rheumatoid arthritis: an education in pathophysiology and therapeutics. Immunol Rev. 2008;223(1):7–19.

18. Pham TN, Rahman P, Tobin YM, Khraishi MM, Hamilton SF, Alderdice C, Richardson VJ. Elevated serum nitric oxide levels in patients with inflammatory arthritis associated with co-expression of inducible nitric oxide synthase and protein kinase C-eta in peripheral blood monocyte-derived macrophages. J Rheumatol. 2003;30(12):2529–34.

19. Suleyman H, Demircan B, Karagoz Y. Anti-inflammatory and side effects of cyclooxygenase inhibitors. Pharmacol Reports. 2007;59(3):247–58.

20. Islam S. Sweetpotato (*Ipomoea batatas* L.) leaf: its potential effect on human health and nutrition. J Food Sci. 2006;71(2):R13-R121.

21. Mohanraj R, Sivasankar S. Sweet potato (*Ipomoea batatas* [L.] Lam)-A valuable medicinal food: a review. J Med Food. 2014;17(7):733–41.

22. Milind P. Monika. Sweet potato as a super-food. Int J Res Ayurveda Pharm. 2015;6(4):557–62.

23. Yoshimoto M, Okuno S, Islam M, Kurata R, Yamakawa O. Polyphenolic content and antimutagenicity of sweetpotato leaves in relation to commercial vegetables. Acta hort. 2003;628(628):677–85.

24. Ishiguro K, Toyama J, Islam M, Yoshimoto M, Kumagai T, Kai Y, Nakazawa Y, Yamakawa O. Suioh, a new sweetpotato cultivar for utilization in vegetable greens. Acta hort. 2004;637:339–45.

25. Islam MS, Yoshimoto M, Yahara S, Okuno S, Ishiguro K, Yamakawa O. Identification and characterization of foliar polyphenolic composition in sweetpotato (Ipomoea batatas L.) genotypes. J Agric Food Chem. 2002;50(13):3718–22.

26. Islam MS, Yoshimoto M, Yamakawa O. Distribution and physiological functions of caffeoylquinic acid derivatives in leaves of sweetpotato genotypes. J Food Sci. 2003;68(1):111–6.

27. Fatima H, Khan K, Zia M, Ur-Rehman T, Mirza B, Haq I-u. Extraction optimization of medicinally important metabolites from *Datura innoxia* Mill.: an in vitro biological and phytochemical investigation. BMC Complement Altern Med. 2015;15(1):376.

28. Sahreen S, Khan MR, Khan RA, Shah NA. Estimation of flavoniods, antimicrobial, antitumor and anticancer activity of *Carissa opaca* fruits. BMC Complement Altern Med. 2013;13(1):372.

29. Sahreen S, Khan MR, Khan RA. Comprehensive assessment of phenolics and antiradical potential of *Rumex hastatus* D. Don. roots. BMC Complement Altern Med. 2014;14(1):47.

30. Phull A-R, Majid M, Haq I-U, Khan MR, Kim SJ. In vitro and in vivo evaluation of anti-arthritic, antioxidant efficacy of fucoidan from *Undaria pinnatifida* (Harvey) Suringar. Int J Biol Macromol. 2017;97:468–80.

31. Suman G, Jamil K. Application of human lymphocytes for evaluating toxicity of anti-cancer drugs. Int J Pharmacol. 2006;2(4):374–81.

32. Waseem D, Butt AF, Haq I-U, Bhatti MH, Khan GM. Carboxylate derivatives of tributyltin (IV) complexes as anticancer and antileishmanial agents. DARU J Pharm Sci. 2017;25(1):8.

33. Dhawan A, Bajpayee M, Parmar D. Comet assay: a reliable tool for the assessment of DNA damage in different models. Cell Biol Toxicol. 2009;25(1):5–32.

34. Leelaprakash G, Dass SM. Invitro anti-inflammatory activity of methanol extract of *Enicostemma axillare*. Int J Drug Develop Research. 2011;3(3):189–96.

35. Reanmongkol W, Noppapan T, Subhadhirasakul S. Antinociceptive, antipyretic, and anti-inflammatory activities of *Putranjiva roxburghii* Wall. leaf extract in experimental animals. J Nat Med. 2009;63(3):290.

36. Zhang R-X, Fan AY, Zhou A-N, Moudgil KD, Ma Z-Z, Lee DY-W, Fong HH, Berman BM, Lao L. Extract of the Chinese herbal formula Huo Luo Xiao LingDan inhibited adjuvant arthritis in rats. J Ethnopharmacol. 2009;121(3):366–71.

37. Han X, Su D, Xian X, Zhou M, Li X, Huang J, Wang J, Gao H. Inhibitory effects of *Saussurea involucrata* (Kar. Et Kir.) Sch.-Bip. On adjuvant arthritis in rats. J Ethnopharmacol. 2016;194:228–35.

38. Attia AM, Ibrahim FA, Abd El-Latif NA, Aziz SW, Elwan AM, Aziz A, Aziz A, Elgendy A, Elgengehy FT. Therapeutic antioxidant and anti-inflammatory effects of laser acupuncture on patients with rheumatoid arthritis. Lasers Surg Med. 2016;48(5):490–7.

39. Shah NA, Khan MR, Ahmad B, Noureen F, Rashid U, Khan RA. Investigation on flavonoid composition and anti free radical potential of *Sida cordata*. BMC Complement Altern Med. 2013;13(1):276.

40. Sajid M, Khan MR, Shah NA, Ullah S, Younis T, Majid M, Ahmad B, Nigussie D. Proficiencies of *Artemisia scoparia* against CCl 4 induced DNA damages and renal toxicity in rat. BMC Complement Altern Med. 2016;16(1):149.

41. Sundaram MS, Hemshekhar M, Santhosh MS, Paul M, Sunitha K, Thushara RM, NaveenKumar SK, Naveen S, Devaraja S, Rangappa KS. Tamarind seed (Tamarindus indica) extract ameliorates adjuvant-induced arthritis via regulating the mediators of cartilage/bone degeneration, inflammation and oxidative stress. Sci Rep. 2015;5:11117.

42. Batool R, Khan MR, Majid M. *Euphorbia dracunculoides* L. abrogates carbon tetrachloride induced liver and DNA damage in rats. BMC Complement Altern Med. 2017;17(1):223.

43. Chitme HR, Patel NP. Antiarthritis activity of *Aristolochia bracteata* extract in experimental animals. Open Nat Prod J. 2009;2:6–15.

44. Lee YH, Rho YH, Choi SJ, Ji JD, Song GG. Association of TNF-alpha–308 G/a polymorphism with responsiveness to TNF-α-blockers in rheumatoid arthritis: a meta-analysis. Rheum int. 2006;27(2):157–61.

45. McInnes IB, Schett G. Cytokines in the pathogenesis of rheumatoid arthritis. Nat Rev Immunol. 2007;7(6):429–42.

46. Umara MI, Altafa R, Iqbalb MA, Sadiqc MB. In vivo experimental models to investigate the anti-inflammatory activity of herbal extracts. Sci International. 2010;22(3):199–203.

47. Sanchez CG. Aging in COPD and idiopathic pulmonary fibrosis. In: Sierra F, Kohanski R, editors. Advances in Geroscience. Cham: Springer; 2016. p. 429–70.

48. Bauerova K, Bezek S. Role of reactive oxygen and nitrogen species in etiopathogenesis of rheumatoid arthritis. Gen Physiol Biophys. 2000;18:15–20.

49. Ullah S, Khan MR, Shah NA, Shah SA, Majid M, Farooq MA. Ethnomedicinal plant use value in the Lakki Marwat District of Pakistan. J Ethnopharmacol. 2014;158 (412–22.

50. Sajid M, Khan MR, Shah SA, Majid M, Ismail H, Maryam S, Batool R, Younis T. Investigations on anti-inflammatory and analgesic activities of *Alnus nitida* Spach (Endl). Stem bark in Sprague Dawley rats. J Ethnopharmacol. 2017;198:407–16.

51. Silva RO, Sousa FBM, Damasceno SR, Carvalho NS, Silva VG, Oliveira FR, Sousa DP, Aragão KS, Barbosa AL, Freitas RM. Phytol, a diterpene alcohol, inhibits the inflammatory response by reducing cytokine production and oxidative stress. Fundam Clin Pharmacol. 2014;28(4):455–64.

52. Zampeli E, Tiligada E. The role of histamine H4 receptor in immune and inflammatory disorders. Brit J Pharmacol. 2009;157(1):24–33.

53. Yong YK, Zakaria ZA, Kadir AA, Somchit MN, Lian GEC, Ahmad Z. Chemical constituents and antihistamine activity of *Bixa orellana* leaf extract. BMC Complement Altern Med. 2013;13(1):32.

54. Jawed H, Shah SUA, Jamall S, Simjee SU. N-(2-hydroxy phenyl) acetamide inhibits inflammation-related cytokines and ROS in adjuvant-induced arthritic (AIA) rats. Int Immunopharmacol. 2010;10(8):900–5.

55. Simoes S, Delgado T, Lopes R, Jesus S, Ferreira A, Morais J, Cruz M, Corvo M, Martins M. Developments in the rat adjuvant arthritis model and its use in therapeutic evaluation of novel non-invasive treatment by SOD in Transfersomes. J Control Release. 2005;103(2):419–34.

56. Kumar V, Al-Abbasi F, Verma A, Mujeeb M, Anwar F. Umbelliferone β-D-galactopyranoside exerts an anti-inflammatory effect by attenuating COX-1 and COX-2. Toxicol Res. 2015;4(4):1072–84.

57. Suresh P, Kavitha CN, Babu SM, Reddy VP, Latha AK. Effect of ethanol extract of Trigonella foenum graecum (Fenugreek) seeds on Freund's adjuvant-induced arthritis in albino rats. Inflammation. 2012;35(4):1314–21.

58. Shin K-M, Kim I-T, Park Y-M, Ha J, Choi J-W, Park H-J, Lee YS, Lee K-T. Anti-inflammatory effect of caffeic acid methyl ester and its mode of action through the inhibition of prostaglandin E 2, nitric oxide and tumor necrosis factor-α production. Biochem Pharmacol. 2004;68(12):2327–36.

59. Guardia T, Rotelli AE, Juarez AO, Pelzer LE. Anti-inflammatory properties of plant flavonoids. Effects of rutin, quercetin and hesperidin on adjuvant arthritis in rat. Il farmaco. 2001;56(9):683–7.

60. Kroes B, Van den Berg A, Van Ufford HQ, Van Dijk H, Labadie R. Anti-inflammatory activity of gallic acid. Planta Med. 1992;58(06):499–504.

61. Hämäläinen M, Nieminen R, Vuorela P, Heinonen M, Moilanen E. Anti-inflammatory effects of flavonoids: genistein, kaempferol, quercetin, and daidzein inhibit STAT-1 and NF-κB activations, whereas flavone, isorhamnetin, naringenin, and pelargonidin inhibit only NF-κB activation along with their inhibitory effect on iNOS expression and NO production in activated macrophages. Mediat Inflamm. 2007;2007:45673.

62. Nakanishi T, Mukai K, Yumoto H, Hirao K, Hosokawa Y, Matsuo T. Anti-inflammatory effect of catechin on cultured human dental pulp cells affected by bacteria-derived factors. Eur J Oral Sci. 2010;118(2):145–50.

63. Funakoshi-Tago M, Nakamura K, Tago K, Mashino T, Kasahara T. Anti-inflammatory activity of structurally related flavonoids, Apigenin, Luteolin and Fisetin. Int Immunopharmacol. 2011;11(9):1150–9.

64. Jiang C-P, He X, Yang X-L, Zhang S-L, Li H, Song Z-J, Zhang C-F, Yang Z-L, Li P, Wang C-Z. Anti-rheumatoid arthritic activity of flavonoids from Daphne genkwa. Phytomedicine. 2014;21(6):830–7.

65. Hasan UH, Uttra AM, Rasool S. Evaluation of in vitro and in vivo anti-arthritic potential of Berberis calliobotrys. Bangla J Pharmacol. 2015;10(4):807–19.

66. Kumari RP, Anbarasu K. Protective role of C-Phycocyanin against secondary changes during sodium selenite mediated cataractogenesis. Nat prod bioprospect. 2014;4(2):81–9.

67. Khan MR, Rizvi W, Khan GN, Khan RA, Shaheen S. Carbon tetrachloride-induced nephrotoxicity in rats: protective role of Digera muricata. J Ethnopharmacol. 2009;122(1):91–9.

68. Kazmi STB, Majid M, Maryam S, Rahat A, Ahmed M, Khan MR, ul Haq I. Quercus dilatata Lindl. Ex Royle ameliorates BPA induced hepatotoxicity in Sprague Dawley rats. Biomed Pharmacother. 2018;102(728–38.

14

Phenolic contents, antimicrobial and antioxidant activity of *Olea ferruginea* Royle (Oleaceae)

Ansar Mehmood[1*] and Ghulam Murtaza[2]

Abstract

Background: *Olea ferruginea* Royle (Oleaceae) has long been used as an important ethnomedicinal plant to cure fever and debility, toothache, hoarseness, throatache and skeleton disorders. In this study, phenolic contents, antimicrobial and antioxidant activities of leaf and bark extracts (chloroform, ethanol and methanol) of *O. ferruginea* were evaluated.

Methods: Total phenolic contents were determined by Folin-Ciocalteu Spectrophotometric method. Antimicrobial activity was examined against *Bacillus subtilis* and *Staphylococcus aureus* (Gram positive), *Escherichia coli* (Gram negative), *Candida albicans* and *Sccharomyces cerevisiae* (yeas strains) by disc diffusion method. Antioxidant activity was observed through DPPH assay.

Results: The higher phenolic content was found in bark extract (376 µg/mg) of *O. ferruginea*. Chloroform extracts was found inactive against tested microorganisms while ethanol and methanol extracts showed pronounced inhibitory activity against both gram positive and gram negative bacteria. Only methanol extract of leaves inhibited the yeast strains. None of the bark extract inhibited the growth of tested yeast strains. The zones of inhibition formed by plant extracts were compared with zones of inhibition of available reference antibiotic discs such as tetracycline, ciprofloxacin and nystatin. Higher antioxidant activity was observed with methanol extracts of leaves and bark of *O. ferruginea*.

Conclusion: These findings show that *O. ferruginea* has potential antimicrobial and antioxidant activities. This study suggests a possible application of olive leaves and bark as sources of natural antimicrobial and antioxidants.

Keywords: Extract, *E. coli*, Ethnopharmacology

Background

Medicinal plants constitute a large group of economically significant plants having raw materials for the synthesis of medicines, flavors, perfumes and cosmetics. The products of these plants serve as valuable foundation of income for small owners and also add valuable foreign exchange for a country by export. No doubt, anti-microbial agents are the most significant therapeutic findings of the twentiethcentury. However, with the extensive use of antibiotics, human is now facing a problem of developing resistance in almost all pathogens [1].

Various type of sources such as microorganisms, plant, animals and oils have been explored to discover the new antimicrobial agents. The systematic screening of such sources like folk medicine result in the finding of innovative effective compounds [2]. Folk medicines are great source not only for curing health of the poor in developing countries but also in developed countries where conventional medicines are predominant for national health care [3]. The pathogens developed resistance to antibiotics which opened the door to use herbal medicines as antimicrobial agents [4].

Plant synthesized and produced different types of secondary metabolites which possess antimicrobial activity [5]. Formerly it was thought that secondary metabolites, not the products of the primary metabolic pathway, have no advantage to the plants who produced them.

* Correspondence: ansar.mehmood321@gmail.com
[1]Department of Botany, University of Poonch, Rawalakot, Azad Jammu and Kashmir 12350, Pakistan
Full list of author information is available at the end of the article

However, now it is believed that they containvigorous functions [6]. The search for new antibiotics which can replace conventional antibiotics is a need of hour. To meet this need present work was carried out to scan the antimicrobial and antioxidant activity of a valuable medicinal plant such as *O. ferruginea.*

Olive tree (*O. ferruginea* Royle), covers 8 million hectares in Mediterranean countries almost 98% of the world crop, is one of the most important fruit trees [7]. These figures show its pronounced economic and social meaning and the probable aids to be derived from exploitation of any of its byproducts [8]. The fruits and oil of *Olea*, important constituents of daily diet in a large part of the world's population, are widely studied for their alimentary use, whereas the leaves contain important secondary metabolites like oleuropein and oleacein, the former responsible for hypoglycemic activity [9] and the latter for hypotensive activity [10]. It was also shown by several studies that leaf extract of olive has the ability to reduce the blood pressure in animals [11], prevent intestinal muscle spasms and relieve arrhythmia [12]. Present work was aimed to investigate the phenolic contents, antimicrobial and antioxidant activity of *O. ferruginea.*

Methods
Plant materials
In this study, *Olea ferruginea* (stem bark and leaves) was selected for its antimicrobial and antioxidant potential. The plant was collected from Kotli in 2017 and identified by a taxonomist Dr. Sajjad Hussain, Department of Botany, University of Poonch Rawalakot. The voucher specimen (KNV 416) was submitted in the Herbarium, University of Poonch Rawalakot. The plant material was obtained in the course of flowering stage. Both bark and leaves were shade dried at room temperature (25 ± 2 °C).

Extraction procedure
After drying, a fine powder of bark and leaves was made using electric grinder. For extraction, Fifty g powder was soaked with 200 ml of chloroform, ethanol and methanol solvents in three separate flasks. The maceration was carried out at room temperature in each solvent for 7 days with constantly shaking after every 24 h. After maceration, the mixture was filtered using Whatmann filter paper in labeled flasks. The filtrate was evaporated at low temperature and pressure by a rotary evaporator to obtain the crude extract [13].

Dilution
Ten mg crude extract was dissolve in 1 ml respective solvents (chloroform, ethanol and methanol) to make 10 mg/ml dilution.

Microorganisms
All the tested bacteria (*Bacillus subtilis, Staphylococcus arureus* and *Escherichia coli*) were obtained from Combined Military Hospital (CMH) Muzaffarabad while the tested yeasts (*Candida albicans* and *Sccharomyces cerevisiae*) were grown in Laboratory, Department of Botany, University of Azad Jammu and Kashmir, Muzaffarabad.

Culture media
Nutrient agar medium (28 g dehydrated nutrient agar in 1000 ml distilled water, warmed and shake) was used for culturing bacterial species. The fungal species were cultured in Sabouraud's dextrose agar (65 g Sabouraud's dextrose agar in 1000 ml distilled water). Both the media were autoclaved for 15 min at 121 °C.

Antimicrobial assay
Disc diffusion essay proposed by [14] was used to test the extracts of plants for their antimicrobial activities. The microorganisms were suspended in 10 ml distilled water by dipping a loop of organism in sterilized labeled test tube. From test tube, 1 ml dilution was transported in the corresponding sterilized petri plates. The dilution and medium were mix in petri plates by gently shaking and kept at room temperature for solidification.

Sterilized filter paper discs of 6 mm in diameter were dipped in each 10 mg/ml crude extracts (chloroform, ethanol and methanol) of *O. ferruginea* and placed on agar medium in petri plates at their labeled positions. Commercially available antibiotics (Tetracyline, ciprolaxacine, and nystatin) were used as positive control and water, chloroform, ethanol and methanol as negative control. The experiment was performed in aseptic environment.

Incubation of plates
The plates containing the bacterial and yeasts culture were incubated at 37 °C for 24 h and 25 °C for 72 h respectively. The zones of inhibition were measured in millimeter by using measuring scale.

Antioxidant activity
To determine antioxidant activity of selected plants, the DPPH (2,2-diphenyl-1-picrylhydrazyl) radical scavenging assay [15] was used to determine the antioxidant activity of different extracts of leaves and bark of *O. ferruginea*. The DPPH solution fades its color when received hydrogen ions from antioxidant, which was initially violet. A stock of DPPH was prepared by adding 7 mg DPPH in 100 ml of methanol. The DPPH solution, methanol and extracts with various concentrations (1.25 mg/ul, 2.5 mg/ul and 5 mg/ul) were added in labeled test tubes for sample and blank reading, mixed well and kept it for 30 min at room temperature. Ascorbic acid was used as control. The optical density was measured against standard at λ_{max} 517 nm by using UV

visible spectrophotometer. The experiments were carried out in triplicate. The percentage radicals scavenging activity was calculated by using following formula

$$\%\text{Inhibition} = \left[\frac{\text{Absorbance of control} - \text{Absorbance of tested sample}}{\text{Absorbance of control}} \right]$$
$$\times 100$$

Where standard is the absorbance of control reaction (containing all reagents except the test compounds). 50% inhibition (IC50) of each extract concentrations against graph of inhibition was calculated by applying SSP10 software.

Phenolic estimation

Folin-Ciocalteu Spectrophotometric method described by Kim et al. [16] was used to determine the total phenolc content of plant extracts on a UV-vis spectrophotometer at 650 nm. Results were expressed as catechol equivalents (µg/mg).

Statistical analysis

A statistical analysis was used to interpret the antimicrobial and antioxidant results. The experiment was conducted in completely randomized design with 3 replicates. The results are presented as means ±standard error of means using MS excel [17].

Results

Antimicrobial activity

Figure 1 shows the antimicrobial activity of crude leaf extracts of O. ferruginea while Fig. 2 shows the antimicrobial activity of crude bark extracts of O. ferrugnea. The antimicrobial activity of negative controls such as water, chloroform, ethanol and methanol is shown in Fig. 3. The chloroform extract from both leaves and bark did not inhibit the growth of any of the tested organisms and found to be inactive. Ethanol leaf extract was less active against B. subtilis i.e. 8.33 ± 0.33 mm while it

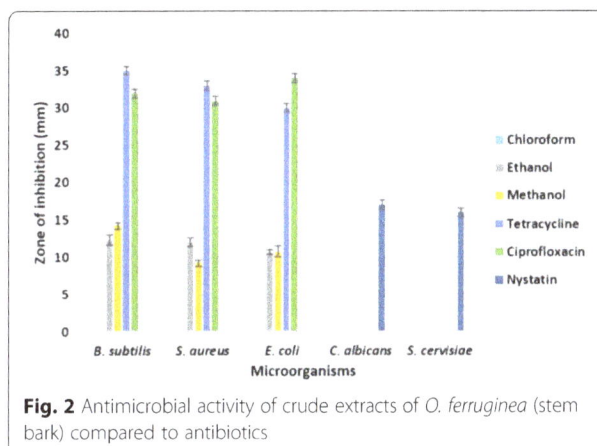

Fig. 2 Antimicrobial activity of crude extracts of O. ferruginea (stem bark) compared to antibiotics

showed appreciable bactericidal activity against S. aureus and E. coli i.e. 11.00 ± 0.58 mm and 10.00 ± 0.58 mm. While C. albicans and S. cerevisiae were resistant to ethanolic leaf extract. Ethanol bark extract showed good inhibitory activity against B. subtilis (12.33 ± 0.67 mm) and S. aureus (12.00 ± 0.58 mm) while it was moderately active against E. coli (10.67 ± 0.33 mm). It was also unable to inhibit the growth of yeast strains.

Methanolic leaf extract induced higher antimicrobial activity against B. subtilis and S. aureus (14.00 ± 0.58 mm, 18.33 ± 0.58 mm) respectively. It also showed a considerable amount of activity against E. coli with zone of inhibition of 11.33 ± 0.33 mm. Methanol leaf extract also inhibited the growth of C. albicans and S. cerevisiae with zones of 9.00 ± 0.58 mm and 9.33 ± 0.33 mm. It was also observed that Gram positive bacteria are more susceptibleto the tested extracts than gram negative bacterium. The highest activity (18.33 ± 0.58 mm) was found of methanol extract of leaves of O. europaea against S. aureus.

Phenolic contents

Tables 1 and 2 shows the total phenolic contents in crude extracts of O. ferruginea and were reported as catechol equivalents (µg/mg). The higher phenolic

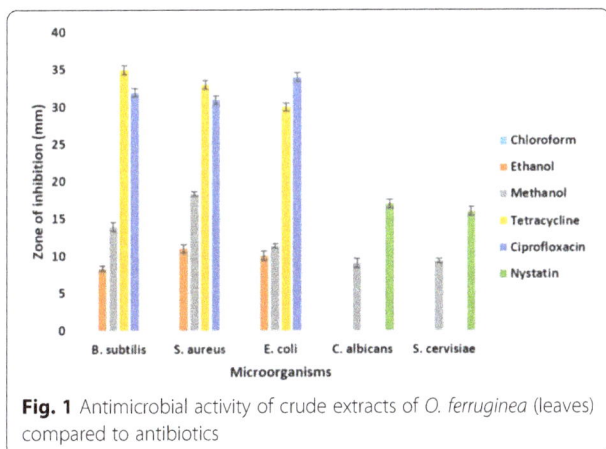

Fig. 1 Antimicrobial activity of crude extracts of O. ferruginea (leaves) compared to antibiotics

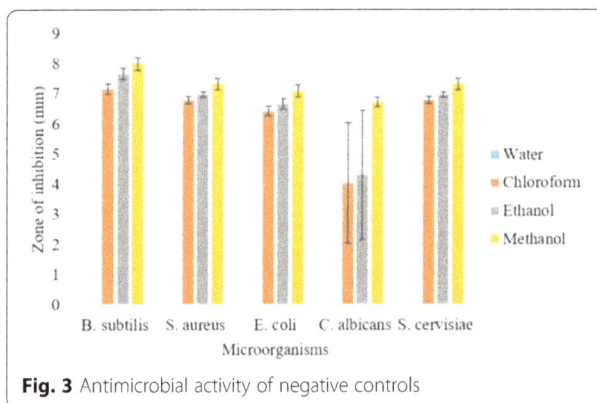

Fig. 3 Antimicrobial activity of negative controls

Table 1 Phenolic content and IC50 value in *O. ferruginea*leaves

Solvent used	Stem bark	
	Phenolic contents (µg/mg)	IC $_{50}$ value (mg/ml)
Chloroform	312	0.84
Ethanol	351	0.56
Methanol	399	0.46

compounds (376 µg/mg) were present in the methanol extract, followed by ethanol (321 µg/mg) and chloroform extract (288 µg/mg) of leaves of *O. ferruginea*. In stem bark extract, highest phenol was reported in methanol (399 µg/mg), followed by ethanol (351 µg/mg) and chloroform (312 µg/mg).

Free radical scavenging activity

Free radical (DPPH) scavenging activity of leaves of *O. ferruginea* is shown in Fig. 4 in the form of percentage inhibition. According to Fig. 4, chloroform, ethanol and methanol showed 22.22 ± 0.03, 42.48 ± 0.05 and 25.26 ± 0.01 free scavenging activity respectively at 1.25 mg/ml. the extracts of 2.50 mg/ml concentration of chloroform, ethanol and methanol revealed 26.68 ± 0.02, 34.03 ± 0.03 and 49.71 ± 0.03 respectively. While chloroform, ethanol and methanol extracts at 5.00 mg/ml concentration showed 40.22 ± 0.06, 60.15 ± 0.03 and 71.24 ± 0.02 activity respectively. Figure 5 shows the results of the free radical (DPPH) scavenging activity in % inhibition of stem bark of *O. ferruginea*. The result suggested that the chloroform, ethanol and methanol extract of leaves exhibited antioxidant activities of 23.56 ± 0.01, 26.05 ± 0.02 and 31.41 ± 0.05 respectively at a concentration of 1.25 mg/ml. At concentration of 2.50 mg/ml, the chloroform, ethanol and methanol extract of leaves showed 29.34 ± 0.06, 35.82 ± 0.06 and 40.67 ± 0.03 antioxidant activity respectively. Similarly chloroform, ethanol and methanol extract at 5.00 mg/ml concentration showed antioxidant activity of 47.33 ± 0.06, 60.72 ± 0.03 and 73.97 ± 0.02 respectively.

Half maximum inhibitory concentration (IC$_{50}$ value)

Tables 1 and 2 also shows the IC$_{50}$ value of chloroform extract (0.8 mg/ml), ethanol (0.55 mg/ml) and methanol extract (0.45 mg/ml) of leaves of *O. ferruginea*. While stem bark showed IC$_{50}$ value of 0.67, 0.46 and

Table 2 Phenolic content and IC$_{50}$ value in *O. ferruginea* stem bark

Solvent used	Leaves	
	Phenolic contents (µg/mg)	IC 50Value (µg/ml)
Chloroform	288	0.67
Ethanol	321	0.47
Methanol	376	0.37

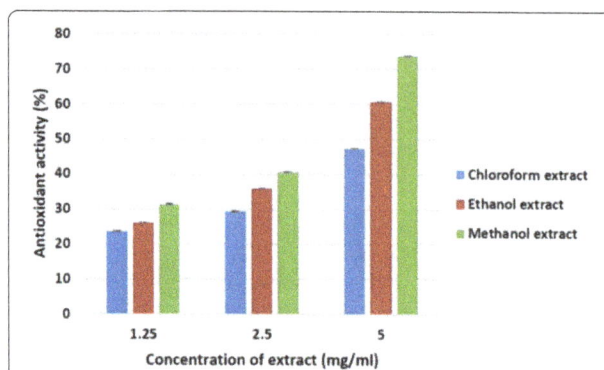

Fig. 4 Antioxidant activity of *O. ferruginea* leaves in different solvents

0.37 mg/ml with chloroform, ethanol and methanol extracts respectively.

Discussion

Medicinal plants are the active source of both traditional as well as modern medicines. The active compounds present in herbal medicines have the compensations of being joined with several other compounds that seem to be inactive. However as compared to isolated and pure active compounds, the bio compounds present in plants give them far superior security and efficiency as a whole [18]. Many studies have been carried out to investigate the antibacterial and antifungal activities of essential oil of olive. The presented work was conducted to observe the antimicrobial activity of medicinal plant as *O. ferruginea* against gram positive bacteria, gram negative bacterium and yeast strains. From the results it was observed that Gram positive bacteria (*B. subtilis and S. aureus*) were more sensitive as compared to gram negative bacterium (*E. coli*) used. The results were well correlated to findings of [19] where gram negative bacterium *E. coli* was also more resistant to the extracts of *S. xanthocarpum*. It was also observed that methanol extract showed highest inhibitory activity because of its high polarity and it allows extracting all the phenolic compounds. In addition, as compared to isolated compounds, extracts can be more

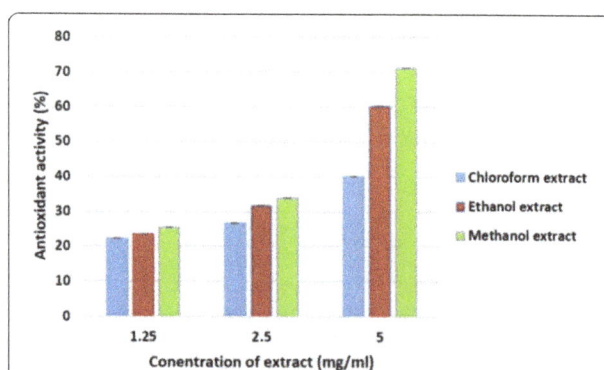

Fig. 5 Antioxidant activity of *O. ferruginea* stem bark in different solvents

beneficial. Since in presence of other compounds in the extracts, an individual bioactive component can change its properties [20]. It was also found that n-hexane fraction of leaf of *O. ferruginea* has higher biological activity against gram positive and gram negative bacteria as compared to chloroform and methanol. While in our study methanol extract was found to have higher antimicrobial activity [21].

It is observed from present results that active antimicrobial biocompounds could be extracted in ethanol and methanol extracts. Except phenolics, bound to insoluble carbohydrates or proteins, most of the compounds extract in methanol or acetone [22]. In present study, ethanolic and methanolic extractions of *O. ferruginea* were found to have acceptable antimicrobial activities with respect to reference antibiotic discs (Fig. 1). It was observed in present study that plant extracts showed high inhibitory activity against bacteria in contrast to fungi. Previously extracts of *Bellis perennis* have also shown more activity towards bacteria [23]. Moreover, methanolic extract was found more active in our studies which is correlated to results of [24], methanol extract of *H. afficinalis* was more active against *P. aeruginosa* and *B. subtillus*. The antimicrobial activity of plants may be the consequence of presence of wide range of bioactive compounds. Plant extracts comprise many polyphenols, flavonoids and alkaloids which could be antimicrobial representatives. Many studies show the association between antimicrobial activities of plants and the phytochemicals present in them. Flavonoids are well known for their antiviral [25], antimicrobial [26] and spasmolytic [27] activities. Likewise, alkaloids extracted from plants have also shown antimicrobial activity [28]. The inhibition of microbial growth may result from the binding of biocompounds to the cell wall.

The antioxidant activity of plants and their natural products is widely evaluated by using scavenging activity for free radicals of 1.1-diphenyl-2-picrylhydrazyl (DPPH).The methanol extract of stem bark of *O. ferruginea* showed higher radical scavenging activity (73.97 ± 0.02) followed by ethanol and chloroform extracts. Overall, methanol extracts have shown higher antioxidant activity. It has already been proven that phenolic compounds are best extracted in ethanol and methanol solvents [29]. Total phenolic content was found higher in methanol extract as compared to ethanol and chloroform extracts. Therefore, it can be easily assume that DPPH free radical scavenging activity is corresponded to present of bioactive compounds like phenols, as methanol extract showed highest antioxidant activity. A significant variation was found in total phenolic content among the different extracts of stem bark and leaf extract of *O. ferruginea*. Free radicals such as superoxide, hydroxyl, peroxyl and singly oxygen play a vital role in many disease conditions. Herbal drugs, comprising free radical scavengers, are getting prominence in treating such diseases.

Many plants shows competent antioxidant properties due to presence of phytochemicals including phenolic compounds [30].

The amount or concentration of substrate causes 50% loss of the DPPH activity is known as its IC50 and it is calculated by plotting a linear regression of antiradical activity in percentage against the amount of compounds tested. Methanol extracts showed being the lowest IC50 values which shows highest antioxidant activity. As compared to leaves extracts, stem bark extracts of *O. ferruginea* exhibited significant activity with low IC50 value. Moreover, a linear relationship was found between the total polyphenol and the reciprocal of IC50 value, indicating that polyphenols are directly proportional to antioxidant activity. Similar results were recorded by [31].

Conclusion

O. ferruginea is known for treating many important infectious diseases including to kill cancerous cells. Different crude extracts of tested plants were prepared by using various solvents with the aim of screening better antimicrobial activities in comparison with some standard antibiotics. Among these, the extract obtained with methanol was found to have a better effectiveness against the tested bacteria and also has highest antioxidant activities. The results of present study support the use of this valuable plant in traditional medicines for treating infectious diseases. Further phytochemicals studies are needed to find the major bioactive compounds responsible for antimicrobial and antioxidant effect of this plant.

Acknowledgments
We are thankful to Combined Military Hospital for providing clinical pathogens.

Authors' contributions
AM carried out the experimental work and wrote the manuscript. GM designed experiment and helped out in data analysis. Both authors have read and approved the manuscript, and ensure that this is the case.

Competing interests
The authors declare that they have no competing interests.

Author details
[1]Department of Botany, University of Poonch, Rawalakot, Azad Jammu and Kashmir 12350, Pakistan. [2]Department of Botany, University of Azad Jammu and Kashmir, Muzaffarabad 13100, Pakistan.

References
1. Peterson LR, Dalhoff A. Towards targeted prescribing: will the cure for antimicrobial resistance be specific, directed therapy through improved diagnostic testing? J Antimicrob Chemotherap. 2004;53:902–5.
2. Janovska D, Kubikova K, Kokoska L. Screening for antimicrobial activity of some medicinal plants species of traditional Chinese medicine. Czech J Food Sci. 2003;21:107–10.
3. Lanfranco G. Invited review article on traditional medicine. Electron J Biotechnol. 1999;2:1–3.

4. Martin F, Oliver AM, Kearney JF. Marginal zone and B1 B cells unite in the early response against T-independent blood-borne particulate antigens. Immunity. 2001;14:617–29.

5. Cowan MM. Plant products as antimicrobial agents. Clin Microbiol Rev. 1999;12:564–82.

6. Upadhyay RK, Dwivedi P, Ahmad S. Screening of antibacterial activity of six plant essential oils against pathogenic bacterial strains. Asian J Med Sci. 2010;2:152–8.

7. Guinda A, Perez-Camino MC, Lanzon A. Supplementation of oils with oleanolic acid from the olive leaf (Olea europaea). Eur J Lipid Sc Technol. 2004;106:22–6.

8. Tabera J, Guinda A, Ruiz-Rodriguez A, Senorans FJ, Ibanez E, Albi T, Reglero G. Countercurrent supercritical fluid extraction and fractionation of high-added-value compounds from a hexane extract of olive leaves. J Agri Food Chem. 2004;52:4774–9.

9. Gonzalez M, Zarzuelo A, Gamez M, Utrilla M, Jimenez J, Osuna I. Hypoglycemic activity of olive leaf. Planta Med. 1992;58:513–5.

10. Hansen K, Adsersen A, Christensen SB, Jensen SR, Nyman U, Smitt UW. Isolation of an angiotensin converting enzyme (ACE) inhibitor from Olea europaea and Olea lancea. Phytomedicine. 1996;2:319–25.

11. Zarzuelo A, Duarte J, Jimenez J, Gonzalez M, Utrilla M. Vasodilator effect of olive leaf. Planta Med. 1991;57:417–9.

12. Benavente-Garcia O, Castillo J, Lorente J, Ortuno A, Del-Rio J. Antioxidant activity of phenolics extracted from Olea europaea L. leaves. Food Chem. 2000;68:457–62.

13. Hussain A, Murtaza G, Mehmood A, Qureshi RA. Conservation of indigenous knowledge of medicinal plants of Western Himalayan region Rawalakot, Azad Kashmir, Pakistan. Pak J Pharm Sci. 2017;30:773–82.

14. Bauer A, Kirby W, Sherris JC, Turck M. Antibiotic susceptibility testing by a standardized single disk method. Amer J Clin Pathol. 1996;45:493.

15. Amarowicz R, Estrella I, Hernández T, Robredo S, Troszyńska A, Kosińska A, Pegg RB. Free radical-scavenging capacity, antioxidant activity, and phenolic composition of green lentil (Lens culinaris). Food Chem. 2010;121:705–11.

16. Kim KT, Yoo KM, Lee JW, Eom SH, Hwang IK, Lee CY. Protective effect of steamed American ginseng (Panax quinquefolius L.) on V79-4 cells induced by oxidative stress. J Ethnopharmacol. 2007;111:443–50.

17. Steel RG, Torrie JH, Dickey DA. Principles and procedures of statistics: a biological approach. New York: McGraw-Hill; 1997.

18. Shariff ZU. Modern herbal therapy for common ailments. Ibadan: Spectrum Books; 2001.

19. Salar RK. Evaluation of antimicrobial potential of different extracts of Solanum xanthocarpum Schrad, and Wendl. Afri J Microbiol Res. 2009;3:97–100.

20. Borchers AT, Keen CL, Gershwin ME. Mushrooms, tumors, and immunity: an update. Experim Biol Med. 2004;229:393–406.

21. Amin A, Khan MA, Shah S, Ahmad M, Zafar M, Hameed A. Inhibitory effects of Olea ferruginea crude leaves extract against some bacterial and fungal pathogen. Pak J Pharm Sci. 2013;26(2):251–4.

22. Van-Sumere C. Phenols and Phenolic Acids. Methods Plant Biochem. 2012;1:29.

23. Avato P, Vitali C, Mongelli P, Tava A. Antimicrobial activity of polyacetylenes from Bellis perennis and their synthetic derivatives. Planta Med. 1997;63:503–7.

24. Jankovsky M, Landa T. Genus Hyssopus L. Recent knowledge. Horticult Sci. 2002;29:119–23.

25. Karamoddini MK. Antiviral activities of aerial subsets of Artemisia species against herpes simplex virus type 1 (HSV1) in vitro. Asian Biomed. 2011;5:63.

26. Maria LA, Maria RF. Studies on the antimicrobial activity and brine shrimp toxicity of Z. tuberculosa extracts and their main constituents. Ann Clin Microbiol Antimicrob. 2009;8:16.

27. Julianeli T, Jackson R, Kelly S, Sílvia S. Selective spasmolytic effect of a new furanoflavoquinone derivative from diplotropin on Guinea-pig trachea. J Chem Pharm Res. 2011;3:249–58.

28. Ahmed EHM, Nour BY, Mohammed YG, Khalid HS. Antiplasmodial activity of some medicinal plants used in Sudanese folk-medicine. Environ Health Insights. 2010;4:1.

29. Siddhuraju P, Becker K. Antioxidant properties of various solvent extracts of total phenolic constituents from three different agroclimatic origins of drumstick tree (Moringa oleifera lam.) leaves. J Agri Food Chem. 2003;51:2144–55.

30. Larson RA. The antioxidants of higher plants. Phytochemistry. 1988;27:969–78.

31. Katsube T, Tabata H, Ohta Y, Yamasaki Y, Anuurad E, Shiwaku K, Yamane Y. Screening for antioxidant activity in edible plant products: comparison of low-density lipoprotein oxidation assay, DPPH radical scavenging assay, and Folin-Ciocalteu assay. J Agri Food Chem. 2004;52:2391–6.

15

Protective effects and mechanisms of *Terminalia catappa* L. methenolic extract on hydrogen-peroxide-induced oxidative stress in human skin fibroblasts

Ya-Han Huang[1], Po-Yuan Wu[2,3], Kuo-Ching Wen[1], Chien-Yih Lin[4*] and Hsiu-Mei Chiang[1*]

Abstract

Background: Oxidative stress plays a crucial role in aging-related phenomenon, including skin aging and photoaging. This study investigated the protective role and possible mechanism of *Terminalia catappa* L. methanolic extract (TCE) in human fibroblasts (Hs68) against hydrogen peroxide (H_2O_2)-induced oxidative damage.

Methods: Various in vitro antioxidant assays were performed in this study. The effect and mechanisms of TCE on oxidative stress-induced oxidative damage were studied by using western blotting.

Results: The IC_{50} of TCE was 8.2 μg/mL for 1,1-diphenyl-2-picrylhydrazyl radical scavenging, 20.7 μg/mL for superoxide anion radical scavenging, 173.0 μg/mL for H_2O_2 scavenging, 44.8 μg/mL for hydroxyl radical scavenging, and 427.6 μg/mL for ferrous chelation activities. Moreover, TCE inhibited the H_2O_2-induced mitogen-activated protein kinase signaling pathway, resulting in the inhibition of c-Jun, c-Fos, matrix metalloproteinase (MMP)-1, MMP-3, MMP-9, and cyclooxygenase-2 expression. TCE also increased hemeoxygenase-1 expression inhibited by H_2O_2. Finally, TCE was demonstrated reverse type I procollagen expression in fibroblasts after H_2O_2 treatment.

Conclusions: According to our findings, TCE is a potent antioxidant and protective agent that can be used in antioxidative stress-induced skin aging.

Keywords: Oxidative stress, Reactive oxygen species, Aging, Hemeoxygenase-1 (HO-1), Extracellular matrix

Background

Aging can be divided into two basic processes: intrinsic aging, which is related to age, and extrinsic aging, which is generally due to long-term exposure to environmental factors, including ultraviolet (UV) light and pollutants. Oxidative stress plays a crucial role in aging-related disorders, including atherosclerosis, cardiovascular diseases and skin aging [1]. High levels of reactive oxygen species (ROS), such as hydrogen peroxide (H_2O_2), superoxide anion, and singlet oxygen, can cause oxidative damage to cellular DNA, protein, and lipids, resulting in the initiation or development of various disorders and diseases

such as cardiovascular diseases, type 2 diabetes mellitus, and cancer [2]. In addition, free transition metal ions combine with H_2O_2 and can cause extensive oxidative damage to biomolecules such as lipids, proteins, and nucleic acids, leading to age-related disorders [3].

Skin aging is characterized by a sagging appearance, wrinkles, and pigmentary changes, and principally manifests as the degradation of extracellular matrix (ECM) proteins, including type I collagen, elastin, proteoglycans, and fibronectin [4, 5]. Type I collagen is the most abundant structural protein in skin connective tissue and is primarily synthesized by fibroblasts, whereas collagen in the dermis is responsible for skin strength and resiliency [6, 7]. Oxidative stress or inflammation can cause collagen degradation resulting in wrinkle formation and sagging skin [8]. In addition, ROS activate the mitogen-activated protein kinase (MAPK) pathway, which subsequently induces

---

* Correspondence: yihlin@asia.edu.tw; hmchiang@mail.cmu.edu.tw
[4]Department of Biotechnology, Asia University, 500 Liufeng Road, Wufeng District, Taichung City 41354, Taiwan
[1]Department of Cosmeceutics, China Medical University, 91 Hsueh-Shih Road, Taichung 40402, Taiwan
Full list of author information is available at the end of the article

the expression and activation of matrix metalloproteinases (MMPs) in human skin [9]. The activation of MAPK and MMPs may cause damage and aging of the skin [10, 11]. Agents that can elevate ECM protein levels or downregulate collagen-degrading enzymes, such as MMPs, may prove useful in the development of effective antiaging agents [12, 13].

Terminalia catappa L. belongs to the family Combretaceae, and in Southeast Asia, it is commonly used as a folk medicine for treating hepatoma and hepatitis [14, 15]. The leaf and bark extracts of *T. catappa* have been reported to exhibit chemopreventive, antioxidant, hepatoprotective, and anti-inflammatory activities [16, 17]. *T. catappa* includes the phytochemicals of flavanoids (rutin, isoorientin, vitexin, and isovitexin), tannins (chebulagic acid, punicalagin, punicalin, and terflavins A and B), and triterpenoids (asiatic acid and ursolic acid) [14, 18]. In addition, the *T. catappa* extract exhibits antifungal and antidepressant activities [19, 20]. Topical application of ointment containing *T. catappa* was shown to promote wound healing in rats [21], and our previous study demonstrated that the *T. catappa* L. hydrophilic extract exerts protective effects on UVB-induced photoaging by inhibiting MMPs expression and upregulating type I procollagen expression [22]. However, the activity and related mechanisms of *T. catappa* against oxidative stress-induced skin damaging are unclear. Therefore, this study investigated the effects of *T. catappa* methanolic extract (TCE) on H_2O_2-induced skin damage and on the protein expression of MAPKs, which activate protein-1 (AP-1), MMPs, and type I procollagen in human skin fibroblasts (Hs68).

Methods
Chemicals
Fetal bovine serum (FBS), penicillin-streptomycin, trypsin-EDTA, and Dulbecco's Modified Eagle's Medium (DMEM) were purchased from Gibco, Invitrogen (Carlsbad, CA, USA). The Bradford reagent was supplied by Bio-Rad Laboratories (Hercules, CA, USA), and Tris and MTT were purchased from USB (Cleveland, OH, USA). Methanol, dimethyl sulfoxide, doxycycline hyclate, calcium chloride ($CaCl_2$), DPPH, DL-dithiothreitol, and all other reagents used in this study were purchased from Sigma-Aldrich Chemicals (St. Louis, MO, USA).

Preparation and quantitation of TCE
T. catappa leaves were collected in Wufeng, Taichung City, Taiwan, as previously described [22]. The leaves were identified by Professor KC Wen, a professor in Department of Cosmeceutics, China Medical University and a voucher specimen of this material (FCRDSAL-Plants-0003) has been deposited in Functional Cosmeceutics Research & Development and Safety Assessment Laboratory, China

Medical University, Taiwan. The dried leaves (150 g) were ground and then extracted twice with 2 L of methanol for 1 h by using ultrasonication. The extraction liquid was filtrated, and the filtrate was evaporated to dryness in a vacuum to obtain TCE.

The total phenolic content of TCE was measured using the Folin–Ciocalteu reaction, as previously described [23]. Briefly, TCE was mixed with the Folin–Ciocalteu phenol reagent and sodium carbonate, and absorbance was measured at 760 nm. The phenolic content is expressed as microgram GAE/microgram *T. catappa* leaf dry weight herein.

The total flavonoid content of TCE was determined using the aluminum chloride colorimetric assay, as described elsewhere [23]. Briefly, TCE was mixed with aluminum chloride hexahydrate, potassium acetate, and deionized water, and the absorbance of the mixture was measured at 405 nm on an enzyme-linked immunosorbent assay (ELISA) reader (Tecan, Grödig, Austria). The flavonoid content is expressed as microgram QE/microgram *T. catappa* leaf dry weight herein.

DPPH radical scavenging activity assay
DPPH was mixed with various concentrations of TCE. The mixture was added to a 96-well microplate and incubated at room temperature for 30 min in the dark. Subsequently, absorbance was measured at 492 nm on the ELISA reader. Ascorbic acid was used as a positive control [24, 25].

Superoxide anion radical scavenging activity assay
Dihydronicotinamide-adenine dinucleotide, phenazine-methosulfate, and nitroblue tetrazolium were prepared in 0.1 M phosphate buffered saline (PBS), after which TCE was added. Absorbance was measured at 560 nm on the ELISA reader.

Determination of peroxide scavenging activity
The peroxide scavenging activity of TCE was spectrophotometrically detected using a previously described method [23, 26]. H_2O_2 was prepared in PBS and mixed with various concentrations of TCE. Then, after incubation, absorption was measured at 230 nm on the ELISA reader.

Hydroxyl radical scavenging activity assay
The hydroxyl radical scavenging activity assay was performed by mixing TCE, ascorbic acid, deoxyribose, iron (III) chloride, EDTA, H_2O_2, a monopotassium phosphate–potassium hydroxide buffer, and distilled water; the mixture was then incubated at 100 °C for 15 min and centrifuged. The absorbance of the supernatant was subsequently measured at 532 nm on a microplate reader (BioTek, Winooski, VT, USA). Mannitol was used as a positive control, and the hydroxyl radical

scavenging activity of TCE was obtained as the percentage inhibition of deoxyribose degradation [3, 27].

Ferrous ion chelating activity assay

Various concentrations of TCE were mixed with an iron (II) chloride solution. The reaction was initiated after ferrozine was added. Absorbance was then spectrophotometrically measured at 562 nm on the microplate reader. The results are expressed as the percentage inhibition of the generation of the ferrozine–ferrous complex herein [24].

Measurement of reducing power

The reducing power of TCE was determined using a previously described method [24, 28]. Various concentrations of TCE were mixed with ferrocyanate and trichloroacetic acid. After centrifugation, the supernatant was mixed with ferric chloride and absorbance was measured at 700 nm. Ascorbic acid and distilled water were used as the positive and negative controls, respectively.

Cell cultures

Hs68, HaCaT cells, and B16F0 cells were purchased from the Bioresource Collection and Research Center in Hsinchu, Taiwan. These cells were maintained in DMEM containing 10% FBS, 100 U/mL penicillin, and 100 U/mL streptomycin in an incubator set at 37 °C.

Cell viability assay for three skin cell lines

To understand the cytotoxicity of TCE on the skin, Hs68, HaCaT cells, and B16F0 cells were applied to study the cell viability. The cells were seeded in the plate, allowed to attach overnight, and were treated with 1 mL of various concentrations of TCE dissolved in DMEM for 24 h. The cytotoxicity of TCE was then evaluated using the MTT assay, as described elsewhere [22].

Fluorescence assay for IntracellularROS generation in fibroblasts

Intracellular ROS generation was measured using a previously detailed method [22]. In brief, fibroblasts were added to a 24-well plate and then incubated with various concentrations of TCE for 24 h. The cells were washed with PBS and incubated with 150 μM H_2O_2 for 1 h. Subsequently, the cells were incubated with 10 μM DCFDA in DMEM for 30 min, after which they were examined under a fluorescence microscope (Leica DMIL, Wetzlar, Germany). Fluorescence (emission wavelength: 520 nm; excitation wavelength: 488 nm) was measured on a microplate reader (Thermo Electron Corporation, Vantaa, Finland).

Western blotting

The cells were incubated with TCE (5–50 μg/mL) for 4 h, followed by incubation with 150 μM H_2O_2 for 1 h. The cells were collected and lysed with protein extraction buffer, as previously described [22]. An equal amount of protein was loaded, separated on 10% sodium dodecyl sulfate polyacrylamide gels, and then electrophoretically transferred to a polyvinylidene difluoride membrane. The membrane was incubated with specific antibodies against MMP-1, – 3, and – 9; type I procollagen; HO-1; MAPKs; c-Jun; c-Fos; and COX-2 (Santa Cruz Biotechnology, Inc., Santa Cruz, CA, USA). The blots were then incubated with anti-immunoglobulin G-horseradish peroxidase and chemiluminescent detection reagent (Amersham Biosciences, Buckinghamshire, United Kingdom). Finally, immunoreactive bands were detected using a chemiluminescent detection system (LAS-4000, Fujifilm, Tokyo, Japan), and the density of the bands was determined using a densitometric program (Multi Gauge V2.2, Fujifilm, Tokyo, Japan).

Statistical analyses

Values are presented as the mean ± standard deviation of at least three independent experiments. The results were analyzed using one-way analysis of variance, followed by Scheffe's test. Statistical significance was set at $p < 0.05$.

Results

Extraction yield and quantitation of TCE

The extraction yield of TCE from leaves was 11.5%. The total phenolic content of the extract was determined using the Folin–Ciocalteu method, and the regression coefficient of the calibration curve was 0.9995. Specifically, the total phenolic content of TCE was 220.2 ± 0.2 μg/mg gallic acid equivalent (GAE). Additionally, the total flavonoid content of TCE was determined using the aluminum chloride colorimetric method, and the regression coefficient of the calibration curve was 0.9991. The total flavonoid content was 109.0 ± 0.8 μg/mg quercetin equivalent (QE). The content of gallic acid was 74.62 μg/mL by HPLC/UV analysis (Additional file 1: S1).

The antioxidant activity of TCE

The antioxidant activity of TCE was study by using free radical scavenging assay and chelating assay. Figure 1a shows the DPPH radical scavenging activity of TCE and 10 μg/mL ascorbic acid (positive control). The results indicated that 10 μg/mL TCE exhibited a scavenging activity of 70.4% ± 4.9%, and that the activity was 99.0% ± 1.6% for the same concentration of ascorbic acid. The IC_{50} of TCE for DPPH scavenging activity was 5.6 μg/mL; in other words, TCE preparations exhibited potent DPPH free radical scavenging activity. As shown in Fig. 1b, the superoxide anion radical scavenging activity was 49.5% ± 0.2% for 250 μg/mL beta hydroxyl acid (BHA) (positive control), and ranged from 73.9% ± 2.1% to 92.4% ± 2.0% for 50–1000 μg/mL TCE. The IC_{50} of TCE

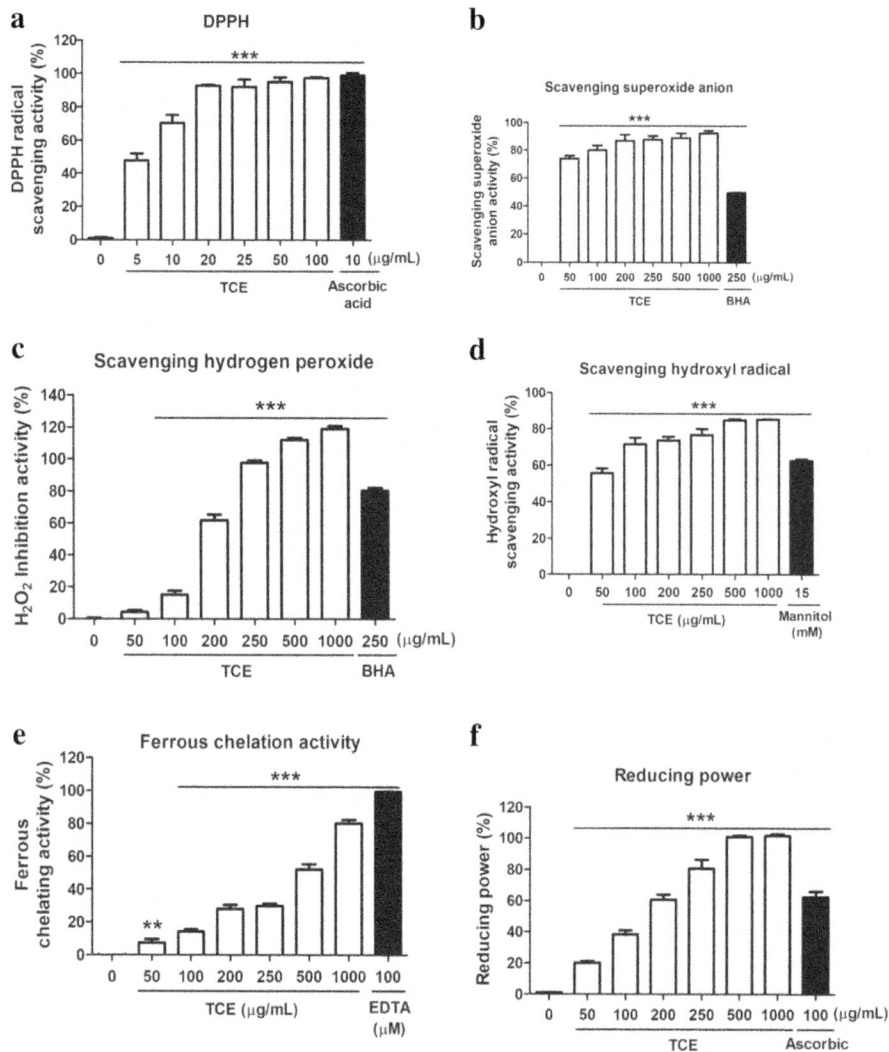

Fig. 1 The aioxidant activity of *Terminalia catappa* L. methenolic extract (TCE). **a** 1,1-diphenyl-2-picrylhydrazyl radical scavenging activity of TCE; **b** Superoxide anion radical scavenging activity of TCE; **c** Peroxide scavenging activity of TCE; **d** Hydroxyl radical scavenging activity of TCE; **e** Ferrous chelating activity of TCE; and **f** Reducing power of TCE. Significant difference versus control (without extract): *$p < 0.05$; **$p < 0.01$; ***$p < 0.001$

for superoxide anion radical scavenging was 20.6 µg/mL. Thus, the superoxide anion radical scavenging activity of TCE was superior to that of BHA. The peroxide scavenging activities of TCE (50–1000 µg/mL) and the positive control BHA (250 µg/mL) are shown in Fig. 1c. Specifically, the peroxide scavenging activity ranged from 4.2% ± 1.2% to 111.8% ± 1.3% for various concentrations of TCE, and was 80.4% ± 1.8% for BHA. Notably, the peroxide scavenging activity of TCE was superior to that of BHA (IC_{50} = 166.1 µg/mL). The hydroxyl radical scavenging activities of TCE (50–1000 µg/mL) and the positive control mannitol (15 mM) are shown in Fig. 1d. Specifically, the hydroxyl radical scavenging activity ranged from 55.7% ± 2.6% to 85.3% ± 0.1% for various concentrations of TCE, and was 62.0% ± 0.9% for mannitol. The IC_{50} of TCE for hydroxyl radical scavenging was 39.6 µg/mL.

Figure 1e shows the metal chelating activities of TCE and the positive control ethylenediaminetetraacetic acid (EDTA). The activities ranged from 7.5% ± 2.1% to 80.0% ± 2.3% for various concentrations of TCE (50–1000 µg/mL), and was 99.4% ± 0.1% for EDTA (100 µM). The IC_{50} of TCE was 427.6 µg/mL for metal chelation. The reducing power ranged from 20.1% ± 1.0% to 101.7% ± 1.2% for 50–1000 µg/mL TCE, whereas the reducing power for 100 µg/mL ascorbic acid (positive control) was 62.6% ± 3.5% (Fig. 1f). The IC_{50} of TCE was 128.5 µg/mL.

TCE inhibited $H_2O_2^-$ induced cytotoxicity and intracellular ROS generation

Human fibroblasts (Hs68), human keratinocytes (HaCaT), and mouse melanoma cells (B16F0) were treated with various concentrations of TCE (5–100 µg/mL), and their cell viability was measured using the 3-(4,5-dimethylthiazol-2-yl)-2,5-diphenyltetrazolium bromide (MTT) assay. As shown in Fig. 2a, the results indicated that TCE did not exhibit cytotoxic effects in the three skin cell lines; these concentrations were thus applied in subsequent experiments.

As shown in Fig. 2b, cell viability was 67.6% ± 1.7% after H_2O_2 treatment. Cell viability ranged from 72.7% ± 1.8% to 81.9% ± 3.9% for 5–50 µg/mL TCE. These results indicated that TCE protects the skin from oxidative stress-induced cytotoxicity.

The 2′,7′-dichlorofluorescin diacetate (DCFDA) fluorescence assay was used to qualitatively characterize intracellular ROS generation. As shown in Fig. 2c, ROS levels were markedly higher in H_2O_2-exposed fibroblasts than in control cells. Moreover, this increase in ROS generation was attenuated in H_2O_2-exposed fibroblasts pretreated with various concentrations of TCE (5–50 µg/mL). ROS generation in H_2O_2-exposed fibroblasts increased to 1.7-fold compared with control cells, and significantly decreased to 1.3-fold compared with control cells. TCE at 50 µg/mL decreased H_2O_2-induced intracellular ROS generation by 23.1%. Thus, TCE protects the skin from ROS damage.

Inhibition of MAPK phosphorylation through TCE

As shown in Fig. 3a, H_2O_2 induced the phosphorylation of p38, extracellular signal–regulated kinase (ERK), and

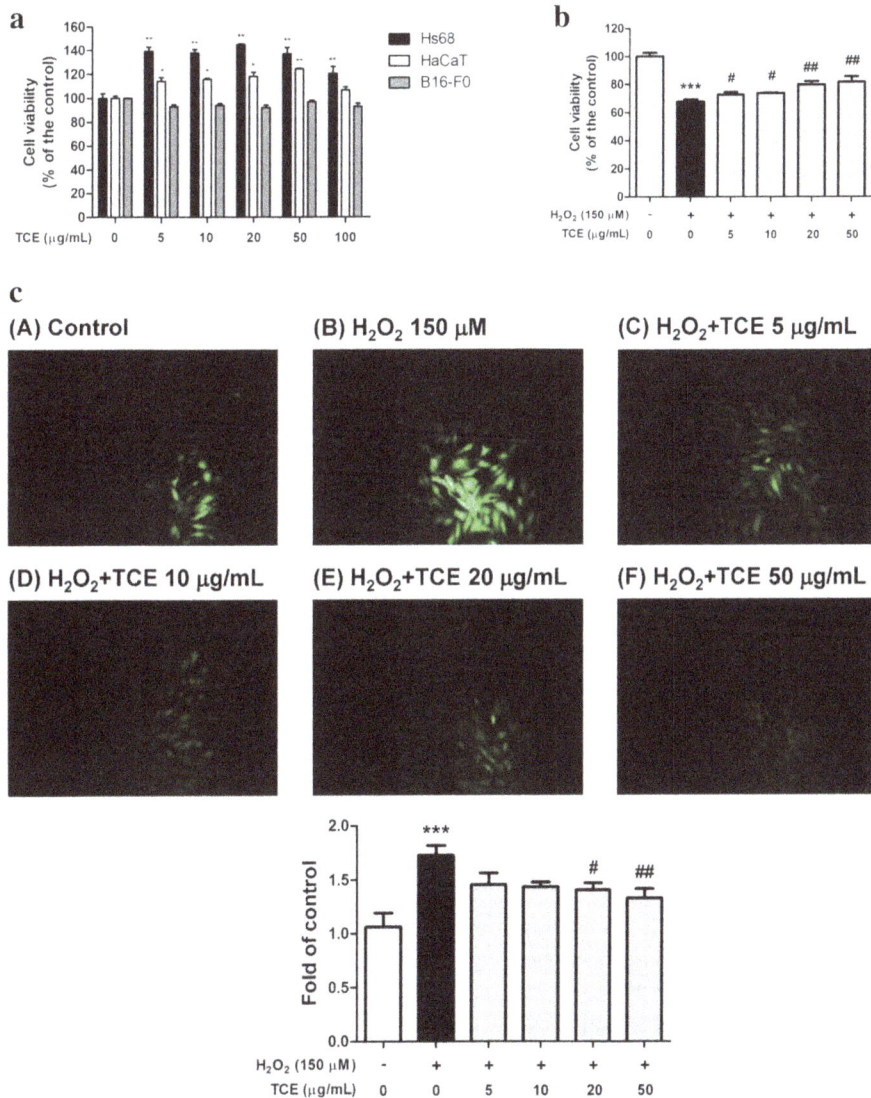

Fig. 2 The cytotoxicity and effect on intracellular oxidative stress in Hs68 of TCE. **a** Cell viability (%) of human fibroblasts (Hs68), human keratinocytes, and mouse melanoma cells treated with TCE; **b** Cell viability of Hs68 after treatment with TCE with or without 150 µM hydrogen peroxide (H_2O_2) exposure. **c** Repressive effect of TCE on H_2O_2-induced intracellular oxidative stress in Hs68. Significant difference versus control: *$p < 0.05$; **$p < 0.01$; ***$p < 0.001$. Significant inhibition versus H_2O_2-exposed group: #$p < 0.05$; ##$p < 0.01$

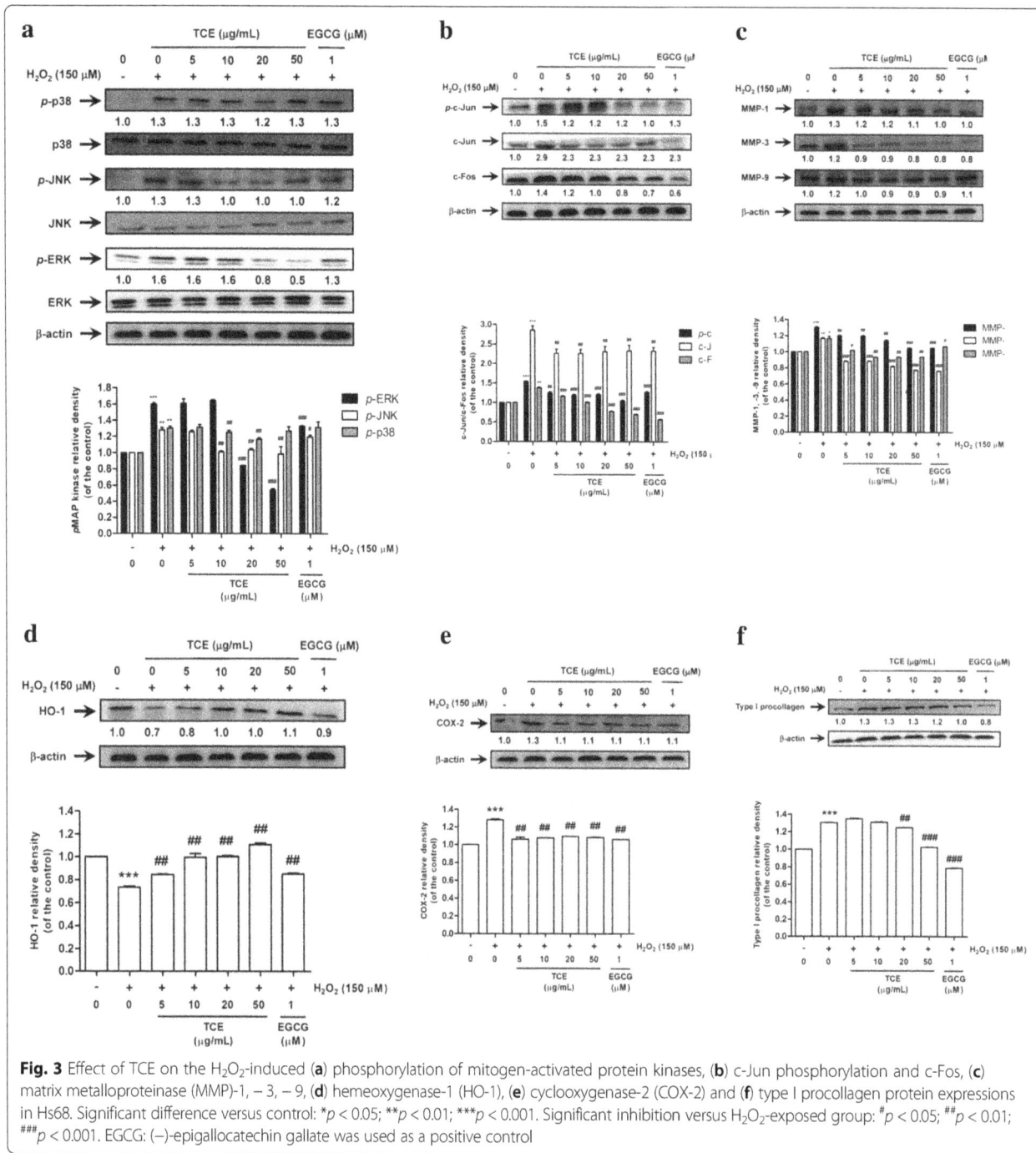

Fig. 3 Effect of TCE on the H₂O₂-induced (**a**) phosphorylation of mitogen-activated protein kinases, (**b**) c-Jun phosphorylation and c-Fos, (**c**) matrix metalloproteinase (MMP)-1, − 3, − 9, (**d**) hemeoxygenase-1 (HO-1), (**e**) cyclooxygenase-2 (COX-2) and (**f**) type I procollagen protein expressions in Hs68. Significant difference versus control: $^*p < 0.05$; $^{**}p < 0.01$; $^{***}p < 0.001$. Significant inhibition versus H₂O₂-exposed group: $^{\#}p < 0.05$; $^{\#\#}p < 0.01$; $^{\#\#\#}p < 0.001$. EGCG: (−)-epigallocatechin gallate was used as a positive control

c-Jun N-terminal kinase (JNK). TCE (5–50 μg/mL) dose-dependently inhibited the phosphorylation of ERK, and the effect was significant in the cells treated with > 20 μg/mL TCE. Similar to the effect on ERK, TCE inhibited JNK and p38 activation, which were significantly suppressed when TCE concentration was 20 μg/mL.

TCE inhibited phosphorylation of AP-1 in Hs68

As shown in Fig. 3b, H₂O₂ increased c-Jun and p-c-Jun expression to 1.5- and 2.9-fold that of the control,

respectively, whereas > 5 μg/mL TCE significantly reduced the effect. In addition, H₂O₂ induced c-Fos expression, but TCE reduced the effect. These results further indicated that TCE protects the skin from oxidative stress-induced damage.

Effect of TCE on MMP expression in Hs68

To examine whether TCE protects H₂O₂-exposed Hs68 from oxidative stress-induced damage, the expression of cellular MMP-1, − 3, and − 9 proteins was measured. As depicted in Fig. 3c, H_2O_2 significantly elevated the expression of MMP-1, – 3, and – 9 proteins by 1.3-, 1.2-, and 1.2-fold compared with controls in Hs68, respectively. By contrast, TCE attenuated H_2O_2-induced MMP expression. Specifically, treatment with > 5 µg/mL TCE significantly reduced H_2O_2-induced MMP-1, – 3, and – 9 expression. These results indicated that TCE prevents the H_2O_2-induced elevation of MMP-1, – 3 and – 9 levels, thus protecting the skin from oxidative stress-induced damage.

Effect of TCE on H_2O_2-induced Hemeoxygenase-1 expression

The hemeoxygenase (HO)-1 gene and protein play a pivotal role in the modulation of antioxidant, anti-inflammatory, and antiapoptotic activities. This study revealed that H_2O_2 significantly reduces HO-1 protein expression in Hs68, whereas TCE treatment dose-dependently increases HO-1 expression (Fig. 3d).

Effect of TCE on H_2O_2-induced Cyclooxygenase-2 expression in Hs68

Cyclooxygenase (COX)-2 levels were 1.3-fold higher in fibroblasts exposed to 150 µM H_2O_2 than in control cells (Fig. 3e). In addition, various concentrations of TCE (5–50 µg/mL) reduced COX-2 expression; the effect was significant in the cells treated with > 5 µg/mL TCE. These results further confirmed that TCE protects the skin from damage by inhibiting inflammation.

Reversal of H_2O_2-induced upregulation of type I procollagen expression in Hs68 through TCE

After treatment with 150 µM H_2O_2, the expression of type I procollagen increased to 1.3-fold compared with that in control cells, whereas TCE inhibited this effect

(Fig. 3f). Notably, treatment of the cells with 50 µg/mL TCE decreased type I procollagen expression to a level similarly expressed in the control cells.

Discussion

Polyphenols are the second most abundant metabolic products in plants. Notably, plants with high polyphenolic content exhibit potent antioxidant activity [29]. Free radical scavenging activity is related to the polyphenic and flavonoid content of plants. In a previous study, the total phenol content of *Rosa hemisphaerica* was 138.3 µg/mg GAE [30]. In the present study, the total phenolic content was 220.2 µg/mg GAE dry leaves, the total flavonoid content was 109.0 µg/mg QE dry leaves, and the IC_{50} of TCE for DPPH radical scavenging was 5.6 µg/mL. In addition, TCE exhibited strong scavenging activity for ROS including superoxide, peroxide, and hydroxyl radicals. Peroxide is the primary product of initial oxidation, and it can react with ferrous ions, producing more toxic hydroxyl radicals. Iron also has high reactivity and is the pivotal factor in lipid peroxidation catalyzed by transition metals [3]. Furthermore, TCE exhibits potent metal chelating activity and reducing power attenuating features; in the present study, TCE attenuated H_2O_2-induced metal chelation, reducing power, ROS generation, and free radical scavenging. Our results suggest that the high polyphenic and flavonoid content of TCE contribute to it potent antioxidant activity.

Molecules such as glutathione, catalase, and HO-1 provide cells, and the body overall, with defense systems against intrinsic and extrinsic oxidative stress. Nuclear factor E2-related factor 2 (Nrf2) and Keap1 are redox-sensitive transcription factors and key intracellular modulators of antioxidant defense against environmental stresses. For

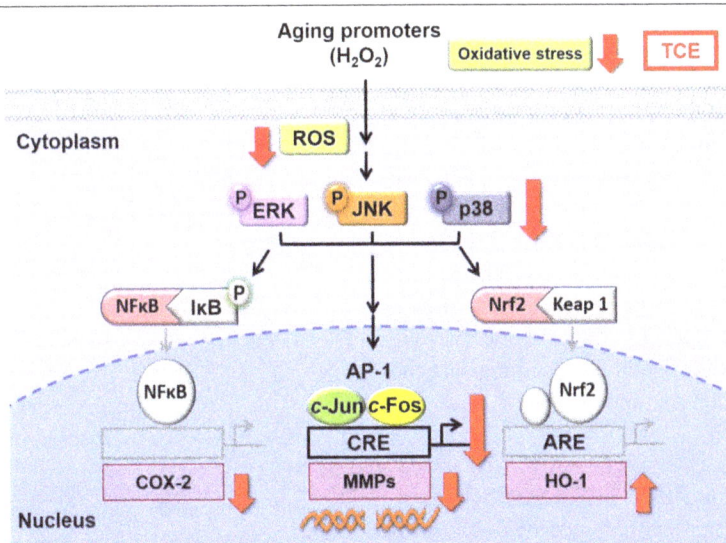

Fig. 4 Scheme for TCE inhibition of oxidative stress-induced skin damage. (↑: upregulation; ↓inhibition)

example, Nrf2 has been reported to protect skin cells from UV- and pollutant-induced oxidative damage and cellular dysfunction [31]. On exposure to oxidative stress, Nrf2 is translocated to the cell nucleus and binds to antioxidant elements, activating phase II detoxification enzymes such as HO-1 and glutathione [32]. In the present study, H_2O_2 was found to reduce HO-1 expression; however, TCE treatment increased HO-1 expression, alleviating H_2O_2-induced oxidative stress in the skin cells. In other words, TCE may repair or protect skin from the damage caused by superoxide peroxide and hydroxyl radicals.

Exposure of the skin to UV induces ROS generation and regulates the expression of genes and proteins, resulting in photodamage and photocarcinogenesis [7]. In addition, H_2O_2 has been reported to cause skin aging by inducing oxidative stress and MMP expression [33], while UVB-induced ROS generation triggers ERK, JNK, and p38 phosphorylation, AP-1 activation, and MMP expression, leading to collagen degradation [7]. In addition, H_2O_2 disrupts transforming growth factor beta transduction and subsequently inhibits collagen biosynthesis, inducing skin aging [8]. In the present study, H_2O_2 was determined to upregulate the phosphorylation of MAPKs, c-Jun, c-Fos, and MMP-1, – 3, and – 9 proteins, whereas TCE inhibited these effects. This finding suggests that TCE activity is dependent on this signaling transduction. MMPs mediate degradation of ECM and play an important role in tissue homeostasis and remodeling including angiogenesis and tissue repair. Over suppression of MMPs may cause abnormal accumulation of ECM.

The results are consistent with those of our previous study, in which the *T. catappa* water extract protected skin from photodamage by inhibiting the MAPK/AP-1/MMP pathway [22]. UVB rays inhibited collagen synthesis and induced collagen degradation, whereas *T. catappa* water extract elevated the collagen content in Hs68 [22]. Similarly, in the present study, H_2O_2 was found to increase the collagen content in Hs68, whereas TCE reversed the effect. One previous study showed that H_2O_2 also reduces mRNA expression of type I collagen (COL1A1) in fibroblasts [34], although these results are inconsistent with those reported elsewhere. For example, researchers demonstrated that H_2O_2 induces oxidative stress damage to cells and the body, which can trigger the repair process of the skin, thereby increasing the collagen content. However, excessive collagen synthesis may cause collagen fibrosis and scleroderma [35]. Overall, our results here indicate that TCE can regulate the collagen content within a normal range.

Conclusion

The present study indicated that TCE with high polyphenic and flavonoid content exhibits potent free radical scavenging and antioxidant activity. Specifically, we determined that TCE protects against H_2O_2-induced skin damage by inhibiting the protein expression of MMP, AP-1, MAPKs, and COX-2 (Fig. 4). The antioxidant and antiaging activities of TCE make it suitable for application in skin care products.

Abbreviations
AP-1: Activate protein-1; BHA: Beta hydroxyl acid; COX: Cyclooxygenase; DCFDA: 2′,7′-dichlorofluorescin diacetate; DMEM: Dulbecco's Modified Eagle's Medium; ECM: Extracellular matrix; EDTA: Ethylenediaminetetraacetic acid; ELISA: Enzyme-linked immunosorbent assay; ERK: Extracellular signal-regulated kinase; FBS: Fetal bovine serum; GAE: Gallic acid equivalent; H_2O_2: Hydrogen peroxide; HO-1: Hemeoxygenase-1; JNK: C-Jun N-terminal kinase; MAPK: Mitogen-activated protein kinase; MMP: Matrix metalloproteinase; MTT: 3-(4,5-dimethylthiazol-2-yl)-2,5-diphenyltetrazolium bromide; Nrf2: Nuclear factor E2-related factor 2; PBS: Phosphate buffered saline; QE: Quercetin equivalent; ROS: Reactive oxygen species; TCE: *Terminalia catappa* L. methanolic extract; UV: Ultraviolet

Acknowledgments
Experiments and data analysis were partly performed at the Medical Research Core Facilities Center, Office of Research & Development, at China Medical University, Taichung, Taiwan, R.O.C. Authors would like to express our very great appreciation to Ms. Jia-Ling Lyu, Ms. Yi-Jung Liu and Mr. Jyun-Shing Wu for their support in data analysis.

Funding
This study was sponsored by China Medical University (CMU103-ASIA-11; CMU105-ASIA-08), Taichung and the Ministry of Science and Technology (MOST 104-2320-B-039-006), Taipei, Taiwan.

Authors' contributions
YHH performed the cell culture and experiments and analyzed the data; PYW, KCW, CYL and HMC conceived the study and participated in its design and coordination; and PYW, KCW, CYL, and HMC wrote and revised the paper. All authors read and approved the final manuscript.

Competing interests
The authors declare that they have no competing interests.

Author details
Department of Cosmeceutics, China Medical University, 91 Hsueh-Shih Road, Taichung 40402, Taiwan. ²Department of Dermatology, China Medical University Hospital, Taichung 40402, Taiwan. ³School of Medicine, China Medical University, 91 Hsueh-Shih Road, Taichung 40402, Taiwan. †Department of Biotechnology, Asia University, 500 Liufeng Road, Wufeng District, Taichung City 41354, Taiwan.

References
1. Chen L, Hu JY, Wang SQ. The role of antioxidants in photoprotection: a critical review. J Am Acad Dermatol. 2012;67(5):1013–24.
2. Gilca GE, Stefanescu G, Badulescu O, Tanase DM, Bararu I, Ciocoiu M. Diabetic cardiomyopathy: current approach and potential diagnostic and therapeutic targets. J Diabetes Res. 2017;2017:1310265.
3. Ak T, Gulcin I. Antioxidant and radical scavenging properties of curcumin. Chem Biol Interact. 2008;174(1):27–37.
4. Lee DH, Oh JH, Chung JH. Glycosaminoglycan and proteoglycan in skin aging. J Dermatol Sci. 2016;83(3):174–81.
5. Uitto J. The role of elastin and collagen in cutaneous aging: intrinsic aging versus photoexposure. J Drugs Dermatol. 2008;7(2 Suppl):s12–6.
6. Fisher GJ, Shao Y, He T, Qin Z, Perry D, Voorhees JJ, Quan T. Reduction of fibroblast size/mechanical force down-regulates TGF-beta type II receptor: implications for human skin aging. Aging Cell. 2016;15(1):67–76.
7. Kammeyer A, Luiten RM. Oxidation events and skin aging. Ageing Res Rev. 2015;21:16–29.

8.   Bosch R, Philips N, Suarez-Perez JA, Juarranz A, Devmurari A, Chalensouk-Khaosaat J, Gonzalez S. Mechanisms of photoaging and cutaneous photocarcinogenesis, and photoprotective strategies with phytochemicals. Antioxidants. 2015;4(2):248–68.

9.   Fisher GJ, Wang ZQ, Datta SC, Varani J, Kang S, Voorhees JJ. Pathophysiology of premature skin aging induced by ultraviolet light. N Engl J Med. 1997;337(20):1419–28.

10. Kuo YH, Chen CW, Chu Y, Lin P, Chiang HM. In vitro and in vivo studies on protective action of n-phenethyl caffeamide against photodamage of skin. PLoS One. 2015;10(9):e0136777.

11. Kuo YH, Lin TY, You YJ, Wen KC, Sung PJ, Chiang HM. Antiinflammatory and antiphotodamaging effects of ergostatrien-3beta-ol, isolated from antrodia camphorata, on hairless mouse skin. Molecules. 2016;21(9). https://doi.org/10.3390/molecules21091213.

12. Bae JS, Han M, Shin HS, Kim MK, Shin CY, Lee DH, Chung JH. *Perilla frutescens* leaves extract ameliorates ultraviolet radiation-induced extracellular matrix damage in human dermal fibroblasts and hairless mice skin. J Ethnopharmacol. 2017;195:334–42.

13. Kanlayavattanakul M, Lourith N. An update on cutaneous aging treatment using herbs. J Cosmet Laser Ther. 2015;17(6):343-52.

14. Chen PS, Li JH, Liu TY, Lin TC. Folk medicine *Terminalia catappa* and its major tannin component, punicalagin, are effective against bleomycin-induced genotoxicity in Chinese hamster ovary cells. Cancer Lett. 2000;152(2):115–22.

15. Kinoshita S, Inoue Y, Nakama S, Ichiba T, Aniya Y. Antioxidant and hepatoprotective actions of medicinal herb, *Terminalia catappa* L. from Okinawa Island and its tannin corilagin. Phytomedicine. 2007;14(11):755–62.

16. Abiodun OO, Rodriguez-Nogales A, Algieri F, Gomez-Caravaca AM, Segura-Carretero A, Utrilla MP, Rodriguez-Cabezas ME, Galvez J. Antiinflammatory and immunomodulatory activity of an ethanolic extract from the stem bark of *Terminalia catappa* L. (Combretaceae): in vitro and in vivo evidences. J Ethnopharmacol. 2016;192:309–19.

17. Anuracpreeda P, Chankaew K, Puttarak P, Koedrith P, Chawengkirttikul R, Panyarachun B, Ngamniyom A, Chanchai S, Sobhon P. The anthelmintic effects of the ethanol extract of Terminalia catappa L. leaves against the ruminant gut parasite, *Fischoederius cobboldi*. Parasitology. 2016;143(4):421–33.

18. Dikshit M, Samudrasok RK. Nutritional evaluation of outer fleshy coat of Terminalia catappa fruit in two varieties. Int J Food Sci Nutr. 2011;62(1):47–51.

19. Chandrasekhar Y, Ramya EM, Navya K, Phani Kumar G, Anilakumar KR. Antidepressant like effects of hydrolysable tannins of Terminalia catappa leaf extract via modulation of hippocampal plasticity and regulation of monoamine neurotransmitters subjected to chronic mild stress (CMS). Biomed Pharmacother. 2017;86:414–25.

20. Tercas AG, Monteiro AS, Moffa EB, Dos Santos JRA, de Sousa EM, Pinto ARB, Costa P, Borges ACR, Torres LMB, Barros Filho AKD, Fernandes ES, Monteiro CA. Phytochemical characterization of *Terminalia catappa* Linn. Extracts and their antifungal activities against Candida spp. Front Microbiol. 2017;8:595.

21. Khan AA, Kumar V, Singh BK, Singh R. Evaluation of wound healing property of *Terminalia catappa* on excision wound models in wistar rats. Drug Res. 2014;64(5):225–8.

22. Wen KC, Shih IC, Hu JC, Liao ST, Su TW, Chiang HM. Inhibitory effects of *Terminalia catappa* on uvb-induced photodamage in fibroblast cell line. Evid Based Complement Alternat Med. 2011;2011:904532.

23. Chiang HM, Chiu HH, Liao ST, Chen YT, Chang HC, Wen KC. Isoflavonoid-rich *Flemingia macrophylla* extract attenuates UVB-induced skin damage by scavenging reactive oxygen species and inhibiting MAP kinase and MMP expression. Evid Based Complement Alternat Med. 2013;2013:12.

24. Moein MR, Moein S, Ahmadizadeh S. Radical scavenging and reducing power of *Salvia mirzayanii* subfractions. Molecules. 2008;3(11):2804–13.

25. Esmaeili MA, Sonboli A. Antioxidant, free radical scavenging activities of *Salvia brachyantha* and its protective effect against oxidative cardiac cell injury. Food Chem Toxicol. 2010;48(3):846–53.

26. Ruch RJ, Cheng SJ, Klaunig JE. Prevention of cytotoxicity and inhibition of intercellular communication by antioxidant catechins isolated from Chinese green tea. Carcinogenesis. 1989;10(6):1003–8.

27. Wen KC, Chiu HH, Fan PC, Chen CW, Wu SM, Chang JH, Chiang HM. Antioxidant activity of *Ixora parviflora* in a cell/cell-free system and in UV-exposed human fibroblasts. Molecules. 2011;16(7):5735–52.

28. Wu PY, Huang CC, Chu Y, Huang YH, Lin P, Liu YH, Wen KC, Lin CY, Hsu MC, Chiang HM. Alleviation of ultraviolet B-induced photodamage by *Coffea arabica* extract in human skin fibroblasts and hairless mouse skin. Int J Mol Sci. 2017;18(4). https://doi.org/10.3390/ijms18040782.

29. Nichols JA, Katiyar SK. Skin photoprotection by natural polyphenols: anti-inflammatory, antioxidant and DNA repair mechanisms. Arch Dermatol Res. 2010;302(2):71–83.

30. Serteser A, Kargioglu M, Gok V, Bagci Y, Ozcan MM, Arslan D. Determination of antioxidant effects of some plant species wild growing in Turkey. Int J Food Sci Nutr. 2008;59(7–8):643–51.

31. Chaiprasongsuk A, Lohakul J, Soontrapa K, Sampattavanich S, Akarasereenont P, Panich U. Activation of Nrf2 reduces UVA-mediated MMP-1 upregulation via MAPK/AP-1 signaling cascades: the photoprotective effects of sulforaphane and hispidulin. J Pharmacol Exp Ther. 2017;360(3):388–98.

32. Kim YG, Sumiyoshi M, Sakanaka M, Kimura Y. Effects of ginseng saponins isolated from red ginseng on ultraviolet B-induced skin aging in hairless mice. Eur J Pharmacol. 2009;602(1):148–56.

33. Park MJ, Bae YS. Fermented *Acanthopanax koreanum* root extract reduces UVB- and H_2O_2-induced senescence in human skin fibroblast cells. J Microbiol Biotechnol. 2016;26(7):1224–33.

34. Park G, Jang DS. Oh MS. *Juglans mandshurica* leaf extract protects skin fibroblasts from damage by regulating the oxidative defense system. Biochem Biophys Res Commun. 2012;421(2):343–8.

35. McGaha TL, Phelps RG, Spiera H, Bona C. Halofuginone, an inhibitor of type-I collagen synthesis and skin sclerosis, blocks transforming-growth-factor-beta-mediated Smad3 activation in fibroblasts. J Investig Dermatol. 2002;118(3):461–70.

Anti-cancer effects of *Kaempferia parviflora* on ovarian cancer SKOV3 cells

Suthasinee Paramee[1,2], Siriwoot Sookkhee[3], Choompone Sakonwasun[3], Mingkwan Na Takuathung[1], Pitchaya Mungkornasawakul[4,5], Wutigri Nimlamool[1] and Saranyapin Potikanond[1*] ⓘ

Abstract

Background: *Kaempferia parviflora* (KP) is an herb found in the north of Thailand and used as a folk medicine for improving vitality. Current reports have shown the anti-cancer activities of KP. However, the anti-cancer effects of KP on highly aggressive ovarian cancer have not been investigated. Therefore, we determined the effects of KP on cell proliferation, migration, and cell death in SKOV3 cells.

Methods: Ovarian cancer cell line, SKOV3 was used to investigate the anti-cancer effect of KP extract. Cell viability, cell proliferation, MMP activity, cell migration, and invasion were measured by MTT assay, cell counting, gelatin zymography, wound healing assay, and Transwell migration and invasion assays, respectively. Cell death was determined by trypan blue exclusion test, AnnexinV/PI with flow cytometry, and nuclear staining. The level of ERK and AKT phosphorylation, and caspase-3, caspase-7, caspase-9 was investigated by western blot analysis.

Results: KP extract was cytotoxic to SKOV3 cells when the concentration was increased, and this effect could still be observed even though EGF was present. Besides, the cell doubling time was significantly prolonged in the cells treated with KP. Moreover, KP strongly suppressed cell proliferation, cell migration and invasion. These consequences may be associated with the ability of KP in inhibiting the activity of MMP-2 and MMP-9 assayed by gelatin zymography. Moreover, KP at high concentrations could induce SKOV3 cell apoptosis demonstrated by AnnexinV/PI staining and flow cytometry. Consistently, nuclear labelling of cells treated with KP extract showed DNA fragmentation and deformity. The induction of caspase-3, caspase-7, and caspase-9 indicates that KP induces cell death through the intrinsic apoptotic pathway. The antitumor activities of KP might be regulated through PI3K/AKT and MAPK pathways since the phosphorylation of AKT and ERK1/2 was reduced.

Conclusions: The inhibitory effects of KP in cell proliferation, cell migration and invasion together with apoptotic cell death induction in SKOV3 cells suggest that KP has a potential to be a new candidate for ovarian cancer chemotherapeutic agent.

Keywords: *Kaempferia parviflora*, Thai black ginger, Ovarian cancer, Anti-cancer activity

Background

Ovarian cancer is one of the three common gynecological cancers worldwide after cervical and uterine cancers [1]. However, it is the most leading cause of death among these three gynecologic cancers [2]. Compared to others, ovarian cancer has the poorest prognosis, with the five-year survival rate of 44% for all stages [3]. Up to 70% of all ovarian cancer cases are high-grade carcinomas which grow aggressively, metastasize rapidly, and have high chromosomal instability [4, 5]. Asymptomatic or non-specific symptoms at an early stage together with poor screening method makes ovarian cancer a late diagnostic tumor. Chemotherapeutic drugs are treatment choices for unresectable tumor. However, they have many side effects including hair loss, fatigue, bone marrow suppression, and bleeding which can lower the quality of patient life [6]. Even though many new chemotherapeutics have been developed, the drugs are less accessible for many patients due to their high cost. We hope that our findings of effective medicinal plant tested in vitro

---

* Correspondence: saranyapin.p@cmu.ac.th; spotikanond@gmail.com
[1]Department of Pharmacology, Faculty of Medicine, Chiang Mai University, Chiang Mai 50200, Thailand
Full list of author information is available at the end of the article

may be an important step valuable for pacing into the next level of drug discovery and to be a complementary option with reasonable cost for patients with ovarian cancer.

Kaempferia parviflora (KP) is a Thai traditional plant in the Zingiberaceae family. It is commonly known as Thai black ginger or in Thai as "Krachai dum". KP has been previously demonstrated to have several pharmacological effects including anti-plasmodial, anti-fungal, anti-mycobacterial [7], and anti-cancer properties [7–9]. We previously described the anti-cancer property of KP against cervical cancer HeLa cells showing the promising possibility that KP may be used as a potential agent for cervical cancer treatment [10]. However, the anti-cancer effects of KP against ovarian cancer have not yet been reported. This leads us to investigate anti-cancer properties of KP against a high-grade ovarian cancer cell line, SKOV3, which is highly resistant to many cytotoxic agents. Since epidermal growth factor receptor (EGFR), is strongly expressed in ovarian cancer [11] and involved in cell proliferation, cell migration, cell survival, and metastasis, we therefore examined the effects of KP on SKOV3 alone and under the influence of EGF to verify whether KP can overcome the EGF-dependent growth and survival signal transduction pathways. Nevertheless, the molecular mechanisms of how KP suppresses tumor growth and survival were also explored. In particular, the effects of KP on the PI3K/AKT and MAPK pathways which are important signal transduction pathways for tumorigenesis [12, 13] were defined.

Methods
Cell culture
Human ovarian cancer SKOV3 cells were obtained from ATCC (ATCC, Manassas, VA, United States) and maintained in (Roswell Park Memorial Institute) RPMI-1640 medium (Gibco, BRL, USA) supplemented with 10% fetal bovine serum (FBS) (Gibco BRL, USA) and antibiotics (100 U/mL penicillin and 100 μg/mL streptomycin) (Caisson, USA) and incubated at 37 °C in a humidified atmosphere, 5% CO_2. The cells were sub-cultured every 2–3 days.

Extraction of *Kaempferia parviflora* rhizomes
The rhizomes of *Kaempferia parviflora* with voucher specimen number (R-CMUKP002) authenticated by Dr. Angkhana Inta and deposited at the Faculty of Science, Chiang Mai University, Thailand, were harvested from the CMU-RSPG Kaempferia housing at Chiang Dao, Chiang Mai Province, Thailand. For the extraction, chopped rhizomes of the plant were extracted with 95% ethanol at room temperature (RT) for 3 days and filtered before concentrated using a rotary evaporator. After solvent evaporation, the plant ethanolic extraction yielded 9.85% dry weight of KP rhizomes. One milliliter of DMSO was

used to dissolve 1 g of KP extract to make a 1 g/mL stock solution. The KP stock was pre-diluted in medium prior to each treatment. Each experiment was performed with three independent batches of KP extract, each assayed in triplicate. The final concentration of DMSO was maintained below 0.5% v/v throughout the experiment.

Cell viability assay
The cytotoxicity of KP on SKOV3 cells was determined by MTT (3-(4, 5-dimethylthiazol-2-yl)-2, 5-diphenyl tetrazolium bromide). Cells were seeded at a density of 1×10^4 cells per well in 96-well plates overnight and treated with KP or DMSO (vehicle control 0.006–0.1%) in quadruplicate. For the treatment group, cells were incubated with complete media containing different concentrations of KP extract, ranging from 0 to 10 mg/mL with or without the presence of 100 ng/ml of EGF. After 24 h, cells were incubated with 0.5 mg/mL MTT reagent (Applichem GmbH, Germany) for 1–3 h. The culture supernatant was aspirated and 100 μl of DMSO was added to each well. The absorbance was measured at 570 nm using Synergy™ H4 Hybrid Multi-Mode Microplate Reader. Cell viability assay was performed in 3 individual experiments.

Cell counting
Cells were seeded in 24-well plates at a density of 0.05×10^6 cells/well in culture media and incubated for 24 h at 37 °C, 5% CO_2. Cells were treated with KP extract at non-toxic concentrations (0.01, 0.025, and 0.05 mg/mL). The total number of cells at different time points (0, 24, 48, 72 and 96 h) was counted using a haemacytometer. The doubling time of the cell was calculated according to the following formula: Doubling time = (Time×log2)/(log(final number)-log(initial number)).

Gelatin zymography
The activity of MMP-2 and MMP-9 was examined using gelatin zymography. The sample culture supernatants of SKOV3 cells (1×10^6 cells in a 3-cm dish) incubated with different concentrations of KP extract (0, 0.01, 0.05, and 0.1 mg/mL) with or without the presence of EGF (100 ng/mL) for 24 h were collected. The sample culture supernatants were separated in 10% sodium dodecyl sulfate polyacrylamide gel electrophoresis (SDS-PAGE) containing 0.1 mg/mL of gelatin B (Bio-Rad Laboratories, Hercules, California, USA) under a non-reducing condition in cold running conditions. After electrophoresis, the gels were incubated with 2.5% Triton X-100 twice (for 30 min each), at RT and washed with 10 mM Tris buffer, pH 8.0 for 2 min. The gels were incubated with 1% gelatinase buffer (50 mM Tris HCl, 10 mM $CaCl_2$, pH 8) overnight at 37 °C. The gels were stained with 0.5% (w/v) Coomassie brilliant blue R250 (Bio-Rad Laboratories) in 50% methanol and

10% glacial acetic acid for 30 min and destained with a destaining solution (10% acetic acid and 50% methanol). Proteolytic activities of MMP-2 and MMP-9 were visualized as clear zone bands on a blue background and analyzed using ImageJ software.

Wound healing assay

SKOV3 cells (0.5×10^6 cells/well) were seeded and cultured in 24-well plates for 24 h. A scratch wound was made by using 200 mL pipette tip. Cells were treated with different concentrations of KP extract (0.01, 0.05, and 0.1 mg/mL) for 24 h. Images of the scratched wounds were captured at different time points (0, 12, and 24 h). The closing of scratched wounds was considered to be the completion of the migration process. The migrated areas were analyzed and determined using the ImageJ software.

Cell migration

A Cell Culture Insert (8 μm) (SPL Life Sciences, South Korea) was used to confirm the effect of KP on suppressing cell migration. Cells at a density of 0.3×10^6 cells/well were seeded in the upper chambers and cultured in serum-free media for 24 h. The next day cells in the upper chamber were treated with different concentrations (0, 0.01, 0.05, and 0.1 mg/mL) of KP in serum free media (SFM), and the upper chambers were put into the (lower) wells containing RPMI with 5% FBS and incubated for 24 h. Absolute methanol was used to fix cells for 5 min at RT, and cells were then stained with 0.5% crystal violet for 30 min. The upper chambers were washed for 3 times with water, and cells attached to the surface inside the chamber were removed with a cotton swab and the stained cells attached at the other site of the chamber were captured and analyzed with the ImageJ software.

Cell invasion assay

The effects of KP on SKOV3 cell invasion were determined using Cell Culture Inserts (SPL life sciences, Korea). The polycarbonate invasion chambers (8 μm pore size) were coated with Matrigel® Matrix (356,234, Lot 4,272,006, Corning, Bedford, USA) per well and incubated at RT for 1–4 h. Cells, at a density of 0.25×10^6 cells per well, were seeded on Matrigel with 0.01 and 0.05 mg/mL of KP in serum-free media and the invasion chambers were put into the wells (the lower) containing RPMI with 10% FBS and incubated for 20 h. Cells were then fixed with absolute methanol for 5 min at RT and stained with 0.5% crystal violet for 15 min. After three washes with water, cells in the invasion chambers were removed with cotton swab and the pictures of the stained cells attached at the other site of the invasion chamber were taken and analyzed with ImageJ software.

Trypan blue exclusion test

Cells were seeded at a density of 0.05×10^6 cells/well in 24-well plates and incubated with different cytotoxic concentrations (0, 0.05, 0.1, and 0.25 mg/mL) of KP extract. Cells were harvested after 3, 6, 12, 24, and 48 h of incubation. Trypan blue solution (Gibco, USA) was added to the cell suspensions in a ratio of 1:1. Total cells and dead cells (stained in blue) were counted using haemacytometer. The percentage of living cells and dead cells was calculated.

Cell apoptosis assay

Cell apoptosis was assessed by annexin-V-FITC/propidium iodide (PI) staining. Cells were seeded at a 0.3×10^6 cells/well density in 3-cm cell culture dishes and cultured for 24 h. Cells were treated with different concentrations of KP extract (0, 0.1, 0.3, and 0.5 mg/mL) for 12 h. Cells were harvested and resuspended in 1X annexin-V binding buffer (50 mM Tris-HCl (pH 7.5), 5 mM EDTA, 0.5 mM DTT, 50% glycerol). Cells were incubated with annexin V-FITC (ImmunoTools, Germany) and propidium iodide (PI) (Sigma Aldrich) for 15 min in the dark at RT before performing flow cytometry.

Nuclear staining

SKOV3 cells were seeded at a density of 0.5×10^6 cells/well on glass coverslips for 24 h. Cells were treated with KP extract at different concentrations (0.1, 0.3, and 0.5 mg/mL) and incubated for 7 h. Cells were fixed with 4% paraformaldehyde/PBS at RT for 15 min. Then, cells were washed thrice and incubated with 5 μg/mL of Hoechst 33342 in PBS (Thermo Fisher Scientific. Thailand) for 1 h. Following staining, the sample slides were washed twice with PBS for 5 min each time, and the sample slides were mounted using Fluoromount media (SouthernBiotech, United States). Cells were observed by a fluorescent microscope, AX70 Olympus R, Japan, with 40X magnification, and micrographs were captured with the DP-BSW Basic Software for the DP71 microscope digital camera.

Western blot analysis

SKOV3 cells were seeded in 3-cm dishes at a density of 0.3×10^6 cells/well for 24 h. The next day, media were changed to SFM and cells were cultured for 24 h. Cells were treated with KP extract at non-toxic concentrations (0.01 and 0.05 mg/mL) for 6 h and 100 ng/mL of EGF was added to the wells 15 min before harvesting cells. Cell lysates were prepared by adding 300 μL of 1X reducing Laemmli buffer and heating at 95 °C for 5 min. Cell lysates were separated by SDS-PAGE for 90 min at 140 V and transferred to PVDF membranes (Immobilon-P; Millipore, Bedford, MA) for 120 min at 100 V. After electrophoresis, membranes were blocked with 5% skim milk in TBS containing 0.1% tween-20 (TBST) at RT for 1 h. The blots were incubated with primary antibodies (1:10000 of anti-β-actin, 1:5000 of anti-pERK1/2, 1:5000 of anti-pAKT, 1:5000 of anti-ERK1/2, 1:5000 of anti-AKT, 1:3000 of caspase-3, or caspase-7, or caspase-9) at 4 °C overnight. Anti-β-actin was obtained from US biological (USA) and the remaining antibodies were purchased from Cell Signaling Technology (USA). The membranes were washed and incubated with an anti-mouse Ig conjugated with IRDye®800CW (1:5000) or an anti-rabbit Ig conjugated with IRDye®680RT (1:5000) at RT for 2 h. The immunoreactive bands were visualized by Odyssey ® CLx Imaging System - LI-COR Biosciences (USA). The bands were analyzed using Image Studio Lite.

Statistical analysis

Data are presented as mean ± SD. Data were analyzed by one-way ANOVA and P-value < 0.05 was considered statically significant.

Results

The effect of KP on SKOV3 cell viability and cell proliferation

To investigate antitumor properties of KP, we first evaluated its cytotoxicity to SKOV3 by using MTT assay. We found that cells treated with KP extract at different concentrations (0.006–1 mg/mL) for 24 h showed significant reduction in cell viability in a concentration-dependent manner from the range of 0.09 mg/mL to 1 mg/mL as shown in Fig. 1a. The half maximal inhibitory concentration (IC50) of KP extract was 0.53 ± 0.08 mg/mL. Since epidermal growth factor receptor (EGFR), which is highly expressed in ovarian cancer cells, is a very important factor for tumor growth [11], we therefore stimulated SKOV3 cells with EGF and performed MTT assay to evaluate whether KP still be able to suppress cell viability. As shown in Fig. 1b, EGF significantly increased cell viability approximately 15%. Interestingly, in the presence of EGF, KP still exhibited strong growth suppression in a concentration-dependent manner. The vehicle control, DMSO, at all concentrations, did not show any cytotoxic effect. The IC50 of KP extract in the presence of EGF was 0.63 ± 0.08 mg/mL which is similar to the IC50 of KP treatment without EGF. We further performed cell counting at 24, 48, 72, 96 h after KP treatment and found that KP extract significantly reduced the number of cells in a concentration-dependent manner (Fig. 2). These observations were still seen in the treatment with the presence of EGF. The number of cell from different time points were used to calculate the doubling time which is the time required for cell dividing from one to two cells. The doubling time of SKOV3 cell was approximately 24 h. Interestingly, cells treated with KP at 0.025 and 0.05 mg/mL significantly increased cell doubling time to 32.6 h, and 31.5 h, respectively.

The effect of KP on inhibiting MMP-9 and MMP-2 activities

We next determined whether KP extract suppresses MMP-9 and MMP-2 activities. Data from zymographic analysis showed that cells treated with KP extract at 0.01 and 0.05 mg/mL reduced MMP-9 activity to 92.52 ± 8.55% and 81.92 ± 5.18% and MMP-2 activity to 88.66 ± 6.17 and 68.83 ± 6.17%, respectively (Fig. 3a and b). EGF at 100 ng/mL strongly increased MMP-2 and MMP-9 activities over 140%. As we expected, KP extract with the presence of EGF was still able to suppress MMP-9 and MMP-2 activities. The percent reduction of MMP-9 activity was 113.97 ± 10.7 and 106.64 ± 9.9 mg/mL and MMP-2 activity was 121.4 ± 4.7and 104.01 ± 10.12 mg/mL for cell treated with KP at 0.01 and 0.05 mg/mL, respectively. The immunoreactive bands of β-actin detected by western indicated the equal amount of cells in all treated groups.

The effect of KP on inhibiting cell migration and invasion

Based on the fact that MMP-9 and MMP-2 are crucial factors for tumor migration and metastasis, we therefore performed wound healing assay to examine cell migration and found that cells treated with KP at 0.01, 0.05, and 0.1 mg/mL effectively reduced the percent of cell migration to 58.30 ± 5.8, 52.91 ± 5.32, and 40.50 ± 9.27%, respectively (Fig. 4a and b). Moreover, we confirmed the ability of KP in inhibiting cell migratory function of SKOV3 cells with Transwell migration assay. The results showed that SKOV3 cells without any treatment could migrate through the upper well to the lower chamber. However, the number of migrated cells was drastically decreased in cells treated with KP extract whereas the vehicle control did not show any inhibitory effect on SKOV3 cell migration (Fig. 4c and d). The effect of KP on cell invasion was determined by using Transwell assay with the presence of matrigel. Similar to cell migration assay, cells treated with KP 0.01 and 0.05 mg/mL showed a decrease in percent cell invasion to 44.42 ± 2.37%, and 30.46 ± 2.23%, respectively (Fig. 4e and f) while the DMSO vehicle did not show significant inhibitory effect on cell invasion.

The effect of KP on inhibiting growth and survival signal transduction pathways

Several signaling molecules are involved in cell growth and survival processes in response to EGF stimulation. Those molecules include ERK1/2 and AKT proteins. We therefore investigated the possible underlying mechanism of KP that suppresses growth in SKOV3 cells. As shown in Fig. 5, we found that cells treated with KP at 0.01 and 0.05 mg/mL exhibited reduction in ERK1/2 phosphorylation to 0.85 ± 0.02 and 0.64 ± 0.031, respectively. Even though EGF strongly activated ERK1/2

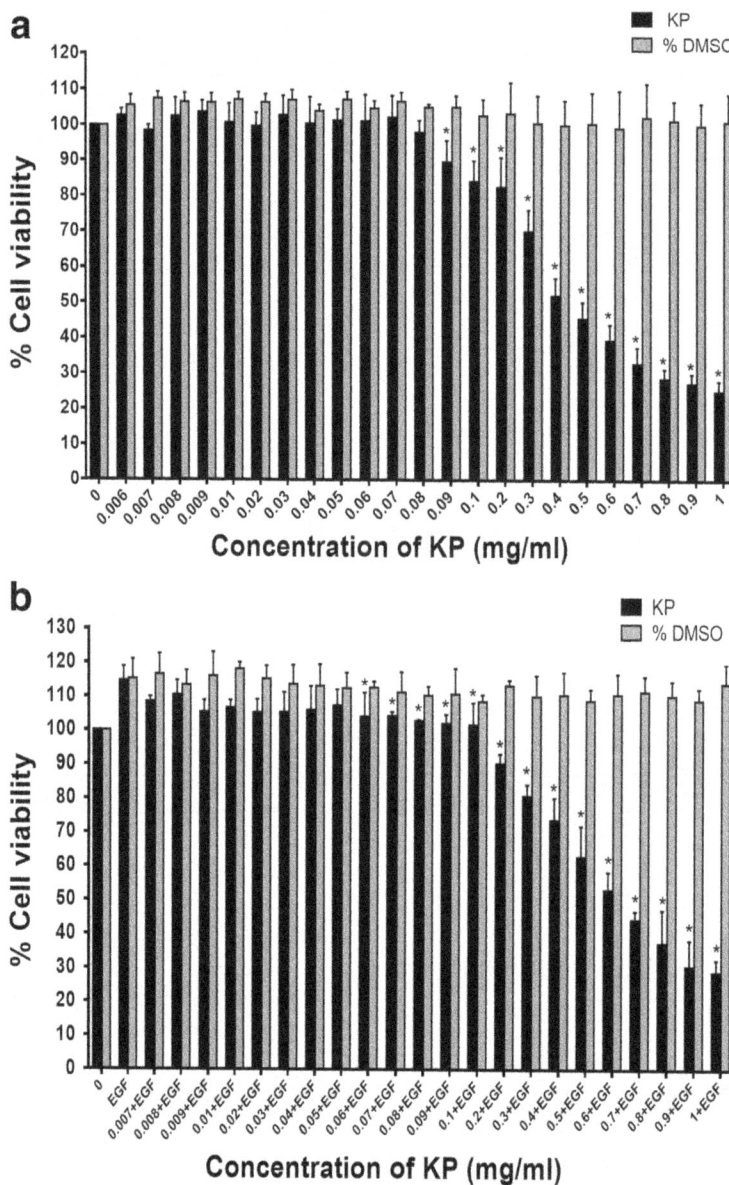

Fig. 1 The cytotoxicity effect of different concentrations of KP ethanol extract on SKOV3 cells without EGF (**a**) and with 100 ng/mL EGF (**b**). All data were from 3 independent experiments and reported as means ± SD of each quadruplicate $^*P < 0.05$ compared to the control (untreated and EGF)

phosphorylation (2.6 fold), KP at 0.01 and 0.05 mg/mL was able to reduce the phosphorylation of ERK1/2 to 2.38 ± 0.22 and 2.21 ± 0.23, respectively. Moreover, KP extract at 0.01 and 0.05 mg/mL reduced the phosphorylation of AKT to 0.87 ± 0.04 and 0.58 ± 0.03 without the presence of EGF and to 0.89 ± 0.04 and 0.7 ± 0.07 with the presence of EGF, respectively.

The effect of KP on inducing apoptotic cell death
Since cell viability assay showed cytotoxicity of KP extract at the concentrations over 0.1 mg/mL. We thus examined whether KP extract increases cell death by using trypan

blue exclusion test. We found that cells treated with KP extract at 0.1 and 0.25 mg/mL significantly increased cell death after 24 h of incubation. The percentage of cell death was 15.67 ± 2% and 26.33 ± 3.5% with KP treatment at 0.1 and 0.25 mg/mL, respectively (Fig. 6a). Importantly, with the presence of EGF 100 ng/mL, KP extract at 0.1 and 0.25 mg/mL was able to induce cell death to 13.17 ± 1.8% and 21.25 ± 2%. In order to confirm whether dead cells were apoptotic cell, fluorescence nuclear staining using Hoechst 33342 was performed after treating cells with KP for 6 h. Figure 6c showed nuclear fragmentation of SKOV3 cells treated with KP extract at 0.3 and 0.5 mg/mL.

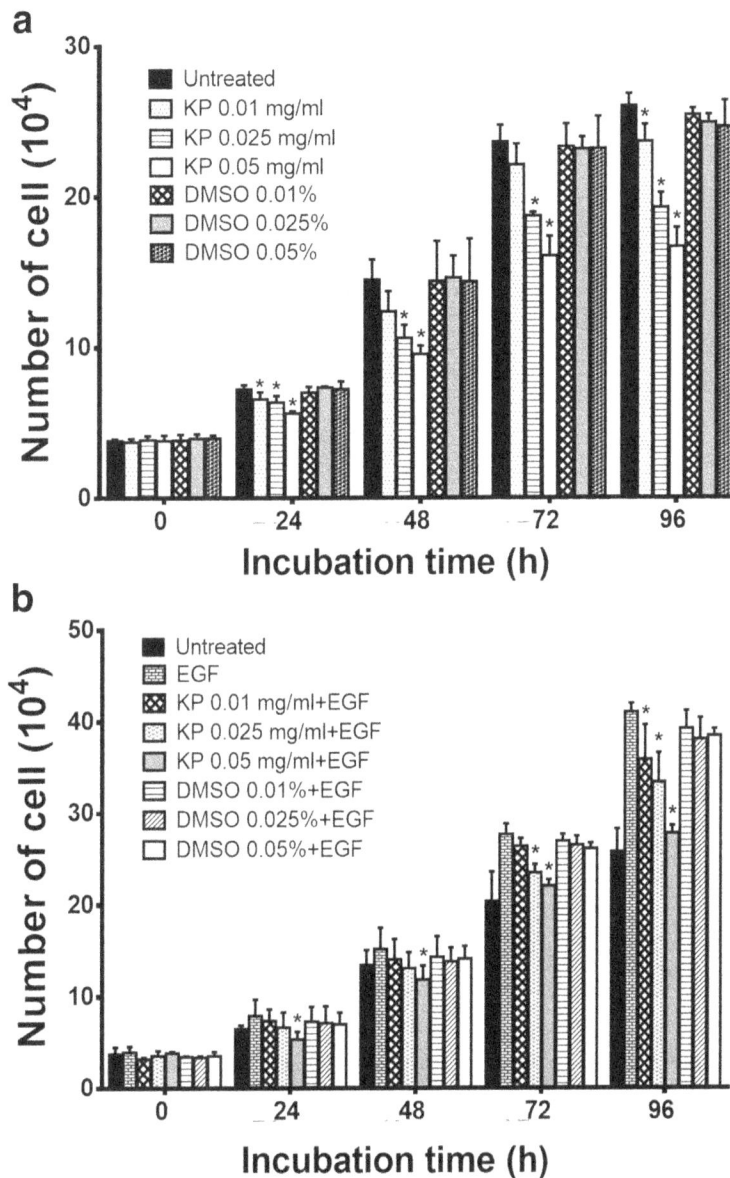

Fig. 2 The number of SKOV3 cells treated with non-toxic concentrations of KP (0.01, 0.025, 0.05 mg/mL) without EGF (**a**) and with 100 ng/mL EGF (**b**) at 24, 48, 72 and 96 h. Data are expressed as mean ± SD ($n = 3$). *$P < 0.05$ as compared to untreated (**a**) or EGF (**b**)

This effect was seen in cells treated with DMSO. Based on this observation, we speculated that KP extract induces cell death via apoptosis machinery. We next determined apoptotic event by performing AnnexinV and PI fluorescent staining and detecting with flow cytometer. We found that cells treated with KP extract at 0.3 and 0.5 mg/mL increased apoptosis to $22.13 \pm 7.6\%$ and $41.13 \pm 19.15\%$, respectively (Fig. 7a, b). We further examined the activation of caspase-9, caspase-3, and caspase-7 by western blot analysis and found that the full length of all caspases was significantly reduced in a concentration-dependent manner (Fig. 7c, d). These data strongly suggest that KP induces cell death via the activation of apoptotic cell death.

Discussion

Ovarian cancer is the most common cause of cancer death among other gynecologic cancers [14]. No obvious symptoms are present at the early stage, thus, most of patients are diagnosed when cancer is in an advanced stage which gives rise to poor response to chemotherapies [15]. Staging is an important factor determining prognosis and clinical outcome. Stage I, is defined as tumor is confined in the ovary. This stage shows overall survival of approximately 84 months. In particular, stage IV has much less overall survival rate of only 10 months [15]. The survival rate is not only related to stages of the disease but also associated with ovarian cell types. Several cell types

A

EGF (100ng/ml)

| KP (mg/ml) | - | 0.01 | 0.05 | - | - | - | 0.01 | 0.05 | - | - |
| DMSO (%) | - | - | - | 0.01 | 0.05 | - | - | - | 0.01 | 0.05 |

MMP-9

MMP-2

β-actin

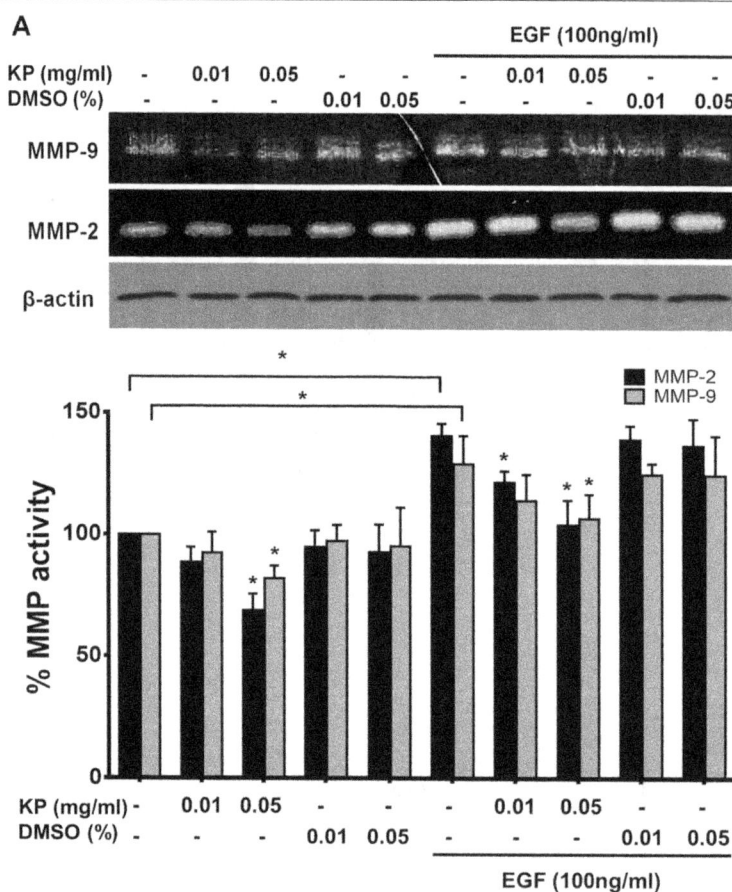

Fig. 3 The effect of KP ethanol extract on MMP-9 and MMP-2 activity. Gelatin zymogram showing MMP9 and MMP2 activities (**a**), Immunoreactive bands of β-actin was used as a loading control. Histogram of MMP-2 and MMP-9 activity is presented as percent of activity (**b**). All data were from 3 independent experiments. $^*P < 0.05$

have been identified in ovarian cancer. The most common histologic subtype is high-grade serous adenocarcinoma which has the worst prognosis [16, 17]. We are particularly interested in using a high-grade serous adenocarcinoma, SKOV3, cell line as a model for investigating anticancer activity of *Kaempferia parviflora* in ovarian cancer.

We first performed cell viability assay to evaluate the cytotoxicity of KP extract in SKOV3 cells. It was found that KP extract decreased cell viability of ovarian cancer in a concentration-dependent manner with IC50 of approximately 0.5 mg/mL, which was slightly higher than the previously reported IC50 of KP in cervical cancer cell line, HeLa [10]. Interestingly, KP extract also strongly exhibited the reduction of ovarian cancer cell viability in the presence of EGF, suggesting that KP has potent cytotoxic effects, which overcome the influence of EGF in maintaining cell viability. We further discovered that treating cells with KP extract at non-toxic concentrations (with or without the presence of EGF) at various time points could significantly inhibit number of cells in a concentration-dependent manner. Therefore, the doubling

time was increased to approximately 1.3–1.4 folds compared to untreated SKOV3 cells. This observation suggests that KP extract may suppress SKOV3 cell proliferation. According to cell viability results, the non-toxic concentrations were chosen for further experiments.

Since SKOV3 cells are known to be a high grade serous adenocarcinoma which has been reported to have high metastatic rate [16, 18]. One major factor that plays important roles in cell invasion and metastasis is matrix metalloproteinase (MMP). Extensive evidence has been shown that the increased MMP level correlates with tumor progression and metastasis, especially in advanced ovarian serous cancers [19, 20]. MMP expression, particularly MMP-2 and MMP-9, has been shown to have clinical association with progression of ovarian cancer [21, 22]. MMPs degrade various components of the extracellular matrix and play a crucial role in tumorigenesis, migration, invasion, and metastasis [23], and inhibition of MMPs by specific inhibitors has been demonstrated to markedly suppress tumor invasion and metastasis [24, 25]. Based on these previous reports, we hypothesized that KP extract

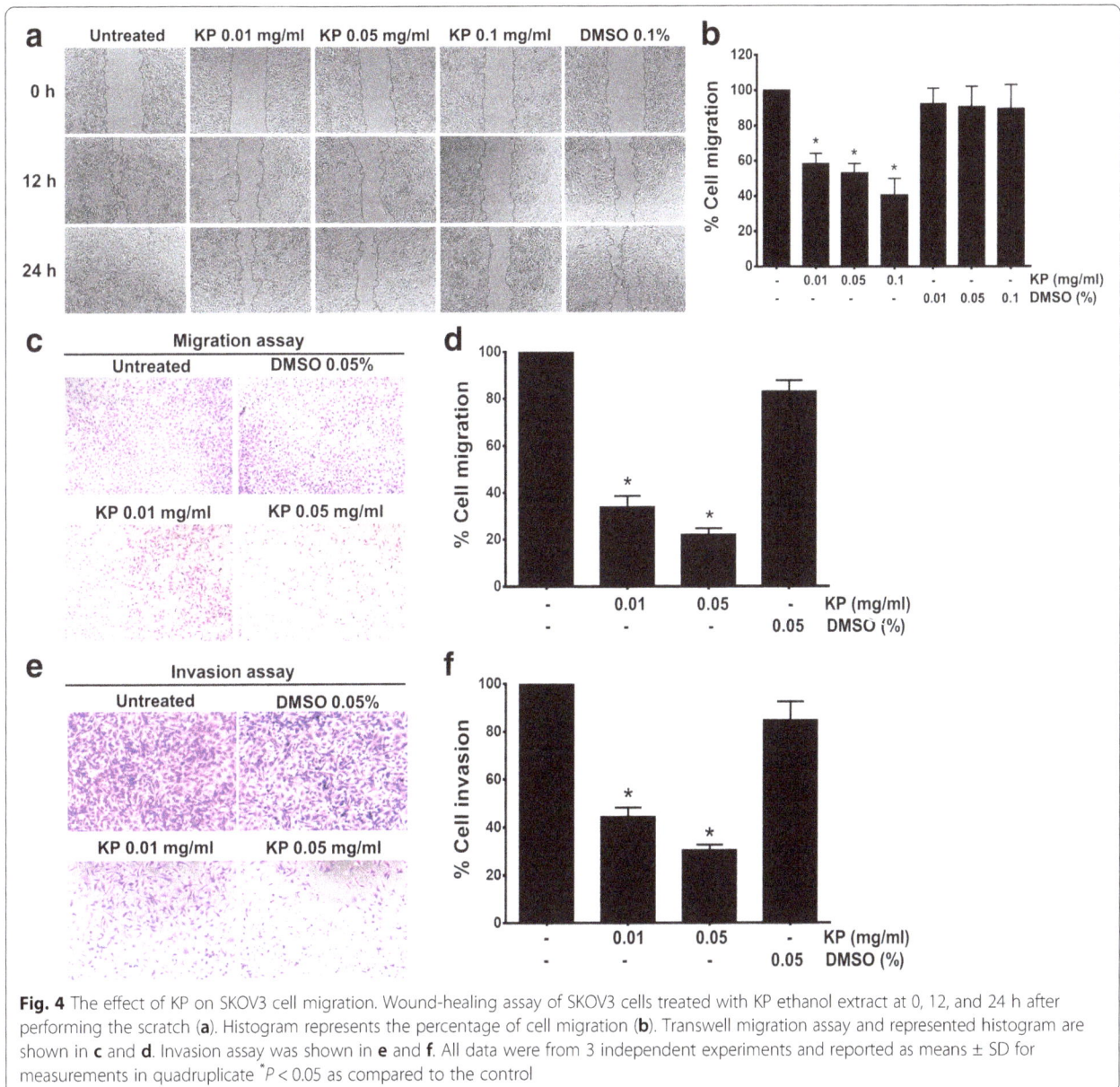

Fig. 4 The effect of KP on SKOV3 cell migration. Wound-healing assay of SKOV3 cells treated with KP ethanol extract at 0, 12, and 24 h after performing the scratch (**a**). Histogram represents the percentage of cell migration (**b**). Transwell migration assay and represented histogram are shown in **c** and **d**. Invasion assay was shown in **e** and **f**. All data were from 3 independent experiments and reported as means ± SD for measurements in quadruplicate *$P < 0.05$ as compared to the control

may be able to modulate the expression of MMPs. Undoubtedly, our zymographic study revealed that KP extract dramatically inhibited the activity of MMP-2 and MMP-9 in a concentration-dependent manner in SKOV3 cells. The ability of KP extract in suppressing the activity of MMPs was independent on the presence of EGF, since KP extract could be able to strongly overcome the effects of EGF. Our findings are in line with our previous studies showing that KP suppressed MMP-2 production in cervical cancer, HeLa cells [10]. Similar observation was reported in colorectal carcinoma cells, where a flavonoid, myricetin, inhibited MMP-2 activity and cell invasion [26]. These let us to believe that KP extract may also be able to reduce cancer cell migration

and invasion. We, therefore, further investigated the effects of KP extract on cell migration and invasion.

Generally, cancer cell migration is involved in altering the cell-matrix interface on the cell surface [27]. The overexpression of MMPs could enhance cell migration [28], whereas the inhibition of MMP activity or overexpression of tissue inhibitor of metalloproteinases (TIMPs) resulted in a decrease in cancer cell migration [29]. Our results from wound healing assays showed that KP extract suppressed cell migration of SKOV3 cells in a concentration-dependent manner. Furthermore, the migratory function of cells was confirmed by Transwell migration showing that KP extract drastically inhibited migration and invasion of SKOV3 cells. The results from invasion assay with the presence of

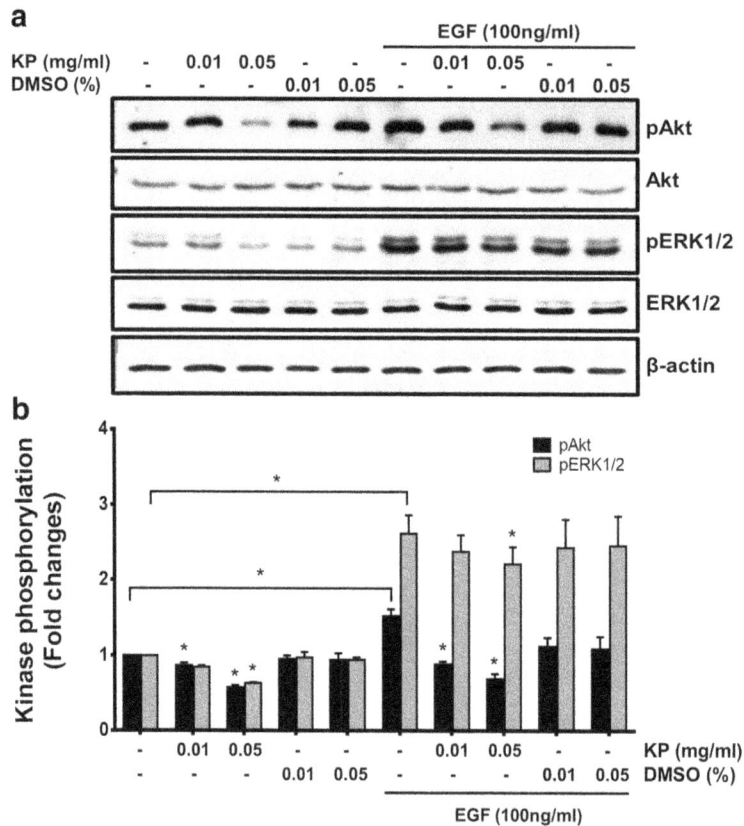

Fig. 5 The effect of KP on the PI3K/AKT and EKR1/2 MAPK signal transduction in SKOV3 cells. The immunoreactive bands of pAKT, AKT, pERK1/2 and ERK1/2 (**a**). Histogram of phosphorylation level of AKT and ERK1/2 (**b**). β-actin was used as a loading control. Data expressed as mean ± SD ($n = 3$). $^*P < 0.05$

matrigel definitively verified that KP extract could be able to suppress invasion of SKOV3 cells. Together, these results strongly suggest that KP possesses the inhibitory effect on migration and invasion of SKOV3. These observations are consistent with the zymography results, suggesting that the reduced activity of MMPs may greatly contribute to the reduction of cancer cell invasion and migration.

Besides the ability of KP extract on an aspect of suppressing ovarian cancer cell metastasis, we would also like to explore its effect on ovarian cancer cell growth and survival. In particular, since SKOV3 cells apparently express EGF receptor (EGFR) [30], we therefore examined whether KP extract can overcome the influence of EGF on activating molecular signal transduction pathways relevant to cell growth and survival. EGFR is involved in cell proliferation, motility, adhesion, angiogenesis, and survival via the activation of phosphatidylinositol-3 kinase (PI3K/AKT) pathway, and the extracellular signal-regulated kinase (ERK) pathway [31]. EGFR is widely expressed in 33–75% of ovarian cancer and has been implicated in the growth and progression of this cancer [32–34]; therefore, EGFR is important to represent a potential target for anticancer drug

development. An example of EGFR-directed monoclonal antibody is cetuximab, which inhibits cell growth in OVCAR-2 cells, whereas the growth of SKOV3 cells is not affected [35]. Another class of EGFR inhibitor is a group of small molecule tyrosine kinase inhibitors that target the receptor catalytic domain of EGFR. Those include gefitinib and erlotinib [36]. AKT and ERK are major downstream signaling molecules of EGFR [37]. Previous evidence demonstrated that KP extract significantly suppressed the phosphorylation of PI3K, AKT, ERK1/2, and Elk1 in HeLa cells [10], thus we hypothesized whether KP extract can suppress the activation of ERK1/2 and AKT signaling in high grade serous ovarian cancers. Our study clearly showed that KP extract markedly suppressed phosphorylation of ERK1/2 and AKT. This observation was still seen when the experiment was performed with the presence of EGF. The present results indicate that KP extract suppresses ERK1/2 pathway which is normally involved in cell proliferation, and the extract suppressed AKT pathway which plays roles in cell survival. A study in *Drosophila* showed that a gain-of-function mutation that results in enhanced ERK1/2 signaling capabilities could support ERK1/2 activation

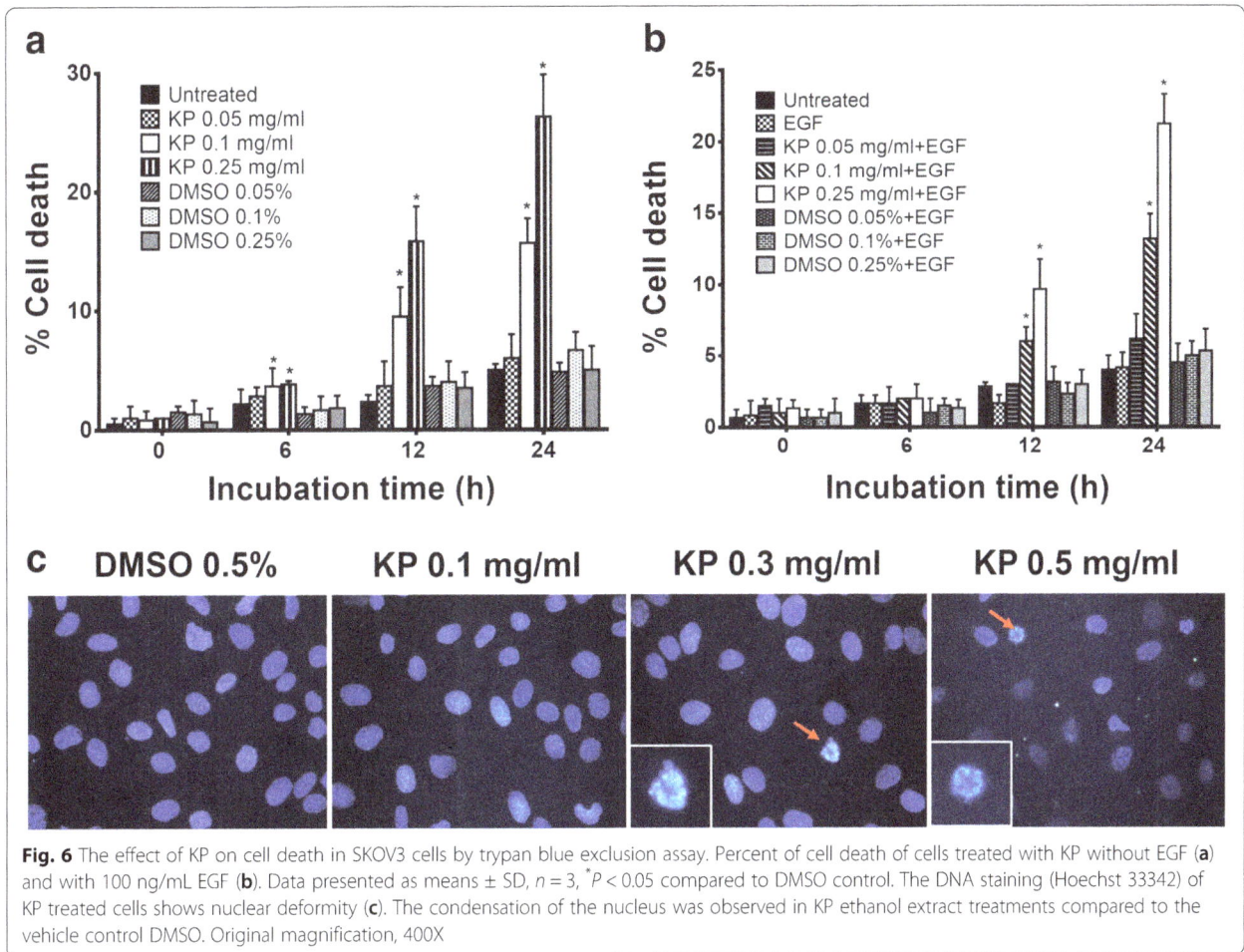

Fig. 6 The effect of KP on cell death in SKOV3 cells by trypan blue exclusion assay. Percent of cell death of cells treated with KP without EGF (**a**) and with 100 ng/mL EGF (**b**). Data presented as means ± SD, $n = 3$, $^*P < 0.05$ compared to DMSO control. The DNA staining (Hoechst 33342) of KP treated cells shows nuclear deformity (**c**). The condensation of the nucleus was observed in KP ethanol extract treatments compared to the vehicle control DMSO. Original magnification, 400X

in the cancer cells [38]. Our findings are supported by recent studies showing that the use of RNA interference to silence ERK1/2 phosphorylation led to the complete suppression of tumor cell proliferation [39]. Since various cancers have aberrant regulation of AKT pathway that leads to prolonged survival of tumor [40], and previous studies showed that the inhibition of AKT activity is useful as a therapeutic approach for the therapy of cisplatin-resistant ovarian cancer because an activation of AKT promotes cisplatin-resistance [41, 42], we hope that KP may be a novel and effective agent that has some potential targets in AKT signaling and therefore may be beneficial for developing a cancer therapeutic means.

One of our key observations was an increase in cell death at 24 h after treatment with KP extract at toxic concentrations. Nuclear fragmentation, which is a result of the cleavage of chromosomal DNA into oligonucleosomal size fragments, is an integral part of apoptosis [43]. The cell apoptosis leads to deformity of nuclear lamina, and consequently increases active caspases [44]. Therefore, to confirm whether these dead cells were apoptotic cells, we stained SKOV3 cells with Hoechst 33342 and observed

nuclear fragmentation of SKOV3 cells treated with KP extract. This finding is consistent with Potikanond et al. (2017) indicating that nuclear deformity and nuclear fragmentation were induced by KP treatment in HeLa cells. In addition, the apoptotic event of KP-treated SKOV3 was further determined by Annexin V/PI and flow cytometry analysis. Clearly, our results showed that KP significantly induced apoptosis in SKOV3 cells in a concentration-dependent manner. To confirm our hypothesis that KP extract induces apoptosis in ovarian cancer cells, we specifically analyzed the key apoptosis execution enzymes, caspase-3, caspase-7, and caspase-9 in SKOV3 cells treated with KP extract. The results showed that the full-length structure of all caspases was reduced in a concentration-dependent manner in SKOV3 cells treated with KP extract, implicating that SKOV3 cell death in KP treatment was possessed through programed cell death signaling pathway.

Conclusions

The current study demonstrated that KP extract has anti-cancer properties against a high grade serous

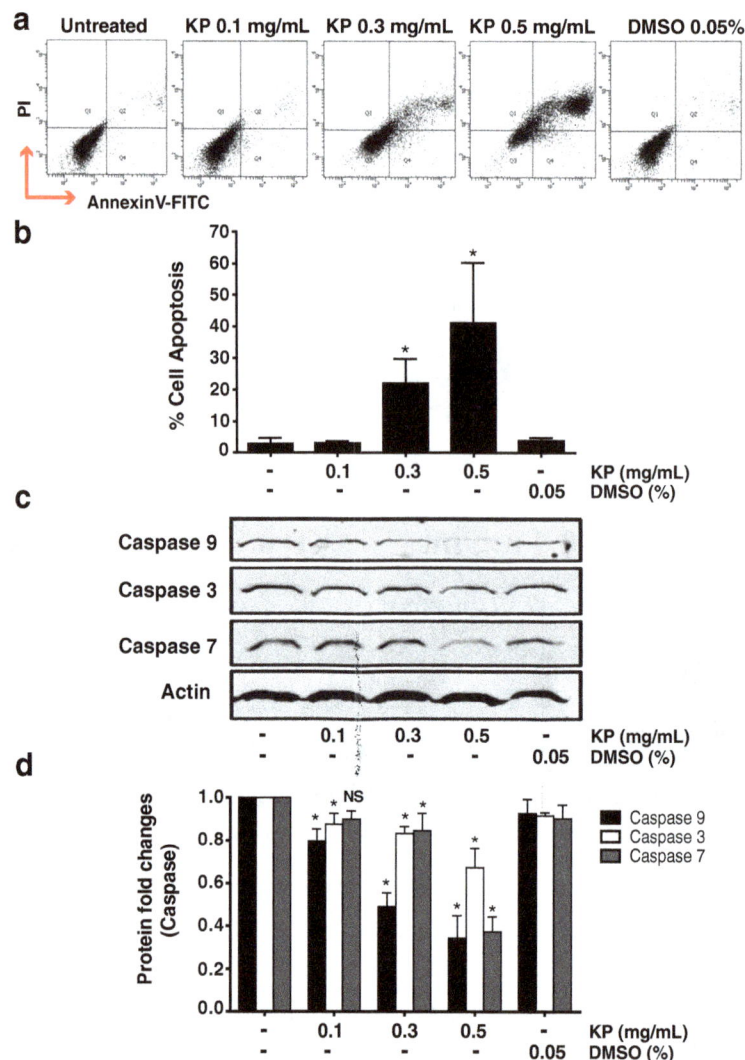

Fig. 7 The effect of KP ethanol extract on apoptosis and caspases in SKOV3 cells. Annexin V-FITC and PI labeling in KP treated cells was measured by flow cytometer (**a**) and histogram of percent of apoptotic cells is shown in **b**. The level of caspase-3, - 9, and -7 by western blotting are shown in **c**. Histogram of relative intensity of full-length of caspase-3, − -9, and -7. β-actin is used as a protein loading control (**d**). These data are represented as mean ± SD of three replicates. $^*P < 0.05$ indicates significant difference compared to control

adenocarcinoma, SKOV3. Specifically, even though SKOV3 cells are every aggressive and resistant to many chemotherapeutic agents, our results showed that KP extract was able to suppress the activity of MMP-2 and MMP-9, migration and invasion, activation of growth and survival signal transduction pathways, and induction of apoptotic cell death. These observations convince us to believe that KP extract is a potential agent to be further developed as an effective therapy for ovarian cancer.

Acknowledgements
We thank Mr.Sathit Monkaew for assistance with laboratory support.

Funding
This work was supported by CMB funding, Faculty of Medicine, Chiang Mai University (SPO) and the Center for Innovation in Chemistry (PERCH-CIC), Commission on Higher Education, Ministry of Education (at Faculty of Science, Mahidol University, Thailand) (SPO). We also are thankful for the supports from the Thailand Research Fund (MRG6080193) (WN) and Plant Genetic Conservation Project under the Royal Initiation of Her Royal Highness Princess Maha Chakri Sirindhorn (RSPG) (SS and CS), and Research Center of Pharmaceutical Nanotechnology, Chiang Mai University (SPO) for partial financial support. The funders had no role in the project design, data collection, interpretation, or decision to publish.

Authors' contributions
Plant cultivation, collection, harvesting, and identification were conducted by SS and CS. PM prepared the plant extract. The experiments, data analysis,

and manuscript writing were conducted by SPA and MNT. SPO and WN funded the research project, designed, performed the experiments, prepared the manuscript, and contributed to the funding of the project. All authors have read and approved the manuscript.

Competing interests

The authors declare that they have no competing interests.

Author details

[1]Department of Pharmacology, Faculty of Medicine, Chiang Mai University, Chiang Mai 50200, Thailand. [2]Graduate School, Chiang Mai University, Chiang Mai 50200, Thailand. [3]Department of Microbiology, Faculty of Medicine, Chiang Mai University, Chiang Mai 50200, Thailand. [4]Department of Chemistry, Faculty of Science, Chiang Mai University, Chiang Mai 50200, Thailand. [5]Environmental Science Program, Faculty of Science, Chiang Mai University, Chiang Mai 50200, Thailand.

References

1. Waldmann A, Eisemann N, Katalinic A. Epidemiology of Malignant Cervical, Corpus Uteri and Ovarian Tumours - Current Data and Epidemiological Trends. Geburtshilfe Frauenheilkd. Thieme Medical Publishers; 2013 [cited 2017 Nov 14];73:123–9.
2. Siegel RL, Miller KD, Jemal A. Cancer statistics, 2017. CA Cancer J Clin. 2017 [cited 2018 May 10];67:7–30.
3. Jelovac D, Armstrong DK. Recent progress in the diagnosis and treatment of ovarian cancer. CA Cancer J Clin. NIH Public Access. 2011;61:183–203.
4. Vang R, Shih I-M, Kurman RJ. Ovarian low-grade and high-grade serous carcinoma: pathogenesis, clinicopathologic and molecular biologic features, and diagnostic problems. Adv Anat Pathol. NIH Public Access. 2009;16:267–82.
5. Kurman RJ. Origin and molecular pathogenesis of ovarian high-grade serous carcinoma. Ann Oncol. 2013;24:x16–21.
6. Mukhtar E, Adhami VM, Mukhtar H. Targeting microtubules by natural agents for cancer therapy. Mol Cancer Ther. NIH Public Access. 2014;13:275–84.
7. Yenjai C, Prasanphen K, Daodee S, Wongpanich V, Kittakoop P. Bioactive flavonoids from Kaempferia parviflora. Fitoterapia. 2004;75:89–92.
8. Patanasethanont D, Nagai J, Matsuura C, Fukui K, Sutthanut K, Sripanidkulchai B, et al. Modulation of function of multidrug resistance associated-proteins by Kaempferia parviflora extracts and their components. Eur J Pharmacol. 2007;566:67–74.
9. Banjerdpongchai R, Chanwikruy Y, Rattanapanone V, Sripanidkulchai B. Induction of apoptosis in the human leukemic U937 cell line by Kaempferia parviflora Wall.ex.Baker extract and effects of paclitaxel and camptothecin. Asian Pac J Cancer Prev. 2009;10:1137–40.
10. Potikanond S, Sookkhee S, Na Takuathung M, Mungkornasawakul P, Wikan N, Smith DR, et al. Kaempferia parviflora extract exhibits anti-cancer activity against HeLa cervical Cancer cells. Front Pharmacol. 2017;8:630.
11. Hudson LG, Zeineldin R, Silberberg M, Stack MS. Activated epidermal growth factor receptor in ovarian cancer. Cancer Treat Res. NIH Public Access. 2009;149:203–26.
12. Catasús L, Bussaglia E, Rodríguez I, Gallardo A, Pons C, Irving JA, et al. Molecular genetic alterations in endometrioid carcinomas of the ovary: similar frequency of beta-catenin abnormalities but lower rate of microsatellite instability and PTEN alterations than in uterine endometrioid carcinomas. Hum Pathol. 2004;35:1360–8.
13. Mandai M, Konishi I, Kuroda H, Komatsu T, Yamamoto S, Nanbu K, et al. Heterogeneous distribution of K-ras-mutated epithelia in mucinous ovarian tumors with special reference to histopathology. Hum Pathol. 1998;29:34–40.
14. Wilailak S. Epidemiologic report of gynecologic cancer in Thailand. J Gynecol Oncol. Korean Society of Gynecologic Oncology and Colposcopy. 2009;20:81.
15. Cristea M, Han E, Salmon L, Morgan RJ. Review: practical considerations in ovarian cancer chemotherapy. Ther Adv Med Oncol. 2010;2:175–87.
16. Anglesio MS, Wiegand KC, Melnyk N, Chow C, Salamanca C, Prentice LM, et al. Type-specific cell line models for type-specific ovarian cancer research. PLoS One. 2013;8:e72162.
17. Reid BM, Permuth JB, Sellers TA. Epidemiology of ovarian cancer: a review. Cancer Biol Med. Chinese Anti-Cancer Association. 2017;14:9–32.
18. Beaufort CM, Helmijr JCA, Piskorz AM, Hoogstraat M, Ruigrok-Ritstier K, Besselink N, et al. Ovarian Cancer cell line panel (OCCP): clinical importance of in vitro morphological subtypes. Pearson R, editor. PLoS One. 2014;9:e103988.
19. Garzetti GG, Ciavattini A, Lucarini G, Goteri G, De Nictolis M, Garbisa S, et al. Tissue and serum metalloproteinase (MMP-2) expression in advanced ovarian serous cystoadenocarcinomas: clinical and prognostic implications. Anticancer Res. 1995;15:2799–804.
20. Fishman DA, Bafetti LM, Banionis S, Kearns AS, Chilukuri K, Stack MS. Production of extracellular matrix-degrading proteinases by primary cultures of human epithelial ovarian carcinoma cells. Cancer. 1997;80:1457–63.
21. Lopata A, Agresta F, Quinn MA, Smith C, Ostor AG, Salamonsen LA. Detection of endometrial cancer by determination of matrix metalloproteinases in the uterine cavity. Gynecol Oncol. Academic Press. 2003;90:318–24.
22. Torng P-L, Mao T-L, Chan W-Y, Huang S-C, Lin C-T. Prognostic significance of stromal metalloproteinase-2 in ovarian adenocarcinoma and its relation to carcinoma progression. Gynecol Oncol. 2004;92:559–67.
23. Bauvois B. New facets of matrix metalloproteinases MMP-2 and MMP-9 as cell surface transducers: outside-in signaling and relationship to tumor progression. Biochim Biophys Acta. Rev. Cancer. 2012;1825:29–36.
24. Liotta LA, Tryggvason K, Garbisa S, Hart I, Foltz CM, Shafie S. Metastatic potential correlates with enzymatic degradation of basement membrane collagen. Nature. Nature Publishing Group. 1980;284:67–8.
25. Stetler-Stevenson WG. The role of matrix metalloproteinases in tumor invasion, metastasis, and angiogenesis. Surg Oncol Clin N Am. 2001;10:383–92.
26. Ko C-H, Shen S-C, Lee TJF, Chen Y-C. Myricetin inhibits matrix metalloproteinase 2 protein expression and enzyme activity in colorectal carcinoma cells. Mol. Cancer Ther. American association for. Cancer Res. 2005;4:281–90.
27. Kim YH, Kwon H-J, Kim D-S. Matrix metalloproteinase 9 (MMP-9)-dependent processing of βig-h3 protein regulates cell migration, invasion, and adhesion. J Biol Chem. American Society for Biochemistry and Molecular Biology. 2012;287:38957–69.
28. Deryugina EI, Luo GX, Reisfeld RA, Bourdon MA, Strongin A. Tumor cell invasion through matrigel is regulated by activated matrix metalloproteinase-2. Anticancer Res. 1997;17:3201–10.
29. George SJ, Johnson JL, Angelini GD, Newby AC, Baker AH. Adenovirus-mediated gene transfer of the human TIMP-1 gene inhibits smooth muscle cell migration and Neointimal formation in human saphenous vein. Hum Gene Ther. 1998;9:867–77.
30. Sewell JM, Macleod KG, Ritchie A, Smyth JF, Langdon SP Targeting the EGF receptor in ovarian cancer with the tyrosine kinase inhibitor ZD 1839 ("Iressa"). Br J Cancer. Nature Publishing Group; 2002;86:456–62.
31. Tanaka Y, Terai Y, Tanabe A, Sasaki H, Sekijima T, Fujiwara S, et al. Prognostic effect of epidermal growth factor receptor gene mutations and the aberrant phosphorylation of Akt and ERK in ovarian cancer. Cancer Biol Ther. 2011;11:50–7.
32. Berchuck A, Rodriguez GC, Kamel A, Dodge RK, Soper JT, Clarke-Pearson DL. Epidermal growth factor receptor expression in normal ovarian epithelium and ovarian cancer: II. Relationship between receptor expression and response to epidermal growth factor. Am J Obstet Gynecol. Mosby. 1991;164:745–50.
33. Psyrri A, Kassar M, Yu Z, Bamias A, Weinberger PM, Markakis S, et al. Effect of epidermal growth factor receptor expression level on survival in patients with epithelial ovarian Cancer. Clin Cancer Res. 2005;11:8637–43.
34. Stadlmann S, Gueth U, Reiser U, Diener P-A, Zeimet AG, Wight E, et al. Epithelial growth factor receptor status in primary and recurrent ovarian cancer. Mod Pathol. Nature Publishing Group. 2006;19:607–10.
35. Bijman MNA, van Berkel MPA, Kok M, Janmaat ML, Boven E. Inhibition of functional HER family members increases the sensitivity to docetaxel in human ovarian cancer cell lines. Anti-Cancer Drugs. 2009;20:450–60.
36. Harari PM. Epidermal growth factor receptor inhibition strategies in oncology. Endocr Relat Cancer. 2004;11:689–708.
37. Bunn PA Jr and Franklin W. Epidermal growth factor receptor expression, signal pathway, and inhibitors in non-small cell lung cancer. Semin Oncol. 2002;29(5Suppl 14):38-44.
38. Bott CM, Thorneycroft SG, Marshall CJ. The sevenmaker gain-of-function mutation in p42 MAP kinase leads to enhanced signalling and reduced sensitivity to dual specificity phosphatase action. FEBS Lett. 1994;352:201–5.

39. Steinmetz R, Wagoner HA, Zeng P, Hammond JR, Hannon TS, Meyers JL, et al. Mechanisms Regulating the Constitutive Activation of the Extracellular Signal-Regulated Kinase (ERK) Signaling Pathway in Ovarian Cancer and the Effect of Ribonucleic Acid Interference for ERK1/2 on Cancer Cell Proliferation. Mol. Endocrinol. [Internet]. Oxford University Press; 2004;18:2570–82.

40. Steelman LS, Stadelman KM, Chappell WH, Horn S, Bäsecke J, Cervello M, et al. Akt as a therapeutic target in cancer. Expert Opin Ther Targets. 2008; 12:1139–65.

41. Yang X, Fraser M, Abedini MR, Bai T, Tsang BK. Regulation of apoptosis-inducing factor-mediated, cisplatin-induced apoptosis by Akt. Br J Cancer. 2008;98:803–8.

42. Peng D-J, Wang J, Zhou J-Y, Wu GS. Role of the Akt/mTOR survival pathway in cisplatin resistance in ovarian cancer cells. Biochem Biophys Res Commun. 2010;394:600–5.

43. Zhang JH, Ming M. DNA fragmentation in apoptosis. Cell Res. [Internet]. Nature Publishing Group. 2000;10:205–11.

44. Elmore S. Apoptosis: a review of programmed cell death. Toxicol Pathol. 2007;35:495–516.

Post-marketing safety surveillance and re-evaluation of Xueshuantong injection

Chunxiao Li[1], Tao Xu[1], Peng Zhou[1], Junhua Zhang[2], Ge Guan[1], Hui Zhang[1], Xiao Ling[1], Weixia Li[1], Fei Meng[1], Guanping Liu[3], Linyan Lv[3], Jun Yuan[4], Xuelin Li[1*] and Mingjun Zhu[1*]

Abstract

Background: Traditional Chinese medicine injections (TCMIs) have been widely used to treat severe and acute diseases due to their high bioavailability, accurate curative effect, and rapid effect. However, incidence rates of adverse drug reactions (ADRs) of TCMIs have also increased in recent years. Xueshuantong injection (XSTI) is a commonly-used TCMI comprised of Panax notoginseng total sapiens for the treatment of stroke hemiplegia, chest pain, and central retinal vein occlusion. Its safety remains uncelar. Therefore, post-marketing safety of XSTI was studied in this research.

Methods: In present study, post-marketing safety surveillance and re-evaluation of XSTI were reported. Thirty thousand eight hundred eighty-four patients in 33 hospitals from 7 provinces participated in this study. Incidence rate, most common clinical manifestations, types, severity, occurrence time, and disposal of ADRs were calculated.

Results: Incidence rate of ADR of XSTI was 4.14‰ and the most common clinical manifestations were skin and its appendages damage. Type A accounts for 95.49% of ADRs of XSTI and most of them (41.41%) were occurred within 24 h after receiving XSTI treatment. Severities of most ADRs of XSTI were moderate reactions (86.72%). Main disposition of ADRs of XSTI was drug withdrawal and symptomatic treatment (54.69%).

Conclusions: Our data provide basis for improvement of instructions of XSTI and clinical safety of XSTI. Post-marketing surveillance of TCMIs in this study is a powerful tool to identify types and manifestations of ADRs to improve safety and effectiveness of drugs in clinical applications.

Trial registration: This protocol has international registration in China clinical trial registration center (ChiCTR~OPC~ 14,005,718) at December 22, 2014.

Keywords: Xueshuantong injection, Post-marketing, ADRs/ADEs, Traditional Chinese medicine injections

Background

Traditional Chinese medicine injection (TCMI) is made by modern technologies and scientific methods to extract and purify effective substances from herbs (or decoction pieces). Compared with other traditional Chinese medicine formulations, injection has advantages of high bioavailability, rapid, and accurate curative effect. Therefore, TCMI is widely used to treat many severe and acute diseases [1–7]. In recent years, with the widespread use of TCMIs, the incidences of adverse drug reactions (ADRs)/adverse drug events (ADEs) has gradually increased [8–10]. However,

safety profile of most TCMIs remains largely unknown currently.

Xueshuantong injection (lyophilized) (XSTI) is a standardized herbal preparation and has been collected by "2012 national essential drugs list" and People's Republic of China Pharmacopoeia, respectively. Notoginseng total saponins, isolated from the root and rhizome of *P. notoginseng*, is the main component of XSTI. XSTI is generally used for treatment of cardiovascular and cerebrovascular disease [11]. Total revenue of XSTI in Chinese market in 2013 was over $700 million [12]. Therefore, the enormous consumption requires stricter and accurate evidence on its safety. However, many reports on the ADRs of XSTI were case reports and there is still lack large sample and high level evidence-based basis for safety of XSTI. Till now,

* Correspondence: lixuelin450000@163.com; zhumingjun317@163.com
[1]The First Affiliated Hospital of Henan University of Chinese Medicine, Zhengzhou 450000, People's Republic of China
Full list of author information is available at the end of the article

evaluation on post-marketing safety of XSTI has not been reported. Therefore, ADRs/ADEs of XSTI were studied in this research using hospital centralized monitoring method.

Hospital centralized monitoring also known as real world study (RWS), is an observational research method by recording detailed ADRs of drugs within a certain range of a hospital or an area in a certain period of time. It is attracting more and more attention in field of global clinical epidemiology due to its broad range of inclusion and exclusion criteria, comprehensive coverage of population, and authenticity [13–15]. A new hospital centralized monitoring method based on hospital information system (HIS) system was established in. our previous study on post-market clinical safety evaluation of TCMI [16]. In present research, post marketing safety (including incidence rate, types, severities, and other information of ADRs/ADEs) of XSTI with 30,884 cases by employing an improved method of hospital-centralized monitoring. This research is the first post-marketing ADRs/ADEs study of XSTI with large scale and multi-center and can provide essential basis for safe clinical use of XSTI.

Methods
Inclusion and exclusion criteria
Inclusion criteria: patients who used XSTI.
Exclusion criteria: patients who did not use XSTI.

Subjects
A total of 30,884 in-patients received XSTI from 33 hospitals in 7 provinces participated in this study between January 1, 2015 and December 31, 2016.

Drug
All three product specification (100 mg、150 mg and 250 mg per bottle) of XSTI were manufactured by Guangxi Wuzhou Pharmaceutical Co., Ltd. (Wuzhou, Guangxi, China). All drugs used in this research were sold on the market and in conformity with the standard of Ministry of Public Health of China.

Method design
This study was not a randomized controlled trial but a centralized monitoring study in hospital and all data were collected from clinical daily treatment without any intervention. Thus this study was not designed entirely according to CONSORT guidelines. We designed the monitoring data collection and quality control method according to other hospital centralized monitoring methods [13–16].

Method of monitoring data collection
The monitoring data were from two parts: monitoring table and hospital information system / laboratory information management system (HIS/LIS). Information in front page of the medical record, doctor's orders and results of laboratory examination were extracted from HIS/LIS system after being approved by ethics committee. To ensure the safety of the patient's personal information all monitors have been trained on information confidentiality. Monitoring table consists of Table A (basic monitoring information including daily dose, frequency, drug combination, etc.) and Table B (ADR/ADE information). Table A was filled by pharmacists within 5 days after the end of medication by "face-to-face" observation. Monitoring Table B was filled once ADR/ADE, especially serious ADR/ADE such as anaphylactic shock, severe allergic reactions, severe mucocutaneous lesions, liver damage, renal damage, and death, was happened. Accordance to requirements of "National ADR Reporting and Monitoring Management Measures", all serious ADRs/ADEs were further investigated by a panel consisting of head of organizer of the project and staffs from sub center and manufacturing enterprise. "Adverse Drug Reaction / Event Report" was written and submitted to official website according to the rules of the CFDA. The overall data collection flow chart is shown in Fig. 1 and ADRs/ADEs processing process is shown in Fig. 2.

Method of monitoring quality control
In order to guarantee the objectivity and accuracy of ADR results, unified training on monitoring plan and ADRs/ADEs judgment was carried out for monitoring personnel and a three-grade evaluation of ADRs / ADEs and third party quality control were conducted in this study. The detailed monitoring process is shown in Fig. 2. Strict selection criteria were set for the screening of participating hospital. Primary quality control monitoring hospital included comprehensive hospital and traditional Chinese medicine hospital. Sub-center monitoring hospitals were all three grade hospital in China and have organized or participated in the evaluation of drug safety. All participating hospitals had a team of clinical pharmacists and collected at least 500 cases within 1 years. There were 7 sub centers in total, and each sub center was responsible for 5–6 hospitals. A contract research organization (CRO) company (Shanghai Yongzheng medical science and Technology Co., Ltd.), was employed to carry on quality management of the study (Fig. 3). Reliability of monitoring reports and research progress of each monitoring hospitals and monitoring centers regularly were judged by CRO company. The hospitals which couldn't complete the monitoring progress on time or their monitoring reports were judged as unqualified more than three times were refused to continue to participate into the research project. The sub center was eliminated when more than half of its monitoring hospitals were eliminated.

Correlation assessment between ADRs and ADEs
Correlation assessment between ADRs and ADEs was conducted according to method recommended by CFDA

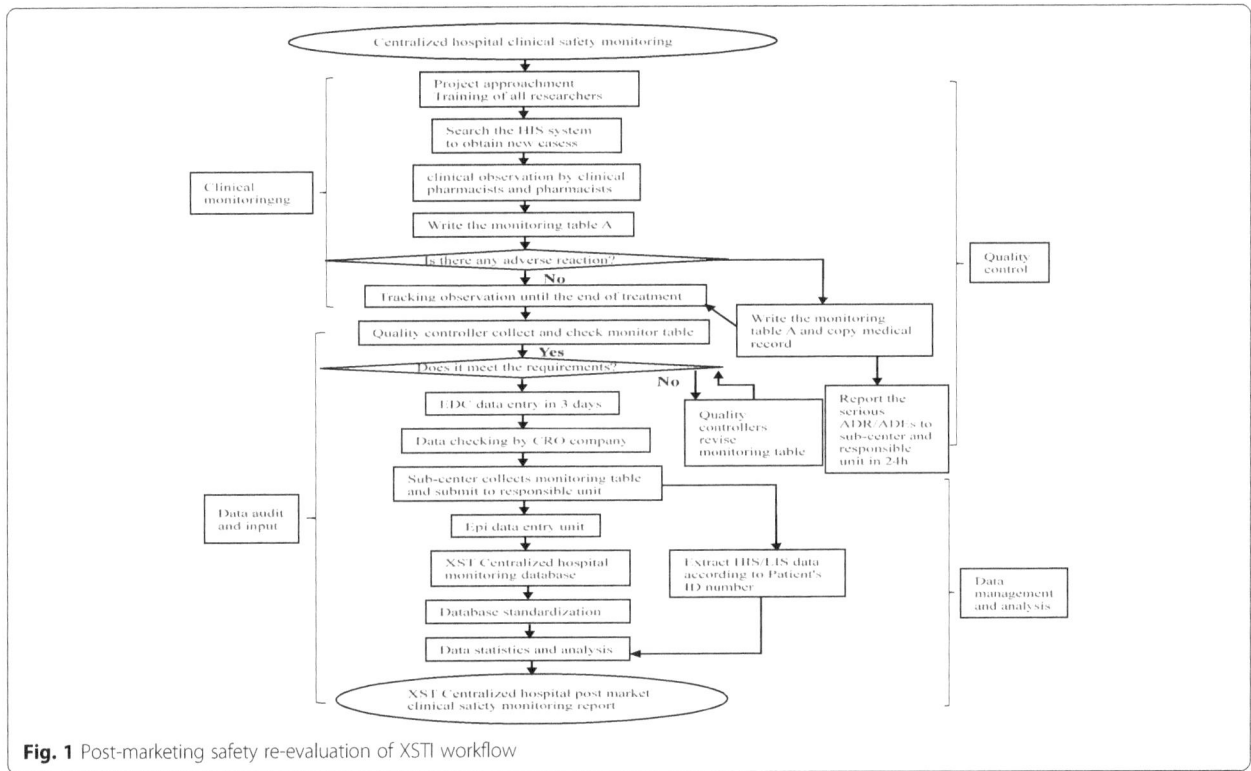

Fig. 1 Post-marketing safety re-evaluation of XSTI workflow

evaluation center of adverse reactions. All ADRs/ADEs were preliminarily classified on basis of their definitions, respectively. ADR is unrelated or unexpected adverse reaction to medication purpose when using approved drugs within normal dosage. It does not include reactions caused by accidental or intentional drug overdoses or improper medications. ADE refers to any injury occurred during drug administration period, whether or not drug usage is the cause of injury. ADR is a special type of ADE for which the causative relationship between drug usage and adverse reaction is identified. Relevance assessment is divided into 6 grades: (1) Certain: the sequence between medication and ADRs' occurrence is reasonable. ADRs could be stopped or quickly reduced or turn better after drug withdrawal. Alternatively, ADRs would be occured again or significantly worse when drug was re-administered. It could also be supported by literatures. Notably, primary disease and other factors should be ruled out. (2) Probable: there is no history of repeating medication, others are same as "Certain". If the investigated drug was administrated in combination with other drugs, the probability of ADR caused by combined drugs could be excluded. (3) Possible: there is close relationship between medication and ADEs' occurrence. It is coincided with common type of ADRs, but there is no reaction data after drug withdrawal, or there are more than one drug leading to ADRs/ADEs, or causative factors of primary disease could not be ruled out. (4) Unlikely: there was no close relationship between medication and ADEs' occurrence. The reactions do not link to ADRs/ADEs of the investigated

drug. Reactions during development of primary disease may display similar clinical manifestations. (5) Pending: There are missing contents of "Monitoring Information Form" and evaluation will not be completed until the supplementary specifications are provided. Thus, it is difficult to determine relationship between cause and effect due to absence in documentation. (6) Unassessable: many items in the "Monitoring Information Form" are unavailable. It is unable to analyze relationship between cause and effect because missing items could not be supplemented [2, 17, 18].

Results
Number of cases of XSTI in each hospital
In this study, a total of 30,884 cases received XSTI from 33 hospitals participated in the monitoring assessment. The number of ADE cases in 33 monitoring hospitals is shown in Table 1.

Association assessment of adverse reactions
In this study, 128 cases were grouped as "probable and possible ". Results of relevance evaluation were shown in Table 2.

Incidence rate and manifestations of ADRs
The ADR incidence of XSTI was 4.14‰. The clinical manifestations were 236 times. The most common clinical manifestations were skin and its appendages damage (52.97%), systemic injury (9.32%), and central and peripheral nervous

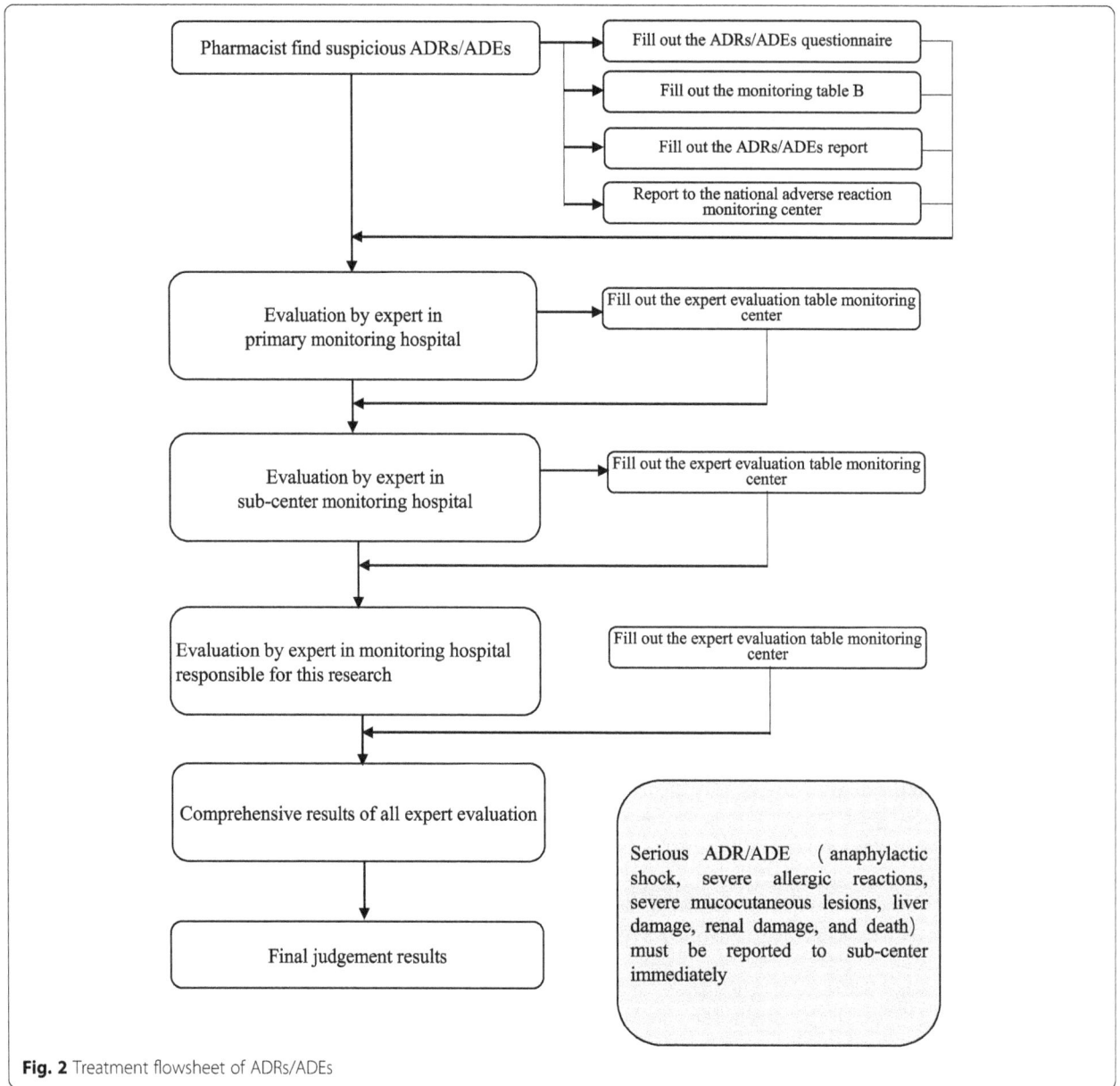

Fig. 2 Treatment flowsheet of ADRs/ADEs

system damage (8.90%). Statistics analysis were shown in Table 3 in detail.

Types of ADRs

ADRs are classified into three types (types A, B, and C) by WHO. Type A reaction caused by the enhancement of pharmacological effect of drugs is dose-related and able to be predicted. Type B reaction is abnormal reaction unrelated to normal pharmacological effect. It is not able to be detected by conventional toxicological screening and hard to make prediction. Type C reaction refers to abnormal reaction other than types A and B. According to above classification, all 128 cases of ADRs were divided into type A, B, and C, respectively as shown in Table 4.

Time of occurrence of ADRs

Time of occurrence of ADRs after injection of XSTI is shown in Table 5 and Table 6. According to the results, most ADRs of XST were occurred rapidly and nearly half cases of ADRs were appeared on the first day of injection (41.41%). There is 25.78% of ADRs were happened 2~ 4 days after injection.

Severity of ADRs

As shown in Table 7, severity of ADRs were classified into three grades: mild (symptoms or signs can be felt and stopping medication or special treatment is no necessary), moderate (symptoms and signs are tolerable and there is no effect on daily life but special treatment is necessary), and severe (symptoms and signs are intolerable and drug

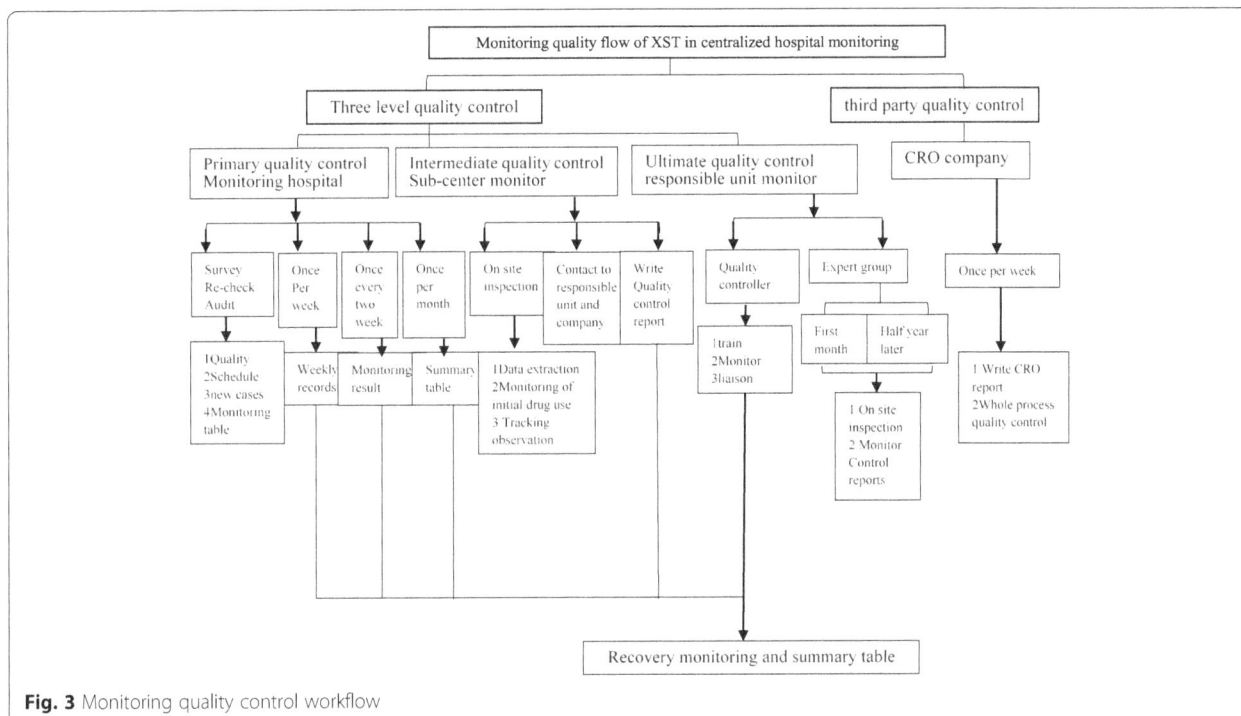

Fig. 3 Monitoring quality control workflow

withdrawal and special treatment are needed). Our results showed that most cases (86.72%) were graded into moderate reactions and 11 cases were classified as mild. In addition, among 6 cases with severe ADRs, 3 cases had severe symptoms, including rash, flushing, shivering, palpitation, high fever, dyspnea, and convulsions.

Disposal of ADRs

In most cases, ADRs need special treatments such as reducing times and dose of usage, withdrawal, symptomatic treatment, or combined together. Special treatments used in this study were listed as follows: withdrawal and symptomatic treatment (54.69%), withdrawal (30.47%), symptomatic treatment (7.03%) (Table 8). In addition, 1.56% of the ADRs did not get any special treatment.

Recovery of ADRs

Among of patients with ADRs, 80 cases were cured, 48 cases got improved, and there was no sequelae and death. Upon recovery time, 12, 26, 17, and 70 cases were improved within 1 h (9.38%), 1 ~ 6 h (20.31%), 6 ~ 24 h (13.28%), or over 24 h (54.69%), respectively. In addition, 3 cases were not recorded in detail.

Discussion

The incidence of ADRs of XSTI was 4.14‰, which was an "occasionally" "level and severe ADRs was 0.19 ‰, which was a "rare" grade and 95.49% of ADRs in this research were type A which can be predicted. 42.97% of ADRs were recovered in 24 h and there was no sequelae

and death. Therefore, XSTI is safe in clinical use according to the incidence, type and recovery of ADRs in this study. Most of ADRs were anaphylaxis which indicated that safety monitoring should be in progress promptly. In addition, ADRs of XSTI could happened throughout the whole course of treatment after administration which indicated that the whole process needs safety monitoring. So far, the description of the XSTI used in the study is not clear about ADRs. The results of this study make clear the manifestations of ADRs of XSTI, which provide a high level evidence-based basis for the improvement of the instructions. In this research, manifestations of ADRs were studied and the most common ADR manifestation of XSTI was skin and its appendages damages which were consistent with other published reports [19]. However, there is no suitable medicine to alleviate the ADRs of cutaneous systems. The main preventive measures by far is washing infusion tube before the injection of different injections to reduce the incidence of ADRs during the combined use of XSTI and other injections. It is generally believed that the skin and its appendages damages were caused by allergies. There is a study using P815 cell degranulation model to screen components of XSTJ [20]. Results showed that XSTI promoted the P815 cell degranulation and the effect may have related to Ginsenoside Rb1 and Rg1. Besides, impurities are difficult to remove in purification and refining processes due to the complex components in traditional Chinese medicine injections, which may also cause anaphylaxis [21–23]. However, few studies on the

Table 1 The number of ADE cases in 33 monitoring hospitals

Hospitals	Number of cases	Constituent ratio (%)
The First Affiliated Hospital of Henan University of TCM	2103	6.81
The Second Affiliated Hospital of Henan University of TCM	1006	3.26
Henan Province People's Hospital	1997	6.47
Luohe Central Hospital	697	2.26
General Hospital of Shenma medical group	1089	3.53
The First Affiliated Hospital of Guangxi University of TCM	1500	4.86
The First people's Hospital of Nanning	1011	3.27
The people's Hospital Guangxi Zhuang Autonomous Region	601	1.95
Nanning Hospital of TCM	607	1.97
The Jiangbin Hospital Guangxi Zhuang Autonomous Region	600	1.94
Wuzhou Red Cross Hospital	812	2.63
Wuzhou People's Hospital	802	2.60
The Second Affiliated Hospital of Tianjin University of TCM	1810	5.86
Peking University Binhai Hospital	515	1.67
Tianjin Huanhu Hospital	1203	3.89
Tianjin First Central Hospital	1213	3.93
Tianjin Hospital of ITCWM Nankai Hospital	802	2.60
Shuguang Hospital of Shanghai University of TCM	501	1.62
Tongji Hospital of Shanghai	501	1.62
Longhua Hospital of Shanghai University of TCM	502	1.63
People's Hospital of Pudong District of Shanghai	504	1.63
West China Hospital of Scichuan University	1504	4.87
Sichuan Cancer Hospital	1001	3.24
The people's Hospital of Dujiangyan	800	2.59
Affiliated Hospital of Chengdu University	603	1.95
Affiliated Hospital of Chengdu University of TCM	1034	3.35
Gansu Province Hospital of TCM	1223	3.96
The Second People's Hospital of Gansu	406	1.31
The People's Hospital of Gansu	807	2.61
Affiliated Hospital of Gansu University of TCM	635	2.06
The First Bethune Hospital of Jilin University	1830	5.93
Affiliated Hospital of Changchun University of TCM	502	1.63
The General Hospital of CNPC in Jilin	163	0.53
Total	30,884	100.00

Table 2 Results of correlation evaluation between ADRs and ADEs of XSTI

Results of correlation evaluation	Number of cases	Constituent ratio (%)
Certain	0	0.00
Probable	53	41.09
Possible	75	58.14
Unlikely	1	0.78
Pending	0	0.00
Unassessable	0	0.00
Total	129	100

Table 3 ADR manifestations of XSTI

Systems/organs	Number of cases/ incidence rate ‰	Constituent ratio (%)	Manifestations (number of cases/frequency‰)
Skin and its appendages	125/4.05	52.97	erythra (61/1.98), pruritus (50/1.62), maculopapule (8/0.26), hyperhidrosis (4/0.13), urticaria (4/0.13)
Systemic injury	22/0.71	9.32	fever (6/0.19), Shiver (6/0.19), edema (4/0.13), Chest pain (2/0.06), anaphylactoid reaction (1/0.03), periorbital edema (1/0.03), hot flush (1/0.03), acratia (1/0.03)
Central and peripheral nervous system damage	21/0.68	8.90	headache (9/0.29), giddy (6/0.19), paresthesia (4/0.13), lower limb spasticity (1/0.03), tremor (1/0.03)
Gastrointestinal system damage	14/0.45	5.93	sicchasia (4/0.13), vomit (2/0.06), hemorrhage of gastrointestinal tract (1/0.03), aggravation of gastrointestinal bleeding (1/0.03), dry lips (1/0.03), Stool discoloration (1/0.03), abdominal pain (1/0.03), discoloration of tongue (1/0.03), flatulence (1/0.03), toothache (1/0.03)
Respiratory system damage	14/0.45	5.93	Chest tightness (10), dyspnea (2), laryngeal spasm (1/0.03), epistaxis (1/0.03)
Extra cardiac vessel damage	10/0.32	4.24	flushing (9/0.29), phlebitis (1/0.03)
Medication site damage	10/0.32	4.24	local numbness (4/0.13), injection site pain (4/0.13), injection site numbness (1/0.03), injection site pruritus (1/0.03)
Urinary system damage	7/0.23	2.97	facial edema (6/0.19), hematuria (1/0.03)
Heart rate and arrhythmia	6/0.19	2.54	palpitation (5/0.16), tachycardia (1/0.03)
Nerve disorders	4/0.13	1.69	feel suffocated (3/0.10), insomnia (1/0.03)
Visual impairment	1/0.03	0.42	abnormal tears (1/0.03)
General cardiovascular system damage	1/0.03	0.42	Hypertension (1/0.03)
latelets and bleeding, coagulopathy	1/0.03	0.42	Gingival bleeding (1/0.03)
Total	236	100.00	

Incidence rate = number of adverse events *1000‰/ total number of cases

anaphylaxis mechanism of XSTI or panax notoginseng saponins and further investigation are needed to explore the ADR mechanism of XSTI. In addition, this study found some ADRs beyond instruction.

By comparison of four methods (hospital-centralized monitoring method, spontaneous reporting method, literature research method, and medical record review method) in our previous study on post-market clinical safety evaluation of TCMI and other reports, hospital centralized monitoring is a scientific, advanced, and feasible tool to assess clinical safety of TCM injection receiving approval [16]. In this study, monitoring method was improved on the basis of classic hospital-centralized monitoring. First, HIS/LIS system was utilized in the study. To analyze the impact factors of the ADRs/ADEs caused by XSTI, a large number of information associated with

ADRs/ADEs were collected. The data collected in the research were composed of general information, medication information and laboratory test data. The general information and medication information such as patients' ID number, gender, age, height, weight, admission diagnosis, allergic history, nationality, dosage, combined administration were mainly collected by monitoring table, while the laboratory test data such as blood routine, urine routine, faecal routine, liver function, renal function, thrombus and hemostasis and other inspection results were all extracted from HIS/LIS. Besides, the missing information in some of the monitoring tables were also supplemented by the HIS system. Secondly, majority of data collection and analyses in this study was performed by clinical pharmacists. Pharmacist plays important role in rational drug applications and improvement of life quality of patients. In one hand, clinical pharmacists are familiar with the treatment process of ADR/ADEs, on the other hand, they can put

Table 4 Comprehensive evaluation of occurrence types of ADR/ADE

Type	Number of cases	Constituent ratio (%)
A	127	95.49
B	6	4.51
C	0	0.00
Total	133	100

Table 5 ADR Occurrence time of XSTI

	occurrence time (hours)				Total
	Day 1	Day 2~4	Day 5~7	>7 Days	
Number of cases	53	33	18	24	128
Constituent ratio (%)	41.41	25.78	14.06	18.72	100.00

Table 6 The time distance of ADR occurrence time and the last medication time of XSTI

	occurrence time (hours)				Total
	<0.5	0.5~1	1~12	12~24	
Number of cases	33	23	53	19	128
Constituent ratio (%)	25.78	17.97	41.41	14.84	100.00

more concentration on the research by comparison with clinician. Altogether, pharmacist is the best candidate for ADE surveillance. Last but not least, strict quality control method was designed in this multi-center research. Three-level quality control method used in this study has been successfully used in our previous post-marketing safety surveillance of Danhong injection. In order to strengthen quality control, third-party quality control, a contract research organization (CRO) company, was employed in this study. Because CRO companies has a large number of professional medical and pharmaceutical experts, they actively participate in many phase II or III clinical trials and undertake supervision as the third party, to guarantee the objectivity of the result in studies. Application of above working model in our study contributed greatly to improve objectivity of results and efficiency of research.

Our study has several shorter. We calculated the incidence, main types, main manifestations and severity classification of ADRs in this article, which reflect the safety of clinical use of XSTI in general, but the main influencing factors of ADRs were not studied in this article. However, all relevant data have been collected and are being analyzed. We will complete this part of study in following researches. In addition, the mechanism of the ADRs in the study is still unknown.

Conclusion

Post-marketing safety surveillance and re-evaluation of XSTI was carried out with 30,884 cases from 33 hospitals in 7 provinces. We obtained incidence rate, types, severities, as well as other information of ADRs/ADEs of XSTI. As far as we know, this research is the first study on the ADR of XSTI using large-scale hospital centralized monitoring method. The results in this study provide a high level

Table 7 The severity classification of ADR of XSTI

Severity classification	Number of cases	Constituent ratio (%)
Mild	11	8.59
Moderate	111	86.72
Severe	6	4.69
Total	128	100.00

Table 8 The disposal of ADR of XSTI

Disposal	Number of cases	Constituent ratio (%)
None	2	1.56
Reduce dripping speed (RDS)	7	5.47
Reduce dose	0	0.00
Drug withdrawal (DW)	39	30.47
Symptomatic treatment (ST)	9	7.03
RDS + DW + ST	1	0.78
DW + ST	70	54.69
Total	128	100.00

evidence-based basis for safety of XSTI. We further founded novel research system and mode of post-marketing safety surveillance and re-evaluation of TCMIs, which also provides a method to dramatically improve rationality and safety of clinical applications of TCMIs.

Acknowledgments
The authors want to thank all volunteers in our research team who participated in this study. We also thank academician Boli Zhang and researcher Weiliang Wong for guidance.

Funding
This work was supported by a grant from the National Science and Technology Major Projects for "Major New Drugs Innovation and Development" (2012ZX09101201).

Authors' contributions
C-XL, TX, PZ and GG were participated in this study as clinical pharmacists and all data were collected by them and C-XL wrote the manuscript. TX, J-HZ and HZ performed the analysis of the data. XL and W-XL were major contributors in writing the manuscript. FM, G-PL, L-YL, JY were major contributors in the data quality control. X-LL and M-JZ designed this research and were corresponding authors of this article. All authors read and approved the final manuscript.

Ethics approval and consent to participate
This study was an observational study. No medical intervention was conducted on the observed objects. The experiment protocol was approved by the Ethical Committee of the First Affiliated Hospital of Henan University of TCM (Approval number 2014HL~053). In addition, this protocol has international registration in China clinical trial registration center (ChiCTR~OPC~14,005,718). Written informed consents were obtained from all participants.

Competing interests
The authors declare that they have no competing interests.

Author details
[1]The First Affiliated Hospital of Henan University of Chinese Medicine, Zhengzhou 450000, People's Republic of China. [2]Evidence-based Medicine Center, Tianjin University of Traditional Chinese Medicine, Tianjin 300000, People's Republic of China. [3]Guangxi Wuzhou Pharmaceutical (group) Co., Ltd, Wuzhou 543000, People's Republic of China. [4]Shanghai Yongzheng Medical Science and Technology Co., Ltd, Shanghai 200000, People's Republic of China.

References

1. National Pharmacopoeia Committee, Chinese Pharmacopoeia. Part 1. Beijing: Chemical Industry Press; 2005: Appendix 13.
2. Ren D-Q, Zhang B-L. Clinical application guide of TCM injections, People's health publishing house. China: Beijing; 2011.
3. Li B, Wang Y, Lu J, et al. Evaluating the effects of Danhong injection in treatment of acute ischemic stroke: study protocol for a multicenter randomized controlled trial. Trials. 2015, 9;16:561.
4. Liu Y, Huang Y, Zhao C, et al. Salvia miltiorrhiza injection on pulmonary heart disease: a systematic review and meta-analysis. Am J Chin Med. 2014; 42(6):1315–31.
5. Yang H, Zhang W, Huang C, et al. A novel systems pharmacology model for herbal medicine injection: a case using Reduning injection. BMC Complement Altern Med. 2014, 4;14:430.
6. Luo J, Shang Q, Han M, et al. Traditional Chinese medicine injection for angina pectoris: an overview of systematic reviews. Am J Chin Med. 2014;42(1):37–59.
7. Fu S, Zhang J, Menniti-Ippolito F, et al. Huangqi injection (a traditional Chinese patent medicine) for chronic heart failure: a systematic review. PloS One. 2011, 6;6(5): 19604.
8. Guo XJ, Ye XF, Wang XX, et al. Reporting patterns of adverse drug reactions over recent years in China: analysis from publications. Expert Opin Drug Saf. 2015;14(2):191–8.
9. Liao X, Robinson N. Methodological approaches to developing and establishing the body of evidence on post-marketing Chinese medicine safety. Chin J Integr Med. 2013;19(7):494–7.
10. Wang L, Yuan Q, Marshall G, et al. Adverse drug reactions and adverse events of 33 varieties of traditional Chinese medicine injections on National Essential medicines list (2004 edition) of China: an overview on published literatures. J Evid Based Med. 2010;3(2):95–104.
11. Wang XM, Wang SX, Wang JX, et al. Neuroprotective effect of xueshuantong for injection (lyophilized) in transient and permanent rat cerebral ischemia model. Evid Based Complement Alternat Med. 2015;2015:134685.
12. Wang FJ, Wang SX, Chai LJ, et al. Xueshuantong injection (lyophilized) combined with salvianolate lyophilized injection protects against focal cerebral ischemia/reperfusion injury in rats through attenuation of oxidative stress. Acta Pharmacol Sin. 2017;36:1–14.
13. Zhao Y, Shi C, Huang P. Analysis of clinical use of post-marketing hospital centralized monitoring of Xiyanping injection. Zhongguo Zhong Yao Za Zhi. 2016;41(4):743–7.
14. Jiang JJ, Xie YM. Discussion on establishment of quality control system for intensive hospital monitoring on traditional Chinese medicine injections. Zhongguo Zhong Yao Za Zhi. 2012;37(18):2689–91.
15. Li X, Tang J, Meng F, et al. Study on 10 409 cases of post-marketing safety Danhong injection centralized monitoring of hospital. Zhongguo Zhong Yao Za Zhi. 2011;36(20):2783–5.
16. Li XL, Tang JF, Li WX, et al. Postmarketing safety surveillance and reevaluation of Danhong injection: clinical study of 30888 cases. Evid Based Complement Alternat Med. 2015;2015:610846.
17. Y.-Y. Wang, A.-P. Lv, and Y.-M. Xie. The key technologies of clinical re-evaluation of post-marketing traditional Chinese medicine, People's medical publishing house, Beijing, China,2011.
18. Baars E-W, Jong M, Nierop AF, et al. Savelkoul, "Citrus/cydonia compositum subcutaneous injections versus nasal spray for seasonal allergic rhinitis: a randomized controlled trial on efficacy and safety,". ISRN Allergy. 2011;2011:836051.
19. He GF, Dou WM. Zeng retrospective analysis on 697 cases of adverse drug reaction of Xueshuantong preparations. Chin J Pharmacoepidemiol. 2016; 11(25):715–8.
20. Li HC, Wu QY, Fu JT, et al. Study on screening method of allergenic ingredients of TCM injections. Pharmacol Clin Chin Mater Med. 2014;01(30):139–41.
21. Feng WW, Zhang Y, Tang JF, et al. Combination of chemical fingerprinting with bioassay, a preferable approach for quality control of safflower injection. Anal Chim Acta. 2018,20;1003:56–63.
22. Zhang L, Ma L, Feng W, et al. Quality fluctuation detection of an herbal injection based on biological fingerprint combined with chemical fingerprint. Anal Bioanal Chem. 2014;406(20):5009–18.
23. Ren Y, Zhang P, Yan D, et al. A strategy for the detection of quality fluctuation of a Chinese herbal injection based on chemical fingerprinting combined with biological fingerprinting. J Pharm Biomed Anal. 2011;56(2):436–42.

Croton gratissimus leaf extracts inhibit cancer cell growth by inducing caspase 3/7 activation with additional anti-inflammatory and antioxidant activities

Emmanuel Mfotie Njoya[1,2]* ⓘ, Jacobus N. Eloff[1] and Lyndy J. McGaw[1]

Abstract

Background: *Croton* species (Euphorbiaceae) are distributed in different parts of the world, and are used in traditional medicine to treat various ailments including cancer, inflammation, parasitic infections and oxidative stress related diseases. The present study aimed to evaluate the antioxidant, anti-inflammatory and cytotoxic properties of different extracts from three *Croton* species.

Methods: Acetone, ethanol and water leaf extracts from *C. gratissimus*, *C. pseudopulchellus*, and *C. sylvaticus* were tested for their free radical scavenging activity. Anti-inflammatory activity was determined via the nitric oxide (NO) inhibitory assay on lipopolysaccharide (LPS)-stimulated RAW 264.7 macrophages, and the 15-lipoxygenase inhibitory assay using the ferrous oxidation-xylenol orange assay. The cytotoxicity of the extracts was determined on four cancerous cell lines (A549, Caco-2, HeLa, MCF-7), and a non-cancerous African green monkey (Vero) kidney cells using the tetrazolium-based colorimetric (MTT) assay. The potential mechanism of action of the active extracts was explored by quantifying the caspase-3/−7 activity with the Caspase-Glo® 3/7 assay kit (Promega).

Results: The acetone and ethanol leaf extracts of *C. pseudopulchellus* and *C. sylvaticus* were highly cytotoxic to the non-cancerous cells with LC_{50} varying between 7.86 and 48.19 μg/mL. In contrast, the acetone and ethanol extracts of *C. gratissimus* were less cytotoxic to non-cancerous cells and more selective with LC_{50} varying between 152.30 and 462.88 μg/mL, and selectivity index (SI) ranging between 1.56 and 11.64. Regarding the anti-inflammatory activity, the acetone leaf extract of *C. pseudopulchellus* had the highest NO inhibitory potency with an IC_{50} of 34. 64 μg/mL, while the ethanol leaf extract of the same plant was very active against 15-lipoxygenase with an IC_{50} of 0.57 μg/mL. A linear correlation ($r < 0.5$) was found between phytochemical contents, antioxidant, anti-inflammatory and cytotoxic activities of active extracts. These extracts induced differentially the activation of caspases − 3 and − 7 enzymes in all the four cancerous cells with the highest induction (1.83-fold change) obtained on HeLa cells with the acetone leaf extract of *C. gratissimus*.

Conclusion: Based on their selective toxicity, good antioxidant and anti-inflammatory activities, the acetone and ethanol leaf extracts of *C. gratissimus* represent promising alternative sources of compounds against cancer and other oxidative stress related diseases.

Keywords: *Croton gratissimus*, Free radicals, Nitric oxide, 15-lipoxygenase, Cytotoxicity, Caspases

* Correspondence: mfotiefr@yahoo.fr
[1]Phytomedicine Programme, Department of Paraclinical Sciences, Faculty of Veterinary Science, University of Pretoria, Private Bag X04, Onderstepoort, Pretoria 0110, South Africa
[2]Department of Biochemistry, Faculty of Science, University of Yaoundé I, P.O. Box 812, Yaoundé, Cameroon

Background

Oxidative stress results from an imbalance between the production of free radicals and the ability of the body to counteract or detoxify their harmful effects through neutralization by antioxidants [1]. The free radical theory of aging developed by Denham Harman is based on the concept that damage accumulates throughout the entire lifespan and causes age dependent disorders including diabetes, atherosclerosis, neurodegenerative diseases and cancer [2, 3]. Cancer development is characterized by redox imbalance with a shift towards oxidative conditions. In fact, free radicals can bind through electron pairing with macromolecules such as proteins, phospholipids and DNA in normal cells to cause protein and DNA damage along with lipid peroxidation [1]. Consequently, the accumulation of these cellular disorders may cause mutation and lead to various disturbances in the cell metabolism, which can result in deregulated cell growth, and finally carcinoma [4]. Antioxidants are helpful in reducing and preventing damage caused by free radicals because of their ability to donate electrons, which neutralize the radicals without forming another. This property has led to the hypothesis that antioxidants, with their ability to decrease the level of free radicals, might lessen the radical damage causing chronic diseases, and even radical damage responsible for aging and cancer. Antioxidant phytochemicals found in vegetables, fruits and medicinal plants have been reported to be responsible for health benefits such as the prevention and treatment of chronic diseases caused by oxidative stress [5]. Many antioxidant phytochemicals have been associated with anti-cancer activities, and this includes curcumin from turmeric, genistein from soybean, tea polyphenols from green tea, resveratrol from grapes, sulforaphane from broccoli, isothiocyanates from cruciferous vegetables, silymarin from milk thistle, diallyl sulfide from garlic, lycopene from tomato, rosmarinic acid from rosemary, apigenin from parsley, and gingerol from gingers [6].

During the last two decades, it has been revealed that oxidative stress can lead to chronic inflammation, which in turn could mediate most chronic diseases including cancer. Chronic inflammation is usually associated with an increased risk of several human cancers [7]. Indeed, the relationship between inflammation and cancer has been suggested by epidemiological and experimental data, and confirmed by the fact that anti-inflammatory therapies were also efficient in cancer prevention and treatment [8, 9].

The genus *Croton* belongs to the family Euphorbiaceae, and is a diverse and complex group of plants ranging from herbs and shrubs to trees. *Croton* species can be found in different parts of the world, and some of the most popular uses include treatment of cancer, constipation, diabetes, digestive problems, dysentery, external wounds, intestinal worms, pain, ulcers and weight loss

[10]. *Croton sylvaticus* Hochst. is a fast-growing and decorative tree, which is widely used in the management of inflammatory conditions, infections and oxidative stress related diseases. In Tanzania and Kenya, the decoction of the leaves and root bark of *C. sylvaticus* is used in traditional medicine against tuberculosis (TB), inflammation, as a purgative, as a wash for body swelling caused by kwashiorkor or by tuberculosis, and for the treatment of malaria [11]. Previous reports showed the acetylcholinesterase inhibitory activity of the ethyl acetate leaf extract of *C. sylvaticus* and isolated compounds [12]. Other compounds isolated from this plant have antiplasmodial activity [13], and low to high toxicity observed in the brine shrimp larval lethality test [11]. *Croton gratissimus* Burch. (synonym *C. zambesicus* Müll.Arg.) is native to tropical west and central Africa, and is used to treat fever, dysentery and convulsions [14]. The leaf decoction is used in Benin as anti-hypertensive, anti-microbial (against urinary infections) and to treat malaria-linked fever [15]. Some compounds, named cembranolides isolated from leaf extracts of *Croton gratissimus*, have moderate activity against ovarian cancer cell lines and *Plasmodium falciparum* [16, 17]. *Croton pseudopulchellus* Pax, originating from southern Africa, is widely distributed in tropical East and West Africa. This *Croton* species is used in southern and central parts of South Africa against TB symptoms such as coughs, fever and blood in sputum [18]. Based on their diverse uses in traditional medicine against various diseases in which excess production of free radicals or inflammation is implicated, the present study aims to evaluate the antioxidant, anti-inflammatory and cytotoxic properties of three *Croton* species extracted using different solvents.

Materials and methods
Plant material and extraction

Fresh leaves of the three *Croton* species were collected at the Lowveld Botanical Gardens, Nelspruit, Mpumalanga (South Africa) in January 2016. The plant materials were dried at room temperature in a well-ventilated room for two weeks. The dried materials were ground to fine powder and stored in honey jars in the dark until use. Herbarium specimens for each of the plant species were prepared, and identification was made by Mrs. Elsa van Wyk and Ms. Magda Nel of the HGWJ Schweickerdt Herbarium (PRU), University of Pretoria. The identification numbers of plant species are presented in Table 1. Powder (100 g) from each plant was extracted by maceration in 1000 mL of different solvents (water, acetone and ethanol). The mixtures were covered and left overnight at room temperature. Each mixture was filtered through Whatman No.1 filter paper into pre-weighed honey jars and the filtrates obtained from acetone and ethanol extraction were concentrated under reduced pressure using a rotary evaporator at 40 °C to obtain a residue which

Table 1 Herbarium specimen identification and yield of crude extracts from the three *Croton* species

Plant name	Family name	Herbarium specimen no.	Yield of extraction (%)		
			Water	Acetone	Ethanol
Croton gratissimus Burch.	Euphorbiaceae	PRU/122516	3.29	5.15	6.23
Croton pseudopulchellus Pax	Euphorbiaceae	PRU/122519	4.65	7.63	8.95
Croton sylvaticus Hochst.	Euphorbiaceae	PRU/122523	4.11	6.18	7.59

constituted the crude extract. The water filtrate was dried in a ventilated oven at 50–55 °C until complete evaporation of water. The extraction process was repeated three times with fresh solvent. The honey jars containing the crude extracts were weighed again to determine the percentage yield of the crude extracts (Table 1). The dried extracts were stored in a cold room (4 °C) until use.

Phytochemical analysis
Total phenolic content
The total phenolic content (TPC) of different extracts was determined using the Folin-Ciocalteu method adapted to a 96-well microplate as described by Zhang et al. [19]. The reaction mixture was prepared by adding respectively 20 μL of each extract (5 mg/mL in DMSO), 100 μL of Folin-Ciocalteu reagent (1 mL of Folin-Ciocalteu reagent in 9 mL of distilled water), and 80 μL 7.5% Na_2CO_3 solution in deionized water. The mixture was then incubated in the dark at room temperature (25 °C) for 30 min, and the absorbance was read at 765 nm on a microplate reader (Epoch, BioTek). The total phenolic content was estimated from a gallic acid (GA) calibration curve (10–100 mg/L; $y = 0.6886x + 0.0884$; $R^2 = 0.9901$), and results were expressed as milligram of gallic acid equivalent (GAE) per gram of extract.

Total flavonoid content
The total flavonoid content (TFC) of different extracts was determined using the aluminium chloride spectrophotometric method based on the formation of aluminium-flavonoid complexes [20]. The reaction mixture was prepared by mixing 2 mL of each extract (0.3 mg in 1 mL of methanol), 0.1 mL of aluminium chloride hexahydrate solution (10% aqueous $AlCl_3$ solution), 0.1 mL of 1 M potassium acetate and 2.8 mL of deionized water. The mixture was shaken and incubated at room temperature (25 °C) for 10 min, and 200 μL of each mixture was transferred to 96-well microplate. The absorbance was measured at 415 nm using a microplate reader (Epoch, BioTek). A calibration curve was plotted from the absorbance of quercetin (0.005–0.1 mg/mL; $y = 9.0545x - 0.0142$; $R^2 = 0.9999$), and the total flavonoid content was expressed as milligram of quercetin equivalent (QE) per gram of extract.

Antioxidant assays
The 2,2-diphenyl-1-picrylhydrazyl (DPPH) assay
The technique described by Brand-Williams et al. [21] with some modifications was applied for the determination of the DPPH scavenging capacity of extracts. Briefly, the extracts (40 μL) were serially diluted with methanol on a 96-well plate, followed by the addition of the DPPH solution (160 μL) prepared at 25 μg/mL. The mixture was incubated at room temperature in the dark for 30 min and the absorbance was measured at 517 nm using a microplate reader (Epoch, BioTek). Ascorbic acid and trolox were used as positive controls, methanol plus DPPH as negative control, and sample without DPPH as blank. The DPPH scavenging capacity was calculated at each concentration according to the formula (1) below:

$$\text{Scavenging capacity (\%)}$$
$$= \frac{\text{Absorbance (control)-Absorbance (sample)}}{\text{Absorbance (control)}} \times 100$$

(1)

The inhibitory concentration (IC_{50}) was determined by plotting a non-linear curve of percentage DPPH scavenging capacity against the logarithm of different concentrations of the extract.

The 2,2'-azino-bis (3-ethylbenzothiazoline-6-sulfonic acid) (ABTS) assay
The method described by Re et al. [22] with some modifications was used for the determination of the ABTS radical scavenging capacity of the extracts. Firstly, the reaction solution was prepared by mixing a solution of ABTS (7 mM) with a solution of potassium persulfate (2.45 mM) at room temperature for 12 to 16 h. The optical density of the reaction solution containing the ABTS radical produced was calibrated to 0.70 ± 0.02 at 734 nm before use. Secondly, the extracts (40 μL) were serially diluted with methanol, followed by the addition of the ABTS radical (160 μL), and the optical density was measured after 5 min at 734 nm using a microplate reader (Epoch, BioTek). Two positive controls (trolox and ascorbic acid) were used. Methanol plus ABTS radical was used as negative control while extract without ABTS was considered as the blank. The percentage of

ABTS scavenging capacity was calculated at each concentration according to the formula (1) above, and the inhibitory concentrations (IC_{50}) values were determined as indicated in the previous paragraph.

Anti-inflammatory assays

Nitric oxide inhibitory assay

The method published by Dzoyem and Eloff [23] was used to determine the nitric oxide inhibitory activity of the extracts. The RAW 264.7 macrophages were obtained from the American Type Culture Collection (ATCC) (Rockville, MD, USA), and were grown at 37 °C with 5% CO_2 in a humidified environment in Dulbecco's Modified Eagle's Medium (DMEM) high glucose (4.5 g/L) containing L-glutamine (4 mM) and sodium pyruvate (Hyclone™) supplemented with 10% (v/v) fetal bovine serum (Capricorn Scientific Gmbh, South America) and 1% penicillin-streptomycin-fungizone (PSF). Nitric oxide (NO) production by RAW 264.7 macrophages was measured using the Griess reagent (Sigma Aldrich, Germany) after 24 h of lipopolysaccharide (LPS) stimulation in the presence or absence of the extracts or quercetin used as positive control. Briefly, the RAW 264.7 macrophages were inoculated at a density of 2×10^4 cells per well in 96 well-microtitre plates, and the cells were left overnight to allow attachment to the bottom of the plate. The cells were treated with different concentrations of the extracts dissolved in DMSO with the final concentration of DMSO not exceeding 0.5%. Thereafter, the cells were stimulated by addition of LPS at a final concentration of 1 µg/mL per well. The cells treated with only LPS were considered as the negative control. After 24 h of incubation at 37 °C with 5% CO_2 in a humidified environment, the supernatant (100 µL) from each well of the 96-well microtitre plates were transferred into new 96-well microtitre plates, and an equal volume of Griess reagent (Sigma Aldrich, Germany) was added. The mixture was left in the dark at room temperature for 15 min, and the absorbance was determined at 550 nm on a microplate reader (Synergy Multi-Mode Reader, BioTek). The quantity of nitrite was determined from a sodium nitrite standard curve. The percentage of NO inhibition was calculated based on the ability of each extract to inhibit nitric oxide production by RAW 264.7 macrophages compared with the control (cells treated with LPS without extract). In addition, the cell viability was determined using the 3-(4,5-dimethythiazol- 2-yl)-2,5-diphenyl tetrazolium bromide (MTT) assay [24]. The culture medium was aspirated from the plates, and replaced by fresh medium (200 µL) with 30 µL of thiazolyl blue tetrazolium bromide (5 mg/mL) dissolved in phosphate buffered saline. After incubation for 4 h, the medium was gently aspirated, and the formazan crystals were dissolved in 50 µL of DMSO and kept in the dark for 15 min at room temperature. The absorbance was measured spectrophotometrically at 570 nm on a microplate reader (Synergy Multi-Mode Reader, BioTek).

Inhibition of soybean 15-lipoxygenase (15-LOX) enzyme

The assay was performed according to the procedure of Pinto et al. [25] with slight modifications to the microtitre plate format. The assay is based on the formation of the complex Fe^{3+}/xylenol orange with absorption at 560 nm. The 15-lipoxygenase (15-LOX) enzyme from soybean (Sigma Aldrich, Germany) was incubated with different concentrations of extracts or quercetin used as standard inhibitor (both serially diluted from 0.78 to 100 µg/mL) at 25 °C for 5 min. The substrate, linoleic acid (final concentration, 140 µM) prepared in Tris-HCl buffer (50 mM, pH 7.4), was added and the mixture was incubated at 25 °C for 20 min in the dark. The assay was terminated by the addition of 100 µL of FOX reagent [sulfuric acid (30 mM), xylenol orange (100 µM), iron (II) sulfate (100 µM) in methanol/water (9:1)]. The negative control was made of the enzyme 15-LOX solution, buffer, substrate and FOX reagent while the blanks contained the enzyme 15-LOX and buffer, but the substrate was added after the FOX reagent. The lipoxygenase inhibitory activity was evaluated by calculating the percentage of the inhibition of hydroperoxide production from the changes in absorbance values at 560 nm after 30 min at 25 °C as indicated in the formula (2) below.

$$\text{Percentage LO X inhibition } (\%) = \frac{\text{Absorbance (control)-Absorbance (sample)}}{\text{Absorbance (control)}} \times 100$$

$$(2)$$

The IC_{50} values of extracts or quercetin, which represent the concentration leading to 50% inhibition were calculated using the non-linear regression curve of the percentage (15-LOX) inhibition against the logarithm of concentrations tested.

Cytotoxicity assay

Cell culture

The four cancer cell lines (MCF-7: human breast adenocarcinoma cells; HeLa: human cervix adenocarcinoma cells; Caco-2: human epithelial colorectal adenocarcinoma cells; A549: human epithelial lung adenocarcinoma cells) were obtained from the American Type Culture Collection (ATCC) (Rockville, MD, USA). These cells were grown at 37 °C with 5% CO_2 in a humidified environment in Dulbecco's Modified Eagle's Medium (DMEM) high glucose (4.5 g/L) containing L-glutamine (4 mM) and sodium pyruvate (Separations, RSA) supplemented with 10% (v/v) fetal bovine serum (Capricorn Scientific Gmbh, South America). Non-cancerous African green monkey (Vero) kidney cells (obtained from ATCC) were maintained at 37 °C and 5% CO_2 in a humidified environment in Minimal Essential Medium (MEM) containing L-glutamine (Lonza, Belgium) supplemented with 5% fetal bovine serum (Capricorn Scientific Gmbh, South America) and 1% gentamicin (Virbac, RSA).

Cell treatment and assay procedure

The cells were seeded at a density of 10^4 cells per well on 96-well microtitre plates, and were left overnight to allow attachment. After this, the cells were treated with different concentrations of extracts dissolved in dimethyl sulfoxide (DMSO), and further diluted in fresh culture medium. In each experiment, the highest concentration of DMSO (negative control) in the medium was 0.5%. After incubation for 48 h at 37 °C with 5% CO_2, the culture medium was discarded, and replaced by fresh medium (200 µL) with 30 µL of thiazolyl blue tetrazolium bromide (5 mg/mL) dissolved in phosphate buffered saline. The medium was gently aspirated after 4 h of incubation, and the formazan crystals were dissolved in 50 µL of DMSO, and kept in the dark for 15 min at room temperature. The absorbance was measured spectrophotometrically at 570 nm on a microplate reader (Synergy Multi-Mode Reader, BioTek). The viability of cells treated with the extracts was calculated for each concentration compared to the negative control. The 50% inhibitory concentrations (IC_{50}) for cancer cell lines and the 50% lethal concentrations (LC_{50}) for the non-cancerous cells were determined by plotting the non-linear regression curve of percentage of cell survival versus the logarithm of concentrations of each extract. The selectivity index (SI) values were calculated for each extract by dividing the LC_{50} of the non-cancerous cell against the IC_{50} of each cancer cell type in the same units.

Evaluation of the induction of apoptosis on cancer cells

The induction of apoptosis by the most active extracts from each plant was evaluated by measuring the caspase 3/7 activity on different cancer cell lines with the Caspase-Glo® 3/7 assay kit (Promega). All four cancer cell lines were seeded at a density of 10^4 cells per well on 96-well microtitre plates, and were allowed to adhere overnight. These cells were treated with the extracts at different concentrations (½ × IC_{50}, IC_{50} and 2 × IC_{50}) or DMSO (0.5%) as negative control, and the plates were incubated at 37 °C with 5% CO_2 for 24 h. After treatment, the Caspase-Glo® 3/7 was prepared according to manufacturer's guidelines, and 100 µL of the reagent was added per well and incubated for 1 h at room temperature in the dark. Following this incubation, the luminescence was measured on a microplate reader (Synergy Multi-Mode Reader, BioTek). The data was analysed, and expressed as percentage of the untreated cells (control) and fold change.

Statistical analysis

All experiments were performed in triplicate, and the results are presented as mean ± standard error of mean (SEM) values. Statistical analysis was carried out with GraphPad Instat 3.0 software. The Student–Newman–Keuls test was used to determine P-values for the differences observed between the extracts while Dunnett's test was used to compare the extracts with the control. Results were considered significantly different when $P < 0.05$.

Results

Yield of extraction and phytochemical content of crude extracts

The voucher specimen numbers (PRU) and the yield of extraction of each plant material in a particular solvent are summarized in Table 1. The highest yield of extraction was observed with *C. pseudopulchellus* with all the three solvents used. Extraction with ethanol had the highest yield of extraction among the plant species. The phytochemical content of all extracts is presented in Table 2, and significant differences have been noted between total phenolic content (TPC) and total flavonoid content (TFC) of the plant materials extracted with the three solvents used. Organic solvents (acetone and ethanol) extracted more of these compounds compared to water. The acetone leaf extract of *C. gratissimus* had the highest TPC with 222.29 mgGAE/g whereas the highest TFC was obtained with the acetone and ethanol leaf extracts of *C. sylvaticus* with 82.76 and 84.54 mgQE/g respectively.

Antioxidant activity of extracts

Two antioxidant assays which involved the measurement of colour disappearance caused by free radicals such as DPPH and ABTS were used. As expected, the free radical scavenging activity of the extracts was concentration-dependent (data not shown) and the IC_{50} values determined are presented in Table 2. The antioxidant activity varies within extracts from the same plant and between extracts from different plants. It should be noted that a lower IC_{50} value indicates a stronger antioxidant potency of the sample tested. Therefore, the ethanol leaf extracts from all the three plants have good antioxidant potency when compared with acetone and water extracts from the same plant. Among all the extracts from the three plants, the ethanol leaf extract of *C. gratissimus* had the highest antioxidant potency with IC_{50} values of 32.18 and 34.95 µg/mL respectively for the DPPH and ABTS radical scavenging activity. Ascorbic acid and trolox, known as potent antioxidant compounds, had the best antioxidant potency with IC_{50} values of 1.92 and 3.92 µg/mL (ascorbic acid); 2.21 and 4.64 µg/mL (trolox) respectively for the DPPH and ABTS radical scavenging activity (Table 2).

Anti-inflammatory activity of extracts

The anti-inflammatory activity of leaf extracts was determined using the nitric oxide (NO) and 15-lipoxygenase (15-LOX) inhibitory assays.

Nitric oxide inhibitory effect of extracts on LPS-stimulated RAW 264.7 macrophages

All the extracts from the three *Croton* species had inhibitory activity on NO production in a concentration-dependent manner (Fig. 1a and b). Water leaf extracts of the three plants had the lowest NO inhibitory effect except for the water extract from *C. gratissimus* that had a good inhibitory

Table 2 Phytochemical content, antioxidant activity, nitric oxide and 15-lipoxygenase inhibition of different extracts from *Croton* species and positive controls

Plant name	Extracts	Phytochemicals		IC$_{50}$ (µg/mL)			
		TPC (mgGAE/g)	TFC (mgQE/g)	DPPH	ABTS	NO	15-LOX
Croton gratissimus	CGA	222.29 ± 3.90^a	43.35 ± 0.26^a	217.64 ± 3.46^a	170.51 ± 4.95^a	49.24 ± 0.93^a	10.97 ± 1.19^a
	CGE	180.61 ± 1.74^b	44.39 ± 0.27^a	32.18 ± 2.11^b	34.95 ± 0.81^b	51.93 ± 0.11^a	2.58 ± 0.02^b
	CGW	121.92 ± 1.78^c	29.50 ± 1.21^b	> 500	> 500	88.90 ± 0.57^b	> 100
Croton pseudopulchellus	CPA	124.05 ± 2.00^c	35.88 ± 0.40^c	220.34 ± 4.98^a	176.94 ± 2.26^a	34.64 ± 0.06^c	2.64 ± 0.23^b
	CPE	84.28 ± 1.52^d	35.62 ± 0.36^c	205.96 ± 3.66^a	144.01 ± 2.28^c	53.49 ± 0.47^a	0.57 ± 0.17^c
	CPW	35.10 ± 1.44^e	15.97 ± 0.87^d	> 500	> 500	> 100	> 100
Croton sylvaticus	CSA	112.34 ± 1.29^c	82.76 ± 1.57^e	285.64 ± 2.81^c	165.84 ± 7.91^a	68.28 ± 0.32^d	11.64 ± 1.26^a
	CSE	180.88 ± 1.93^b	84.54 ± 1.85^e	252.19 ± 2.11^c	134.96 ± 7.83^c	78.91 ± 2.19^d	2.12 ± 0.37^b
	CSW	99.27 ± 0.18^f	26.06 ± 0.96^b	> 500	> 500	> 100	> 100
Positive controls	Ascorbic acid	ND	ND	1.92 ± 0.08^d	3.92 ± 0.24^d	ND	ND
	Trolox	ND	ND	2.21 ± 0.24^d	4.64 ± 0.46^d	ND	ND
	Quercetin	ND	ND	ND	ND	5.82 ± 0.63^e	24.60 ± 0.49^d

Data are presented as means of triplicate measurements ± standard error, superscript letters a-f represent statistical difference between data obtained, and for each parameter within a column of the above table, data with different letters mean significantly different at p < 0.05 while data with same letters are statistically not different.; ND = Not Determined. IC$_{50}$: concentration required to inhibit the activity by 50% compared to untreated controls. CGA, CGE and CGW represent respectively acetone, ethanol and water extracts of *Croton gratissimus*. CPA, CPE and CPW represent respectively acetone, ethanol and water extracts of *Croton pseudopulchellus*. CSA, CSE and CSW represent respectively acetone, ethanol and water extracts of *Croton sylvaticus*. TPC: total phenolic content (mg of gallic acid equivalent per gram of extract) and TFC: total flavonoid content (mg of quercetin equivalent per gram of extract). DPPH: 2,2-diphenyl-1-picrylhydrazyl radical, ABTS: 2,2'-azino-bis (3-ethylbenzothiazoline-6-sulfonic acid) radical, NO: nitric oxide, 15-LOX: 15-lipoxygenase

activity. Acetone and ethanol leaf extracts of the plants had the highest NO inhibitory activity compared with their respective water leaf extracts. The IC$_{50}$ values were calculated, and are presented in Table 2. Acetone leaf extracts from the three plants had the lowest IC$_{50}$ values, which are not significantly different from the IC$_{50}$ values obtained for the ethanol leaf extracts. However, the acetone leaf extract of *C. pseudopulchellus* had an IC$_{50}$ value (34.64 µg/mL) significantly (P < 0.05) lower than the IC$_{50}$ of the ethanol extract (53.49 µg/mL) from the same plant. The acetone leaf extract of *C. pseudopulchellus* therefore had the highest NO inhibitory potency. Quercetin, used as positive control, had the highest NO inhibitory potency with IC$_{50}$ of 5.82 µg/mL.

The cell viability of LPS-stimulated RAW 264.7 macrophages after treatment with the extracts and quercetin is presented in Fig. 1c. The acetone and ethanol leaf extracts as well as quercetin were slightly cytotoxic on LPS-stimulated RAW 264.7 macrophages with percentage of cell viability varying between 62 and 96%. The water leaf extracts were less cytotoxic with cell viability greater than 76% at the highest concentration (100 µg/mL) tested.

Lipoxygenase inhibitory activity of extracts

The ferrous oxidation-xylenol orange (FOX) assay was used to determine the 15-lipoxygenase inhibitory activity of different extracts from the three *Croton* species, and the IC$_{50}$ values were determined using the non-linear regression curves (Additional file 1: Figure S1) and the results are presented in Table 2. All the extracts except the water extracts had better inhibitory activity against 15-lipoxygenase when

compared to the positive control (quercetin). The IC$_{50}$ values of the active extracts (acetone and ethanol) from the three plants varied between 0.57 and 11.64 µg/mL which is significantly (P < 0.05) different from quercetin (24.60 µg/mL). Ethanol leaf extracts were more active than acetone leaf extracts from the same plant species, thus suggesting that ethanol extracted more anti-lipoxygenase compounds than acetone. The highest lipoxygenase inhibitory activity was obtained with the ethanol leaf extract of *C. pseudopulchellus* (IC$_{50}$ of 0.57 µg/mL).

Selective cytotoxic effect of extracts on a non-cancerous cell versus cancerous cells

Different extracts were tested for cytotoxicity against four cancerous (A549, Caco-2, HeLa and MCF-7) cell types as well as the non-cancerous African green monkey (Vero) kidney cells, and the graphs of cell viability against the concentrations tested are presented in Additional file 2: Figure S2, Additional file 3: Figure S3, Additional file 4: Figure S4, Additional file 5: Figure S5 and Additional file 6: Figure S6 respectively. The LC$_{50}$ and IC$_{50}$ values of extracts were determined from concentration-dependent graphs, and are presented in Table 3. Water leaf extracts had the lowest cytotoxic effect on both non-cancerous and cancerous cells with LC$_{50}$ or IC$_{50}$ greater than 533.33 µg/mL and 200 µg/mL, respectively. An exception was observed with the water leaf extract of *C. sylvaticus* that had good cytotoxicity (IC$_{50}$ of 45.62 µg/mL) on MCF-7 cells with a promising selectivity index greater than 21.92 (see Table 3). On the other hand, ethanol leaf extracts of *C. pseudopulchellus* and *C. sylvaticus* were more cytotoxic on both

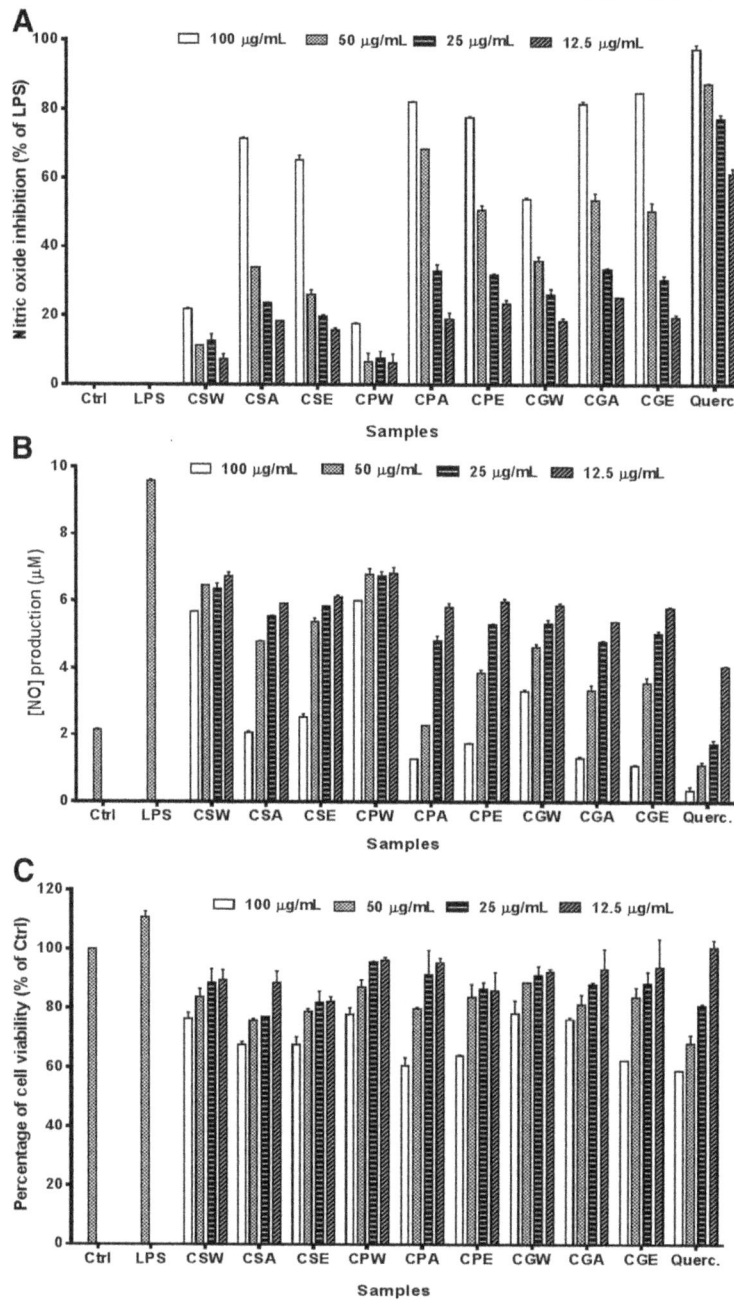

Fig. 1 Activities of the extracts from three *Croton* species on the percentage of nitric oxide inhibition (**a**), nitric oxide production (**b**) and cell viability (**c**) on LPS-stimulated RAW 264.7 macrophages. Data are presented as means of triplicate measurements ± standard error. CSA, CSE and CSW represent respectively acetone, ethanol and water extracts of *Croton sylvaticus*. CPA, CPE and CPW represent respectively acetone, ethanol and water extracts of *Croton pseudopulchellus*. CGA, CGE and CGW represent respectively acetone, ethanol and water extracts of *Croton gratissimus*. Ctrl: control group (0.5% DMSO); LPS: lipopolysaccharide

non-cancerous and cancerous cells with lowest LC_{50} or IC_{50} values obtained against all cell lines. Acetone and ethanol leaf extracts of *C. pseudopulchellus* and *C. sylvaticus* had the highest cytotoxic activity on the non-cancerous cells with LC_{50} varying between 7.86 and 48.19 μg/mL while the acetone and ethanol extracts of *C. gratissimus* were less cytotoxic on these cell lines with LC_{50} varying between 152.30 and 462.88 μg/mL. The selectivity index (SI) values indicated that the acetone and ethanol extracts of *C. gratissimus* were most selective with SI ranging between 1.91 and 6.25 (see Table 3). In addition, the ethanol leaf extract and acetone leaf extract of *C. sylvaticus* were highly selective against A549 and MCF-7 cells with SI of 4.70 and 2.12, respectively. The same observation was made with the acetone leaf extract of *C. pseudopulchellus* which had

Table 3 Cytotoxic effect (IC_{50} and LC_{50}) and the selectivity index (SI) of different extracts from *Croton* species and reference drug (doxorubicin hydrochloride) on cancerous cell lines versus a non-cancerous cell line

Plant Name	Extracts	LC_{50} (µg/mL) Vero	IC_{50} (µg/mL) and Selectivity index = LC_{50}/IC_{50} A549	SI	Caco-2	SI	HeLa	SI	MCF-7	SI
Croton gratissimus	CGA	462.88 ± 7.71^a	97.46 ± 2.20^a	4.75	74.05 ± 5.79^a	6.25	78.21 ± 0.17^a	5.91	83.74 ± 2.06^a	5.52
	CGE	152.30 ± 3.68^b	79.60 ± 2.32^b	1.91	48.46 ± 3.47^b	3.14	73.78 ± 4.12^a	2.06	39.75 ± 2.49^b	3.83
	CGW	533.33 ± 13.21^a	> 200	<2.66	> 200	<2.66	> 200	<2.66	> 200	<2.66
Croton pseudopulchellus	CPA	48.19 ± 5.27^c	36.54 ± 1.81^c	1.31	112.74 ± 4.26^c	0.42	128.69 ± 21.97^b	0.37	24.65 ± 2.37^c	1.95
	CPE	7.86 ± 1.47^d	23.78 ± 1.41^d	0.33	36.24 ± 2.34^d	0.21	63.79 ± 1.02^c	0.12	13.54 ± 1.18^d	0.58
	CPW	> 1000	> 200	ND	> 200	ND	> 200	ND	> 200	ND
Croton sylvaticus	CSA	27.92 ± 0.62^e	32.78 ± 2.55^c	0.85	150.63 ± 8.79^e	0.18	169.09 ± 13.05^b	0.16	13.13 ± 2.76^d	2.12
	CSE	8.23 ± 0.44^d	1.75 ± 0.62^e	4.70	103.73 ± 1.47^c	0.08	106.52 ± 4.50^b	0.07	6.02 ± 1.60^e	1.36
	CSW	> 1000	> 200	ND	> 200	ND	> 200	ND	45.62 ± 5.69^b	>21.92
Doxorubicin (µM)		1.90 ± 0.15^f	1.30 ± 0.06^f	1.46	1.08 ± 0.18^f	1.75	2.17 ± 0.08^d	0.87	1.11 ± 0.03^f	1.71

Data are presented as means of triplicate measurements ± standard error; superscript letters a-f represent statistical difference between data obtained, and for each cell line within a column of the above table, data with different letters mean significantly different at p < 0.05 while data with same letters are statistically not different. ND = Not Determined. IC_{50}: concentration required to inhibit the cell growth by 50% compared to untreated controls. SI is the selectivity index which is determined for each extract by dividing the LC_{50} on the non-cancerous cell by the IC_{50} on each cancer cell in the same units. CGA, CGE and CGW represent respectively acetone, ethanol and water extracts of *Croton gratissimus*. CPA, CPE and CPW represent respectively acetone, ethanol and water extracts of *Croton pseudopulchellus*. CSA, CSE and CSW represent respectively acetone, ethanol and water extracts of *Croton sylvaticus*

SI of 1.31 and 1.95 against A549 and MCF-7 cells, respectively. On the contrary, the ethanol leaf extract of *C. pseudopulchellus* was less selective on non-cancerous cells with the lowest SI values ranging between 0.12 and 0.58 against all cancerous cells. Similarly, acetone and ethanol leaf extracts of *C. sylvaticus* were less selective with SI varying between 0.07 and 0.18 against Caco-2 and HeLa cells. Doxorubicin hydrochloride, the positive control, was highly cytotoxic on all cells with SI ranging between 0.87 and 1.75.

Induction of caspase-dependent apoptosis by active extracts on cancerous cells

In this assay, acetone leaf extracts of the three *Croton* species were used based on their high selectivity indexes or lower cytotoxicity to non-cancerous cells compared to other extracts. The activation of caspase-3 and -7 enzymes was differentially observed in all the four cancerous cells treated with the active extracts compared to the untreated controls (see Fig. 2). Caspase – 3 and – 7 enzymes were better activated after treatment with acetone leaf extracts of the three plants on HeLa and MCF-7 cells. The activation of these enzymes was also observed on A549 and Caco-2 cells only after treatment with the acetone leaf extracts of *C. pseudopulchellus* and *C. gratissimus* (Fig. 2b and c). These two extracts significantly ($P < 0.05$) induced caspase – 3 and – 7 activity in all cancerous cells at concentrations of ½ x IC_{50} (1.24 to 1.56-fold change). A non-significant increase of the activity of caspase – 3 and – 7 was noted after treatment with acetone leaf extracts of *C. sylvaticus* on A549 and MCF-7 cells (1.10 to 1.13-fold change). The acetone leaf extract of *C. gratissimus* induced activation of caspase – 3 and – 7 activity in a concentration-dependent manner on HeLa cells (Fig. 2c), and the highest induction (1.83-fold change) was obtained at the concentration of 2 x IC_{50}.

Discussion

Our study aimed to evaluate the antioxidant, anti-inflammatory and cytotoxic activities of three *Croton* species. The ethanol leaf extracts of the three plants were highly active in all experiments (except the NO inhibitory activity) compared to acetone and water leaf extracts. These results suggested that the antioxidant, anti-inflammatory and cytotoxic compounds extracted from the three plants are more concentrated in the ethanol leaf extract than in the acetone or water leaf extracts. We also investigated the potential relationship between the antioxidant, anti-inflammatory and cytotoxic activities of the active ethanol and acetone extracts. This relationship was analysed by determining the Pearson correlation coefficients (r) after plotting a linear curve with IC_{50} values of each cancer cell on the y-axis against phytochemical content or IC_{50} values of the antioxidant power (DPPH, ABTS) and anti-inflammatory activity (NO, 15-LOX) on the x-axis (Table 4). A linear correlation (r<0.5) existed between antioxidant, anti-inflammatory and cytotoxic activities, although this correlation was considered to be less strong. In fact, free radicals are well known to play a major role in the development of oxidative stress that can lead to many illnesses including cardiovascular diseases, diabetes, inflammation, degenerative diseases, and cancer [26]. Nitric oxide (NO), a molecule playing a crucial role in inflammatory response, can react with free radicals such as superoxides to produce peroxynitrites that can cause irreversible damage to cell membranes leading to the promotion of tumor growth and proliferation [27]. In addition, natural inhibitors of lipoxygenases have been shown to suppress carcinogenesis and tumor growth in a number of experimental models [28]. Moreover, several scientific reports have suggested that antioxidant and anti-inflammatory agents could be beneficial in the prevention and treatment of cancer [29]. Our results therefore suggest that the antioxidant

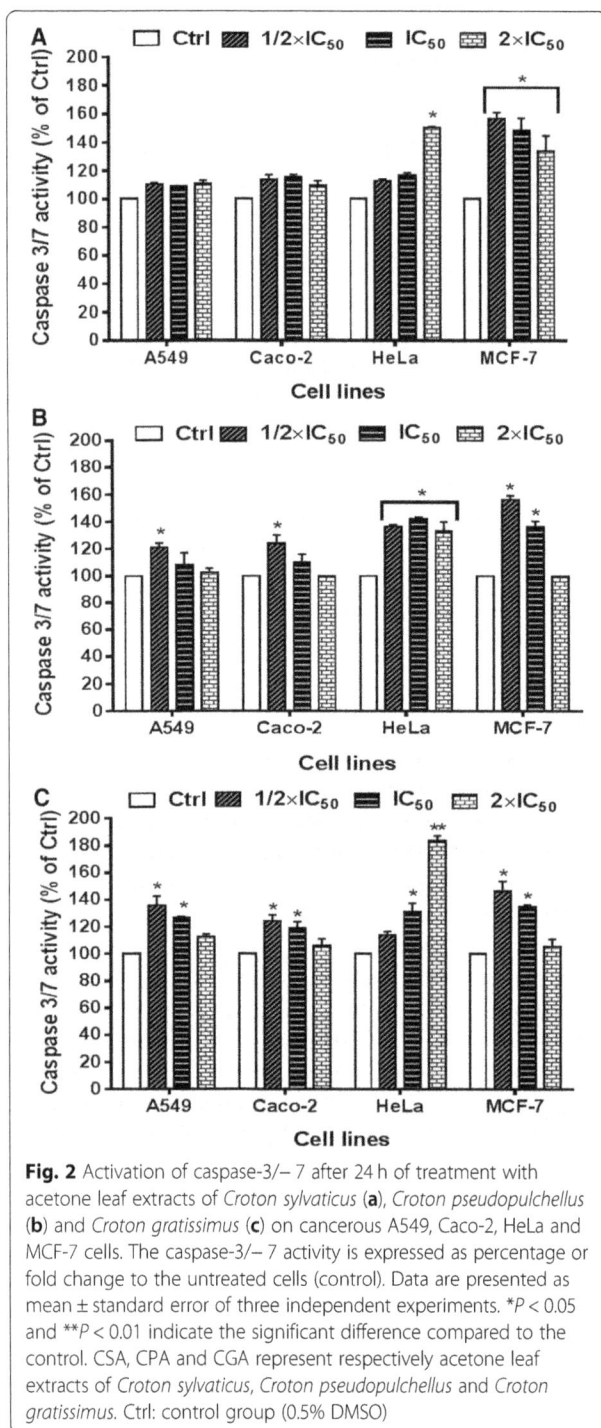

Fig. 2 Activation of caspase-3/– 7 after 24 h of treatment with acetone leaf extracts of *Croton sylvaticus* (**a**), *Croton pseudopulchellus* (**b**) and *Croton gratissimus* (**c**) on cancerous A549, Caco-2, HeLa and MCF-7 cells. The caspase-3/– 7 activity is expressed as percentage or fold change to the untreated cells (control). Data are presented as mean ± standard error of three independent experiments. *$P < 0.05$ and **$P < 0.01$ indicate the significant difference compared to the control. CSA, CPA and CGA represent respectively acetone leaf extracts of *Croton sylvaticus*, *Croton pseudopulchellus* and *Croton gratissimus*. Ctrl: control group (0.5% DMSO)

Table 4 Correlation between phytochemical content, antioxidant, anti-inflammatory and antiproliferative activity of active extracts

Cell lines	Pearson correlation coefficient (r)					
	TPC	TFC	DPPH	ABTS	NO	15-LOX
A549	0.3530	0.2404	0.2850	0.4030	0.2525	0.1935
Caco-2	0.0143	0.4529	0.4545	0.2758	0.2820	0.2798
HeLa	0.0920	0.3724	0.3582	0.2043	0.2847	0.2251
MCF-7	0.3111	0.2399	0.0800	0.0003	0.2027	0.2341

Correlation coefficients were determined by plotting a linear curve with IC_{50} values of extracts obtained for each cancer cell on the y-axis against the corresponding phytochemical content or IC_{50} values of the antioxidant power (DPPH, ABTS) and anti-inflammatory activity (NO, 15-LOX) on the x-axis. NO: nitric oxide, 15-LOX: 15-lipoxygenase. TPC: total phenolic content, TFC: total flavonoid content, DPPH: 2,2-diphenyl-1-picrylhydrazyl radical, ABTS: 2,2'-azino-bis (3-ethylbenzothiazoline-6-sulfonic acid) radical

potential, phenolics (which also include flavonoids) may have cytotoxic activity against different human cancer cells with little or no effect on normal cells. This selectivity in the cytotoxicity properties of phenolics has strengthened interest in formulating novel and less toxic anticancer products based on these types of compounds [30, 31].

The goal of any chemotherapeutic treatment is to selectively attenuate or destroy pathogenic micro-organisms or cancerous cells with minimal side effects to the host cells [32]. This principle, known as selective toxicity, is the key to all chemotherapeutic treatment. In this study, the acetone and ethanol extracts of *C. gratissimus* were more selective with SI ranging between 1.91 and 6.25, and it therefore indicates that these extracts may be useful in the search for anticancer compounds. A cembranolide isolated from stem bark of *Croton gratissimus* had moderate activity against PEO1 and PEO1TaxR ovarian cancer cell lines [16]. In the present work, four cancerous (A549, Caco-2, HeLa, MCF-7) cells and a non-cancerous (Vero) cell line were used to evaluate the antiproliferative activity of the crude extracts from three *Croton* species. The use of these cancerous cells with the non-cancerous (Vero) cell line as cell models has been reported for comparison and determination of the selectivity indexes [33, 34]. However, the cytotoxic effect on this non-cancerous (Vero) cell line of animal origin needs to be confirmed on other non-cancerous cells of human origin. The selective toxicity of acetone and ethanol extracts of *C. gratissimus* also suggested that the active compounds interact with special cancer-associated receptors or cancer cell special molecule (not found in non-cancerous cells), thus activating some mechanisms that cause cancer cell death [35]. The activation of caspase – 3 and – 7 enzymes was observed in all four of the cancer cell types treated with the active extracts compared to the untreated cells, which therefore reveals that apoptosis has taken place in the treated cells. Indeed, caspases – 3, and – 7 are known as "executioners" of apoptosis since they serve as substrates for initiator caspases in extrinsic or intrinsic apoptotic pathways [36]. It will be important to comprehensively investigate the mechanism of the

or anti-inflammatory activities of extracts may contribute moderately to their cytotoxic activity. Phenolics and flavonoids are known for their contribution either directly or indirectly to the cytotoxic activity. In our study, we noted that the acetone and ethanol extracts of *C. gratissimus* which had the highest total phenolic contents (222.29 and 180.61 mgGAE/g respectively) were selectively cytotoxic to cancerous cells compared to non-cancerous. Indeed, due to their anti- and pro-oxidant activity, and this aspect will be addressed once the compounds responsible for the activity have been isolated. The aim of the current study was to explore the possibility that extracts have inhibitory activity on cancer cell growth.

According to the United States National Cancer Institute, a crude extract is generally considered to have in vitro cytotoxic activity if the IC$_{50}$ is lower than 30 μg/mL [37]. Based on this statement, acetone and ethanol extracts of *C. pseudopulchellus* and *C. sylvaticus* were considered as more active on both cancerous A549 and MCF-7 cells. Differences in the selectivity indexes of these extracts on these two cancerous cells may be ameliorated through the isolation of active compounds which might reduce the toxic effects of the crude extracts. Studies are ongoing to isolate active compounds from these active extracts.

Conclusion

In summary, due to their selective toxicity between noncancerous and cancerous cells, with beneficial antioxidant and anti-inflammatory activities, the acetone and ethanol leaf extracts of *Croton gratissimus* may be useful against cancer and other oxidative stress related diseases. The isolation of active compounds from this extract will be of great interest to fully understand the mechanism of anticancer activity. In addition, acetone and ethanol extracts of *C. pseudopulchellus* and *C. sylvaticus*, which were cytotoxic to both cancerous and non-cancerous cells, may be further explored as sources of new cytotoxic compounds.

Additional files

Additional file 1: Figure S1. Non-linear regression curves for IC$_{50}$ determination of different extracts from *Croton* species in 15-lipoxygenase (15-LOX) inhibitory assay. CSA and CSE represent respectively acetone, ethanol and water extracts of *Croton sylvaticus*. CGA and CGE represent respectively acetone, ethanol and water extracts of *Croton gratissimus*. CPA and CPE represent respectively acetone, ethanol and water extracts of *Croton pseudopulchellus*.

Additional file 2: Figure S2. Concentration-dependent graph of A549 cell viability of different extracts from *Croton* species. Extracts were tested at concentrations between 200 and 6.25 μg/mL; Ctrl: 0.5% DMSO.

Additional file 3: Figure S3. Concentration-dependent graph of Caco-2 cell viability of different extracts from *Croton* species. Extracts were tested at concentrations between 200 and 6.25 μg/mL; Ctrl: 0.5% DMSO.

Additional file 4: Figure S4. Concentration-dependent graph of HeLa cell viability of different extracts from *Croton* species. Extracts were tested at concentrations between 200 and 6.25 μg/mL; Ctrl: 0.5% DMSO.

Additional file 5: Figure S5. Concentration-dependent graph of MCF-7 cell viability of different extracts from *Croton* species. Extracts were tested at concentrations between 200 and 6.25 μg/mL; Ctrl: 0.5% DMSO.

Additional file 6: Figure S6. Concentration-dependent graph of Vero cell viability of different extracts from *Croton* species. Extracts were tested at concentrations between 1000 and 50 μg/mL Ctrl: 0.5% DMSO.

Abbreviations
ABTS: 2,2′-azino-bis (3-ethylbenzothiazoline-6-sulfonic acid; ATCC: American type culture collection; DMSO: Dimethyl sulphoxide; DPPH: 2,2-diphenyl-1-picrylhydrazyl; FOX: Ferrous oxidation-xylenol orange; GAE: Gallic acid equivalent; IC$_{50}$: Inhibitory concentration to 50% of cells; LC$_{50}$: Lethal concentration to 50% of cells; LOX: Lipoxygenase; LPS: Lipopolysaccharide; MEM: Minimal essential medium; MTT: 3-(4,5-dimethylthiazol-2-yl)-2,5-diphenyltetrazolium bromide; NO: Nitric oxide; QE: Quercetin equivalent; TFC: Total flavonoid content; TPC: Total phenolic content

Acknowledgements
Authors thank Dr. Tshepiso J. Makhafola from the University of South Africa for providing the cancerous cell lines. EMN is very grateful to the University of Pretoria for the postdoctoral fellowship.

Funding
This work was supported by the National Research Foundation (NRF), South Africa through the Incentive Funding for Rated Researchers (Lyndy J. McGaw). The funder had no implication in the design of the study, collection, analysis and interpretation of data; and in writing the manuscript; and the decision to submit the article for publication.

Authors' contributions
EMN initiated the project, conducted the assays and wrote the manuscript, JNE contributed to initiating the project and editing the manuscript, LJM supervised the research and edited the manuscript. All authors have read and approved the final manuscript.

Competing interests
The authors declare that they have no competing interests. Prof Jacobus N Eloff is a Section Editor and Prof Lyndy J McGaw is an Associate Editor of BMC Complementary and Alternative medicine.

References
1. Gęgotek A, Nikliński J, Žarković N, Žarković K, Waeg G, Łuczaj W, Charkiewicz R, Skrzydlewska E. Lipid mediators involved in the oxidative stress and antioxidant defence of human lung cancer cells. Redox Biol. 2016;9:210–9.
2. Liochev SI. Reactive oxygen species and the free radical theory of aging. Free Radic Biol Med. 2013;60:1–4.
3. Rahman K. Studies on free radicals, antioxidants, and co-factors. Clin Interv Aging. 2007;2(2):219–36.
4. Islam S, Samima N, Muhammad AK, Sakhawat Hossain A, Farhadul I, Proma K, Haque Mollah MN, Mamunur R, Golam S, Md Aziz AR, et al. Evaluation of antioxidant and anticancer properties of the seed extracts of *Syzygium fruticosum* Roxb. Growing in Rajshahi, Bangladesh. BMC Complement Altern Med. 2013;13.
5. Zhang Y-J, Gan R-Y, Li S, Zhou Y, Li A-N, Xu D-P, Li H-B. Antioxidant phytochemicals for the prevention and treatment of chronic diseases. Molecules. 2015;20:21138–56.
6. Wang H, Khor TO, Shu L, Su ZY, Fuentes F, Lee JH, Kong AN. Plants vs. cancer: a review on natural phytochemicals in preventing and treating cancers and their druggability. Anti Cancer Agents Med Chem. 2012;12(10):1281–305.
7. Bartsch H, Nair J. Chronic inflammation and oxidative stress in the genesis and perpetuation of cancer: role of lipid peroxidation, DNA damage, and repair. Langenbeck's Arch Surg. 2006;91:499–510.
8. Gonda TA, Tu S, Wang TC. Chronic inflammation, the tumor microenvironment and carcinogenesis. Cell Cycle. 2009;8:2005–13.
9. Reuter S, Gupta SC, Chaturvedi MM, Aggarwal BB. Oxidative stress, inflammation, and cancer: how are they linked? Free Radic Biol Med. 2010; 49(11):1603–16.
10. Salatino A, Salatino MLF, Negri G. Traditional uses, chemistry and pharmacology of Croton species (Euphorbiaceae). J Braz Chem Soc. 2007;18(1):11–33.
11. Kapingu MC, Mbwambo ZH, Moshi MJ, Magadula JJ. Brine shrimp lethality of alkaloids from *Croton sylvaticus* Hoechst. East and Central African Journal of Pharmaceutical Sciences. 2012;15:35–7.

12. Ndhlala AR, Aderogba MA, Ncube B, Van Staden J. Anti-oxidative and cholinesterase inhibitory effects of leaf extracts and their isolated compounds from two closely related Croton species. Molecules. 2013;18:1916–32.

13. Langat M, Mulholland DA, Crouch N. New diterpenoids from *Croton sylvaticus* and *Croton pseudopulchellus* (Euphorbiaceae) and antiplasmodial screening of ent-kaurenoic acid. Planta Med 2008, 74(09):PB126.

14. Ngadjui BT, Abegaz BM, Keumedjio F, Folefoc GN, Kapche GW. Diterpenoids from the stem bark of Croton zambesicus. Phytochemistry. 2002;60(4):345–9.

15. Block S, Stevigny C, De Pauw-Gillet MC, de Hoffmann E, Llabres G, Adjakidje V, Quetin-Leclercq J. Ent-trachyloban-3beta-ol, a new cytotoxic diterpene from Croton zambesicus. Planta Med. 2002;68(7):647–9.

16. Mulholland DA, Langat MK, Crouch NR, Coley HM, Mutambi EM, Nuzillard JM. Cembranolides from the stem bark of the southern African medicinal plant, *Croton gratissimus* (Euphorbiaceae). Phytochemistry. 2010;71:1381–6.

17. Langat MK, Crouch NR, Smith PJ, Mulholland DA. Cembranolides from the leaves of *Croton gratissimus*. J Nat Prod. 2011;74:2349–55.

18. Lall N, Meyer JJ. In vitro inhibition of drug-resistant and drug-sensitive strains of *Mycobacterium tuberculosis* by ethnobotanically selected south African plants. J Ethnopharmacol. 1999;66(3):347–54.

19. Zhang Q, Zhang J, Shen J, Silva A, Dennis D, Barrow C. A simple 96-well microplate method for estimation of total polyphenol content in seaweeds. J Appl Phycol. 2006;18:445–50.

20. Lin J, Tang C. Determination of total phenolic and flavonoid contents in selected fruits and vegetables, as well as their stimulatory effects on mouse splenocyte proliferation. Food Chem. 2007;101:140–7.

21. Brand-Williams W, Cuvelier ME, Berset C. Use of a free radical method to evaluate antioxidant activity. Lebensmittel Wissenschaftund Technologie. 1995;28(1):25–30.

22. Re R, Pellegrini N, Proteggente A, Pannala A, Yang M, Rice-Evans C. Antioxidant activity applying an improved ABTS radical cation decolourization assay. Free Radic Biol Med. 1999;28:1057–60.

23. Dzoyem JP, Eloff JN. Anti-inflammatory, anticholinesterase and antioxidant activity of leaf extracts of twelve plants used traditionally to alleviate pain and inflammation in South Africa. J Ethnopharmacol. 2015;160:194–201.

24. Mosmann T. Rapid colorimetric assay for cellular growth and survival: application to proliferation and cytotoxicity assays. J Immunol Methods. 1983;65(1–2):55–63.

25. Pinto MC, Tejeda A, Duque AL, Macias P. Determination of lipoxygenase activity in plant extracts using a modified ferrous oxidation-xylenol orange assay. J Agric Food Chem. 2007;55(15):5956–9.

26. Ravipati AS, Zhang L, Koyyalamudi SR, Jeong SC, Reddy N, Bartlett J, Smith PT, Shanmugam K, Munch G, Wu MJ, et al. Antioxidant and anti-inflammatory activities of selected Chinese medicinal plants and their relation with antioxidant content. BMC Complement Altern Med. 2012;12:173.

27. Choudhari SK, Chaudhary M, Bagde S, Amol R Gadbail AR, Joshi V. Nitric oxide and cancer: a review. World Journal of Surgical Oncology. 2013; 11((118)):11.

28. Goossens L, Pommery N, Henichart JP. COX-2/5-LOX dual acting anti-inflammatory drugs in cancer chemotherapy. Curr Top Med Chem. 2007; 7(3):283–96.

29. Dufour D, Pichette A, Mshvildadze V, Hébert M-EB, Lavoie S, Longtin A, Laprise C, Legault J. Antioxidant, anti-inflammatory and anticancer activities of methanolic extracts from *Ledum groenlandicum* Retzius. J Ethnopharmacol. 2007;111:22–8.

30. Sak K. Cytotoxicity of dietary flavonoids on different human cancer types. Pharmacogn Rev. 2014;8(16):122–46.

31. Batra P, Sharma A. Anti-cancer potential of flavonoids: recent trends and future perspectives. 3 Biotech. 2013;3:439–59.

32. Wink M. Medicinal plants: a source of anti-parasitic secondary metabolites. Molecules. 2012;17(11):12771–91.

33. Namvar F, Baharara J, Mahdi AA. Antioxidant and anticancer activities of selected Persian gulf algae. Ind J Clin Biochem. 2014;29(1):13–20.

34. Sasipawan M, Natthida W, Sahapat B. Anticancer effect of the extracts from *Polyalthia evecta* against human hepatoma cell line (HepG2). Asian Pac J Trop Biomed. 2012;2(5):368–74.

35. Chow KH, Sun RW, Lam JB, Li CK, Xu A, Ma DL, Abagyan R, Wang Y, Che CM. A gold(III) porphyrin complex with antitumor properties targets the Wnt/beta-catenin pathway. Cancer Res. 2010;70(1):329–37.

36. Olsson M, Zhivotovsky B. Caspases and cancer. Cell Death Differ. 2011;18(9):1441–9.

37. Singh G, Passsari AK, Leo VV, Mishra VK, Subbarayan S, Singh BP, Kumar B, Kumar S, Gupta VK, Lalhlenmawia H, et al. Evaluation of phenolic content variability along with antioxidant, antimicrobial, and cytotoxic potential of selected traditional medicinal plants from India. Front Plant Sci. 2016;7:407.

19

Aloe-emodin induces apoptosis in human oral squamous cell carcinoma SCC15 cells

Qihong Li[1†] ⓘ, Jun Wen[2†], Kaitao Yu[1], Yao Shu[1], Wulin He[2], Hongxing Chu[2], Bin Zhang[3*] and Cheng Ge[1*]

Abstract

Background: Oral and pharyngeal cancer is the most common malignant human cancers. Chemotherapy is an effective approach for anti-oral cancer therapy, while the drug tolerance and resistance remain a problem for oral cancer patients. Aloe-emodin, rhein and physcion are classified as anthraquinones, which are the main pharmacodynamic ingredients of *Rheum undulatum L.*. This study was undertaken to investigate whether aloe-emodin, rhein and physcion show inhibiting growth and inducing apoptosis in oral squamous cell carcinoma SCC15 cells. We found that aloe-emodin show inhibiting growth and inducing apoptosis in oral squamous cell carcinoma SCC15 cells, we also investigated the underlying mechanisms of apoptosis induced by aloe-emodin.

Methods: Thiazolyl blue tetrazolium bromide (MTT) test was used to detect cell proliferation. Cell apoptosis was detected by flow cytometry. We also used western blot analysis to detect the potential mechanisms of apoptosis.

Results: Aloe-emodin, rhein and physcion inhibit the proliferation of SCC15 cells and the order of inhibition level are aloe-emodin > Rhein > Physcion, the half maximal inhibitory concentrations (IC_{50}) value of aloe-emodin was 60.90 μM at 48 h of treatment. Aloe-emodin treatment resulted in a time- and dose-dependent decrease in cell viability and increased the apoptotic cell ratio. The results of western blotting showed the expression levels of caspase-9 and caspase-3 proteins increased following aloe-emodin treatment.

Conclusions: Our results revealed that aloe-emodin treatment could inhibit cell viability of SCC15 cells and the potential mechanism of inhibition might be through the induction of apoptosis by regulation of the expression levels of caspase-9 and caspase-3. This indicates that aloe-emodin may be a good agent for anti-oral cancer drug exploring.

Keywords: Aloe-emodin, Anthraquinone, Apoptosis, Oral squamous cell carcinoma, SCC15 cells

Background

Oral and pharyngeal cancer is the sixth most common malignant human cancers worldwide [1]. Despite advancements in cancer treatment, the 5-year survival rate of oral cancer patient is less than 50% [2, 3]. Chemotherapy is an effective and useful approach for anti-oral cancer therapy, meanwhile, the drug tolerance and resistance remains an issue for oral cancer patients. Thus, a better and safe chemical molecular for this disease therapy is to develop.

With the aim of developing novel anti-oral cancer drugs, we devoted our attention to natural compounds that have been used to treat a variety of cancer diserases. Aloe-emodin, rhein and physcion (Fig. 1) derived from *Rheum undulatum L.* have potent biological effects. Despite much evidence suggesting that aloe-emodin, rhein and physcion show anticancer activity in many cancer cell lines, such as against human hepatoblastoma cell, colorectal cancer cells and human melanoma cells [4–6], there is not enough information to show that these compounds. Against the human oral cancer cells.

Therefore, in this study, we examined the effect of aloe-emodin, rhein and physcion on the growth of human oral squamous cell carcinoma cell line SCC15. The results demonstrated that aloe-emodin, rhein and physcion inhibit the proliferation of SCC15 cells and the order of

* Correspondence: binzhangfmmu@163.com; gechengde@163.com
†Qihong Li and Jun Wen contributed equally to this work.
3Department of Stomatology, Chinese PLA General Hospital, 28 Fuxing Road, Beijing 100853, China
1Department of Stomatology, 307 Hospital, PLA, 8 Dongda Street, Beijing 100071, China
Full list of author information is available at the end of the article

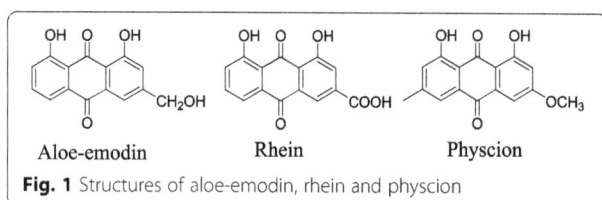

Fig. 1 Structures of aloe-emodin, rhein and physcion

inhibition level is aloe-emodin > rhein > physcion. Our results showed that aloe-emodin could induce SCC15 cells apoptosis, moreover, the expression levels of caspase-9 and caspase-3 increased suggesting that the potential mechanism of aloe-emodin induces apoptosis might by regulating the caspases in SCC15 cells.

Methods
Reagents and chemicals
Dulbecco's modified Eagle's medium (DMEM), phosphate buffered saline (PBS), and fetal bovine serum (FBS) were purchased from Gibco (Thermo Fisher Scientific, NY, USA). 96-Well plates were purchased from Corning Costar (Corning Inc., NY, USA). Aloe-emodin (Cat No. 110795–201710), rhein (Cat No. 110757–201607), physcion (Cat No. 110758–201616) (> 98% pure, free of endotoxin) were purchased from National Institutes for Food and Drug Control (Beijing, China), which were dissolved in DMSO and passed through a 0.22 μm filter (Pall Life Sciences, MI, USA) for sterilization and diluted with culture medium to final concentrations before treatment. In all experiments, the final DMSO concentration did not exceed 1‰ (v/v), so as not to affect cell growth. Thiazolyl blue tetrazolium bromide (MTT) was purchased from Sigma Sigma-Aldrich Co. (St. Louis, MO, USA). Caspase-3 (8G10) Rabbit mAb (Cat No. 9665), Caspase-9 antibody (human specific) (Cat No. 9502), β-actin (13E5) Rabbit mAb (Cat No. 4970), anti-rabbit IgG, HRP-linked antibody (Cat No.7074) were obtained from Cell Signaling Technology (Danvers MA USA).

Cell culture and chemical treatment
Human oral squamous cell carcinoma cell line SCC15 was donated by Zhang Xin-yan, professor of Capital medical university school of stomatology (Beijing, China), which was obtained from the American Type Culture Collection (Manassas VA) and stored in our laboratory. The cells were cultured in DMEM containing with 10% FBS, 100 U/ml penicillin, 100 μg/ml streptomycin and incubated at 37 °C in a humidified atmosphere containing 5% CO_2.

Cell viability assay
Cell viability was evaluated by MTT assay [7]. SCC15 cells were seeded at 1×10^4 cells/ml in 96-well plates

and cultured for 24 h. After treatment with various concentrations of the test compounds for 24 h, 48 h or 72 h, 0.5 mg/ml MTT was added and incubated with cells for 4 h at 37 °C under 5% CO_2. The medium was removed and DMSO (150 μl) was added to each well. The optical density (OD) was measured at 492 nm by a Microplate Reader (Multiskan MK3, Thermo). The percentage of cell viability was calculated according to the following formula: (OD value of the control cells − OD value of the treated cells) / OD value of the control cells × 100%. By definition, the viability of the control cells from the untreated cultures was defined as 100%. The IC_{50} value was calculated by Graph Pad Prism 6.0.

Apoptosis analysis by flow cytometry
Apoptosis was measured using flow cytometry to quantify the levels of detectable phosphatidylserine on the outer membrane of apoptotic cells [8]. Aloe-emodin induces apoptosis of the cells was measured using an Annexin V-Fluorescein isothiocyanate (FITC)/ propidium iodide (PI) apoptosis detection kit (Solarbio life Sciences, Beijing, China) according to the manufacturer's protocol. In brief, SCC15 cells treated with or without aloe-emodin for 24 h or 48 h were collected by trypsinization and washed twice with cold PBS. After centrifugation, the cell pellets were resuspended in a 500 μl binding buffer solution. Then, 5 μl of Annexin V-FITC and 5 μl of PI solutions were added and the mixtures were further incubated in the dark for 30 min at room temperature. The Annexin V-FITC and PI fluorescence of cultured cells were analyzed by flow cytometry (Becton Dickinson FACSCalibur, USA).

Western blot assay
SCC15 (2×10^6) cells were plated in 100 mm culture dishes and cultured for 48 h. After treatment with various concentrations of aloe-emodin for 48 h, the cells were harvested and washed twice with cold PBS. Protein extracts of cells were prepared by lysing cells in RIPA buffer (Beyotime, Shanghai China) and 1 mM PMSF (Beyotime, Shanghai China) for 30 min at 4 °C. After centrifuged, the protein concentration on supernatant was determined with bicinchoninic acid (BCA) assary (Biomed Beijng China). For each sample, equal amounts of cell lysates (containing 25 μg) were loaded on a 10.0% SDS polyacrylamide gel electrophoresis, and transferred to a PVDF membrane (0.45 μm, BioRad, Cal, USA). Membranes were blocked with blocking buffer (TBST (Beyotime, Shanghai China) and 5% non-fat milk (w/v) for 1 h at the RT. Then, the membranes were incubated with primary antibodies overnight at 4 °C. Thereafter, the membranes were washed with TBST buffer and incubated with anti-rabbit secondary antibodies for 1 h at RT. The signals were detected by an Enhanced

Chemiluminescence (ECL) system (Tanon, Shanghai, China) according to the manufacturer's instructions.

Statistical analysis

All data and results were confirmed by at least three independent experiments and were expressed as mean ± standard deviation (SD). Students't-test was used to analyze cell apoptosis, one-way ANOVA followed by Dunnett's multiple-comparison was used for densitometry analysis of western blots. Calculations were carried out using SPSS version 19.0 and $P < 0.05$ was considered statistically significant.

Results

Aloe-emodin reduces viability on SCC15 cell lines

The SCC15 cells were treated with various concentrations of aloe-emodin, rhein, physcion respectively. The results showed aloe-emodin, rhein, physcion all inhibited the proliferation of SCC15 cells. The viability of SCC15 cells were reduced to 85.44% with 12.5 μM ranging to 21.79% with 200 μM at 48 h, and the IC_{50} value was 60.90 μM, while the IC_{50} value of rhein was 160.7 μM and physcion was 486.1 μM. The inhibition effects were in the order of aloe-emodin > rhein > physcion (Fig. 2a). The IC_{50} values of rehin and physcion are at high concentrations (> 160 μM) suggesting that the two compounds were of limited value as anti-cancer agents for high dose for oral cancer theaphy. Therefore, aloe-emodin with low IC_{50} value (60.90 μM) was selected for further assessment in SCC15 cells. The number of viable SCC15 cells treated with aloe-emodin decreased in a dose- and time-dependent manner compared to control cells (Fig. 2b).

Aloe-emodin induces apoptosis in SCC15 cells

To detect whether aloe-emodin induced apoptosis in SCC15 cells, an Annexin V-PI dual staining assay was conducted. The SCC15 cells was treated with 50 μM aloe-emodin for 24 h and 48 h, with the result that apoptotic cell population (early and late stage apoptotic cells) was higher than in the untreated control group.

The ratio of apoptosis of SCC15 cells in Aloe-emodin treated group was 13.91% in 24 h and 24.1% in 48 h respectively, while the ration of apoptotic cell was 4.32%, 7.42% in the control group respectively (Fig. 3) (*P < 0.05, **P < 0.01).

Involvement of caspase-9 and caspase-3 in aloe-emodin induced apotosis

To determine the underlying mechanism by which aloe-emodin induced apoptosis in SCC15 cells, the expression of cell apoptosis molecules caspase-9 and caspase-3 proteins were measured. We found that the expression levels of caspase-9 and caspase-3 increased following aloe-emodin treatment (0, 25 and 50 μM for 48 h) (Fig. 4). These results indicated that aloe-emodin may induces apoptosis by regulating caspase-9 and caspase-3 in SCC15 cells.

Discussion

Over the past several decades, many studies have reported that natural products derived from medicinal herbs have various potent biological advantages against various types of cancer [9, 10]. Aloe-emodin, rhein and physcion, the anthraquinone anaglogues, are derived from *Rheum undulatum L.* and exhibit anti-inflammatory, anti-bacterial, and anti-tumor properties [11]. Oral squamous cell carcinoma has been reported that the prognosis for patients diagnosed is very poor, less than 50% survive for five years or more and incidence rate is to be younger than other tumors worldwide [12]. Many reports have showed that aloe-emodin, rhein and physcion exhibit anti-proliferative effect and induction of apoptosis in various cancer cells [5, 6, 9]. However, there is no available information to show the effect of aloe-emodin, rhein and physcion against the growth of human oral squamous cell carcinoma SCC15 cells. Herein, we revealed that aloe-emodin, rhein and physcion could exerts anti-proliferative effects on SCC15 cells in vitro, aloe-emodin was selected in further bioactive assessment for the low IC_{50} value, the

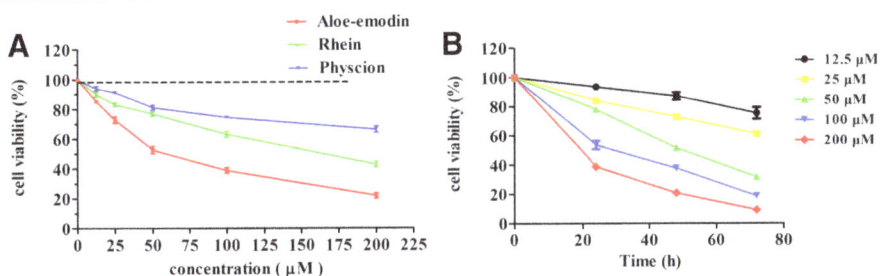

Fig. 2 Effects of indicated compounds on the cell viability of the SCC15 cells. **a** Exponentially growing of SCC15 cells was treated with aloe-emodin, rhein and physcion in various concentrations (0, 12.5, 25, 50, 100 and 200 μM) for 48 h. **b** SCC15 cells were treated with 12.5, 25, 50, 100 and 200 μM of aloe-emodin for various times (24 h, 48 h, 72 h). The cell viability was determined using MTT assay. Each bar represents the mean ± SD

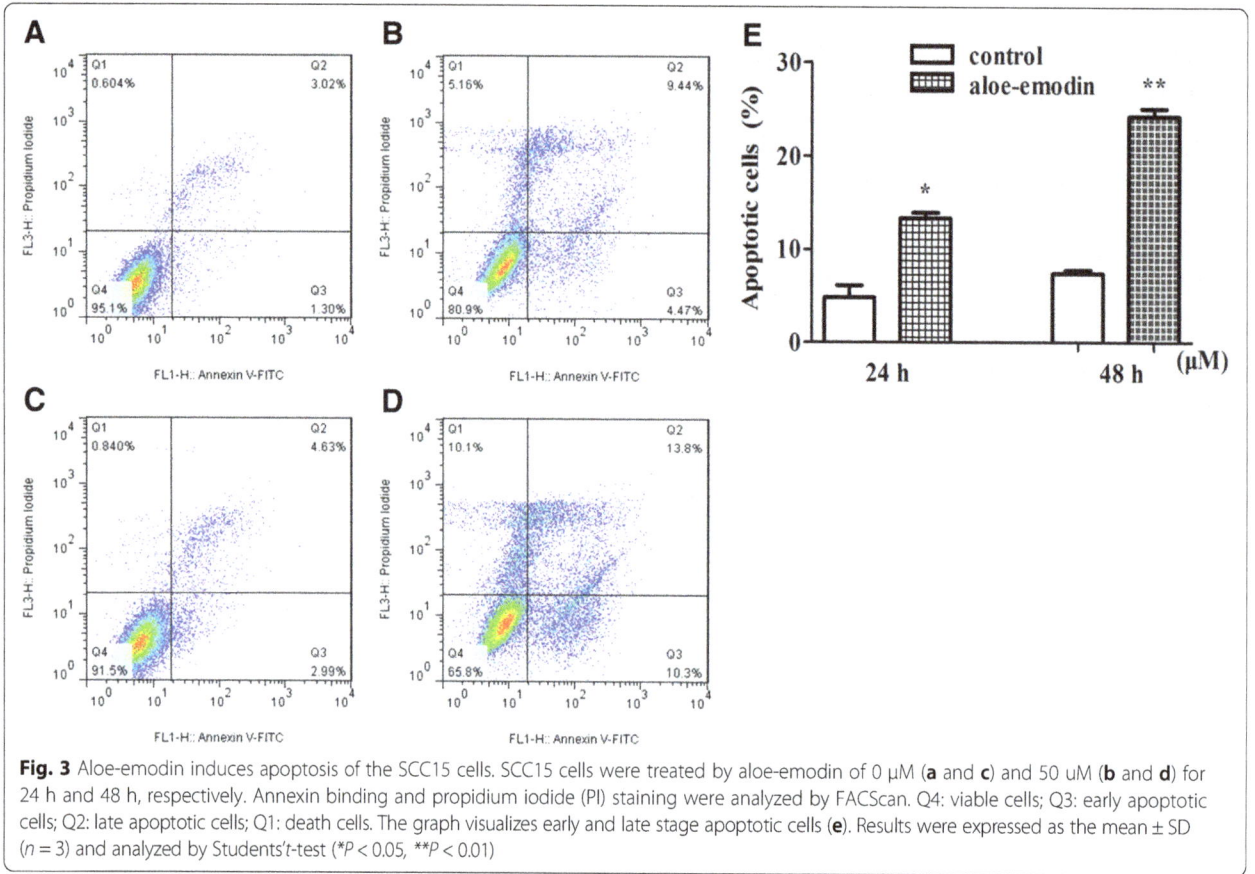

Fig. 3 Aloe-emodin induces apoptosis of the SCC15 cells. SCC15 cells were treated by aloe-emodin of 0 μM (**a** and **c**) and 50 uM (**b** and **d**) for 24 h and 48 h, respectively. Annexin binding and propidium iodide (PI) staining were analyzed by FACScan. Q4: viable cells; Q3: early apoptotic cells; Q2: late apoptotic cells; Q1: death cells. The graph visualizes early and late stage apoptotic cells (**e**). Results were expressed as the mean ± SD ($n = 3$) and analyzed by Students't-test (*$P < 0.05$, **$P < 0.01$)

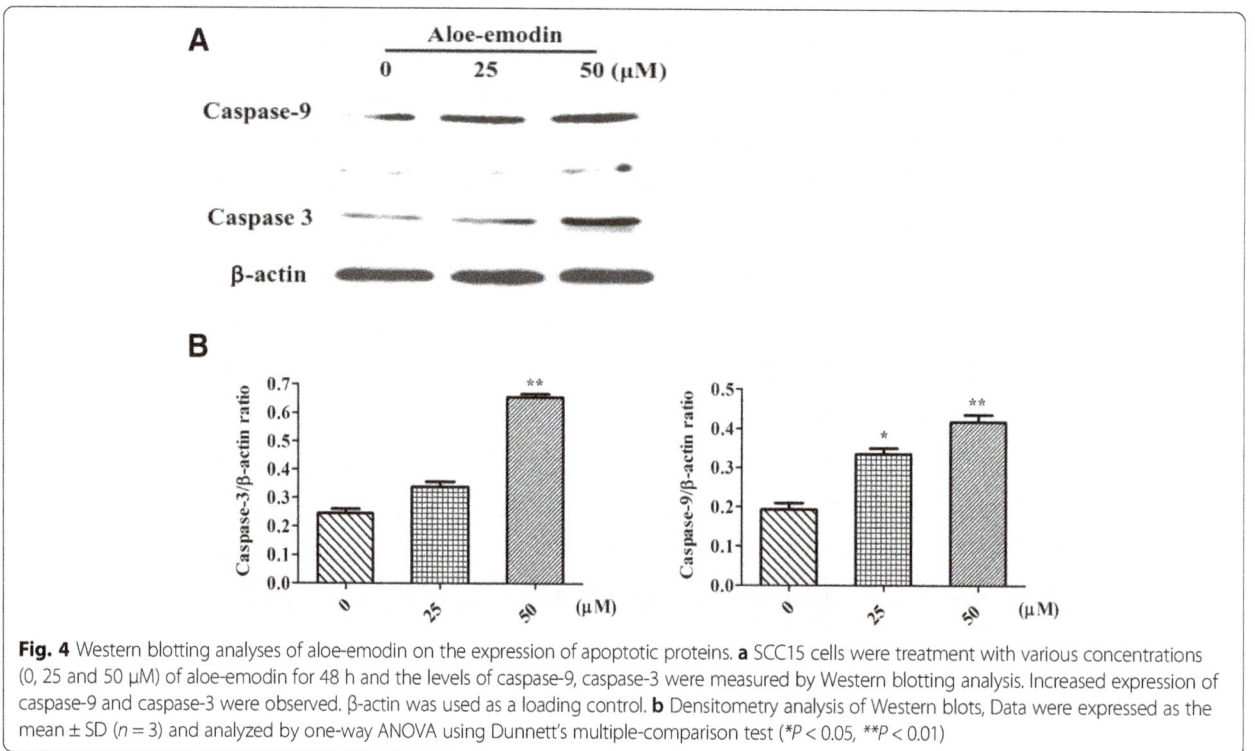

Fig. 4 Western blotting analyses of aloe-emodin on the expression of apoptotic proteins. **a** SCC15 cells were treatment with various concentrations (0, 25 and 50 μM) of aloe-emodin for 48 h and the levels of caspase-9, caspase-3 were measured by Western blotting analysis. Increased expression of caspase-9 and caspase-3 were observed. β-actin was used as a loading control. **b** Densitometry analysis of Western blots, Data were expressed as the mean ± SD ($n = 3$) and analyzed by one-way ANOVA using Dunnett's multiple-comparison test (*$P < 0.05$, **$P < 0.01$)

results demonstrated that aloe-emodin in a time- and dose-dependent decrease in SCC15 cells viability.

Apoptosis plays a critical role in regulating cell death, we detected apoptotic rates using flow cytometry. The apoptotic rate is tested using Annexin V with PI staining. The caspases have been identified to play a vital role in the mechanism of apoptosis [12, 13]. The caspase-3 is considered to be the most important of the executioner caspases, activated caspase-3 can cleave multiple structural and regulatory proteins, that ultimately cause the morphological and biochemical changes seen in apoptotic cells [14]. Caspase-9 is the upstream caspase, the apoptosis process starts with the activation of caspase 9, in turn, activates caspase-3 almost simultaneously, which then activate other caspases, resulting in cell apoptosis. In the present study, we found that the expression levels of caspase-9 and caspase-3 proteins increased, these results may indicate that aloe-emodin induces apoptosis via activation caspase-9 and caspase-3 in SCC15 cells.

Conclusion

In conclusion, the present study demonstrated that aloe-emodin inhibits the proliferation and induces the apoptosis in SCC15 cells, moreover, we reveal the potential mechanism of apoptosis effect and results indicate that aloe-emodin may be a good entity for anti-oral cancer drug exploring. However, confirmation the results of aloe-emodin against in other OSCC cell lines are necessary and further in vivo studies are required.

Abbreviations
BCA: Bicinchoninic acid; DMEM: Dulbecco's modified Eagle's medium; ECL: Enhanced Chemiluminescence; FBS: Fetal bovine serum; FITC: Fluorescein isothiocyanate; IC_{50}: Half maximal inhibitory concentrations; MTT: Thiazolyl blue tetrazolium bromide; OD: Optical density; PBS: Phosphate buffered saline; PI: Propidium iodide; RL: Rheum undulatum L

Acknowledgments
Thanks to Dr. Zhang Xin-yan for her kindly supply us the Human oral squamous cell carcinoma cell line SCC15.

Funding
This work was supported by Beijing NOVA Program Z141107001814013 (used for cell culture, drug assays), National Natural Science Foundation of China 81602534(used for Western blot analysis), Beijing Natural Science Foundation 7172154 (used for flow cytometry test), Military Youth Cultivation Fund 16QNP134 (used for data analysis) and Military Youth Cultivation Fund 15QNP088 (used for data analysis)..

Authors' contributions
QHL and JW carried out the Cell culture, drug assays. KTY and YS carried out the Western blot analysis. WLH and HXC performed and the flow cytometry test. QHL wrote the paper. BZ and CG conceived of the study, and participated in its design and coordination and helped to draft the manuscript. All authors have reviewed and approved the final version of the manuscript.

Consent for publication
Not applicable.

Competing interests
The authors declare that they have no competing interests.

Author details
[1]Department of Stomatology, 307 Hospital, PLA, 8 Dongda Street, Beijing 100071, China. [2]Stomatological Hospital, Southern Medical University, No. 366, South Jiangnan Avenue, Guangzhou 510280, China. [3]Department of Stomatology, Chinese PLA General Hospital, 28 Fuxing Road, Beijing 100853, China.

References
1. Shiga K, Tateda M, Katagiri K, Nakanome A, Ogawa T, Asada Y, Kato K, Kobayashi T. Distinct features of second primary malignancies in head and neck cancer patients in Japan. The Tohoku J Exp Med. 2011;225(1):5–12.
2. Sudbø J, Reith A. Retracted: the evolution of predictive oncology and molecular-based therapy for oral cancer prevention. Int J Cancer. 2005; 115(3):339–45.
3. Cowden Dahl KD, Symowicz J, Ning Y, Gutierrez E, Fishman DA, Adley BP, Stack MS, Hudson LG. Matrix metalloproteinase 9 is a mediator of epidermal growth factor-dependent e-cadherin loss in ovarian carcinoma cells. Cancer Res. 2008;68(12):4606–13.
4. Cui Y, Lu P, Song G, Liu Q, Zhu D, Liu X. Involvement of PI3K/Akt, ERK and p38 signaling pathways in emodin-mediated extrinsic and intrinsic human hepatoblastoma cell apoptosis. Food Chem Toxicol. 2016;92:26–37.
5. Chen X, Gao H, Han Y, Ye J, Xie J, Wang C. Physcion induces mitochondria driven apoptosis in colorectal cancer cells via down regulating EMMPRIN. Eur J Pharmacol. 2015;764:124–33.
6. Tabolacci C, Cordella M, Turcano L, Rossi S, Lentini A, Mariotti S, Nisini R, Sette G, Eramo A, Piredda L, Maria RD, Facchiano F, Beninati S. Aloe-emodin exerts a potent anticancer and immunomodulatory activity on BRAF-mutated human melanoma cells. Eur J Pharmacol. 2015;762:283–92.
7. Lin SR, Fu YS, Tsai MJ, Cheng H, Weng CF. Natural compounds from herbs that can potentially execute as autophagy inducers for cancer therapy. Int J Mol Sci. 2017;18:1412.
8. Xu XF, Zhang TL, Jin S, Wang R, Xiao X, Zhang WD, Wang PY, Wang XJ. Ardipusilloside I induces apoptosis by regulating Bcl-2 family proteins in human mucoepidermoid carcinoma Mc3 cells. BMC Complement Altern Med. 2013;13:322.
9. Treasure J. Herbal medicine and cancer: an introductory overview. Semin Oncol Nurs. 2005;21:177–83.
10. Cao YJ, Pu ZJ, Tang YP, Shen J, Chen YY, Kang A, Zhou GS, Duan JA. Advances in bio-active constituents, pharmacology and clinical applications of rhubarb. Chin Med. 2017;12(1):36.
11. Cragg GM, Newman DJ. Plants as a source of anticancer agents. J Ethnopharmacol. 2005;100(1–2):72–9.
12. Wu JY, Yi C, Chung HR, Wang DJ, Chang WC, Lee SY, Lin CT, Yang YC, Yang WC. Potential biomarkers in saliva for oral squamous cell carcinoma. Oral Oncol. 2010;46:226–31.
13. Susan E. Apoptosis: a review of programmed cell death. Toxicol Pathol. 2007;35(4):495–516.
14. Slee EA, Adrain C, Martin SJ. Executioner caspase-3, –6, and –7 perform distinct, non-redundant roles during the demolition phase of apoptosis. J Biol Chem. 2001;276:7320–6.

20

Study of the anti-allergic and anti-inflammatory activity of *Brachychiton rupestris* and *Brachychiton discolor* leaves (Malvaceae) using in vitro models

Amany A. Thabet[1†], Fadia S. Youssef[1†], Michal Korinek[2,3,4,5], Fang-Rong Chang[2,6], Yang-Chang Wu[2,7,8], Bing-Hung Chen[3,8,9], Mohamed El-Shazly[1,10*], Abdel Nasser B. Singab[1*] and Tsong-Long Hwang[4,5,11,12,13*] (iD)

Abstract

Background: *Brachychiton rupestris* and *Brachychiton discolor* (Malvaceae) are ornamental trees native to Australia. Some members of *Brachychiton* and its highly related genus, *Sterculia*, are employed in traditional medicine for itching, dermatitis and other skin diseases. However, scientific studies on these two genera are scarce. Aiming to reveal the scientific basis of the folk medicinal use of these plants, the cytotoxicity, anti-inflammatory and anti-allergic activities of *Brachychiton rupestris* and *Brachychiton discolor* leaves extracts and fractions were evaluated. Also, phytochemical investigation of *B. rupestris* was performed to identify the compounds exerting the biological effect.

Methods: Extracts as well as fractions of *Brachychiton rupestris* and *Brachychiton discolor* were tested for their cytotoxicity versus hepatoma HepG2, lung A549, and breast MDA-MB-231 cancer cell lines. Assessment of the anti-allergic activity was done using degranulation assay in RBL-2H3 mast cells. Anti-inflammatory effect was tested by measuring the suppression of superoxide anion production as well as elastase release in fMLF/CB-induced human neutrophils. Phytochemical investigation of the *n*-hexane, dichloromethane and ethyl acetate fractions of *B. rupestris* was done using different chromatographic and spectroscopic techniques.

Results: The tested samples showed no cytotoxicity towards the tested cell lines. The nonpolar fractions of both *B. rupestris* and *B. discolor* showed potent anti-allergic potency by inhibiting the release of β-hexosaminidase. The dichloromethane fraction of both species exhibited the highest anti-inflammatory activity by suppressing superoxide anion generation and elastase release with IC_{50} values of 2.99 and 1.98 μg/mL, respectively for *B. rupestris*, and 0.78 and 1.57 μg/mL, respectively for *B. discolor*. Phytochemical investigation of various fractions of *B. rupestris* resulted in the isolation of β-amyrin acetate (1), β-sitosterol (2) and stigmasterol (3) from the *n*-hexane fraction. Scopoletin (4) and β-sitosterol-3-*O*-β-D-glucoside (5) were obtained from the dichloromethane fraction. Dihydrodehydrodiconiferyl alcohol 4-*O*-β-D-glucoside (6) and dihydrodehydrodiconiferyl alcohol 9-*O*-β-D-glucoside (7) were separated from the ethyl acetate fraction. Scopoletin (4) showed anti-allergic and anti-inflammatory activity.

Conclusions: It was concluded that the nonpolar fractions of both *Brachychiton* species exhibited anti-allergic and anti-inflammatory activities.

Keywords: Anti-allergic, Anti-inflammatory, *Brachychiton discolor*, *Brachychiton rupestris*, Cytotoxicity, Phytochemistry

* Correspondence: mohamed.elshazly@pharma.asu.edu.eg;
dean@pharma.asu.edu.eg; htl@mail.cgu.edu.tw
†Amany A. Thabet and Fadia S. Youssef contributed equally to this work.
[1]Department of Pharmacognosy, Faculty of Pharmacy, Ain Shams University, African Union Organization Street, Abbassia, Cairo 11566, Egypt
[4]Graduate Institute of Natural Products, College of Medicine, Chang Gung University, Taoyuan 33302, Taiwan
Full list of author information is available at the end of the article

Background

Allergy is one of the most popular diseases worldwide and its great prevalence makes allergic disorder a growing global concern [1]. Allergic reaction can be defined as the development of signs and symptoms of hypersensitivity reactions upon exposure to certain allergenic substances resulting in massive production of allergen-specific IgE and allergen-specific T-cell populations [2]. Allergic reaction can be a life-threatening condition especially in anaphylaxis and severe asthma or it can be a chronic condition that interferes with the quality of life such as in eczema and allergic rhinitis [3].

Inflammation is another common disorder which is an innate immune response from the host defense mechanism. It consists of a series of complex biological processes aiming to combat infection and tissue injury. These processes lead to accumulation of plasma and blood cells in the tissue in addition to the release of inflammatory mediators aiming to reestablish tissue structures and function [4, 5]. Untreated inflammation can lead to a chronic condition which is characterized as a very long-term inflammation affecting the remodeling of tissue for many weeks and even years. It is considered as a main cause in the development of a various life threatening disorders, such as neurodegenerative diseases and cancers [4].

Non-steroidal anti-inflammatory drugs (NSAIDs) constitute the commonly adopted classes for the alleviation of inflammation and related conditions. Meanwhile, their intolerable side effects represented by gastrointestinal ulcers, and perforation with concomitant bleeding are the main obstacles facing their therapeutic usage [6]. On the contrary, nature continues to serve as a rich and appealing source of novel, safer, and cheaper bioactive molecules in comparison to many synthetic drugs. A plethora of plant extracts, as well as isolated compounds, possess notable anti-allergic and anti-inflammatory activities, as previously reported [5, 7–11].

Malvaceae, the mallows, is a family that comprises more than 200 genera and 2300 species. A great diversity of phytoconstituents such as triterpenes, flavonoids, coumarins, as well as alkaloids was previously reported in the members of this family [12, 13]. *Brachychiton* (Malvaceae) is a small genus native to Australia comprising of 30 species [14, 15]. Recently, *Brachychiton* has been considered as a separate genus from *Sterculia* as proved by the detailed investigation of its follicles, seed coats and embryo [14]. Members of the *Brachychiton* genus were used as food by Australian Aborigines and some are used as ornamental trees or shrubs [16, 17]. Different members of the genus possess several interesting biological effects such as antioxidant, antibacterial, anti-hyperglycemic, hepatoprotective and anti-schistosomal activities [18–21]. Phytochemical studies of various members of *Brachychiton* sp.

resulted in the identification of various classes of compounds such as flavonoids, coumarins, triterpenes, sterols, and alkaloids [22–24]. *Brachychiton rupestris* is commonly known as "Queensland bottle tree" because it is native to Queensland and has a bottle shaped trunk. *B. discolor* (synonym *B. luridus*) is commonly called the lacebark tree [25–27]. The mucilage and ethyl acetate fraction of *B. rupestris* leaves were previously investigated for their in vivo anti-hyperglycemic effect and the phytochemical investigation of this species led to the isolation and identification of flavonoid aglycones and glycosides from the leaves [20, 28]. However, no complete phytochemical study was done on this species. Regarding *B. discolor*, two complete phytochemical studies were reported on this species where many classes of compounds were reported from the leaves, seeds and roots including triterpenes, flavonoids, phenolic acids, coumarins and alkaloids [23, 24].

Tracing current literature, nothing was found regarding the anti-allergic and anti-inflammatory effects of *B. rupestris*. However, different studies were carried out confirming the anti-allergic and anti-inflammatory activities of several triterpenes such as β-amyrin, oleanolic acid and lupeol [29–33] which were also isolated from *B. discolor* [23, 24]. Another species (*B. populneus*) was reported to be effective in relieving pain and skin diseases in folk medicine [34]. Furthermore, many members of the related genus, *Sterculia*, are popular in folk medicine for alleviating itching, dermatitis, boils, inflammations and other skin diseases [35–40]. Herein, we investigated the anti-allergic and anti-inflammatory activities of the methanol extracts and fractions of both *B. rupestris* and *B. discolor* leaves. The cytotoxic effect of *B. rupestris* and *B. discolor* leaves extracts and fractions was also evaluated to ascertain their safety. Additionally, the isolation and structural elucidation of the major constituents from the bioactive fractions of *B. rupestris* was achieved within this work.

Methods

Plant materials

The leaves of *B. rupestris* (T.Mitch.ex Lindl) K.Schum and *B. discolor* F.Muell were obtained from El-Orman Botanical Garden, Giza, Egypt, in summer 2014. The plants were generously authenticated by Prof. Dr. Mohamed El-Gibaly, Department of Botany, National Research Center (NRC), Giza, Egypt. Voucher specimens (PHG-P-BR-248 and PHG-P-BL-249) for *B. rupestris* and *B. discolor* (*B. luridus*), respectively were kept at the Pharmacognosy Department, Faculty of Pharmacy, Ain Shams University.

Extraction and fractionation

Total amount of 3.05 kg of *B. rupestris* air-dried leave were crushed, macerated in 29 L of distilled methanol for three times and filtered. Subsequently, the obtained filtrate was evaporated in vacuo at low temperature (45 °C) till dryness and then subjected to lyophilization to give 333.56 g of the total methanol extract. A portion of the extract (300 g) was successively partitioned with *n*-hexane (37.9 L), dichloromethane (4.8 L) and ethyl acetate (5.2 L) to give 54.35, 8.54 and 5.91 g, respectively along with the remaining hydromethanolic fraction estimated as 191.5 g.

Similarly, for *B. discolor*, the crushed air-dried leaves 600 g were macerated in distilled methanol (6 L × 3), filtered, and evaporated at 45 °C under reduced pressure till dryness to yield 36 g of the total methanol extract. Then, 11 g of the total extract were fractionated using 430 mL of *n*-hexane, 300 mL of dichloromethane and 300 mL of ethyl acetate successively to give 1.3, 1.2, and 0.9 g of the dried residues, respectively.

Biological investigations
In vitro assessment of the cytotoxic activity

Cell culture The cytotoxicity of *B. rupestris* and *B. discolor* total extracts as well as their obtained fractions was examined on A549 (adenocarcinoma human alveolar basal epithelial cells), HepG2 (human liver cancer cell line) and MDA-MB-231 (invasive ductal carcinoma) cells. Cells were preserved in Dulbecco's modified Eagle's medium-high glucose powder (DMEM) containing 10% heat-inactivated fetal bovine serum (FBS), 1 mM sodium pyruvate, 100 μg/mL streptomycin, 100 U/mL penicillin, and 2 mM L-glutamine. Cells were cultured in culture dishes (Cellstar) that were kept in a humidified chamber supplied with 5% (*v/v*) CO_2 at 37 °C. Then the cells were maintained as a monolayer culture adopting serial subculturing. Cells growing in the logarithmic phase were employed in all experiments [41].

Cytotoxicity assay MTT (methylthiazoltetrazolium) assay was employed to evaluate the cytotoxic activity of the tested samples against human cancer cells [42, 43]. Trypsinized cell suspensions were freshly prepared and then planted in a 96-well culture plate followed by overnight incubation. Tested samples were prepared in dimethyl sulfoxide (DMSO) to form stock solutions of 1 mg/mL. Cells were treated with the tested samples using different concentrations (2.5–20 μg/mL) then incubated for 72 h at 37 °C under 5% CO_2. After the incubation, and removal of the cells medium, 100 μL of MTT solution was added to each well followed by incubation of the cells for 1 h. The formed formazan crystals were dissolved in DMSO after the removal of the medium to measure absorbance at 550 nm. The percentage of cell viability was calculated by the following formula:

$$\%\text{cell viability} = \frac{\text{O.D of treated cells–O.D of culture medium}}{\text{O.D of untreated cells–O.D of culture medium}} \times 100$$

Where O.D = optical density

Cytotoxicity was expressed as % cell inhibition. Doxorubicin was used as the positive control.

In vitro assessment of the anti-allergic activity

Chemicals and reagents DMEM, dexamethasone, *p*-nitrophenyl-*N*-acetyl-D-glucosaminide (*p*-NAG), MTT (3-(4,5-dimethylthiazol-2-yl)-2,5-diphenyltetrazolium bromide), penicillin and streptomycin, calcium ionophore A23187, mouse anti-DNP (dinitrophenyl) IgE antibody, and DMSO were purchased from Sigma-Aldrich (St. Louis, MO, USA). Moreover, FBS was obtained from Hyclone (Logan, UT, USA). Dinitrophenyl-conjugated bovine serum albumin (DNP-BSA) was purchased from Merck (Kenilworth, NJ, USA). Additional chemicals as well as reagents were purchased at the highest possible purity.

Cell culture The mucosal mast cell-derived rat basophilic leukemia (RBL-2H3) cell line was obtained from the American Type Culture Collection. Cells were grown in DMEM medium accompanied with 10% FBS in addition to 100 U/mL penicillin plus 100 μg/mL streptomycin. Cells were cultured in 10 cm cell culture dishes (Cellstar) at 37 °C with 5% CO_2 in air.

Cell viability assay MTT assay was used to assess the toxic effects of samples on RBL-2H3 cells [44] and was done as previously mentioned [42, 43]. All experiments were done in triplicates. DMSO served as the negative control not affecting the growth of RBL-2H3 cells. Triton X-100 (0.5% solution) was employed as the positive control resulting in the death of all cells in a well.

Degranulation β-hexosaminidase assay induced by A23187 A23187-induced degranulation in RBL-2H3 cells was evaluated by a *β*-hexosaminidase activity assay as previously reported employing certain modifications [45, 46]. RBL-2H3 cells were seeded into 96-wells plate using a density of 2×10^4 cells/well and were incubated at 37 °C for 5 h in 5% CO_2. Cells were washed with PBS (phosphate buffered saline) and then various concentrations of samples or medium (untreated control) were added to each well (100 μL), and the treated cells were incubated at 37 °C in 5% CO_2 for 20 h. The cells were stimulated by calcium ionophore A23187 (1 μM) diluted in Tyrode's buffer (135 mM NaCl, 1.8 mM $CaCl_2$, 5 mM KCl, 1.0 mM $MgCl_2$, 5.6 mM glucose, 20 mM HEPES at pH 7.4), and kept at 37 °C in 5% CO_2 for 1 h. For the total amount of *β*-hexosaminidase release, the unstimulated cells were lysed using 0.5% Triton X-100. Untreated unstimulated cells represented spontaneous β-hexosaminidase release. The control wells were represented by the stimulated untreated cells. The cells supernatants (50 µL) were incubated with equal volume of 1 µM of p-NAG (50 µL), a substrate for β-hexosaminidase, prepared in 0.05 M citrate buffer (pH 4.5) for 1 h at 37 °C. The reaction was stopped by 100 µL of stop buffer (0.1 M Na_2/NaHCO$_3$, pH 10.0). Microplate reader was used to measure the absorbance at 405 nm. The inhibition percentage of β-hexosaminidase release from RBL-2H3 cells was calculated using the following equation:

$$\text{Inhibition (\%)} = \left[1 - \frac{(\text{ODsample} - \text{ODspontaneous})}{(\text{ODcontrol} - \text{ODspontaneous})}\right] \times 100$$

Dexamethasone (10 nM) was employed as the positive control.

Degranulation β-hexosaminidase assay induced by IgE β-Hexosaminidase release from the activated RBL-2H3 cells was measured as previously reported [45, 47], with some modifications. The inhibition percentage of antigen-induced β-hexosaminidase release from RBL-2H3 cells was assessed in a similar way as described above in the degranulation A23187-induced β-hexosaminidase assay, except of the stimulation process. The cells were sensitized with anti-DNP IgE (0.1 µg/mL) for at least 2 h and then washed with pre-warmed Tyrode's buffer, followed by stimulation by antigen DNP-BSA (100 ng/mL). Dexamethasone (10 nM) was employed as the positive control.

In vitro assessment of the anti-inflammatory activity

Preparation of human neutrophils Blood was withdrawn from 20 to 35 years old healthy human donors adopting a protocol approved by the institutional review board at Chang Gung Memorial Hospital. Isolation of neutrophils was done employing a standard method which was previously reported [48].

Measurement of superoxide generation

Ferricytochrome c (0.5 mg/mL) and Ca^2 (1 mM) were incubated with neutrophils at 37 °C for 2 min, followed by the treatment with the tested samples for 5 min. Cells activation was done using formyl-methionyl-leucyl-phenylalanine (fMLF, 100 nM)/cytochalasin B (CB, 1 µg/mL) for 10 min. The absorbance was detected at 550 nm in a double-beam spectrophotometer Hitachi U-3010. Superoxide inhibition was determined by lowering ferricytochrome c as reported previously [48, 49]. The differences in absorbance between the measurements in the presence of superoxide (100 U/mL) and its absence divided by the extinction coefficient for the reduction of

ferricytochrome c ($\varepsilon = 21.1/\text{mM}/10$ mm) were used as the basis for calculations. Genistein was adopted as the positive control [50, 51].

Measurement of elastase release

The release of elastase was determined by assessing the degranulation of azurophilic granules [48, 49]. An elastase substrate MeO-Suc-Ala-Ala-Pro-Val-p-nitroanilide (100 µM) was equilibrated with neutrophils at 37 °C for 2 min, followed by incubation with drugs for 5 min. Activation of the cells was done using 100 nM fMLF and 0.5 µg/mL CB, and then the variations in absorbance were detected at 405 nm. The results are shown as the percentage of the initial rate of elastase release in the fMLF/CB-activated, drug-free control system. Genistein was employed as the positive control [50, 51].

Statistical analysis

Results are represented as mean ± SD value of at least three independent measurements unless otherwise specified. The 50% inhibitory concentration (IC$_{50}$) was determined using the dose-response curve which was constructed by plotting the percentage of inhibition versus concentrations (linear function, Microsoft Office). Statistical analysis was done using one-way analysis of variance (ANOVA) followed by Dunnet's test (GraphPad Prism 6.0, GraphPad Software, Sand Diego, CA, USA, anti-allergic assay) or Student's t-test (Sigma Plot, Systat software, Systat Software Inc., San Jose, CA, USA, anti-inflammatory assay). Values which show $*p < 0.05$, $**p < 0.001$ are statistically significant.

Phytochemical investigations
General experimental procedures

^{1}H and ^{13}C (APT) NMR analyses were done using a Bruker Ascend 400/R spectrometer (Burker Avance III, Fallanden Switzerland) at the Center for Drug Discovery, Research and Development, Faculty of Pharmacy, Ain Shams University using 400 and 100 MHz the operating frequencies. Chemical shifts were reported in δ ppm and were related to that of the solvents. Dissolution of the tested samples was done using various deuterated solvents (Sigma Aldrich, Germany) in 3 mm NMR tubes (Bruker). Spectra were recorded at 25 °C; δ ppm relative to tetramethylsilane (Me$_4$Si) as the internal standard. Two-dimensional (2D) NMR experiments (^{1}H, ^{1}H-^{1}H COSY; ^{1}H-^{13}C HSQC; ^{1}H-^{13}C HMBC) were done using the pulse sequences from the Bruker user library. Waters Xevo TQD mass spectrometer supplied with UPLC Acquity mode (*Milford*, USA) was employed to carry out ESI-MS analysis. Normal phase column chromatography was done using silica gel (Kieselgel 60, 70–230, and 230–400 mesh, Merck KGaA, Darmstadt, Germany). TLC analysis was done utilizing normal phase silica gel precoated plates F_{254} (Merck, Germany). Detection of TLC spots was done using UV light at 254 nm and 365 nm as well as by spraying with 10% H_2SO_4 with subsequent heating on a hot plate at 100 °C.

Isolation of the secondary metabolites from the bioactive fractions

The *n*-hexane fraction (33 g) of *B. rupestris* was chromatographed on silica gel (600 g) employing *n*-hexane:EtOAc with increasing polarity to give 23 major fractions. Fraction II was further eluted with a mixture of *n*-hexane: EtOAc (9.0:1.0) from which compound 1 (40 mg) was precipitated as a white amorphous powder. A mixture of compounds 2 and 3 (60 mg) was precipitated from fraction III as white crystalline needles using the solvent system *n*-hexane:EtOAc (9.0:1.0) as illustrated in Fig. 1.

The dichloromethane fraction of *B. rupestris* (6 g) was chromatographed on silica gel (300 g) using mixtures of CH_2Cl_2:CH_3OH with increasing polarity as eluents to afford 26 major fractions. Fraction VI (70 mg) was further eluted with dichloromethane and was subjected to silica gel column using a mixture of CH_2Cl_2:CH_3OH to give seven subfractions. Subfraction 7 (30 mg) was eluted with a mixture of CH_2Cl_2:CH_3OH (9.9:0.1) and purified over preparative TLC which resulted in the separation of compound 4 (8 mg) that showed strong fluorescent yellow color. Fraction XV

was eluted using a mixture of CH_2Cl_2:CH_3OH (9.6:0.4) from which compound 5 (50 mg) was precipitated as a yellow powder as shown in Fig. 2.

The EtOAc fraction (4 g) was applied on the top of 150 g Diaion HP column using water, 50% methanol, 100% methanol as the mobile phases. The 50% methanol fraction (2 g) was the most promising fraction after comparing its TLC with the other fractions and was applied on the top of 40 g Sephadex® LH 20 and eluted using water and methanol of decreasing polarity to give 16 fractions. Fraction V (70 mg) and fraction VI (50 mg) were eluted using water 100% and were purified over preparative TLC using CH_2Cl_2:CH_3OH (8.5:1.5) as the mobile phase to separate compounds 6 (6 mg) and 7 (5 mg), respectively (Fig. 3).

Spectroscopic data of compounds 1–7
β-Amyrin acetate (1)

It was isolated as a white amorphous powder; with R_f = 0.530 in *n*-hexane:EtOAc (9.5:0.5). ^{1}H NMR (400 MHz, CDCl$_3$), ^{13}C NMR (100 MHz, CDCl$_3$) and 2D NMR spectroscopic data are displayed in the Additional file 1: Figure S1).

β-Sitosterol (2) and Stigmasterol (3)

They were isolated as white crystalline needles; showing R_f = 0.206 in *n*-hexane:EtOAc (9:1). ^{1}H-NMR (400 MHz, CDCl$_3$), ^{13}C NMR (100 MHz, CDCl$_3$) and 2D NMR spectral data are displayed in the Additional file 1: Figure S2.

Scopoletin (4)

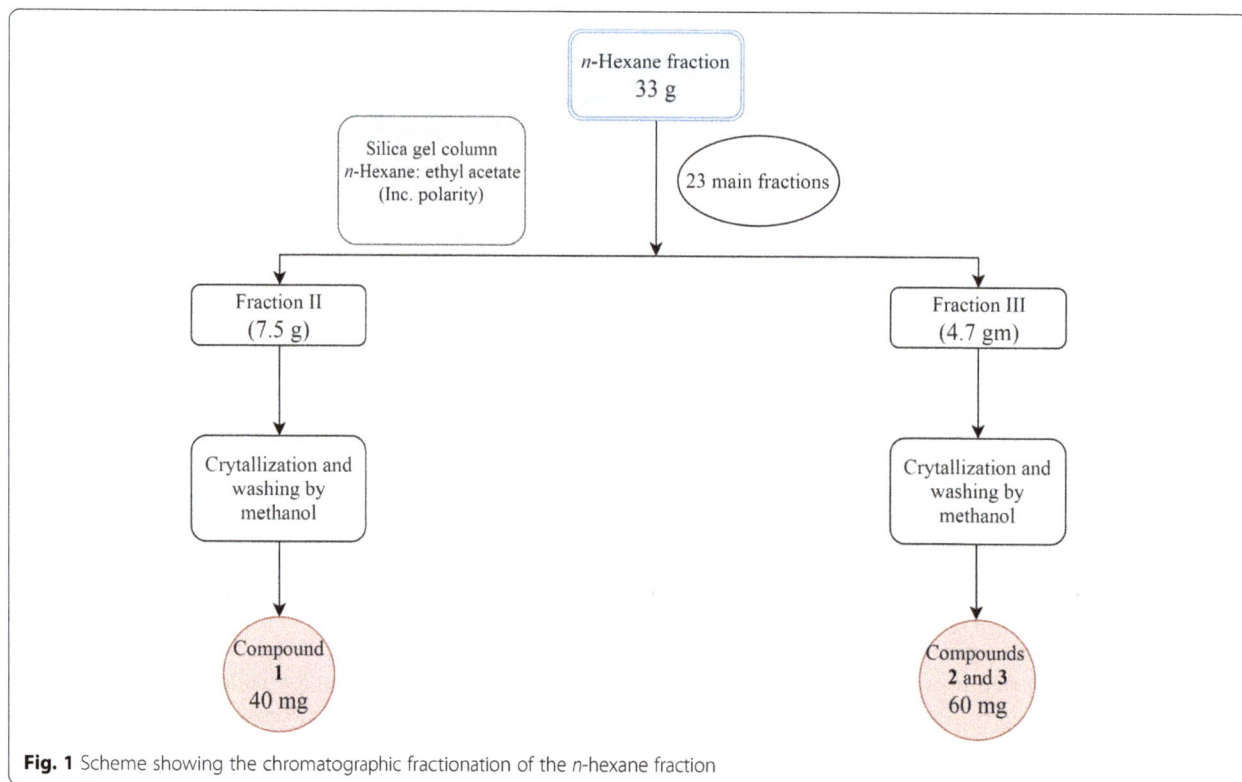

Fig. 1 Scheme showing the chromatographic fractionation of the *n*-hexane fraction

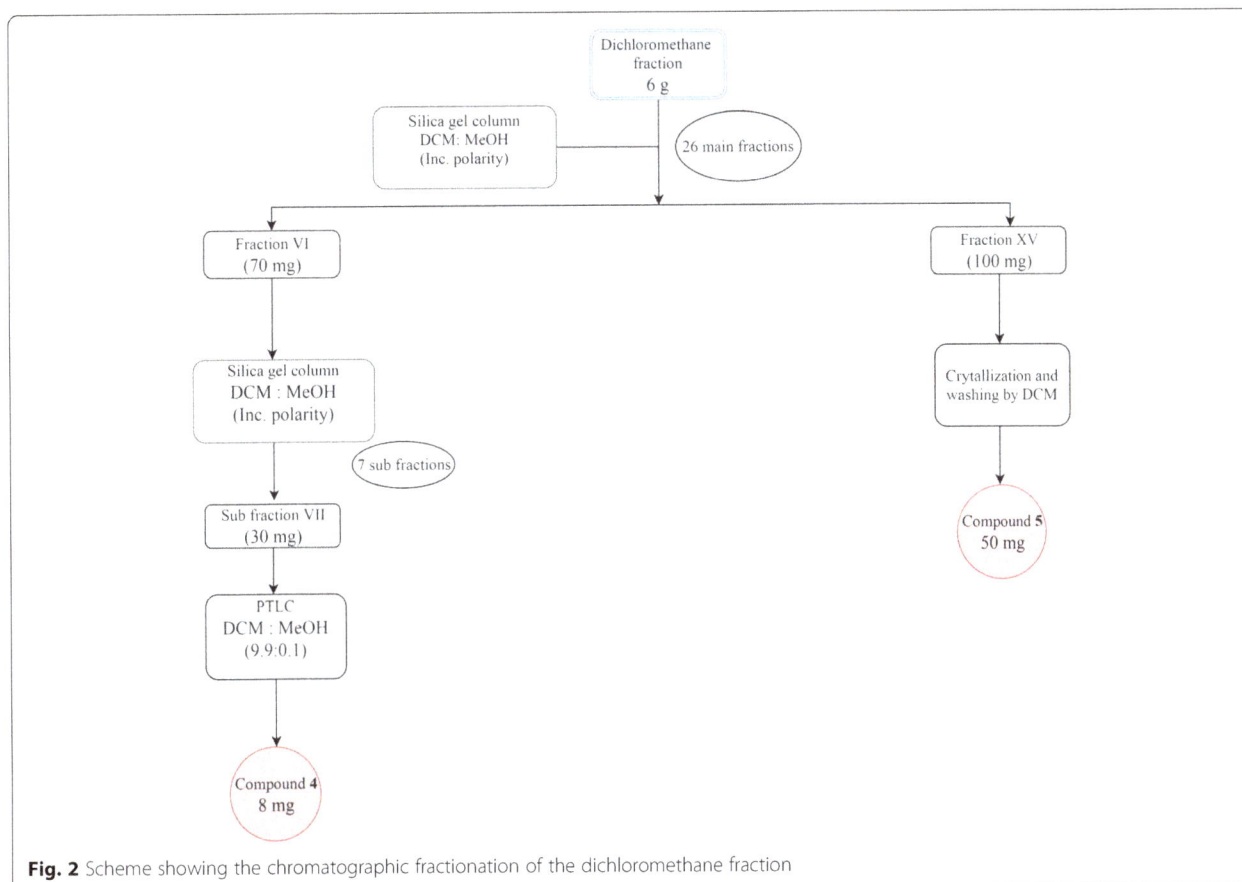

Fig. 2 Scheme showing the chromatographic fractionation of the dichloromethane fraction

It was obtained as a yellow powder; with $R_f = 0.630$ in CH_2Cl_2:CH_3OH (9.9:0.1). ^{1}H-NMR (400 MHz, CD$_3$OD) (δ ppm): 7.75 (1H, d, $J = 9.1$, H-4), 6.80 (1H, s, H-5), 6.45 (1H, s, H-8), 5.85 (1H, d, $J = 9.1$ Hz, H-3), 3.81 (3H, s, 6-OCH$_3$). ^{13}C NMR data (100 MHz, CD$_3$OD) (δ ppm): 166.26 (C-2), 153.86 (C-7), 151.4 (C-6), 146.99 (C-4), 107.65 (C-5), 105.50 (C-3), 104.59, (C-8), 56.03 (6-OCH$_3$). It exhibited a deprotonated molecular ion peak at m/z 190.8 [M-H]$^-$ in ESI-MS negative ion mode, corresponding to the molecular formula $C_{10}H_8O_4$ (Additional file 1: Figure S3).

β-Sitosterol-3-O-β-D-glucoside (**5**)

It was isolated as a buff amorphous powder; with $R_f = 0.630$ in CH_2Cl_2:CH_3OH (9.2:0.8). ^{1}H-NMR (400 MHz, DMSO-d_6), ^{13}C NMR (100 MHz, DMSO-d_6) and 2D NMR spectroscopic data are displayed in the Additional file 1: Figure S4.

Dihydrodehydrodiconiferyl alcohol 4-O-β-D-glucoside (**6**)

It was obtained as a yellowish white amorphous powder; with $R_f = 0.259$ in CH_2Cl_2:CH_3OH (8.5:1.5). ^{1}H-NMR (400 MHz, CD$_3$OD), ^{13}C NMR data (100 MHz, CD$_3$OD) are illustrated in Table 4, (Additional file 1: Figure S5).

Dihydrodehydrodiconiferyl alcohol 9-O-β-D-glucoside (**7**)

It was obtained as a yellowish white amorphous powder; with $R_f = 0.304$ in CH_2Cl_2:CH_3OH (8.5:1.5). ^{1}H-NMR

(400 MHz, CD$_3$OD), ^{13}C NMR (100 MHz, CD$_3$OD) and 2D NMR spectroscopic data are displayed in Table 4 and the Additional file 1: Figure S6.

Results

In vitro assessment of the cytotoxic activity of *B. rupestris* and *B. discolor*

The cytotoxicity of the total methanol extracts and fractions of both *B. rupestris* and *B. discolor* was evaluated versus HepG2, A549 and MDA-MB-231 cancer cells using doxorubicin as the positive control. Extracts and fractions of both species at 20 µg/mL exhibited no cytotoxic activity against any of the tested cell lines. Noteworthy to mention that doxorubicin showed 91.28, 97.69 and 98.05% cell growth inhibition against HepG2, MDA-MB-231 and A549, respectively at 2 µg/mL. The results are illustrated in Table 1. Together with the nontoxic effects of all samples towards RBL-2H3 mast cells (see the following section, and Table 2) the results suggested that both species extracts and fractions exhibited no cytotoxicity against the tested cancer cell lines.

In vitro assessment of the anti-allergic activity of *B. rupestris* and *B. discolor*

The anti-allergic activity of the total methanol extracts and fractions of both *B. rupestris* and *B. discolor* was

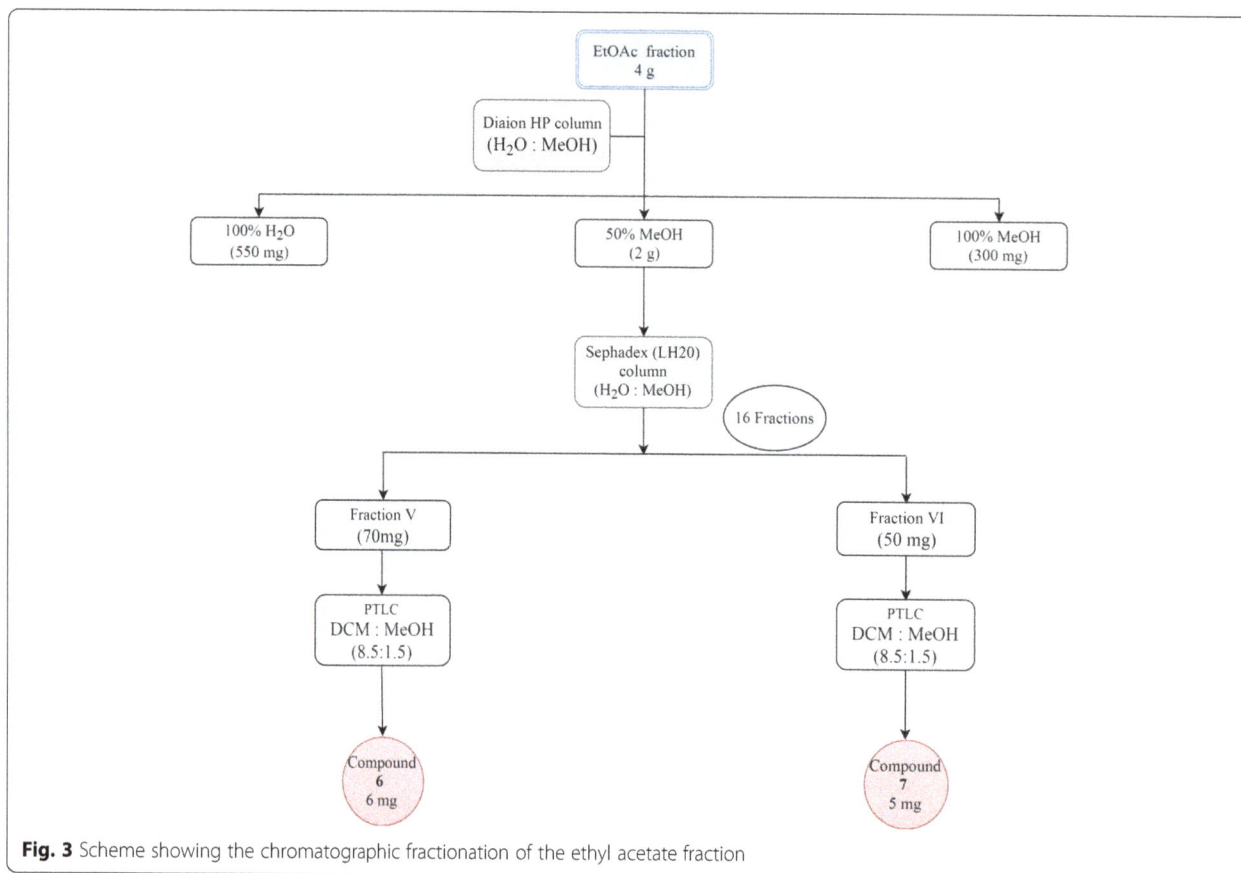

Fig. 3 Scheme showing the chromatographic fractionation of the ethyl acetate fraction

assessed using degranulation assay in RBL-2H3 mast cell model and the results are presented in Table 2. Initially, the cytotoxic effect of all samples was tested against RBL-2H3 cells using MTT viability assay. All samples were found to be nontoxic at 100 μg/mL. The samples were subjected to the anti-allergic assay by evaluating their inhibitory effect on β-hexosaminidase release in RBL-2H3 cells induced by calcium ionophore, A23187. According to our results, B. rupestris and B. discolor crude methanol extracts (BRT 25.7% and BDT 16.0% inhibition) and nonpolar n-hexane (BRH 39.0%, BDH 30.3% inhibition) and dichloromethane fractions (BRD 19.0%; and BDD 44.0% inhibition) exhibited significant inhibition of β-hexosaminidase release in A23187-induced degranulation assay at 100 μg/mL (Table 2). Dexamethasone, a positive control, showed 62.0% inhibition of β-hexosaminidase release at 10 nM.

In vitro assessment of the anti-inflammatory activity of B. rupestris and B. discolor

Similarly, the anti-inflammatory activity was determined for the total methanol extracts and fractions of B. rupestris and B. discolor and the results are presented in Table 3. Both Brachychiton species exhibited a promising inhibitory activity on superoxide anion production as well as elastase release in fMLF-activated human neutrophils indicating their potential applications for the alleviation of both acute and chronic inflammatory disorders. All samples inhibited superoxide anion generation showing IC_{50} values between 0.78 and 6.25 μg/mL in addition

Table 1 In vitro cytotoxicity of different extracts and fractions of B. rupestris and B. discolor against HepG2, MDA-MB-231 and A549 cell lines

Cell line	BRT	BRH	BRD	BRE	BRR	BDT	BDH	BDD	BDE	doxorubicin
HepG2	1.28	−2.078	−8.02	−8.43	−13.74	1.66	−7.43	−16.18	−6.62	91.28 ± 0.3
MDA-MB-231	−15.86	−9.70	−18.83	−25.52	−23.30	−6.19	−6.73	13.17	−20.64	97.69 ± 0.4
A549	0.44	−0.81	7.85	−8.37	−0.89	12.59	8.18	14.99	−6.52	98.05 ± 0.0

Results are presented as growth inhibition percentage at concentration of 20 μg/mL, mean (n = 1). Doxorubicin (2 μg/mL) was used as the reference drug, mean ± SD (n = 2). BRT: B. rupestris total methanol extract; BHT: B. rupestris n-hexane fraction; BRD: B. rupestris dichloromethane fraction; BRE: B. rupestris ethyl acetate fraction; BRR: B. rupestris remaining MeOH(aq) fraction; BDT: B. discolor total methanol extract; BDH: B. discolor n-hexane fraction; BDD: B. discolor dichloromethane fraction; BDE: B. discolor ethyl acetate fraction

Table 2 Anti-allergic activity of *B. rupestris* and *B. discolor* extracts and fractions

Sample	% viability, RBL-2H3[a]	% inhibition of A23187-induced β-hexosaminidase release[b]	
	100 µg/mL	10 µg/mL	100 µg/mL
BRT	99.0 ± 1.7	3.0 ± 5.2	25.7 ± 2.1[**]
BRH	96.7 ± 4.0	3.3 ± 5.8	39.0 ± 13.1[**]
BRD	95.3 ± 8.1	4.3 ± 7.5	19.0 ± 4.4[*]
BRE	97.7 ± 4.0	2.0 ± 3.5	7.0 ± 5.2
BRR	99.0 ± 1.7	4.3 ± 5.1	3.7 ± 6.4
BDT	99.0 ± 1.7	3.7 ± 6.4	16.0 ± 5.0[*]
BDH	99.7 ± 0.6	4.3 ± 7.5	30.3 ± 3.1[**]
BDD	100.0 ± 0.0	0.0 ± 0.0	44.0 ± 7.8[**]
BDE	100.0 ± 0.0	1.7 ± 2.9	0.3 ± 0.6

[a]The cytotoxicity of samples towards RBL-2H3 cells was evaluated using MTT viability assay and none of the samples showed any toxicity; results are presented as mean ± SD ($n = 3$)
[b]Dexamethasone (10 nM) was used as the positive control and inhibited 62.0 ± 9.5%[**] of A23187-induced β-hexosaminidase release in RBL-2H3 cells. Results are presented as mean ± SD ($n = 3$); *$p < 0.05$, **$p < 0.001$ compared with the control value (A23187 only)
BRT *B. rupestris* total methanol extract, BRH *B. rupestris* n-hexane fraction, BRD *B. rupestris* dichloromethane fraction, BRE *B. rupestris* ethyl acetate fraction, BRR *B. rupestris* remaining MeOH(aq) fraction, BDT *B. discolor* total methanol extract, BDH *B. discolor* n-hexane fraction, BDD *B. discolor* dichloromethane fraction, BDE *B. discolor* ethyl acetate fraction

Table 3 Effect of the total extracts and fractions of *B. rupestris* and *B. discolor* on superoxide anion generation and elastase release in fMLF/CB-induced human neutrophils

Sample	Superoxide anion generation[a] IC_{50} (µg/mL)[b]	Elastase release[a] IC_{50} (µg/mL)[b]
BRT	4.92 ± 1.47	3.82 ± 0.55
BRH	5.69 ± 0.80	3.73 ± 1.16
BRD	2.99 ± 0.73	1.98 ± 1.54
BRE	6.25 ± 3.10	2.71 ± 0.79
BRR	3.01 ± 1.91	> 10[c]
BDT	4.73 ± 0.97	5.37 ± 1.23
BDH	6.25 ± 2.18	6.04 ± 2.32
BDD	0.78 ± 0.29	1.57 ± 0.84
BDE	5.22 ± 1.35	2.95 ± 1.08
genistein	0.41 ± 0.09	4.41 ± 1.99

[a]IC_{50} values, results are presented as mean ± SD ($n = 3$), compared with the control value (formyl-methionyl-leucyl-phenylalanine/cytochalasin B, fMLF/CB)
[b]Concentration necessary for 50% inhibition (IC_{50})
[c]BRR exerted significant inhibitory activity in superoxide anion generation (49.6 ± 2.9%, **$p < 0.001$) at 10 µg/mL. BRT *B. rupestris* total methanol extract, BRH *B. rupestris* n-hexane fraction, BRD *B. rupestris* dichloromethane fraction, BRE *B. rupestris* ethyl acetate fraction, BRR *B. rupestris* remaining MeOH(aq) fraction, BDT *B. discolor* total methanol extract, BDH *B. discolor* n-hexane fraction, BDD *B. discolor* dichloromethane fraction, BDE *B. discolor* ethyl acetate fraction

to inhibition of elastase release showing IC_{50} values ranging from 1.57 to > 10 µg/mL (Table 3). The most potent fractions, dichloromethane fractions of *B. rupestris* (BRD) and *B. discolor* (BDD) inhibited superoxide anion generation with IC_{50} values 2.99 µg/mL (BRD) and 0.78 µg/mL (BDD), and inhibited elastase release with IC_{50} values 1.98 µg/mL (BRD) and 1.57 µg/mL (BDD). Such activities indicated comparable or even better inhibitory potential than that of genistein (superoxide IC_{50} 0.41 µg/mL and elastase IC_{50} 4.41 µg/mL), a known anti-inflammatory natural product [50, 51]. The dichloromethane fractions (BRD and BDD) were capable of almost completely abolishing oxidative burst and degranulation in fMLF-activated human neutrophils at 10 µg/mL (data not shown). Meanwhile, the ethyl acetate fraction of both species showed anti-inflammatory activity by inhibiting elastase release showing IC_{50} values of 2.71 µg/mL for *B. rupestris* (BRE) and 2.95 µg/mL for *B. discolor* (BDE).

Phytochemical investigations

In-depth phytochemical investigation was performed on the most bioactive fractions of *B. rupestris* leaves including the *n*-hexane, the dichloromethane and ethyl acetate fractions that showed the highest anti-allergic and anti-inflammatory activities. Three compounds were isolated and structurally elucidated from the *n*-hexane fraction which were β-amyrin acetate (**1**) [29], β-sitosterol (**2**) [52], stigmasterol (**3**) [52]. Meanwhile, two compounds were obtained from the dichloromethane fraction including scopoletin (**4**) [53, 54] and β-sitosterol-3-O-β-D-glucoside (**5**) [55] which were isolated for the first time from *B. rupestris* leaves. Furthermore, two neolignans were obtained from the ethyl acetate fraction, dihydrodehydrodiconiferyl alcohol 4-O-β-D-glucoside (**6**) [56] and dihydrodehydrodiconiferyl alcohol 9-O-β-D-glucoside (**7**) [57] which were isolated for the first time from the genus (Fig. 4). Their structures were fully elucidated using 1D and 2D NMR techniques and they were further ascertained by comparing their data with previously reported data in literature.

Dihydrodehydrodiconiferyl alcohol 4-O-β-D-glucoside (**6**) was isolated as a yellowish white amorphous powder. ^{1}H-NMR of (**6**) revealed the presence of a 1,2,4-trisubstituted benzene ring with signals at δ_H 7.03 (d, $J = 1.84$ Hz), 7.14 (d, $J = 8.43$ Hz) and 6.93 (dd, $J = 8.31$, 2.03 Hz) for H-2, H-5 and H-6, respectively, each integrated for one proton. Also, a 1,2,3,5-tetrasubstituted benzene ring was presented by two broad singlet signals at δ_H 6.73 (H-2') and 6.72 (H-6'). The spectrum revealed the existence of a hydroxypropyl group showing three signals at δ_H 2.63 (t, H-7'), 1.82 (m, H-8'), 3.57 (t, H-9'). Furthermore, a methine-methine-methylene group (CH-CH-CH$_2$) appeared at δ_H 5.56 (d, $J = 5.85$, H-7), 3.44 (m, H-8), 3.80, 3.75 (m, m, H-9). The presence of β-D-glucose was

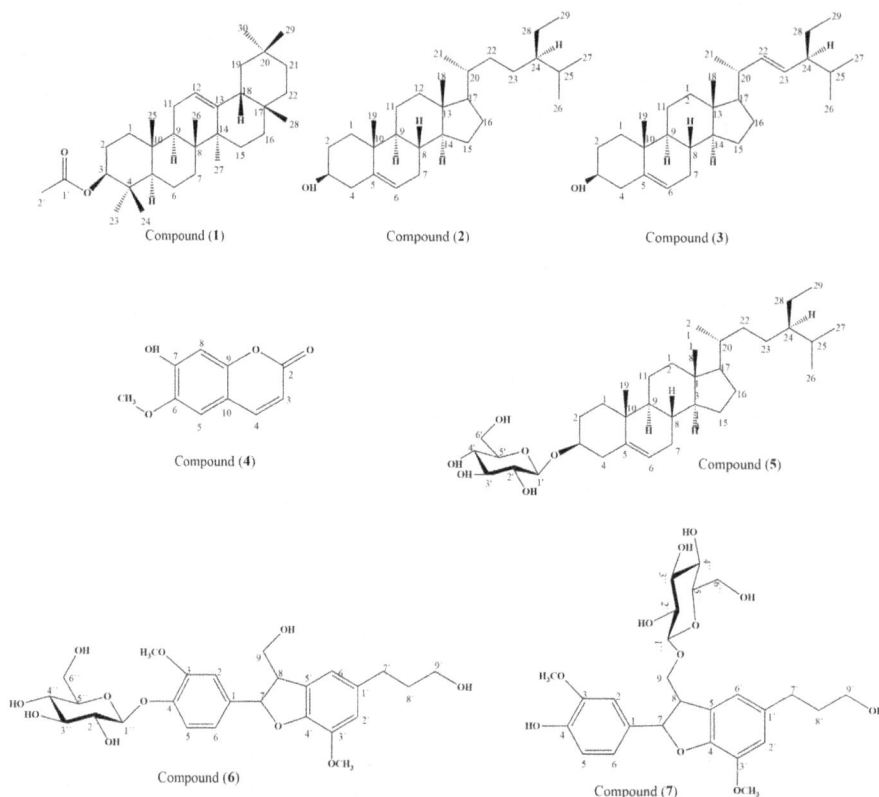

Fig. 4 Structures of identified compounds from *n*-hexane, dichloromethane and ethyl acetate fractions of *B. rupestris*

proposed by the appearance of anomeric proton at δ_H 4.88 and other sugar protons at 3.39–3.85. Two singlet signals each integrated for three protons at δ_H 3.87 and 3.83 were attributed to two methoxy groups. ^{13}C-NMR spectrum of compound (**6**) showed the presence of five aromatic methines and seven quaternary aromatic carbons signals attributed to two benzene rings at δ_C 111.19, 117.95, 119.37, 114.19, 118.04, 137.09, 150.9, 147.6, 138.37, 145.24, 147.6, 129.58. Downfield shifts of C-3 (150.9), C-4 (147.6), C-3′ (145.24), C-4′ (147.6) indicated their attachment to oxygenated functional groups. A signal at δ_C 102.78 was attributed to the anomeric carbon of glucose unit and the other sugar carbons appeared at 74.90, 77.84, 71.34, 78.19 and 62.51. The two signals at δ_C 56.79 and 56.71 represented two methoxy groups. Other aliphatic signals appeared at δ_C 88.48, 65.07, 62.22, 55.68, 35.84 and 32.89. The HMBC spectrum showed that the methoxy group at δ_C 56.79 was placed at C-3 (150.9) and the methoxy group at δ_C 56.71 was placed at C-3′ (145.24). Also, it showed a correlation between C-6, C-2 with H-7; C-6′, C-2′ with H-7′; and C-9′ with H-7′. The correlation between C-4 with H-1″ supported the presence of the sugar at C-4. From the displayed data (Table 4) and through comparison with the previously reported literature [56], compound (**6**) was identified as

dihydrodehydrodiconiferyl alcohol 4-*O*-β-D-glucoside which was the first time to be reported in the genus.

Dihydrodehydrodiconiferyl alcohol 9-*O*-β-D-glucoside (**7**) was isolated as a yellowish white amorphous powder. The ^{1}H-NMR and ^{13}C-NMR data for this compound were similar to compound (**6**) suggesting the same neolignan nucleus; the two compounds differ in the position of the glucose moiety. The HMBC spectrum revealed the correlation between C-9 with H-1″ which supported the attachment of the sugar at C-9. The downfield shift of C-9 at δ_C 72.46 also supported the attachment of the sugar at C-9 [57] (Table 4).

In vitro assessment of the cytotoxic activity of the isolated compounds

Additionally, the cytotoxic activity of the compounds obtained from the *n*-hexane and dichloromethane fractions of *B. rupestris* was examined using different concentrations (20, 10, 5, 2.5 µg/mL) of these compounds on the same cell lines utilized in the determination of the cytotoxic effect of the total extracts and subsequent fractions. The isolated compounds showed no cytotoxicity against hepatoma HepG2, breast MDA-MB-231 and lung A549 cancer cell lines with growth inhibition below 20%. The results are illustrated in Table 5.

Table 4 ¹H- and ¹³C-NMR spectroscopic data for 6 and 7

	Dihydrodehydrodiconiferyl alcohol 4-O-β-D-glucoside (6)		Dihydrodehydrodiconiferyl alcohol 9-O-β-D-glucoside (7)	
	δ_C	δ_H (Mult, Int), J in Hz	δ_C	δ_H (Mult, Int), J in Hz
1	137.09		134.67	
2	111.19	7.03 (d, 1H), 1.84	110.71	7.02 (d, 1H), 2.01
3	150.9		149.05	
4	147.6		147.48	
5	117.95	7.14 (d, 1H), 8.43	116.08	6.78 (d, 1H), 8.09
6	119.37	6.93 (dd, 1H), 8.31, 2.03	119.72	6.89 (dd, 1H), 8.28, 2
7	88.48	5.56 (d, 1H), 5.85	88.98	5.62 (d, 1H), 6.21
8	55.68	3.44 (m, 1H)	53.28	3.69 (m, 1H)
9	65.07	3.80, 3.75 (m, m, 2H)	72.46	4.23, 3.79 (dd, m, 2H)
3-OCH₃	56.79	3.87 (s, 3H)	56.44	3.85 (s, 3H)
1'	138.37		136.64	
2'	114.19	6.73 (s, 1H)	114.19	6.75 (s, 1H)
3'	145.24		145.21	
4'	147.6		147.48	
5'	129.58		129.56	
6'	118.04	6.72 (s, 1H)	118.21	6.80 (s, 1H)
7'	32.89	2.63 (t, 2H)	32.89	2.65 (t, 2H)
8'	35.84	1.82 (m, 2H)	35.82	1.84 (m, 2H)
9'	62.22	3.57 (t, 2H)	62.23	3.59 (t, 2H)
3'-OCH₃	56.71	3.83 (s, 3H)	56.77	3.88 (s, 3H)
1"	102.78	4.88 (covered by solvent, 1H)	104.57	4.38 (d, 1H), 7.79
2"	74.90	3.48 (m, 1H)	75.18	3.25 (m, 1H)
3"	77.84	3.39 (m, 1H)	78.07	3.31 (m, 1H)
4"	71.34	3.39 (m, 1H)	71.66	3.31 (m, 1H)
5"	78.19	3.39 (m, 1H)	78.26	3.31 (m, 1H)
6"	62.51	3.85, 3.69 (m, 2H)	62.81	3.88, 3.70 (m 2H)

NMR data (δ) were measured ¹H-NMR (400 MHz, CD₃OH) and ¹³C-NMR data (100 MHz, CD₃OH)

Doxorubicin was employed as a positive control and exhibited a strong cytotoxic effect against HepG2 (IC$_{50}$ 0.49 µg/mL), MDA-MB-231 (IC$_{50}$ 0.68 µg/mL) and A549 (IC$_{50}$ 0.13 µg/mL) cells.

In vitro assessment of the anti-allergic activity of the isolated compounds

To ascertain, whether the isolated compounds might be responsible for the anti-allergic activity observed in *Brachychiton* sp. crude extracts and nonpolar fractions, the isolated compounds were subjected to degranulation assay in RBL-2H3 mast cell model. The results are presented in Table 6. MTT viability assay was used to evaluate the potential toxic effects against RBL-2H3 cells. A mixture of β-sitosterol (**2**) and stigmasterol (**3**) (200 and 100 µg/mL) was considered toxic (viability below 85%). According to our results, scopoletin (**4**) showed 23.0% inhibition of A23187-induced and 30.0% of antigen-

induced degranulation at 500 µM. Dihydrodehydrodiconiferyl alcohol 9-O-β-D-glucoside (**7**) showed only weak inhibitory effect in the A23187-induced assay (16.3% at 100 µM and 18.0% at 500 µM). Dexamethasone (10 nM) was utilized as the positive control and inhibited β-hexosaminidase release by 93.7%.

In vitro assessment of the anti-inflammatory activity of the isolated compounds

The anti-inflammatory effect of the isolated compounds was determined to understand whether any of these compounds might be accountable for the potent activity of *B. rupestris* crude extract and its fractions. The results are illustrated in Table 7. According to the results, scopoletin (**4**) was found to significantly inhibit elastase release in fMLF-induced human neutrophils by 22.8% at 10 µM. Genistein, natural tyrosine kinase inhibitor [50, 51], was used as the positive control and caused significant

Table 5 Cytotoxic activity of the isolated compounds

Cell line	Conc. (µg/mL)	% Inhibition	
		β-amyrin acetate (1)	Scopoletin (4)
HepG2	20	12.1 ± 3.4	11.4 ± 2.1
	10	16.0 ± 0.3	6.5 ± 1.2
	5	20.4 ± 2.3	0.9 ± 0.1
	2.5	8.23 ± 0.7	5.9 ± 1.2
MDA-MB-231	20	−19.6 ± 1.2	8.2 ± 1.0
	10	−13.9 ± 1.2	6.0 ± 0.3
	5	−5.5 ± 1.2	10.7 ± 9.8
	2.5	7.0 ± 0.1	15.5 ± 0.3
A549	20	2.2 ± 0.5	7.9 ± 0.4
	10	9.0 ± 1.0	14.9 ± 0.4
	5	10.8 ± 0.5	14.6 ± 0.5
	2.5	0.4 ± 0.7	14.3 ± 0.7

Results are presented as cell growth inhibition percentage at concentrations of 2.5 to 20 µg/mL, mean ± SD ($n = 3$). Doxorubicin was used as the positive control and exerted significant cell viability inhibitory effects against HepG2 (IC_{50} 0.49 µg/mL), MDA-MB-231 (IC_{50} 0.68 µg/mL)

suppression of superoxide anion generation (IC_{50} 1.16 µM) and elastase release (IC_{50} 21.51 µM).

Discussion

RBL-2H3 are mast cells that greatly affect the development of allergic response [58]. Upon activation by antigen or A23187 (calcium ionophore), mast cells produce histamine in addition to other mediators that immediately initiate hypersensitivity reactions. β-Hexosaminidase represents an important mast cells degranulation marker that is commonly used for the assessment of anti-allergic activity [59].

The anti-allergic activity of the crude extracts as well as n-hexane and dichloromethane fractions of B. rupestris and B. discolor leaves (Table 2) might be attributed

to the presence of many active constituents from their non-polar fractions. Sterols, sterol glycosides, coumarin, and triterpenes were isolated and identified in B. rupestris leaves. Lanosterol, lupeol, β-amyrin, β-amyrin acetate and oleanolic acid were previously reported from B. discolor leaves by Kassem et al. [23]. These triterpenes were reported to exert a potent anti-allergic activity [60–62] including β-amyrin that was previously documented to exhibit mast cell membrane stabilization [30]. The anti-allergic activity of triterpenes might be attributed to the suppression of secretion of histamine and interleukins (IL-2, IL-4) from mast cells [62]. Also, β-sitosterol was reported to possess anti-allergic activity and might have therapeutic potential in allergic asthma [63, 64]. It was suggested that β-sitosterol and its glycoside inhibited the release of IL-4 so it could act as an immune modulator to relieve symptoms associated with seasonal allergic response [65]. However, we did not observe any significant effect of either β-amyrin acetate (1), the mixture of β-sitosterol (2) and stigmasterol (3) or β-sitosterol glycoside (5) in degranulation assay using the RBL-2H3 mast cell model (Table 6). Meanwhile, scopoletin (4) and dihydrodehydrodiconiferyl alcohol 9-O-β-D-glucoside (7) showed inhibitory activity on degranulation in RBL-2H3 cells.

Regarding the in vitro anti-inflammatory activity, neutrophils exert a vital role in host's defenses versus the attack by microorganisms and in the pathogenesis of various inflammatory diseases [66]. In response to stimuli, such as fMLF, the activated neutrophils secrete a series of inflammatory mediators such as superoxide anion (O_2^{-}) and elastase which are major contributors to the destruction of tissue in inflammatory response [67]. We observed that the crude extracts and fractions of B. rupestris and B. discolor leaves (Table 3) exerted potent anti-inflammatory activity in human neutrophils. Many studies supported the anti-inflammatory activity

Table 6 Anti-allergic activity of compounds isolated from B. rupestris

Sample	% viability, RBL-2H3[a]		% inhibition of A23187-induced β-hexosaminidase release[b]		
	100 µM	500 µM	10 µM	100 µM	500 µM
β-amyrin acetate (1)	98.3 ± 2.9	[c]	0.3 ± 0.6	0.7 ± 1.2	[c]
scopoletin (4)	96.0 ± 4.0	93.7 ± 6.5	3.7 ± 4.7	13.7 ± 8.0	23.0 ± 8.0[**d]
β-sitosterol-3-O-β-D-glucoside (5)	96.0 ± 1.0	[c]	5.0 ± 5.6	7.7 ± 3.8	[c]
dihydrodehydrodiconiferyl alcohol 4-O-β-D-glucoside (6)	97.3 ± 2.5	[e]	7.0 ± 10.4	12.7 ± 7.6	[e]
dihydrodehydrodiconiferyl alcohol 9-O-β-D-glucoside (7)	97.7 ± 2.1	95.3 ± 4.2	3.3 ± 4.2	16.3 ± 5.5[*]	18.0 ± 8.7[*]

A mixture of β-sitosterol (2) and stigmasterol (3) was toxic towards RBL-2H3 cells at the concentration of 200 µg/mL (73.7 ± 11.7% viability) and 100 µg/ml (78.7 ± 11.6% viability) and inactive at the concentration of 10 µg/mL (5.0% ± 5.0% inhibition) in A23187-induced degranulation assay
[a]The cytotoxicity of samples to RBL-2H3 was evaluated using MTT viability assay; results are presented as mean ± SD ($n = 3$)
[b]Dexamethasone (10 nM) was used as the positive control and inhibited 93.7 ± 1.5%[**] of A23187-induced β-hexosaminidase release in RBL-2H3 cells. Results are presented as mean ± SD ($n = 3$); [*]$p < 0.05$, [**]$p < 0.001$ compared with the control value (A23187 only)
[c]Precipitate was formed upon the addition into the medium at the concentration of 500 µM, therefore the result could not be justified
[d]Scopoletin (500 µM) exerted 30.0 ± 7.1% inhibition of antigen-induced β-hexosaminidase release (mean ± SD, $n = 2$)
[e]Dihydrodehydrodiconiferyl alcohol 4-O-β-D-glucoside was not tested at the concentration of 500 µM, however, it was nontoxic towards RBL-2H3 cells (96.0 ± 6.9% viability) and inactive in A23187-induced degranulation assay (10.0 ± 4.6% inhibition) at the concentration of 200 µM

Table 7 Effect of pure compounds on superoxide anion generation and elastase release in fMLF/CB-induced human neutrophils

Sample	Superoxide anion generation[a] IC$_{50}$ (µM)[b]	Elastase release[a] IC$_{50}$ (µM)[b]
β-amyrin acetate (1)	> 10	> 10
scopoletin (4)	> 10	> 10[c]
β-sitosterol-3-O-β-D-glucoside (5)	> 10	> 10
dihydrodehydrodiconiferyl alcohol 4-O-β-D-glucoside (6)	> 10	> 10
dihydrodehydrodiconiferyl alcohol 9-O-β-D-glucoside (7)	>1[d]	>1[d]
genistein	1.16 ± 0.12	21.51 ± 6.50

[a]IC$_{50}$ values, results are presented as mean ± SD ($n = 3$–4), compared with the control value (formyl-methionyl-leucyl-phenylalanine/cytochalasin B, fMLF/CB)
[b]Concentration necessary for 50% inhibition (IC$_{50}$)
[c]Scopoletin (4) exerted significant inhibitory activity in elastase release assay (22.8 ± 15.3%, *$p < 0.05$) at 10 µM
[d]Dihydrodehydrodiconiferyl alcohol 9-O-β-D-glucoside (10) was used at the final concentration of 1 µM due to solubility issues

of sterols and their glycosides [68–70]. They induce immunomodulatory response that affects inflammatory mediators [71, 72]. They were also reported to possess potent in vivo anti-inflammatory activity with the concomitant reduction of edema and inflammation in rats [73]. Various studies confirmed the anti-inflammatory activity of triterpenes including *β-amyrin and β-amyrin acetate* [29, 74–76]. Coumarins also were found to have anti-inflammatory activity by inhibiting different inflammatory mediators such as cyclooxygenase-2, nitric oxide, tumor necrosis factor-α and interleukins [77–79]. Neolignans were reported to exert anti-inflammatory effects by suppressing superoxide anion generation and elastase release [80], they also exhibited nitric oxide (NO) and tumor necrosis factor-α (TNF-α) inhibitory effects [81]. However, according to our results, only scopoletin (**4**) exerted mild inhibition of elastase release. All other isolated compounds including dihydrodehydrodiconiferyl alcohol glycosides (**6** and **7**) were inactive in fMLF-activated human neutrophils.

Conclusions

The total extract and fractions of *B. rupestris* and *B. discolor* were nontoxic against hepatoma, breast and lung cancer cell lines. The crude extracts as well as the *n*-hexane and dichloromethane fractions of *B. rupestris* and *B. discolor* exhibited significant anti-allergic as well as anti-inflammatory activities. The phytochemical study of the leaves of *B. rupestris* resulted in the isolation of compounds from different chemical classes, including triterpene, sterols, sterol glycoside, coumarin and neolignans. All the tested compounds were nontoxic against the tested cancer cell lines. Among the isolated

compounds, scopoletin exerted anti-allergic effects and mild anti-inflammatory activity by reducing elastase release in human neutrophils. However, the bioactivity of *B. rupestris* extracts and fractions was much more potent compared with any of the isolated compounds. Thus, leaves of *B. rupestris* and *B. discolor* are worth to be considered for further development and research based on their anti-allergic and anti-inflammatory activities. In vivo evaluation of the anti-allergic and anti-inflammatory activities is highly recommended for the active fractions of both *Brachychiton* species.

Abbreviations

ANOVA: One-way analysis of variance; APT: Attached proton test; *B*: *Brachychiton*; BHT: tert-Butyl-1-hydroxytoluene; BDD: *Brachychiton discolor* leaves dichloromethane fraction; BDE: *Brachychiton discolor* leaves ethyl acetate fraction; BDH: *Brachychiton discolor* leaves *n*-hexane fraction; BDT: *Brachychiton discolor* leaves total extract; BRD: *Brachychiton rupestris* leaves dichloromethane fraction; BRE: *Brachychiton rupestris* leaves ethyl acetate fraction; BRH: *Brachychiton rupestris* leaves *n*-hexane fraction; BRR: *B. rupestris* remaining fraction; BRT: *Brachychiton rupestris* leaves total extract; CDCL$_3$: Deuterated chloroform; CD$_3$OD: Deuterated methanol; ^{13}C-NMR: Carbon-13 Nuclear Magnetic Resonance; *d*: doublet; *dd*: doublet of doublet; DMEM: Dulbecco's modified Eagle's medium; DMSO: Dimethylsulfoxide; DMSO-d6: Deuterated dimethylsulfoxide-d6; 2D-NMR: Two-dimensional nuclear magnetic resonance spectroscopy; DNP: Dinitrophenyl; DNP-BSA: Dinitrophenyl-conjugated bovine serum albumin; ESI-MS: Electro-Spray Ionization Mass Spectrometry; EtOAc: Ethyl acetate; FBS: Fetal bovine serum; fMLF/CB: formyl-methionyl-leucyl-phenylalanine/cytochalasin B; ^{1}H-^{1}H COSY: ^{1}H-^{1}H Correlated spectroscopy; HMBC: Heteronuclear Multiple-Bond Correlation Spectroscopy; ^{1}H-NMR: Proton Nuclear Magnetic Resonance; HSQC: Heteronuclear Single Quantum Coherence; IC$_{50}$: The half maximal inhibitory concentration; *m*: multiplet; MTT: (3-(4,5-dimethylthiazol-2-yl)-2,5-diphenyltetrazolium bromide); *p*-NAG: *p*-Nitrophenyl-N-acetyl-D-glucosaminide; PTLC: Preparative thin layer chromatography; *q*: quartet; R$_f$: Retardation factor; *s*: Singlet; S.D.: Standard deviation; SEM: Standard error of mean; *t*: Triplet; TLC: Thin Layer Chromatography; UPLC: Ultra Performance Liquid Chromatography

Acknowledgements

We are grateful to the Center for Research Resources and Development, Kaohsiung Medical University for providing instrumentation support and to Ms. Shu-Li Chen for kind assistance in cytotoxicity measurements. Also, we would like to thank the Center for Drug Discovery, Research and Development at Faculty of Pharmacy, Ain Shams University for the analyses of the isolated compounds.

Funding

This research was financial supported by the grants from the Ministry of Science and Technology (MOST 107–2911-I-037-502, MOST 106–2320-B-037-007-MY3, MOST 106–2320-B-255-003-MY3 and MOST 104–2320-B-255-004-MY3), Ministry of Education (EMRPD1G0231), Kaohsiung Medical University (106CM-KMU-02, KMU-DK107003, KMU-M106009), and Chang Gung Memorial Hospital (CMRPF1F0011~ 3, CMRPF1F0061~ 3, CMRPF1G0241~ 3, and BMRP450), Taiwan. The funders had no role in study design, data collection and analysis, decision to publish, or preparation of the manuscript.

Authors' contributions

AAT and FSY performed extraction, isolation and identification of pure compounds and shared writing the whole manuscript. MK, YCW, and BHC carried out the cytotoxic and anti-allergic studies, interpreted the results and edited the manuscript. ME, FRC and ANBS formulated the research hypothesis, supervised the biological part and shared in critical revision of the manuscript and the whole work. TLH contributed to the anti-inflammatory assays. All authors participated in interpretations of results, read and approved the final manuscript.

Competing interests
The authors declare that they have no competing interests.

Author details
[1]Department of Pharmacognosy, Faculty of Pharmacy, Ain Shams University, African Union Organization Street, Abbassia, Cairo 11566, Egypt. [2]Graduate Institute of Natural Products, College of Pharmacy, Kaohsiung Medical University, Kaohsiung 80708, Taiwan. [3]Department of Biotechnology, College of Life Science, Kaohsiung Medical University, Kaohsiung 80708, Taiwan. [4]Graduate Institute of Natural Products, College of Medicine, Chang Gung University, Taoyuan 33302, Taiwan. [5]Research Center for Chinese Herbal Medicine, Research Center for Food and Cosmetic Safety, and Graduate Institute of Health Industry Technology, College of Human Ecology, Chang Gung University of Science and Technology, Taoyuan 33302, Taiwan. [6]National Research Institute of Chinese Medicine, Ministry of Health and Welfare, Taipei 11221, Taiwan. [7]Research Center for Natural Products & Drug Development, Kaohsiung Medical University, Kaohsiung 80708, Taiwan. [8]Department of Medical Research, Kaohsiung Medical University Hospital, Kaohsiung 80708, Taiwan. [9]The Institute of Biomedical Sciences, National Sun Yat-sen University, Kaohsiung 80424, Taiwan. [10]Department of Pharmaceutical Biology, Faculty of Pharmacy and Biotechnology, German University in Cairo, Cairo 11835, Egypt. [11]Department of Anesthesiology, Chang Gung Memorial Hospital, Taoyuan 33305, Taiwan. [12]Chinese Herbal Medicine Research Team, Healthy Aging Research Center, Chang Gung University, Taoyuan 33302, Taiwan. [13]Department of Chemical Engineering, Ming Chi University of Technology, New Taipei City 24301, Taiwan.

References
1. Kawai M, Hirano T, Higa S, Arimitsu J, Maruta M, Kuwahara Y, et al. Flavonoids and related compounds as anti-allergic substances. Allergol Int. 2007;56:113–23.
2. Galli SJ, Tsai M, Piliponsky AM. The development of allergic inflammation. Nature 2008;454:445–454.
3. Broide DH. Immunomodulation of allergic disease. Annu Rev Med. 2009;60: 279–91.
4. Baek K-S, Yi Y-S, Son Y-J, Yoo S, Sung NY, Kim Y, et al. In vitro and in vivo anti-inflammatory activities of Korean red ginseng-derived components. J Ginseng Res. 2016;40:437–44.
5. Wang Y-T, Zhu L, Zeng D, Long W, Zhu S-M. Chemical composition and anti-inflammatory activities of essential oil from Trachydium roylei. J Food Drug Anal. 2016;24:602–9.
6. Shaikh RU, Pund MM, Gacche RN. Evaluation of anti-inflammatory activity of selected medicinal plants used in Indian traditional medication system in vitro as well as in vivo. J Tradit Complement Med. 2016;6:355–61.
7. Andhare RN, Raut MK, Naik SR. Evaluation of antiallergic and anti-anaphylactic activity of ethanolic extract of Sanseveiria trifasciata leaves (EEST) in rodents. J Ethnopharmacol. 2012;142:627–33.
8. Sato A, Zhang T, Yonekura L, Tamura H. Antiallergic activities of eleven onions (Allium cepa) were attributed to quercetin 4'-glucoside using QuEChERS method and Pearson's correlation coefficient. J Funct Foods. 2015;14:581–9.
9. Shi Y-H, Zhu S, Ge Y-W, He Y-M, Kazuma K, Wang Z, et al. Monoterpene derivatives with anti-allergic activity from red peony root, the root of Paeonia lactiflora. Fitoterapia. 2016;108:55–61.
10. Singh B, Nadkarni JR, Vishwakarma RA, Bharate SB, Nivsarkar M, Anandjiwala S. The hydroalcoholic extract of Cassia alata (Linn.) leaves and its major compound rhein exhibits antiallergic activity via mast cell stabilization and lipoxygenase inhibition. J Ethnopharmacol. 2012;141:469–73.
11. Tian J, Che H, Ha D, Wei Y, Zheng S. Characterization and anti-allergic effect of a polysaccharide from the flower buds of Lonicera japonica. Carbohydr Polym. 2012;90:1642–7.
12. Silva FV, Oliveira IS, Figueiredo KA, Melo Júnior FB, Costa DA, Chaves MH, et al. Anti-inflammatory and antinociceptive effects of Sterculia striata a. St.-Hil. & Naudin (Malvaceae) in rodents. J Med Food. 2014;17:694–700.
13. Dai Y, Harinantenaina L, Brodie PJ, Callmander MW, Randrianasolo S, Rakotobe E, et al. Isolation and synthesis of two antiproliferative calamenene-type sesquiterpenoids from Sterculia tavia from the Madagascar rain forest. Bioorg Med Chem. 2012;20:6940–4.
14. Guymer GP. A taxonomic revision of Brachychiton (Sterculiaceae). Aust Syst Bot. 1988;1:199–323.
15. Wilkie P, Clark A, Pennington RT, Cheek M, Bayer C, Wilcock CC. Phylogenetic relationships within the subfamily Sterculioideae (Malvaceae/Sterculiaceae-Sterculieae) using the chloroplast gene ndhF. Syst Bot. 2006;31:160–70.
16. Salem MZM, Ali HM, Mansour MM. Fatty acid methyl esters from air-dried wood, bark, and leaves of Brachychiton diversifolius R. Br: antibacterial, antifungal, and antioxidant activities. Bioresources. 2014;9:3835–45.
17. Rao KS. Characteristics and fatty acid composition of Brachychiton species seeds and the oils (Sterculiaceae). J Agric Food Chem. 1991;39:881–2.
18. Abdel-Megeed A, Salem MZ, Ali HM, Gohar YM. Brachychiton diversifolius as a source of natural products: antibacterial and antioxidant evaluation of extracts of wood branches. J Pure Appl Microbiol. 2013;7:1843–50.
19. Yousif F, Hifnawy MS, Soliman G, Boulos L, Labib T, Mahmoud S, et al. Large-scale in vitro screening of Egyptian native and cultivated plants for schistosomicidal activity. Pharm Biol. 2007;45:501–10.
20. Thabet AA, Youssef FS, El-Shazly M, El-Beshbishy HA, Singab ANB. Validation of the antihyperglycaemic and hepatoprotective activity of the flavonoid rich fraction of Brachychiton rupestris using in vivo experimental models and molecular modelling. Food Chem Toxicol. 2018;114:302–10.
21. Kassem HA, Eid HH, Abdel-Latif HA. Phytochemical and hypoglycemic studies of the leaves of Brachychiton australis (Schott & Endl.) a. Terrac. Grown in Egypt. Bull Fac Pharm Cairo Univ. 2001;40:85–91.
22. De Laurentis N, Armenise D, Milillo M, Matrella R. Chemical investigation of Sterculia acerifolia leaves. Riv Ital EPPOS. 2003;13:21–30.
23. Kassem HA. Study of further phytoconstituents of Brachychiton discolor F.J. Muell. cultivated in Egypt. Bull Fac Pharm Cairo Univ. 2007;45:155–60.
24. Kassem HA, Aziz WM. A Pharmacognostical study of Brachychiton discolor F. J.Muell. Cultivated in Egypt. Az Pharm Sci. 2002;29:196–219.
25. Chapman AD. Australian plant name index: Australian Biological Resources Study Canberra; 1991.
26. The International Plant Names Index. 2012. http://www.ipni.org. Accessed 24 Sept 2018.
27. The Plant List. Version 1. 2010. http://www.theplantlist.org. Accessed 24 Sept 2018.
28. Desoky E, Youssef S. Hypoglycaemic effect of Sterculia rupestris and a comparative study of its flavonoids with Sterculia diversifolia. Bull Fac Pharm Cairo Univ. 1997;35:257–61.
29. Okoye NN, Ajaghaku DL, Okeke HN, Ilodigwe EE, Nworu CS, Okoye FB. Beta-Amyrin and alpha-amyrin acetate isolated from the stem bark of Alstonia boonei display profound anti-inflammatory activity. Pharm Biol. 2014;52:1478–86.
30. Oliveira FA, Lima-Junior RCP, Cordeiro WM, Vieira-Júnior GM, Chaves MH, Almeida FRC, et al. Pentacyclic triterpenoids, α, β-amyrins, suppress the scratching behavior in a mouse model of pruritus. Pharmacol Biochem Behav. 2004;78:719–25.
31. Ayeleso TB, Matumba MG, Mukwevho E. Oleanolic acid and its derivatives: biological activities and therapeutic potential in chronic diseases. Molecules. 2017;22:1915.
32. Córdova C, Gutiérrez B, Martínez-García C, Martín R, Gallego-Muñoz P, Hernández M, et al. Oleanolic acid controls allergic and inflammatory responses in experimental allergic conjunctivitis. PLoS One. 2014;9:e91282.
33. Geetha T, Varalakshmi P. Anti-inflammatory activity of lupeol and lupeol linoleate in rats. J Ethnopharmacol. 2001;76:77–80.
34. Khan AS. Antipyretic and analgesic activities of some economically important woody plants. In: Medicinally important trees: Springer; 2017. p. 159–85.
35. Mujumdar AM, Naik DG, Waghole RJ, Kulkarni DK, Kumbhojka MS. Pharmacological studies on Sterculia foetida leaves. Pharm Biol. 2000;38:13–7.
36. Raja T. Evaluation of anticonvulsant effect of Sterculia foetida (Pinari) in pentylenetetrazole (PTZ) and MES induced convulsions in albino rats. World J Pharm Pharm Sci. 2014;3:1898–907.
37. Babalola IT, Adelakun EA, Wang Y, Shode FO. Anti-TB activity of Sterculia setigera Del., leaves (Sterculiaceae). J Pharmacogn. Phytochemistry. 2012;1: 19–26.
38. Tor-Anyiin T, Akpuaka M, Oluma H. Phytochemical and antimicrobial studies on stem bark extract of Sterculia setigera, Del. Afr J Biotechnol. 2011;10: 11011–5.
39. Hossain MM, AIH E, Akbar MA, Ganguly A, Rahman SA. Evaluation of analgesic activity of Sterculia villosa Roxb.(Sterculiaceae) bark in swiss-albino mice. Dhaka Univ J Pharm Sci. 2013;12:125–9.
40. Hossain MF, Talukder B, Rana MN, Tasnim R, Nipun TS, Uddin SN, et al. In vivo sedative activity of methanolic extract of Sterculia villosa Roxb. Leaves. BMC Complement Altern Med. 2016;16:398.

41. Sobeh M, Mamadalieva NZ, Mohamed T, Krstin S, Youssef FS, Ashour ML, et al. Chemical profiling of *Phlomis thapsoides* (Lamiaceae) and *in vitro* testing of its biological activities. Med Chem Res. 2016;25:2304–15.

42. Van de Loosdrecht AA, Nennie E, Ossenkoppele GJ, Beelen RH, Langenhuijsen MM. Cell mediated cytotoxicity against U 937 cells by human monocytes and macrophages in a modified colorimetric MTT assay: a methodological study. J Immunol Methods. 1991;141:15–22.

43. Marks DC, Belov L, Davey MW, Davey RA, Kidman AD. The MTT cell viability assay for cytotoxicity testing in multidrug-resistant human leukemic cells. Leuk Res. 1992;16:1165–73.

44. Chen B-H, Wu P-Y, Chen K-M, Fu T-F, Wang H-M, Chen C-Y. Antiallergic potential on RBL-2H3 cells of some phenolic constituents of *Zingiber officinale* (ginger). J Nat Prod. 2009;72:950–3.

45. Korinek M, Tsai YH, El-Shazly M, Lai KH, Backlund A, Wu SF, et al. Anti-allergic hydroxy fatty acids from *Typhonium blumei* explored through ChemGPS-NP. Front Pharmacol. 2017;8:356.

46. Matsuda H, Tewtrakul S, Morikawa T, Nakamura A, Yoshikawa M. Anti-allergic principles from Thai zedoary: structural requirements of curcuminoids for inhibition of degranulation and effect on the release of TNF-α and IL-4 in RBL-2H3 cells. Bioorg Med Chem. 2004;12:5891–8.

47. Chen B-H, Hung M-H, Chen JY-F, Chang H-W, Yu M-L, Wan L, et al. Anti-allergic activity of grapeseed extract (GSE) on RBL-2H3 mast cells. Food Chem. 2012;132:968–74.

48. Chung Y-M, Chang F-R, Tseng T-F, Hwang T-L, Chen L-C, Wu S-F, et al. A novel alkaloid, aristopyridinone a and anti-inflammatory phenanthrenes isolated from *Aristolochia manshuriensis*. Bioorg Med Chem Lett. 2011;21: 1792–4.

49. Yang SC, Chung PJ, Ho CM, Kuo CY, Hung MF, Huang YT, et al. Propofol inhibits superoxide production, elastase release, and chemotaxis in formyl peptide-activated human neutrophils by blocking formyl peptide receptor 1. J Immunol. 2013;190:6511–9.

50. Mócsai A, Jakus Z, Tibor Vántus T, Berton G, Lowell GA, Ligeti E. Kinase pathways in chemoattractant-induced degranulation of neutrophils: the role of p38 mitogen-activated protein kinase activated by Src family kinases. J Immunol. 2000;164:4321–31.

51. Liou JR, El-Shazly M, Du YC, Tseng CN, Hwang TL, Chuang YL, et al. 1,5-Diphenylpent-3-en-1-ynes and methyl naphthalene carboxylates from *Lawsonia inermis* and their anti-inflammatory activity. Phytochemistry. 2013; 88:67–73.

52. Youssef FS, Ashour ML, Sobeh M, El-Beshbishy HA, Singab ANB, Wink M. *Eremophila maculata*- isolation of a rare naturally-occurring lignan glycoside and the hepatoprotective activity of the leaf extract. Phytomedicine. 2016; 23:1484–93.

53. Dubey H, Ticari J. Flavonoids and other constituents of *Sterculia* genus. J Indian Chem Soc. 1991;68:426–7.

54. Anjaneyulu A, Raju S. Terpenoids and phenolics from the bark and heartwood of *Sterculiaurens* ROXB. J Indian Chem Soc. 1987;64:323–4.

55. Khan NMU, Hossain MS. Scopoletin and ß-sitosterol glucoside from roots of *Ipomoea digitata*. J Pharmacogn. 2015;4:05–7.

56. H-x K, Y-g X, B-y Y, Wang Q-h, S-w L. Lignan constituents from *Chloranthus japonicus* Sieb. Arch Pharm Res. 2009;32:329–34.

57. Lee S, Song I-H, Lee J-H, Yang W-Y, Oh K-B, Shin J. Sortase a inhibitory metabolites from the roots of *Pulsatilla koreana*. Bioorg Med Chem Lett. 2014;24:44–8.

58. De Souza Santos M, Jonis Andrioli W, Freire de Morais Del Lama MP, Kenupp Bastos J, NPD N, Zumstein Georgetto Naal RM. *In vitro* anti-allergic activity of the fungal metabolite pyridovericin. Int Immunopharmacol. 2013; 15:532–8.

59. Korinek M, Chen KM, Jiang YH, El-Shazly M, Stocker J, Chou CK, et al. Anti-allergic potential of *Typhonium blumei*: inhibition of degranulation *via* suppression of PI3K/PLCgamma2 phosphorylation and calcium influx. Phytomedicine. 2016;23:1706–15.

60. Ryu SY, Oak MH, Yoon SK, Cho DI, Yoo GS, Kim TS, et al. Anti-allergic and anti-inflammatory triterpenes from the herb of *Prunella vulgaris*. Planta Med. 2000;66:358–60.

61. Yoshikawa M, Nakamura S, Kato Y, Matsuhira K, Matsuda H. Medicinal flowers. XIV. New acylated oleanane-type triterpene oligoglycosides with antiallergic activity from flower buds of chinese tea plant (*Camellia sinensis*). Chem Pharm Bull. 2007;55:598–605.

62. Chen M-L, Hsieh C-C, Chiang B-L, Lin B-F. Triterpenoids and polysaccharide fractions of *Ganoderma tsugae* exert different effects on antiallergic activities. Evid Based Complement Altern Med. 2015;2015:1–10.

63. Nirmal SA, Patel AP, Bhawar SB, Pattan SR. Antihistaminic and antiallergic actions of extracts of *Solanum nigrum* berries: possible role in the treatment of asthma. J Ethnopharmacol. 2012;142:91–7.

64. Mahajan SG, Mehta AA. Suppression of ovalbumin-induced Th2-driven airway inflammation by beta-sitosterol in a Guinea pig model of asthma. Eur J Pharmacol. 2011;650:458–64.

65. Bouic P, Lamprecht JH. Plant sterols and sterolins: a review of their immune-modulating properties. Altern Med Rev. 1999;4:170–7.

66. Hwang TL, Yeh SH, Leu YL, Chern CY, Hsu HC. Inhibition of superoxide anion and elastase release in human neutrophils by 3'-isopropoxychalcone *via* a cAMP-dependent pathway. Br J Pharmacol. 2006;148:78–87.

67. Mantovani A, Cassatella MA, Costantini C, Jaillon S. Neutrophils in the activation and regulation of innate and adaptive immunity. Nat Rev Immunol. 2011;11:519–31.

68. Kim JA, Son JH, Song SB, Yang SY, Kim YH. Sterols isolated from seeds of *Panax ginseng* and their antiinflammatory activities. Pharmacogn Mag. 2013;9:182.

69. Kaith BS, Kaith NS, Chauhan NS. Anti-inflammatory effect of *Arnebia euchroma* root extracts in rats. J Ethnopharmacol. 1996;55:77–80.

70. Vassallo A, De Tommasi N, Merfort I, Sanogo R, Severino L, Pelin M, et al. Steroids with anti-inflammatory activity from *Vernonia nigritiana* Oliv. & Hiern. Phytochemistry. 2013;96:288–98.

71. Bouic PJ. The role of phytosterols and phytosterolins in immune modulation: a review of the past 10 years. Curr Opin Clin Nutr Metab Care. 2001;4:471–5.

72. Lee J-H, Lee JY, Park JH, Jung HS, Kim JS, Kang SS, et al. Immunoregulatory activity by daucosterol, a β-sitosterol glycoside, induces protective Th1 immune response against disseminated candidiasis in mice. Vaccine. 2007; 25:3834–40.

73. Correa G, Abreu VDC, Martins D, Takahashi JA, Fontoura H, Cara DC, et al. Antiinflamatory and antimicrobial activities of steroids and triterpenes isolated from aerial parts of *Justicia acuminatissima* (Acanthaceae). Int J Pharm Pharm Sci. 2014;6:75–81.

74. de Almeida PD, Boleti AP, Rudiger AL, Lourenco GA, da Veiga Junior VF, Lima ES. Anti-inflammatory activity of triterpenes isolated from *Protium paniculatum* oil-resins. Evid Based Complement Altern Med. 2015;2015:293768.

75. Romero-Estrada A, Maldonado-Magaña A, González-Christen J, Bahena SM, Garduño-Ramírez ML, Rodríguez-López V, et al. Anti-inflammatory and antioxidative effects of six pentacyclic triterpenes isolated from the Mexican copal resin of *Bursera copallifera*. BMC Complement Altern Med. 2016;16:422.

76. Thirupathi A, Silveira PC, Nesi RT, Pinho RA. Beta-Amyrin, a pentacyclic triterpene, exhibits anti-fibrotic, anti-inflammatory, and anti-apoptotic effects on dimethyl nitrosamine-induced hepatic fibrosis in male rats. Hum Exp Toxicol. 2017;36:113–22.

77. Wei W, Wu X-W, Deng G-G, Yang X-W. Anti-inflammatory coumarins with short- and long-chain hydrophobic groups from roots of *Angelica dahurica* cv. Hangbaizhi. Phytochemistry. 2016;123:58–68.

78. Azelmat J, Fiorito S, Taddeo VA, Genovese S, Epifano F, Grenier D. Synthesis and evaluation of antibacterial and anti-inflammatory properties of naturally occurring coumarins. Phytochem Lett. 2015;13:399–405.

79. Kang K-H, Kong C-S, Seo Y, Kim M-M, Kim S-K. Anti-inflammatory effect of coumarins isolated from *Corydalis heterocarpa* in HT-29 human colon carcinoma cells. Food Chem Toxicol. 2009;47:2129–34.

80. Shih H-C, Kuo P-C, Wu S-J, Hwang T-L, Hung H-Y, Shen D-Y, et al. Anti-inflammatory neolignans from the roots of *Magnolia officinalis*. Bioorg Med Chem. 2016;24:1439–45.

81. Peng Y, Lou L-L, Liu S-F, Zhou L, Huang X-X, Song S-J. Antioxidant and anti-inflammatory neolignans from the seeds of hawthorn. Bioorg Med Chem Lett. 2016;26:5501–6.

Evaluation of the effect of *Lactobacillus reuteri* V3401 on biomarkers of inflammation, cardiovascular risk and liver steatosis in obese adults with metabolic syndrome

Carmen Tenorio-Jiménez[1], María José Martínez-Ramírez[1,2], Mercedes Tercero-Lozano[3], Carmen Arraiza-Irigoyen[1], Isabel Del Castillo-Codes[3], Josune Olza[4,5,6,7], Julio Plaza-Díaz[4,5,6], Luis Fontana[4,5,6], Jairo H. Migueles[8], Mónica Olivares[9], Ángel Gil[4,5,6,7] and Carolina Gomez-Llorente[4,5,6,7*] [iD]

Abstract

Background: Obesity is characterized by increased fat mass and is associated with the development of insulin resistance syndrome (IRS), usually known as metabolic syndrome. The alteration of the intestinal microbiota composition has a role in the development of IRS associated with obesity, and probiotics, which are live microorganisms that confer a health benefit to the host, contribute to restore intestinal microbiota homeostasis and lower peripheral tissue insulin resistance. We aim to evaluate the effects of the probiotic strain *Lactobacillus reuteri* (*L. reuteri*) V3401 on the composition of intestinal microbiota, markers of insulin resistance and biomarkers of inflammation, cardiovascular risk, and hepatic steatosis in patients with overweight and obesity exhibiting IRS.

Methods/design: We describe a randomized, double-blind, crossover, placebo-controlled, and single-centre trial. Sixty participants (aged 18 to 65 years) diagnosed with IRS will be randomized in a 1:1 ratio to receive either a daily dose of placebo or 5×10^9 colony-forming units of *L. reuteri* V3401. The study will consist of two intervention periods of 12 weeks separated by a washout period of 6 weeks and preceded by another washout period of 2 weeks. The primary outcome will be the change in plasma lipopolysaccharide (LPS) levels at 12 weeks. Secondary outcomes will include anthropometric parameters, lipid profile, glucose metabolism, microbiota composition, hepatic steatosis, and inflammatory and cardiovascular biomarkers. Blood and stool samples will be collected at baseline, at the midpoint (only stool samples) and immediately after each intervention period. Luminex technology will be used to measure interleukins. For statistical analysis, a mixed ANOVA model will be employed to calculate changes in the outcome variables.

(Continued on next page)

* Correspondence: gomezll@ugr.es
[4]Department of Biochemistry and Molecular Biology II, University of Granada, Granada, Spain
[5]Institute of Nutrition and Food Technology "José Mataix", Centre of Biomedical Research, University of Granada, Campus de la Salud, 18100 Armilla, Granada, Spain
Full list of author information is available at the end of the article

(Continued from previous page)

Discussion: This is the first time that *L. reuteri* V3401 will be evaluated in patients with IRS. Therefore, this study will provide valuable scientific information about the effects of this strain in metabolic syndrome patients.

Trial registration: The trial has been retrospectively registered in ClinicalTrials.gov on the 23rd November 2016 (ID: NCT02972567), during the recruitment phase.

Keywords: Human adults, Insulin resistance syndrome, *Lactobacillus reuteri* V3401, Non-alcoholic fatty liver disease, Obesity, Probiotics

Trial status

Currently, the trial is ongoing and the analyses of the data and biomarkers continuing.

Background

Obesity is a chronic, low-grade systemic inflammatory disease that is complex and multifactorial, with both genetic and environmental factors involved. This condition and its comorbidities have reached epidemic proportions, both in developed and developing countries [1]. Obesity is associated with the development of insulin resistance syndrome (IRS), commonly referred to as metabolic syndrome. IRS is defined by the presence of impaired glucose metabolism, hypertriglyceridemia, low concentrations of serum high-density lipoprotein (HDL) and other alterations associated with an increased risk of cardiovascular disease (CVD). IRS is a key factor in the development of type 2 diabetes mellitus (DM2), CVD and non-alcoholic fatty liver disease (NAFLD) [2]. Clinical management of IRS remains a public health challenge. Indeed, current treatment is based on changes in lifestyle through hygienic-dietary measures (diet and exercise) combined with medical therapy, if necessary, to treat the components of IRS separately and not as a whole entity.

In recent years, it has become clear that the alteration of the intestinal microbiota composition can contribute to the development of insulin resistance associated with obesity [3–5]. In this sense, a decreased *Bacteroidetes/ Firmicutes* ratio has been described in obese compared to lean individuals [6]. Furthermore, an aberrant intestinal microbiota is able to promote a state of low-grade systemic inflammation, insulin resistance and increased CVD risk through mechanisms that include exposure to bacterial products. In particular, lipopolysaccharide (LPS) produces metabolic endotoxaemia capable of modulating pro-inflammatory cytokines and altering glucose and lipid metabolism in the liver and adipose tissue [7, 8]. In addition, it has been reported that high concentrations of serum LPS-binding protein (LBP) are associated with obesity, IRS and DM2 [9].

Probiotics are live microorganisms that confer a health benefit on the host when administered in adequate amounts. They can modulate the gut microbiota and the immune system. The strains most frequently used as probiotics belong to the *Bifidobacterium* and *Lactobacillus* genera [10]. In this regard, our group has reported that the administration of 9×10^9 cfu (colony-forming units)/day of three probiotics strains (*Lactobacillus paracasei* CNCM I-4034, *Lactobacillus rhamnosus* CNCM I-4036 and *Bifidobacterium* breve CNCM I-4035) to healthy subjects during 30 days induced significant colon microbiota modifications [11].

This fact opens the possibility of a new approach in the treatment of IRS, not with drugs but with functional foods containing probiotics [12]. Intervention studies to determine the effect of probiotics on the components of IRS are limited and often contradictory, mainly due to differences in the design of the study protocol and in the selection of the probiotic strain because the effects observed are strain dependent.

In this sense, it has been described that *Lactobacillus reuteri (L. reuteri)* V3401 (CECT 8605) successfully reduces the absorption of cholesterol by intestinal epithelial cells in in vitro and in vivo assays. This cholesterol-absorbing capacity may be induced through an increase in lytic activity specific to *L. reuteri* V3401 [13]. In an animal model, mice fed a hypercholesterolemic diet supplemented with 2×10^9 cfu of *L. reuteri* V3401/day for 57 days exhibited reduced serum cholesterol levels compared to hypercholesterolemic mice that did not receive the probiotic supplement. Moreover, the animals supplemented with the probiotic strain showed glycemic values similar to those of normocholesterolemic mice [13]. These results suggest that this strain might be adequate for the treatment of dyslipidaemia [13]. We therefore hypothesize that *L. reuteri* V3401 may provide a beneficial effect on IRS treatment, and we aim to study *L. reuteri* V3401 effects in a crossover clinical double-blind, randomized, placebo-controlled trial in IRS patients.

Method/design

Aim of the study

The main objective is to evaluate the effects of *L. reuteri* V3401 on the composition of intestinal microbiota, anthropometric parameters, and biomarkers of insulin resistance (inflammation, cardiovascular risk, and hepatic steatosis) in IRS patients.

Lactobacillus reuteri V3401 characteristics

Lyophilized *L. reuteri* V3401 capsules will be specially prepared for the trial. The capsules will contain 5×10^9 cfu, in agreement with previous data obtained from studies in animals [13]. The placebo will contain maltodextrin and will also be supplied in capsules. Capsules for the probiotic and placebo will be indistinguishable in shape, colour, and organoleptic conditions, and will be provided by Biosearch Life.

Study design

The study is a randomized, double-blind, crossover, controlled, and single-center trial. The trial will be conducted by members of both the Endocrinology and Nutrition Department and the Gastroenterology Department of Complejo Hospitalario de Jaén (Spain). Participants will be instructed to follow a prebiotic- and probiotic-free diet two weeks before the beginning of the intervention and during the study. The study will be performed as shown in Fig. 1. Blood samples, as well as the food and physical activity questionnaire will be analysed by the members of the University of Granada at the University facilities. Microbial DNA isolated from faecal samples will be sequenced in the facilities of the Hospital Universitario San Cecilio (Granada, Spain).

The protocol (PROSIR version 2) will be approved by the local Ethics Committee of Granada and Jaen (CEI-Granada and CEI Jaén with references CEI- Jaen 25,022,016 and CEI-Granada 28,022,016, respectively), and conducted according to the standards given in the Declaration of Helsinki and the Good Clinical Practice Guidelines [14]. All investigators participating in the trial are appropriately qualified.

The Standard Protocol Items: Recommendations for Interventional Trials (SPIRIT) guidelines for this study protocol has been included as an Additional file 1.

Participants, interventions, and outcomes
Inclusion criteria

Individuals aged 18 to 65 years newly-diagnosed with IRS, according to the criteria of the International Diabetes Federation (IDF), and without any previous treatment for the metabolic syndrome, will participate in the study. The prescription of any treatment not allowed during the course of the study, according to exclusion criteria, will be considered a reason for dropping out. Before starting the trial, written informed consent will be provided by all patients.

Exclusion criteria

The use of hypoglycaemic treatment, lipid-lowering medications and treatment with drugs that increase liver enzymes, treatment with specific anti-hypertensives (beta-blockers, angiotensin 2 receptor antagonists, angiotensin-converting enzyme inhibitors) will be considered as an exclusion criteria. Moreover, the exclusion criteria include the presence of kidney disease; diabetes; acute liver injury or severe cirrhosis; immune deficiency conditions; elevated values of C-reactive protein; pregnancy or breastfeeding; history of drug or alcohol abuse; or participation in a study of an investigational medication within the past 30 days.

Recruitment

A total of 60 subjects are expected to be recruited from the Endocrine and Nutrition Clinic at Complejo

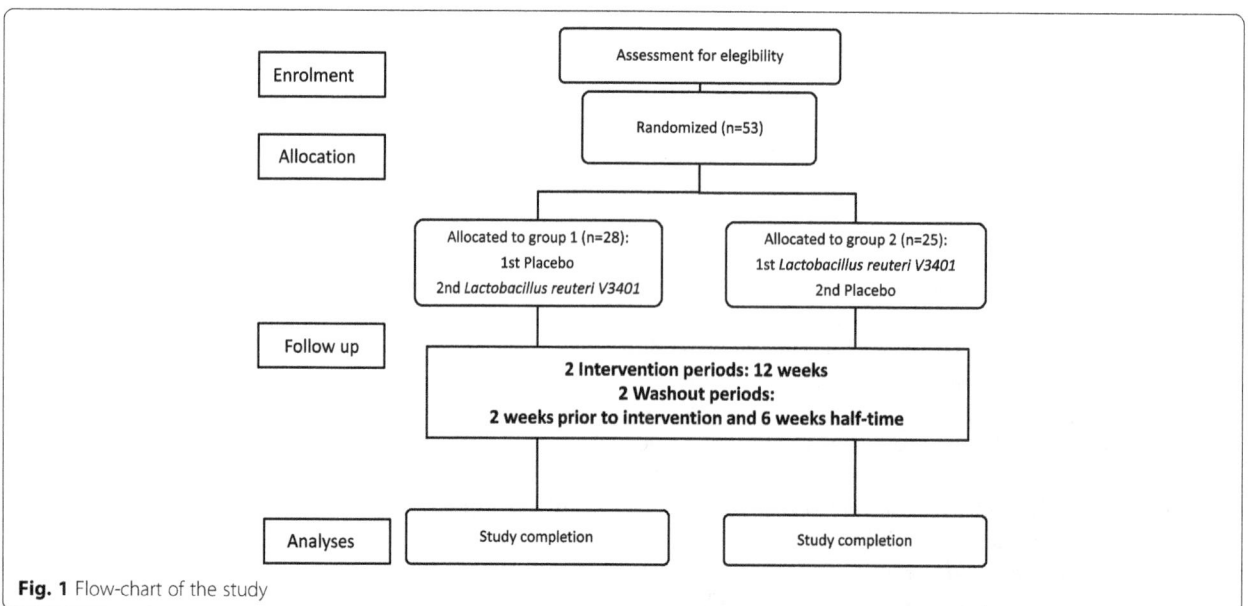

Fig. 1 Flow-chart of the study

Hospitalario de Jaén (Spain) by the physician responsible, through the local newspaper and using advertisement posts at different locations at the hospital facilities.

Randomization, allocation, and blinding

Patients will be randomly allocated in a 1:1 ratio to receive a capsule containing either lyophilized *L. reuteri* V3401 or placebo once daily with food for 12 weeks. A stratified block-randomization method of a software program for sequence generation will be used. After a 6-week washout, participants will crossover to receive the alternative intervention for another 12 weeks. Subjects and investigators will be blinded to the treatment allocation during the course of the intervention. The blind will be broken following consultation with the sponsor.

The capsules will be prepared in special containers with the random number label. Capsules will be delivered at the beginning of each intervention and six weeks later to ensure probiotic viability.

Intervention

We will conduct a standard semi-structured clinical interview with clinical assessment. Subsequently, we will audit the clinical reports to extract relevant information (Additional file 2). In addition, a physical examination, and a complete blood test will be also conducted prior to inclusion in the study. Participants meeting the inclusion criteria will be randomly assigned to the probiotic or placebo group. During the intervention, participants will be asked to ingest a capsule per day with food. Capsules will be administered over two periods of 12 weeks. During the washout period, participants will not receive dietary recommendations. Clinical follow-up visits will be scheduled at the beginning, midpoint, and end of each interventional period. At each visit, anthropometric parameters will be registered, and possible adverse effects will be recorded (Table 1).

The data and samples will be collected in the Complejo Hospitalario de Jaén by qualified personal, and will be codified according to the biobank of the Public Health System of Andalusia (BSSPA) guidelines. All samples will be managed and processed in accordance with BSSPA protocols. All samples will be centralized at the BSSPA facilities.

Dietary and physical activity control

Participants will be provided with a list of local foods to avoid due to their potential probiotic or prebiotic content. Subjects will be asked to complete a three-day dietary record at the beginning, midpoint, and end of each intervention period. Energy and dietary intakes will be assessed from the 3-day records using the EvalFINUT software (http://www.finut.org/evalfinut/). Additionally, subjects will complete the Food Frequency Questionnaire (FFQ)

at the beginning of each intervention period. Participants will receive nutritional counselling on a healthy Mediterranean diet providing approximately 25 kcal/kg/day to achieve and maintain 7% loss of initial body weight and increase moderate-intensity physical activity (such as brisk walking) for at least 150 min/week following the guidelines of the American Diabetes Association for the prevention or delay of DM2 [15]. Likewise, physical activity will be monitored through the International Physical Activity Questionnaire (IPAQ) at the beginning, midpoint, and end of each intervention period. In the following visits, an intensive lifestyle intervention programme will be carried out to reinforce the behaviour.

Outcome measures

Clinical and anthropometric parameters (weight, height, waist circumference and blood pressure) will be recorded. A hepatic ultrasound (US) test will also be performed at the beginning of the two intervention periods, as well as at the end of the intervention periods. US diagnostic criteria for diagnosis and grading of hepatic steatosis will be used [16]. Smoking habits and anxiolytic and antihistaminic drug intake will also be recorded.

Blood samples will be collected after 12 h of fasting at the beginning and at the end of each intervention period (t0, t12, t18 and t30). Stool samples will also be taken at baseline and at 6, 12, 18, 24, and 30 weeks (t0, t6, t12, t18, t24, and t30, respectively). Serum will be collected by centrifugation of blood samples for the determination of biochemical and inflammation biomarkers. Faecal samples will be collected and kept at $-80\,°C$ until analysis. All samples will remain frozen at $-80\,°C$ in the BSSPA Platform.

Primary outcome

The primary outcome will be the change in plasma lipopolysaccharide (LPS) concentration. The determination of LPS concentration and LPS-binding lipoprotein (LBP) will be performed by a simple ELISA (Cloud-Clone Corp., Houston, USA).

Secondary outcomes

Body Mass Index (BMI) and waist circumference will be registered at the beginning, midpoint, and end of each intervention period by qualified staff. Systolic and diastolic blood pressures will be determined three times at 5-min intervals while volunteers are seated using a standardized mercury sphygmomanometer; the final two measurements will be averaged for the analysis.

Serum glucose, insulin, Homeostasis Model Assessment (HOMA) index, cholesterol, LDL, HDL, triacylglycerols, glutamate-pyruvate transaminase (GPT), glutamate-oxaloacetate transaminase (GOT), gamma-glutamyltransferase

Table 1 Detailed study procedures

Visits (V) / Week (W)			V1 (W-2)	V2 (W0)	V3 (W6)	V4 (W12)	Washout	V5 (W18)	V6 (W24)	V7 (W30)
Screening analysis			X							
Demographics/ general information			X							
Informed content form			X							
Randomization and allocation			X							
Treatment distribution			X							
Blood test				X		X		X		X
Stools collection				X	X	X		X	X	X
Hepatic ultrasound				X		X				X
Assessments	General outcomes	Clinical interview		X	X	X		X	X	X
		Blood pressure and anthropometry		X	X	X		X	X	X
		3-day dietary record		X		X		X		X
		Food Frequency Questionnaire (FFQ)		X		X		X		X
		Physical activity questionnaire (IPAQ)		X		X		X		X
	Primary outcomes	Plasma LPS		X		X		X		X
	Secondary outcomes	Blood Pressure		X	X	X		X	X	X
		HOMA		X		X		X		X
		Lipid profile		X		X		X		X
		Inflammatory markers		X		X		X		X
		Hepatic steatosis markers		X		X		X		X

(γ-GT), glycated haemoglobin, and C-reactive protein will be determined before and at the end of each intervention period by standard methods.

Inflammatory and CDV biomarkers, including adiponectin, resistin, myeloperoxidase (MPO), plasminogen activator inhibitor-1 (PAI-1), tumour necrosis factor-alpha (TNF-α), interleukin-6 (IL-6), interleukin-8 (IL-8), soluble intercellular adhesion molecule-1 (sICAM-1) and soluble vascular adhesion molecule-1 (sVCAM-1), will be measured using MILLIPLEXMAP test kits (Milliplex Map Kit, Millipore Corp, Billerica, MA). Arginase, prolidase and retinol binding protein-4 will be measured as hepatic steatosis markers. The arginase and prolidase activity will be measured according to Palomero-Rodriguez et al. [17] and Kayadibi et al. [18], respectively, whereas RBP-4 will be determined by ELISA technology (AdipoGen Inc).

For the study of intestinal microbiota composition, a 16S metagenomics sequencing will be performed. In brief, faecal DNA will be extracted using a commercial isolation kit (QIAamp DNA Stool Mimi Kit, Qiagen). The variable V3 and V4 regions of the 16S rRNA gene will be PCR-amplified and sequenced on an Illumina MiSeq platform at Hospital Universitario San Cecilio, Spain, following the Illumina recommendations.

Withdrawal, dropout, discontinuation, and compliance
Withdrawal will be allowed at any time during the trial. Participants may be advised to discontinue the trial if there is no compliance or if a severe adverse event occurs. Women will be advised not to become pregnant during the study. Participants will be instructed to return the unconsumed capsules when collecting the follow-up doses. Participants whose compliance with treatments or placebo is ≤80% of the total, those who

become pregnant and those who develop diabetes will be considered dropouts.

Adverse events and safety monitoring

All *Lactobacillus* strains are considered safe by the EFSA (European Food Safety Authority). However, each participant will be monitored for abdominal discomfort, diarrhoea, bloating, constipation and nausea/vomiting, among other possible effects, during each visit, and all unexpected adverse events will be reported by participants and written on the individual case report form by the investigator.

Sample size and power analysis

Based on the range and median value of LPS [8] and assuming a power of 80% and a significance level of 5%, the minimum number of subjects will be 21 per arm. To avoid possible bias caused by gender and taking into account withdrawal, we will be recruiting a total of 60 subjects. Missing data will be considered as unavailable data.

Statistical analysis

Data analyses will be performed at the end of the intervention, therefore, a replacement or substitution of a withdrawal subject is not planned; therefore, the missing data will be considered unavailable data.

The normality of variables will be assessed. Variables not following a normal distribution will be transformed. Normal variables will be expressed as the mean and standard error of the mean. An intention-to-treat analysis will be performed for the analysis of efficacy. In order to determine differences in basal characteristics, a paired *t-test* will be used. Carryover effects will be assessed by three-way ANOVA. A general lineal model for repeated measurements will be performed to evaluate differences between variables at the beginning, midpoint, and end of each intervention period. Two-way ANOVA will be used to determine the influence of treatment (probiotic or placebo) and time on the continuous dependent variables. Statistical analyses will be performed using IBM SPSS statistics v22.

Discussion

The present study has been designed to demonstrate whether a probiotic strain, *L. reuteri* V3401, is capable of reducing the IRS components together with healthy lifestyle recommendations (hypocaloric diet and physical activity).

Currently, altered intestinal microbiota is considered a new player in IRS based on its capacity to promote a state of low-grade systemic inflammation, insulin resistance and increased cardiovascular risk through mechanisms that include exposure to bacterial products such as LPS, a component of the outer membrane of gram-negative bacteria. It is currently accepted that the increase in serum levels of LPS produces a metabolic endotoxaemia capable of modulating pro-inflammatory cytokines, as well as glucose and lipid metabolism in the liver and adipose tissue. There is scientific evidence to support the contribution of LPS in DM2 and obesity [7]. Additionally, on the basis of studies in both animals and humans, dietary intake appears to be a major regulator of the structure and function of the gut microbiota [19]. Therefore, promoting changes in the gut microbiota combined with an adequate Mediterranean diet might play an important role in ensuring the efficacy and success of reducing IRS components and avoiding DM2 development.

However, a relatively small number of randomized, clinically controlled studies assessing the beneficial effects of probiotics on metabolic syndrome parameters have been reported. When looking for a specific clinical response, special care must be taken when selecting the strain because probiotic effects are strain specific [12]. The effects of probiotics are explained by their contribution to the intestinal microbiota composition, maintenance of gut barrier function and their immunomodulation capacity [10, 12].

As mentioned above, the most commonly used strains of probiotics are *Bifidobacterium* and *Lactobacillus* spp. The consumption of *L. acidophilus* NCFM has been described to preserve insulin sensitivity without affecting systemic inflammation [20]. Furthermore, *L. reuteri* LR6 has been shown to decrease total cholesterol values and increase HDL-cholesterol levels in the plasma of rats fed a hypercholesterolemic diet [21]. In humans, enrichment of gut microbiota with *L. reuteri* SD5865 has been reported to increase insulin secretion, possibly due to augmented incretin release, although this strain does not seem to affect insulin sensitivity or body fat distribution [22]. However, in a correlation study, Million et al. detected *L. reuteri* in 20% of their study population, with occurrence increasing along with BMI values (7, 8, 34 and 22% for anorexic, lean, overweight and obese individuals, respectively) [23].

To the best of our knowledge, no studies have tested the possible beneficial effect of *L. reuteri* V3401 in patients with IRS. Based on the background provided above, we propose to study the *L. reuteri* V3401 strain by means of an intervention study in subjects with IRS who will follow a healthy lifestyle (hypocaloric diet and physical activity).

Abbreviations
BMI: Body Mass Index; Cfu: Colony forming units; CVD: Cardiovascular disease; DM2: Diabetes mellitus 2; EFSA: European Food Safety Authority; FFQ: Food Frequency Questionnaire; GOT: Glutamate-oxalacetate transaminase; GPT: Glutamate-pyruvate transaminase; HDL: Serum high-density lipoprotein; HOMA: Homeostasis Model Assessment; IDF: International Diabetes Federation; IL-6: Interleukin-6; IL-8: Interleukin-8; IPAQ: International Physical Activity Questionnaire; IRS: Insulin resistance syndrome; LBP: Serum LPS binding protein; LPS: Lipopolysaccharide; MPO: Myeloperoxidase; NAFLD: Non-alcoholic fatty liver disease; PAI-1: Plasminogen activator inhibitor-1; sICAM-1: Soluble intracellular adhesion molecule-1; sVCAM-1: Vascular adhesion molecule-1; TNF-α: Tumor necrosis factor-alpha; US: Ultrasound; γ-GT: Gamma-glutamyltransferase

Acknowledgements
This paper will be part of Carmen Tenorio Jimenez's doctorate, which is being completed as part of Programa de Doctorado en Seguridad de los Alimentos at the University of Jaén, Spain.

Funding
This study is part of the project titled "Guía para la sustanciación de declaraciones de salud en alimentos: funciones inmune, cognitiva y síndrome metabólico". The PROSIR study has been supported by the company Biosearch life, Spain, through grant #3006 managed by Fundación General Empresa-Universidad de Granada, Spain.

Authors' contributions
CTJ, MJMR (physician responsible for the intervention), LF, AG, MO and CGLL contributed to the conception and design the study. MTL, CAI, IDC will participate in the clinical study as a part of the medical team. JHM will be responsible for the IPAQ analysis. All authors have read and approved the final version of the manuscript. All the authors will have access to the final database for analysing results. CGLL, AG, JO, JPD will be responsible for the data analysis and the statistical analysis. CTJ and CGLL wrote the manuscript. All authors have read and approved the final manuscript.

Ethics approval and consent to participate
The study protocol and written informed consent were approved by the Institutional Review Board of the Jaén Hospitals (Comité de Ética de la Investigación de Jaén, Ref. 25/02/2016) and from the Review Board of the Granada Hospitals (Comité de Ética de la Investigación Biomédica de la Provincia de Granada, CEI-GRANADA, Ref.28/01/2016). Written informed consent will be obtained from each patient, according to the BSSPA procedures. Data anonymity will be used during the entire process. Finally, the clinical data of the subjects will be kept in the Complejo Hospitalario de Jaén facilities.

Competing interests
MO who participated in study is the Research Director of the Department of Research and Development at Biosearch life. The funding has no role in the recruitment, biological sample analysis, statistical analysis, data interpretation. None of the authors has any conflict of interest.

Author details
[1]Unidad de Gestión Clínica de Endocrinología y Nutrición. Complejo Hospitalario de Jaén, Jaén, Spain. [2]Departamento de Ciencias de la Salud. Facultad de Ciencias de la Salud, Universidad de Jaén, Jaén, Spain. [3]Unidad de Gestión Clínica de Aparato Digestivo. Complejo Hospitalario de Jaén, Jaén, Spain. [4]Department of Biochemistry and Molecular Biology II, University of Granada, Granada, Spain. [5]Institute of Nutrition and Food Technology "José Mataix", Centre of Biomedical Research, University of Granada, Campus de la Salud, 18100 Armilla, Granada, Spain. [6]Instituto de Investigación Biosanitaria, ibs.GRANADA, Granada, Spain. [7]CIBER Physiopathology of Obesity and Nutrition CB12/03/30028 (CIBEROBN), Instituto de Salud Carlos III, Madrid, Spain. [8]PROFITH "PROmoting FITness and Health through physical activity" Research Group, Department of Physical Education and Sports, Faculty of Sport Sciences, University of Granada, Ctra. Alfacar s/n, 18011 Granada, Spain. [9]Biosearch Life, Granada, Spain.

References
1. Kushner RF, Kahan S. Introduction: the state of obesity in 2017. Med Clin North Am. 2018;102(1):1–11.
2. Alberti KGMM, Eckel RH, Grundy SM, Zimmet PZ, Cleeman JI, Donato KA, Fruchart JC, James WP, Loria CM, Smith SC Jr. Harmonizing the metabolic syndrome: a joint interim statement of the international diabetes federation task force on epidemiology and prevention; National Heart, Lung, and Blood Institute; American Heart Association; world heart federation; international atherosclerosis society; and International Association for the Study of obesity. Circulation. 2009;120(16):1640–5.
3. Bäckhed F, Ding H, Wang T, Hooper LV, Koh GY, Nagy A, et al. The gut microbiota as an environmental factor that regulates fat storage. Proc Natl Acad Sci U S A. 2004;101(44):15718–23.
4. Bäckhed F, Manchester JK, Semenkovich CF, Gordon JI. Mechanisms underlying the resistance to diet-induced obesity in germ-free mice. Proc Natl Acad Sci. 2007;104(3):979–84.
5. Turnbaugh PJ, Ley RE, Mahowald MA, Magrini V, Mardis ER, Gordon JI. An obesity-associated gut microbiome with increased capacity for energy harvest. Nature. 2006;444(7122):1027–131.
6. Turnbaugh PJ, Hamady M, Yatsunenko T, Cantarel BL, Duncan A, Ley RE, Sogin ML, Jones WJ, Roe BA, Affourtit JP, Egholm M, Henrissat B, Heath AC, Knight R, Gordon JI. A core gut microbiome in obese and lean twins. Nature. 2009;457(7228):480–4.
7. Cani PD, Amar J, Iglesias MA, Poggi M, Knauf C, Bastelica D, Neyrinck AM, Fava F, Tuohy KM, Chabo C, Waget A, Delmée E, Cousin B, Sulpice T, Chamontin B, Ferrières J, Tanti JF, Gibson GR, Casteilla L, Delzenne NM, Alessi MC, Burcelin R. Metabolic Endotoxemia initiates obesity and insulin resistance. Diabetes. 2007;56(7):1761–72.
8. Lassenius MI, Pietiläinen KH, Pussinen PJ, Syrjänen J, Forsblom C, Pörsti I, Rissanen A, Kaprio J, Mustonen J, Groop PH, Lehto M. Bacterial endotoxin activity in human serum is associated with dyslipidemia insulin resistance, obesity, and chronic inflammation. Diabetes Care. 2011;34:1809–15.
9. Sun L, Yu Z, Ye X, Zou S, Li H, Yu D, Wu H, Chen Y, Dore J, Clément K, Hu FB, Lin X. A marker of endotoxemia is associated with obesity and related metabolic disorders in apparently healthy Chinese. Diabetes Care. 2010; 33(9):1925–32.
10. Bermudez-Brito M, Plaza-Díaz J, Muñoz-Quezada S, Gómez-Llorente C, Gil A. Probiotic mechanisms of action. Ann Nutr Metab. 2012;61(2):160–74.
11. Plaza-Díaz J, Fernández-Caballero JÁ, Chueca N, García F, Gómez-Llorente C, Sáez-Lara MJ, Fontana L, Gil Á. Pyrosequencing analysis reveals changes in intestinal microbiota of healthy adults who received a daily dose of immunomodulatory probiotic strains. Nutrients. 2015;7(6):3999–4015.
12. Miglioranza Scavuzzi B, Miglioranza LH d S, Henrique FC, Pitelli Paroschi T, Lozovoy MAB, Simão ANC, Dichi I. The role of probiotics on each component of the metabolic syndrome and other cardiovascular risks. Expert Opin Ther Targets. 2015;19(8):1127–38.
13. Sañudo Otero AI, Criado García R, Rodríguez Nogales A, Garach Domech A, Olivares Martín M, Gálvez Peralta JJ, De La Escalera Hueso S, Duarte Pérez JM, Zarzuelo Zurita A, Bañuelos Hortigüela O. Probiotic strains having cholesterol absorbing capacity, methods and uses thereof. Google Patents; 2016. https://encrypted.google.com/patents/EP3031930A1?cl=en&hl=es Accessed 14 Jan 2018.
14. Vijayananthan A, Nawawi O. The importance of good clinical practice guidelines and its role in clinical trials. Biomed Imaging Interv J. 2008;4(1):e5.
15. American Diabetes Association. 5. Prevention or Delay of Type 2 Diabetes: Standards of Medical Care in Diabetes-2018. Diabetes Care. 2018;41 Suppl 1: 51–4.
16. Csendes P, Paolinelli P, Busel D, Venturelli V, Rodríguez J. Higado graso: Ultrasonido y correlación anatomopatológica. Rev Chil Radiol. 2004;10:50–2.
17. Palomero Rodríguez MA, García Navas R, Laporta Báez Y, Al Kassam Martínez D, de Vicente Sánchez J, Cacharro Moras LM, Sánchez Conde P,

Mollinedo F, Muriel Villoria C. Relationship between arginase activity and the storage time of packed red blood cells. Rev Esp Anestesiol Reanim. 2012;59(6):315–20.

18. Kayadibi H, Gültepe M, Yasar B, Ince AT, Ozcan O, Ipcioglu OM, Kurdas OO, Bolat B, Benek YZ, Guveli H, Atalay S, Ozkara S, Keskin O. Diagnostic value of serum prolidase enzyme activity to predict the liver histological lesions in non-alcoholic fatty liver disease: a surrogate marker to distinguish steatohepatitis from simple steatosis. Dig Dis Sci. 2009;54(8):1764–71.

19. Lynch SV, Pedersen O. The human intestinal microbiome in health and disease. N Engl J Med. 2016;375(24):2369–79.

20. Andreasen AS, Larsen N, Pedersen-Skovsgaard T, Berg RM, Møller K, Svendsen KD, Jakobsen M, Pedersen BK. Effects of lactobacillus acidophilus NCFM on insulin sensitivity and the systemic inflammatory response in human subjects. Br J Nutr. 2010;104(12):1831–8.

21. Singh TP, Malik RK, Katkamwar SG, Kaur G. Hypocholesterolemic effects of Lactobacillus reuteri LR6 in rats fed on high-cholesterol diet. Int J Food Sci Nutr. 2015;66(1):71–5.

22. Simon MC, Strassburger K, Nowotny B, Kolb H, Nowotny P, Burkart V, Zivehe F, Hwang JH, Stehle P, Pacini G, Hartmann B, Holst JJ, MacKenzie C, Bindels LB, Martinez I, Walter J, Henrich B, Schloot NC, Roden M. Intake of lactobacillus reuteri improves incretin and insulin secretion in glucose-tolerant humans: a proof of concept. Diabetes Care. 2015;38(10):1827–34.

23. Million M, Angelakis E, Maraninchi M, Henry M, Giorgi R, Valero R, Vialettes B, Raoult D. Correlation between body mass index and gut concentrations of lactobacillus reuteri, Bifidobacterium animalis, Methanobrevibacter smithii and Escherichia coli. Int J Obes Nat. 2013;37(11):1460–6.

Permissions

All chapters in this book were first published in CAM, by BioMed Central; hereby published with permission under the Creative Commons Attribution License or equivalent. Every chapter published in this book has been scrutinized by our experts. Their significance has been extensively debated. The topics covered herein carry significant findings which will fuel the growth of the discipline. They may even be implemented as practical applications or may be referred to as a beginning point for another development.

The contributors of this book come from diverse backgrounds, making this book a truly international effort. This book will bring forth new frontiers with its revolutionizing research information and detailed analysis of the nascent developments around the world.

We would like to thank all the contributing authors for lending their expertise to make the book truly unique. They have played a crucial role in the development of this book. Without their invaluable contributions this book wouldn't have been possible. They have made vital efforts to compile up to date information on the varied aspects of this subject to make this book a valuable addition to the collection of many professionals and students.

This book was conceptualized with the vision of imparting up-to-date information and advanced data in this field. To ensure the same, a matchless editorial board was set up. Every individual on the board went through rigorous rounds of assessment to prove their worth. After which they invested a large part of their time researching and compiling the most relevant data for our readers.

The editorial board has been involved in producing this book since its inception. They have spent rigorous hours researching and exploring the diverse topics which have resulted in the successful publishing of this book. They have passed on their knowledge of decades through this book. To expedite this challenging task, the publisher supported the team at every step. A small team of assistant editors was also appointed to further simplify the editing procedure and attain best results for the readers.

Apart from the editorial board, the designing team has also invested a significant amount of their time in understanding the subject and creating the most relevant covers. They scrutinized every image to scout for the most suitable representation of the subject and create an appropriate cover for the book.

The publishing team has been an ardent support to the editorial, designing and production team. Their endless efforts to recruit the best for this project, has resulted in the accomplishment of this book. They are a veteran in the field of academics and their pool of knowledge is as vast as their experience in printing. Their expertise and guidance has proved useful at every step. Their uncompromising quality standards have made this book an exceptional effort. Their encouragement from time to time has been an inspiration for everyone.

The publisher and the editorial board hope that this book will prove to be a valuable piece of knowledge for researchers, students, practitioners and scholars across the globe.

List of Contributors

Maria Fernanda Taviano, Manuela D'Arrigo and Natalizia Miceli
Dipartimento di Scienze Chimiche, Biologiche, Farmaceutiche ed Ambientali, University of Messina, Polo Annunziata, Viale Annunziata, 98168 Messina, Italy

Paola Dugo and Luigi Mondello
Dipartimento di Scienze Chimiche, Biologiche, Farmaceutiche ed Ambientali, University of Messina, Polo Annunziata, Viale Annunziata, 98168 Messina, Italy
Scienze dell'Alimentazione e della Nutrizione Umana, Università Campus Biomedico di Roma, via Àlvaro del Portillo 21, 00128 Rome, Italy
Chromaleont s.r.l., c/o Dipartimento di Scienze Chimiche, Biologiche, Farmaceutiche ed Ambientali, University of Messina, Polo Annunziata, Viale Annunziata, 98168 Messina, Italy

Khaled Rashed
Pharmacognosy Department, National Research Centre, 33 El-Bohouth st. Dokki, Giza, Egypt

Angela Filocamo
Foundation "Prof. Antonio Imbesi", University of Messina, Piazza Pugliatti 1, 98122 Messina, Italy.
Dipartimento di Scienze Chimiche, Biologiche, Farmaceutiche ed Ambientali, University of Messina, Polo Annunziata, Viale Annunziata, 98168 Messina, Italy

Francesco Cacciola and Carlo Bisignano
Dipartimento di Scienze Biomediche, Odontoiatriche e delle Immagini Morfologiche e Funzionali, University of Messina, Via Consolare Valeria, 98125 Messina, Italy

Rosaria Acquaviva
Dipartimento di Scienze del Farmaco, sezione Biochimica, Viale Andrea Doria 6, 95123 Catania, Italy

Seon-Ok Lee and Hyuk Ji
Department of Science in Korean Medicine, Graduate School, Kyung Hee University, Hoegi-dong, Dongdaemun-gu, 130-701 Seoul, Republic of Korea

Eun-Ok Lee and Hyo-Jeong Lee
Department of Science in Korean Medicine, Graduate School, Kyung Hee University, Hoegi-dong, Dongdaemun-gu, 130-701 Seoul, Republic of Korea
Department of Cancer Preventive Material Development, Graduate School, Kyung Hee University, Hoegi-dong, Dongdaemun-gu, 130-701 Seoul, Republic of Korea
College of Korean Medicine, Kyung Hee university, 1 Hoegi-dong, Dondaemun-gu, 130-701 Seoul, Republic of Korea

Sung-Ji Kim
Department of Cancer Preventive Material Development, Graduate School, Kyung Hee University, Hoegi-dong, Dongdaemun-gu, 130-701 Seoul, Republic of Korea

Ju-Sung Kim
Major of Plant Resources and Environment, College of Applied Life Sciences, 102 Jeju National University, Jeju-si, Jeju-do 690-756, Korea

Uswa Ahmad
Department of Food Science, Nutrition & Home Economics, Government College University, Allama Iqbal Road, Faisalabad 38000, Pakistan

Rabia Shabir Ahmad
Department of Food Science, Nutrition & Home Economics, Government College University, Allama Iqbal Road, Faisalabad 38000, Pakistan
Institute of Home and Food Sciences, Government College University, Faisalabad 38000, Pakistan

Bayan Al-Dabbagh, Ismail A. Elhaty, Reem Al Sakkaf and S. Salman Ashraf
Department of Chemistry, College of Science, UAE University, Al Ain, UAE

Ala'a Al Hrout
Department of Biology, College of Science, UAE University, Al Ain, UAE

Amr Amin
Department of Biology, College of Science, UAE University, Al Ain, UAE
Zoology Department, Cairo University, Giza, Egypt

Raafat El-Awady
Department of Pharmacy Practice and Pharmacotherapeutics, Sharjah Institute for Medical Research and College of Pharmacy, University of Sharjah, Sharjah, UAE

Shimaa Ibrahim Abdelmenym Mohamed
Drug and Herbal Research Centre, Faculty of Pharmacy, Universiti Kebangsaan Malaysia, Jalan Raja Muda Abdul Aziz, 50300 Kuala Lumpur, Malaysia

Ibrahim Jantan
Drug and Herbal Research Centre, Faculty of Pharmacy, Universiti Kebangsaan Malaysia, Jalan Raja Muda Abdul Aziz, 50300 Kuala Lumpur, Malaysia
School of Pharmacy, Taylor's University, Lakeside Campus, 47500 Subang Jaya, Selangor, Malaysia

Mohd Azlan Nafiah
Department of Chemistry, Faculty of Science and Mathematics, Universiti Pendidikan Sultan Idris, 35900 Tanjung Malim, Perak, Malaysia

Mohamed Ali Seyed
Faculty of Medicine, University of Tabuk, Tabuk 71491, Saudi Arabia

Kok Meng Chan
Faculty of Health Sciences, Universiti Kebangsaan Malaysia, Jalan Raja Muda Abdul Aziz, 50300 Kuala Lumpur, Malaysia

Gulzar Ahmad Bhat
Department of Zoology, HNB Central University Garhwal, Srinagar, Uttarakhand 249161, India

Haseeb A. Khan and Abdullah S. Alhomida
Department of Biochemistry, College of Science, King Saud University, Riyadh 11451, Saudi Arabia

Poonam Sharma
Department of Zoology, Indira Gandhi National Tribal University, (A Central University), Amarkantak, M.P 484887, India

Rambir Singh
Department of Biomedical Sciences, Bundelkhand University, Jhansi, India

Bilal Ahmad Paray
Zoology Department, College of Science, King Saud University, Riyadh 11451, Saudi Arabia

Pengyu Wang
Institute of Chinese Materia Medica, Henan University, Kaifeng 475004, Henan, China

Changyang Ma and Wenyi Kang
Institute of Chinese Materia Medica, Henan University, Kaifeng 475004, Henan, China
Kaifeng Key Laboratory of Functional Components in Health Food, Kaifeng 475004, Henan, China

Hemavathy Harikrishnan, Md. Areeful Haque and Endang Kumolosasi
Drug and Herbal Research Center, Faculty of Pharmacy, Universiti Kebangsaan Malaysia, Jalan Raja Muda Abdul Aziz, 50300 Kuala Lumpur, Malaysia

Ibrahim Jantan
Drug and Herbal Research Center, Faculty of Pharmacy, Universiti Kebangsaan Malaysia, Jalan Raja Muda Abdul Aziz, 50300 Kuala Lumpur, Malaysia
School of Pharmacy, Taylor's University, Lakeside Campus, 47500 Subang Jaya, Selangor, Malaysia

Sa-Haeng Kang, Ji-Yoon Cha, Sung-Woo Hwang, Hoon-Yeon Lee, Min Park, Bo-Ri Lee and Young-Mi Lee
Department of Oriental Pharmacy, College of Pharmacy, Wonkwang-Oriental Medicines Research Institute, Wonkwang University, Iksan, Jeollabuk-do 54538, South Korea

Yong-Deok Jeon, Min-Kyoung Shin and Jong-Sik Jin
Department of Oriental Medicine Resources, Chonbuk National University, 79 Gobongro, Iksan, Jeollabuk-do 54596, South Korea

Su-Jeong Kim and Sang-Min Shin
Laboratory of YOUCEL, YOUCEL, INC, 78 Iksandaero, Iksan, Jeollabuk-do 54526, South Korea

Dae-Ki Kim
Department of Immunology and Institute of Medical Science, Jeonbuk National University Medical School, Jeonju, Jeollabuk-do 54896, South Korea

Chiara Bernardini, Augusta Zannoni, Martina Bertocchi, Irvin Tubon, Mercedes Fernandez and Monica Forni

Department of Veterinary Medical Sciences – DIMEVET, University of Bologna, Via Tolara di Sopra 50, Ozzano Emilia, 40064 Bologna, Italy

Ali M. El-Halawany and Hossam M. Abdallah
Department of Natural Products, Faculty of Pharmacy, King Abdulaziz University, Jeddah 21589, Saudi Arabia
Department of Pharmacognosy, Faculty of Pharmacy, Cairo University, Cairo 11562, Egypt

Ahmed R. Hamed
Phytochemistry Department and Biology Unit lab 610, Central Laboratory for the Pharmaceutical and Dug Industries Research Division, National Research Centre, Giza, Dokki 12622, Egypt

Hany Ezzat Khalil
Department of Pharmacognosy, Faculty of Pharmacy, Minia University, Minia 61519, Egypt
Department of Pharmaceutical Sciences, College of Clinical Pharmacy, King Faisal University, Al-Ahsa, Saudi Arabia

Ameen M. Almohammadi
Department of Clinical Pharmacy, Faculty of Pharmacy, King Abdulaziz University, Jeddah 21589, Saudi Arabia

Hau Van Doan, Siriporn Riyajan, Roongtip Iyara and Nuannoi Chudapongse
School of Preclinical Sciences, Institute of Science, Suranaree University of Technology, Nakhon Ratchasima 30000, Thailand

Muhammad Majid, Bakht Nasir, Syeda Saniya Zahra and Ihsan-ul Haq
Department of Pharmacy, Faculty of Biological Sciences, Quaid-i-Azam University, Islamabad 45320, Pakistan

Muhammad Rashid Khan and Bushra Mirza
Department of Biochemistry, Faculty of Biological Sciences, Quaid-i-Azam University, Islamabad 45320, Pakistan

Ansar Mehmood
Department of Botany, University of Poonch, Rawalakot, Azad Jammu and Kashmir 12350, Pakistan

Ghulam Murtaza
Department of Botany, University of Azad Jammu and Kashmir, Muzaffarabad 13100, Pakistan

Ya-Han Huang, Kuo-Ching Wen and Hsiu-Mei Chiang
Department of Cosmeceutics, China Medical University, 91 Hsueh-Shih Road, Taichung 40402, Taiwan

Po-Yuan Wu
Department of Dermatology, China Medical University Hospital, Taichung 40402, Taiwan
School of Medicine, China Medical University, 91 Hsueh-Shih Road, Taichung 40402, Taiwan

Chien-Yih Lin
Department of Biotechnology, Asia University, 500 Liufeng Road, Wufeng District, Taichung City 41354, Taiwan

Mingkwan Na Takuathung, Wutigri Nimlamool and Saranyapin Potikanond
Department of Pharmacology, Faculty of Medicine, Chiang Mai University, Chiang Mai 50200, Thailand

Suthasinee Paramee
Department of Pharmacology, Faculty of Medicine, Chiang Mai University, Chiang Mai 50200, Thailand
Graduate School, Chiang Mai University, Chiang Mai 50200, Thailand

Siriwoot Sookkhee and Choompone Sakonwasun
Department of Microbiology, Faculty of Medicine, Chiang Mai University, Chiang Mai 50200, Thailand

Pitchaya Mungkornasawakul
Department of Chemistry, Faculty of Science, Chiang Mai University, Chiang Mai 50200, Thailand
Environmental Science Program, Faculty of Science, Chiang Mai University, Chiang Mai 50200, Thailand

Chunxiao Li, Tao Xu, Peng Zhou, Ge Guan, Hui Zhang, Xiao Ling, Weixia Li, Fei Meng, Xuelin Li and Mingjun Zhu
The First Affiliated Hospital of Henan University of Chinese Medicine, Zhengzhou 450000, People's Republic of China

Junhua Zhang
Evidence-based Medicine Center, Tianjin University of Traditional Chinese Medicine, Tianjin 300000, People's Republic of China

Guanping Liu and Linyan Lv
Guangxi Wuzhou Pharmaceutical (group) Co., Ltd, Wuzhou 543000, People's Republic of China

Jun Yuan
Shanghai Yongzheng Medical Science and Technology Co., Ltd, Shanghai 200000, People's Republic of China

Jacobus N. Eloff and Lyndy J. McGaw
Phytomedicine Programme, Department of Paraclinical Sciences, Faculty of Veterinary Science, University of Pretoria, Private Bag X04, Onderstepoort, Pretoria 0110, South Africa

Emmanuel Mfotie Njoya
Phytomedicine Programme, Department of Paraclinical Sciences, Faculty of Veterinary Science, University of Pretoria, Private Bag X04, Onderstepoort, Pretoria 0110, South Africa
Department of Biochemistry, Faculty of Science, University of Yaoundé I, Yaoundé, Cameroon

Qihong Li, Kaitao Yu, Yao Shu and Cheng Ge
Department of Stomatology, 307 Hospital, PLA, 8 Dongda Street, Beijing 100071, China

Jun Wen, Wulin He and Hongxing Chu
Stomatological Hospital, Southern Medical University, No. 366, South Jiangnan Avenue, Guangzhou 510280, China

Bin Zhang
Department of Stomatology, Chinese PLA General Hospital, 28 Fuxing Road, Beijing 100853, China

Amany A. Thabet, Fadia S. Youssef and Abdel Nasser B. Singab
Department of Pharmacognosy, Faculty of Pharmacy, Ain Shams University, African Union Organization Street, Abbassia, Cairo 11566, Egypt

Mohamed El-Shazly
Department of Pharmacognosy, Faculty of Pharmacy, Ain Shams University, African Union Organization Street, Abbassia, Cairo 11566, Egypt
Department of Pharmaceutical Biology, Faculty of Pharmacy and Biotechnology, German University in Cairo, Cairo 11835, Egypt

Michal Korinek
Graduate Institute of Natural Products, College of Pharmacy, Kaohsiung Medical University, Kaohsiung 80708, Taiwan

Department of Biotechnology, College of Life Science, Kaohsiung Medical University, Kaohsiung 80708, Taiwan

Graduate Institute of Natural Products, College of Medicine, Chang Gung University, Taoyuan 33302, Taiwan
Research Center for Chinese Herbal Medicine, Research Center for Food and Cosmetic Safety, and Graduate Institute of Health Industry Technology, College of Human Ecology, Chang Gung University of Science and Technology, Taoyuan 33302, Taiwan

Fang-Rong Chang
Graduate Institute of Natural Products, College of Pharmacy, Kaohsiung Medical University, Kaohsiung 80708, Taiwan
National Research Institute of Chinese Medicine, Ministry of Health and Welfare, Taipei 11221, Taiwan

Yang-Chang Wu
Graduate Institute of Natural Products, College of Pharmacy, Kaohsiung Medical University, Kaohsiung 80708, Taiwan
Research Center for Natural Products & Drug Development, Kaohsiung Medical University, Kaohsiung 80708, Taiwan
Department of Medical Research, Kaohsiung Medical University Hospital, Kaohsiung 80708, Taiwan

Bing-Hung Chen
Department of Biotechnology, College of Life Science, Kaohsiung Medical University, Kaohsiung 80708, Taiwan
Department of Medical Research, Kaohsiung Medical University Hospital, Kaohsiung 80708, Taiwan
The Institute of Biomedical Sciences, National Sun Yat-sen University, Kaohsiung 80424, Taiwan

Tsong-Long Hwang
Graduate Institute of Natural Products, College of Medicine, Chang Gung University, Taoyuan 33302, Taiwan
Research Center for Chinese Herbal Medicine, Research Center for Food and Cosmetic Safety, and Graduate Institute of Health Industry Technology, College of Human Ecology, Chang Gung University of Science and Technology, Taoyuan 33302, Taiwan
Department of Anesthesiology, Chang Gung Memorial Hospital, Taoyuan 33305, Taiwan

Chinese Herbal Medicine Research Team, Healthy Aging Research Center, Chang Gung University, Taoyuan 33302, Taiwan

Department of Chemical Engineering, Ming Chi University of Technology, New Taipei City 24301, Taiwan

Carmen Arraiza-Irigoyen and Carmen Tenorio-Jiménez
Unidad de Gestión Clínica de Endocrinología y Nutrición. Complejo Hospitalario de Jaén, Jaén, Spain

María José Martínez-Ramírez
Unidad de Gestión Clínica de Endocrinología y Nutrición. Complejo Hospitalario de Jaén, Jaén, Spain
Departamento de Ciencias de la Salud. Facultad de Ciencias de la Salud, Universidad de Jaén, Jaén, Spain

Mercedes Tercero-Lozano and Isabel Del Castillo-Codes
Unidad de Gestión Clínica de Aparato Digestivo. Complejo Hospitalario de Jaén, Jaén, Spain

Julio Plaza-Díaz and Luis Fontana
Department of Biochemistry and Molecular Biology II, University of Granada, Granada, Spain
Institute of Nutrition and Food Technology "José Mataix", Centre of Biomedical Research, University of Granada, Campus de la Salud, 18100 Armilla, Granada, Spain
6Instituto de Investigación Biosanitaria, ibs. GRANADA, Granada, Spain

Josune Olza, Ángel Gil and Carolina Gomez-Llorente
Department of Biochemistry and Molecular Biology II, University of Granada, Granada, Spain
Institute of Nutrition and Food Technology "José Mataix", Centre of Biomedical Research, University of Granada, Campus de la Salud, 18100 Armilla, Granada, Spain
6Instituto de Investigación Biosanitaria, ibs. GRANADA, Granada, Spain
CIBER Physiopathology of Obesity and Nutrition CB12/03/30028 (CIBEROBN), Instituto de Salud Carlos III, Madrid, Spain

Jairo H. Migueles
PROFITH "PROmoting FITness and Health through physical activity" Research Group, Department of Physical Education and Sports, Faculty of Sport Sciences, University of Granada, Ctra. Alfacar s/n, 18011 Granada, Spain

Mónica Olivares
Biosearch Life, Granada, Spain

Index

A

Alloxan, 32, 58, 60, 65, 111-114, 116-117, 119

Angiogenesis, 34, 43, 46, 95-96, 99, 101, 103, 154, 164, 167

Anti-cancer Activity, 21, 156, 167

Anti-tumor, 2, 23, 44-45, 191

Antibacterial Mechanism, 67, 74

Antioxidant Activity, 1, 3, 6, 8, 10-12, 14, 21, 33, 35-38, 40, 42-43, 87-89, 93-94, 111-112, 114-115, 118-119, 123, 129, 138, 141-142, 144-146, 149, 153-154, 182-183, 188

Apoptosis, 34, 40, 43, 45-47, 49, 55-56, 58, 76, 102, 110, 130, 132, 139, 156, 158, 161, 165-168, 182, 185-186, 189-193

Artemia Salina Leach, 1, 4, 9

B

Barleria Cristata, 104-105, 110, 138

C

Cancerous Cell, 178, 182, 185, 187

Caspase, 58, 156, 159, 161, 165-166, 178, 182, 185-186, 189-193

Cell Culture, 13, 35, 78, 88, 96, 99, 105-106, 154, 157-158, 181, 190, 193, 196

Chelerythrine, 67-74

Chemoprevention, 44, 104-105, 109

Chemotherapy, 34, 43, 46, 58, 104, 167, 188-189

Chrysophyllum Cainito, 111-112, 119-120

Croton Gratissimus, 178-180, 183-188

Cucumis Sativus L, 95-96, 98-102

Cytokine, 56-58, 76, 78, 80, 86, 97-98, 101, 139

Cytotoxic Activity, 46, 56, 184, 186, 196, 199, 202, 204

Cytotoxicity, 10, 35, 78, 80, 87, 89, 94-96, 98, 104, 106, 108, 110, 131, 149-151, 155, 157, 159-160, 162, 178, 181, 183, 186, 188, 194, 196, 199-201, 204-205, 207

D

Dendritic Cell, 52, 57-58

Detoxification, 12-14, 18, 20-21, 104-105, 109, 154

Diabetes Mellitus, 22-23, 32, 59, 63-65, 111-112, 116, 118, 120, 147, 209, 214

E

Endothelium, 95, 99, 101-103

Escherichia Coli, 1, 3-4, 6, 8-9, 11, 48, 76, 141-142, 215

Ethnopharmacology, 141

Euphorbia Supina, 87, 93-94

Extracellular Matrix, 98-99, 101, 130-131, 136, 147, 154-155, 167

F

Fasting Blood Glucose, 22-24, 28-29, 31, 59-60, 64, 111

Fermentation, 12, 20

Ficus Vasta Forssk, 1-2, 10

Fisetin, 12-13, 16-21, 140

Fustin, 12-13, 16, 18-20

G

Glucagon-like Peptide, 59, 61, 65-66

Glucose Uptake, 111, 113-115, 117-120

H

Hemeoxygenase, 95, 101, 147, 152-154

I

Immune Response, 45-46, 48, 55, 57, 76, 134, 137, 195, 207

Immunotherapy, 45-46, 57-58

Inflammation, 40, 58, 74-76, 84, 86, 93, 95-96, 101, 110, 121-122, 125-128, 131, 133-135, 138-140, 147, 153, 178-179, 185, 187-188, 195, 205-211, 213-214

Insulin, 22, 24, 28, 30-32, 59-66, 111, 113-120, 208-211, 213-215

Interleukin, 45-46, 57-58, 75-76, 85, 101-103, 121, 136, 212, 214

Ipomoea Batatas, 121-122, 130, 136, 139

K

Kaempferia Parviflora, 156-157, 162, 167

L

Lipopolysaccharide, 53-56, 75-76, 86, 95-96, 102, 178, 181, 184, 187, 208-209, 214

Lipoxygenase, 36, 178, 181-183, 186-188, 206

Liver Glycogen, 22, 24, 28, 31, 61-63

M

Macrophage, 57, 76, 78, 84, 86, 102

Melanin Synthesis, 87, 89-90, 94

Melanogenesis, 87, 90-94

Menadione, 104, 106, 108, 110

Menadione Cytotoxicity, 104

Momordica Charantia, 59-65, 86

Moraceae, 1-2, 43

Mushroom Tyrosinase, 89-91, 93

N

Neutrophils, 58, 76, 86, 122, 134, 194, 197, 201, 203-205, 207

Non-alcoholic Fatty Liver, 12, 16, 20, 209, 214-215

O

Olea Ferruginea Royle, 141

Ovarian Cancer, 46, 58, 156-157, 161-162, 164-168, 179, 186

Oxidative Stress, 1, 3, 8, 11, 21, 32, 34, 42, 44, 63, 65, 105, 118-119, 121-122, 136, 138-139, 146-147, 151-154, 177-179, 185, 187

P

Peroxisome, 12, 14, 20, 118, 120

Phenolic Compound, 6

Phenolic Profile, 1-2, 10-11

Phyllanthus Amarus, 45-51, 57-58, 75, 79-86

Q

Quinonereductase, 104-105

R

Random Blood Glucose, 22, 24-25, 27, 31

Reactive Oxygen Species, 30, 33, 43, 110-111, 117, 122, 139, 147, 154-155, 187

Rhazya Stricta, 33-34, 39, 41-44

S

Staphylococcus Aureus, 4, 67-68, 70, 74, 141

Stevia Rebaudiana, 22-23, 28, 31-32

Stevioside, 22-23, 25, 28, 30-32

T

Toddalia Asiatica, 67, 74

Traditional Medicine, 12, 33, 96, 119, 145, 178-179, 194

Tumor Lysate, 45-57

Tyrosinase, 87-94

V

Vascular Integrity, 95

X

Xueshuantong Injection, 169, 177

.

www.ingramcontent.com/pod-product-compliance
Lightning Source LLC
Chambersburg PA
CBHW082052190326
41458CB00010B/3511